CARDIOVASCULAR PHARMACOLOGY OF
5-HYDROXYTRYPTAMINE

Developments in
Cardiovascular Medicine

VOLUME 106

CARDIOVASCULAR PHARMACOLOGY OF 5-HYDROXYTRYPTAMINE

Prospective Therapeutic Applications

edited by

P. R. SAXENA

Department of Pharmacology, Erasmus University,
Rotterdam, The Netherlands

D. I. WALLIS

Department of Physiology, University of Wales,
College of Cardiff, Cardiff, U.K.

W. WOUTERS and P. BEVAN

Department of Pharmacology, Duphar B.V., Weesp,
The Netherlands

Kluwer Academic Publishers

DORDRECHT/BOSTON/LONDON

Library of Congress Cataloging-in-Publication Data

```
Cardiovascular pharmacology of 5-hydroxytryptamine : prospective
  therapeutic applications / edited by P.R. Saxena ... [et al.].
      p.   cm. -- (Developments in cardiovascular medicine ; v. 106)
   Includes bibliographical references.
   ISBN 978-94-010-6701-0 (U.S.)
   1. Serotonin--Physiological effect.  2. Serotonin--Therapeutic
use--Testing.  3. Cardiovascular system--Effect of drugs on.
I. Saxena, Pramod R.  II. Series.
   [DNLM: 1. Cardiovascular System--drug effects.  2. Serotonin-
-pharmacology.  3. Serotonin--therapeutic use.   W1 DE997VME v. 106
 / QV 126 C267]
RM666.S46C37   1990
615'.71--dc20
DGPO/DLC
for Library of Congress                                    89-20120
```

ISBN-13: 978-94-010-6701-0   e-ISBN-13: 978-94-009-0479-8
DOI: 10.1007/978-94-009-0479-8

Published by Kluwer Academic Publishers,
P.O. Box 17, 3300 AA Dordrecht, The Netherlands.

Kluwer Academic Publishers incorporates
the publishing programmes of
D. Reidel, Martinus Nijhoff, Dr W. Junk and MTP Press.

Sold and distributed in the U.S.A. and Canada
by Kluwer Academic Publishers,
101 Philip Drive, Norwell, MA 02061, U.S.A.

In all other countries, sold and distributed
by Kluwer Academic Publishers Group,
P.O. Box 322, 3300 AH Dordrecht, The Netherlands.

printed on acid-free paper

Preface

Many of the advances result from the use of drugs as tools to pharmacologically dissect or isolate different components of a system, be it at the molecular, receptor or tissue level. Indeed, much of the current resurgence of interest in 5-hydroxytryptamine (5-HT; serotonin) can be ascribed to the availability of several such new, relatively potent and specific compounds.

In this book the editors have attempted to synthesise a multi-disciplinary view of the cardiovascular pharmacology of 5-HT. Biochemistry, molecular biology and receptor pharmacology are used to introduce the reader to latest developments relevant to an understanding of the physiological role 5-HT plays in controlling the cardiovascular system. And, as the title of the book implies, the contributions have not been restricted to the basic sciences. Increased understanding of the basic principles and the presence of new exciting drug candidates encourages us to make predictions as to the therapeutic applications of drugs interacting with 5-HT in the cardiovascular system. Much of the book is then devoted to exploring cardiovascular pathologies and the way in which 5-HT-related drugs might correct or prevent them. In this context, experience is drawn from both animal studies and clinical trials.

Interest in 5-HT in general, and 5-HT in relation to the cardiovascular system in particular, has exploded in recent years and information on the subject seems to be growing exponentially. This book represents a photograph taken half way in 1989 and cannot hope to cover all the latest developments. Nevertheless, the editors have strived to produce a volume both wide-ranging and didactic which will remain useful and relevant for some years yet to those newly interested in the field as well as affectionados.

This book is based on an international symposium held in Amsterdam under the joint auspices of the SEROTONIN CLUB, the DUTCH PHARMACOLOGICAL SOCIETY and the ERASMUS UNIVERSITY ROTTERDAM. The meeting was supported by generous support from Janssen pharmaceutica, Duphar, Glaxo, ICI, Sandoz, Dutch Heart Foundation, Upjohn, Dutch Migraine Foundation, Erasmus University Foundation, Wellcome Foundation and Beecham.

P. R. Saxena, D. I. Wallis, W. Wouters, P. Bevan

Table of contents

RECEPTORS

NEUROPHYSIOLOGY AND NEUROPHARMACOLOGY

List of contributors

ANGUS, James A., Baker Medical Research Institute, Prahran, Victoria 3181, Australia.

APPERLEY, E., Pharmacology Division, Glaxo Group Research Ltd., Park Road, Ware, Herts SG12 0DP, U.K.

BANERJEE, Ajay K., Laboratory Animal Centre, Faculty of Medicine and Health Science, Erasmus University Rotterdam, P.O. Box 1738, 3000 DR Rotterdam, The Netherlands.

BERGEIJK, Leo van, Department of Internal Medicine and Intensive Care, Regional Hospital Almelo, P.O. Box 7600, 7600 SZ Almelo, The Netherlands.

BLACKBURN, Thomas P., ICI Pharmaceuticals, Alderely Park, Macclesfield, Cheshire, SK10 4TG, U.K.

BLANDINA, Patrizio, Department of Pharmacology, Mount Sinai School of Medicine, New York, NY 10029-6574, U.S.A.

BLAUW, Gerard Jan, Department of Nephrology and Hypertension, University Hospital Leiden, Leiden, The Netherlands.

BOONEN, H. C. M., Department of Pharmacology, University of Limburg, Maastricht, The Netherlands.

BRANCHEK, A., Department of Anatomy and Cell Biology, Columbia University, College of Physicians & Surgeons, 630 W 168th Street, New York, NY 10032, U.S.A.

BROUGHTON, Archer, Baker Medical Research Institute, Prahran, Victoria 3181, Australia.

BROWN, A. M., Department of Pharmacology, Smith Kline & French Research Ltd., The Frythe, Welwyn, Herts AL6 9AR, U.K.

CHANG, Jing-Yu, Department of Medical Cell Research, Section of Neurobiology, University of Lund, Biskopsgatan 5, S-223 62 Lund, Sweden.

CHERQUI, Claudie, INSERM U 228, Faculté de Médecine Broussais Hôtel-Dieu, 15 rue de l'Ecole de Médecine, 75270 Paris Cédex 06, France.

CLARKE, Dave E., Department of Pharmacology, University of Houston, Houston, TX 77204-5515, U.S.A.

COCKS, Thomas M., Baker Medical Research Institute, Prahran, Victoria 3181, Australia.

COHEN, Marlene L., Lilly Research Laboratories, Eli Lilly and Company, Lilly Corporate Center, Indianapolis, Indiana 46285, U.S.A.

COOTE, John H., Department of Physiology, The Medical School, University of Birmingham, Birmingham B15 2TJ, U.K.

CRAIG, D. A., Department of Pharmacology, University of Houston, Houston, TX 77204-5515, U.S.A

DABIRE, H., INSERM U 228, Faculté de Médecine Broussais Hôtel-Dieu, 15 rue de l'Ecole de Médecine, 75270 Paris Cédex 06, France.

DAVIES, M., Psychiatric Research Unit, CMR Building, University of Saskatchewan, Saskatoon, Saskatchewan, Canada.

DE CHAFFOY DE COURCELLES, D., Department of Biochemistry, Janssen Research Foundation, B-2340 Beerse, Belgium.

DE CLERCK, F., Department of Haematology, Janssen Research Foundation, B-2340 Beerse, Belgium.

DE MEY, J. G. R., Department of Pharmacology, University of Limburg, Maastricht, The Netherlands.

DE VOOGD, J. M., Clinical Research Department, Duphar b.v., P.O. Box 2, 1380 AA Weesp, The Netherlands.

DHASMANA, Mohan K., Department of Anaesthesiology, Faculty of Medicine and Health Sciences, Erasmus University Rotterdam, P.O. Box 1738, 3000 DR Rotterdam, The Netherlands.

DROUILLAT, Madeleine, Insitut de Recherches Servier, 11 rue des Moulineaux, 92150 Suresnes, France.

EENS, A., Department of Biochemical Pharmacology, Janssen Research Foundation, B-2340 Berrse, Belgium.

ELLIOTT, P., Department of Physiology, University of Wales College of Cardiff, Cardiff CF1 1SS, U.K.

EMERIT, M. B., INSERM U.228, Neurobiologie Cellulaire et Fonctionell, Faculté de Médecine Pitié-Salpêtrière, 91, boulevard de l'Hôpital, 75634 Paris Cedex 13, France.

FENIUK, Wasyl, Pharmacology Division, Glaxo Group Research Ltd., Ware, Herts SG12 0DJ, U.K.

FINK, K., Institute of Pharmacology and Toxicology, University of Bonn, Reuterstrasse 2b, D-5300 Bonn 1, Federal Republic of Germany.

FOZARD, John R., Preclinical Research Department, Sandoz Ltd., CH-4002 Basel, Switzerland.

GALLISSOT, S., INSERM U.288, Neurobiologie Cellulaire et Fonctionell, Faculté de Médecine Pitié-Salpêtrière, 91, boulevard de l'Hôpital, 75634 Paris Cedex 13, France.

GANONG, William F., Department of Physiology, University of California, San Francisco, CA 94143-0444, U.S.A.

GERSHON, Michael D., Department of Anatomy and Cell Biology, Columbia University, College of Physicians & Surgeons, 630 W 168th Street, New York, NY 10032, U.S.A.

GOLDFARB, Joseph, Department of Pharmacology, Mount Sinai School of Medicine, New York, NY 10029-6574, U.S.A.

GÖTHERT, Manfred, Institute of Pharmacology and Toxicology, University of Bonn, Reuterstrasse 2b, D-5300 Bonn 1, Federal Republic of Germany.

GOZLAN, H., INSERM U.288, Neurobiologie Cellulaire et Fonctionell,

Faculté de Médecine Pitié-Salpêtrière, 91, boulevard de l'Hôpital, 75634 Paris Cedex 13, France.

GRAHAM, David, Department of Biology, Laboratoires d'Etudes et de Recherches Synthélabo (L.E.R.S.), 58, rue de la Glacière, 75013 Paris, France.

GREEN, Jack P., Department of Pharmacology, Mount Sinai School of Medicine, New York, NY 10029-6574, U.S.A.

HAMON, Michel, INSERM U.288, Neurobiologie Cellulaire et Fonctionell, Faculté de Médecine Pitié-Salpêtrière, 91, boulevard de l'Hôpital, 75634 Paris Cedex 13, France.

HARDEBO, Jan Erik, Department of Medical Cell Research, Section of Neurobiology, University of Lund, Biskopsgatan 5, S-223 62 Lund, Sweden.

HARTIG, Paul R., The Neurogenetic Corporation, 215 College Road, Paramus, NJ 07652, U.S.A.

HAWORTH, Stephen J., ICI Pharmaceuticals, Alderely Park, Macclesfield, Cheshire, SK10 4TG, U.K.

HUMPHREY, Pat P. A., Pharmacology Division, Glaxo Group Research Ltd., Park Road, Ware, Herts SG12 0DP, U.K.

JANSSENS, P. A. J., Janssen Research Foundation, B-2340 Beerse, Belgium.

JANSSENS, W. J., Janssen Research Foundation, B-2340 Beerse, Belgium.

JESSUP, Carol L., ICI Pharmaceuticals, Alderely Park, Macclesfield, Cheshire, SK10 4TG, U.K.

KAUMANN, A. J., Department of Pharmacology, Smith Kline & French Research Ltd., The Frythe Welwyn, Herts AL6 9AR, U.K. and Clinical Pharmacology Unit, Addenbrooke's Hospital, Cambridge CB2 2QQ, U.K.

LANGER, Salomon Z., Department of Biology, Laboratoire d'Etudes et de Recherches Synthélabo (L.E.R.S.), 58, rue de la Glacière, 75013 Paris, France.

LAUBIE, M., Insitut de Recherches Servier, 11 rue des Moulineaux, 92150 Suresnes, France.

LEFF, P., Fisons plc, Bakewell Road, Loughborough, Leicestershire LE12 3BB, U.K.

LEYSEN, J. E., Department of Biochemical Pharmacology, Janssen Research Foundation, B-2340 Beerse, Belgium.

MacLENNAN, S. J., Analytical Pharmacology Group, Wellcome Research Laboratories, Beckenham, Kent BR3 3BS, U.K.

MARTIN, Graham R., Analytical Pharmacology Group, Wellcome Research Laboratories, Beckenham, Kent BR3 3BS, U.K.

MAWE, Gary M., Department of Anatomy and Cell Biology, Columbia University, College of Physicians & Surgeons, 630 W 168st Street, New York, NY 10032, U.S.A.

McCALL, Robert B., Cardiovascular Diseases Research, The Upjohn Company, Kalamazoo, Michigan 49001, U.S.A.

McQUEEN, Daniel S., Department of Pharmacology, University of Edinburgh Medical School, 1 George Square, Edinburgh EH8 9JZ, U.K.

MESTIKAWY, El, INSERM U.228, Neurobiologie Cellulaire et Fonctionell, Faculté de Médecine Pitié-Salpêtrière, 91, boulevard de l'Hôpital, 75634 Paris Cedex 13, France.

MIR, Anis K., Preclinical Research, Sandoz Ltd., CH-4002 Basel, Switzerland.

MOLDERINGS, G., Institute of Pharmacology and Toxicology, University of Bonn, Reuterstrasse 2b, D-5300 Bonn 1, Federal Republic of Germany.

MORTON, Pamela B., ICI Pharmaceuticals, Alderely Park, Macclesfield, Cheshire, SK10 4TG, U.K.

MYLECHARANE, Ewan J., Department of Pharmacology, University of Sydney, N.S.W. 2006, Australia.

NIELSEN, T. H., Department of Neurology, Bispebjerg Hospital and Gentofte Hospital, DK-2400 Copenhagen, Denmark.

ORNSTEIN, A. G., Department of Pharmacology, University of Houston, Houston, TX 77204-5515, U.S.A.

OWMAN, Christer, Department of Medical Cell Research, Section of Neurobiology, University of Lund, Biskopsgatan 5, S-223 62 Lund, Sweden.

PERREN, M. J., Pharmacology Division, Glaxo Group Research Ltd., Park Road, Ware, Herts SG12 DP, U.K.

PRAGER, G., Institute for Cardiology and Clinical Research, 8400 Regensburg, Federal Republic of Germany.

RAMAGE, Andrew G., Academic Department of Pharmacology, Royal Free Hospital School of Medicine, Hampstead, London NW3 2PF, U.K.

ROBERTS, Malcolm H. T., Department of Physiology, University of Wales College of Cardiff, Cardiff CF1 ISS, U.K.

SAXENA, Pramod R., Department of Pharmacology, Faculty of Medicine and Health Sciences, Erasmus University Rotterdam, P.O. Box 1738, 3000 DR Rotterdam, The Netherlands.

SCHALEKAMP, Maarten A. D. H., Department of Internal Medicine I, Faculty of Medicine and Health Sciences, Erasmus University Rotterdam, P.O. Box 1738, 3000 DR Rotterdam, The Netherlands.

SCHLICKER, E., Institute of Pharmacology and Toxicology, University of Bonn, Reuterstrasse 2b, D-5300 Bonn 1, Federal Republic of Germany.

SCHMITT, Henri, INSERM U.228, Faculté de Médecine Broussais Hôtel-Dieu, 15 rue de l'Ecole de Médecine, 75270 Paris Cédex 06, France.

TFELT-HANSEN, Peer, Department of Neurology, Bispebjerg Hospital, DK-2400 Copenhagen, Denmark.

UITENDAAL, M. P., Department of Pharmacology, University of Limburg, Maastricht, The Netherlands.

VAN BRUMMELEN, Peter, Division of Cardiology, Kantonspital and Department of Clinical Research, F. Hoffmann-La Roche & Co., Ltd., Basel, Switzerland.

VAN NUETEN, Jan M., Janssen Research Foundation, B-2340 Beerse, Belgium.

VAN ZWIETEN, Pieter, Department of Pharmacology and Pharmacotherapy, Academic Medical Centre, Amsterdam, The Netherlands.

VANHOUTTE, Paul M., Department of Physiology and Biophysics, Mayo Clinic, 200 First Street S. W., Rochester, MN 55905, U.S.A.

VERBEUREN, Tony J., Fondax, Groupe de Recherches Servier, 7 rue Ampère, 92800 Puteaux, France.

VRIJDAG, M. J. J. F., Department of Pharmacology, University of Limburg, Maastricht, The Netherlands.

WALLIS, David I., Department of Physiology, University of Wales College of Cardiff, Cardiff CF1 1SS, U.K.

WENTING, Gert-Jan, Department of Internal Medicine I, Faculty of Medicine and Health Sciences, Erasmus University Rotterdam, P.O. Box 1738, 3000 DR Rotterdam, The Netherlands

WILLIAMS, Christine, ICI Pharmaceuticals, Alderly Park, Macclesfield, Cheshire, SK10 4TG, U.K.

WOITTIEZ, Arend J. J., Department of Internal Medicine and Intensive Care, Regional Hospital Almelo, P.O. Box 7600, 7600 SZ Almelo, The Netherlands.

WOLTHUIS, Jot, Department of Internal Medicine and Intensive Care, Regional Hospital Almelo, P.O. Box 7600, 7600 SZ Almelo, The Netherlands.

WRIGHT, Christine E., Baker Medical Research Institute, Prahran, Victoria 3181, Australia.

WYNANTS, J., Department of Biochemistry, Janssen Research Foundation, B-2340 Beerse, Belgium.

Biochemistry

Biochemistry

I. The distribution and biochemistry of 5-hydroxytryptamine in the cardiovascular system

TONY J. VERBEUREN

1. Introduction

In most plants and animals, significant levels of 5-HT are present. In mammals, the enterochromaffin cells of the gastrointestinal mucosa, the brain, the pineal gland and the platelets contain important concentrations of 5-HT. The indoleamine has also been detected in peripheral nerves of the gut, in lung, kidney, spleen, thyroid, mast cells, heart and blood vessels of different species. It is well accepted that 5-HT has a role as a neurotransmitter in the brain and as a precursor of melatonin in the pineal gland; its precise function in the other tissues in which it is present has yet to be elucidated.

In the past decade, an overwhelming amount of information describing the interacting of 5-HT with its different receptors and/or binding sites, both centrally and peripherally, has become available; particularly the discovery of new, potent and specific drugs that interfere with the different actions of 5-HT has stimulated much scientific research. Although a role for 5-HT in cardiovascular functioning appears evident, I was surprised to discover, while preparing a review on the biochemistry of 5-HT in peripheral tissues [1] that so many questions about its storage, synthesis, release and metabolism in the heart and the blood vessel wall remain to be answered. The present chapter is aimed to summarize our current knowledge on the distribution and the biochemistry of 5-HT in the cardiovascular system; in the first part of the chapter the general aspects of the biosynthesis and the metabolism of 5-HT will be briefly discussed.

2. Synthesis and metabolism of 5-HT: general aspects

2.1. Synthesis

With the exception of the platelets, 5-HT is synthesized in most tissues in which it is stored. The biosynthesis of 5-HT, schematically represented in

P.R. Saxena, D.I. Wallis, W. Wouters and P. Bevan (eds), Cardiovascular Pharmacology of 5-Hydroxytryptamine, pp. 3—13.
© 1990 *Kluwer Academic Publishers, Dordrecht* —

Figure 1, starts with the hydroxylation of the essential amino acid L-tryptophan; this first, rate limiting, step is catalyzed by the enzyme tryptophan hydroxylase and results in the formation of 5-hydroxytryptophan which is transformed to 5-HT in a reaction catalyzed by the non-specific enzyme aromatic L-amino acid decarboxylase. In man, about 2% of the ingested tryptophan is utilized for the daily synthetis of approximately 10 mg of 5-HT. For a detailed review of the activities and the regulation of the enzymes contributing to the biosynthesis of 5-HT, the reader is referred to a recent review by Tyce [2].

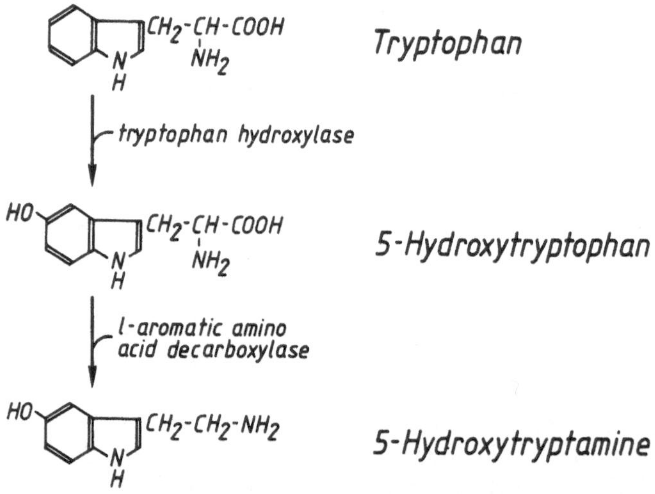

Figure 1. Biosynthesis of 5-hydroxytryptamine.

2.2. *Metabolism*

The principal metabolic pathway of 5-HT is the oxidative deamination by monoamine oxidase which results in the production of 5-hydroxyindoleacetic acid (5-HIAA) (Figure 2). Monoamine oxidase is present both intra — and extraneuronally and the enzyme has a high activity in the liver. Two iso-enzymes contribute to its activity: type A and type B [3—5]. Besides 5-HT, monoamine oxidase catalyzes the deamination of several other biogenic amines such as dopamine, noradrenaline, tyramine and tryptamine.

In a first step, the deamination of 5-HT leads to the formation of 5-hydroxyindoleacetaldehyde which, in most cases, is oxidized to 5-HIAA by the enzyme aldehyde dehydrogenase. 5-hydroxyindoleacetaldehyde can also be reduced to 5-hydroxtryptophol; this metabolite has been detected in several peripheral tissues such as the liver [2].

Besides metabolism by monoamine oxidase, 5-HT is also inactivated by O-sulphation, glucuronidation, N-acetylation, O-methylation and N-methyla-

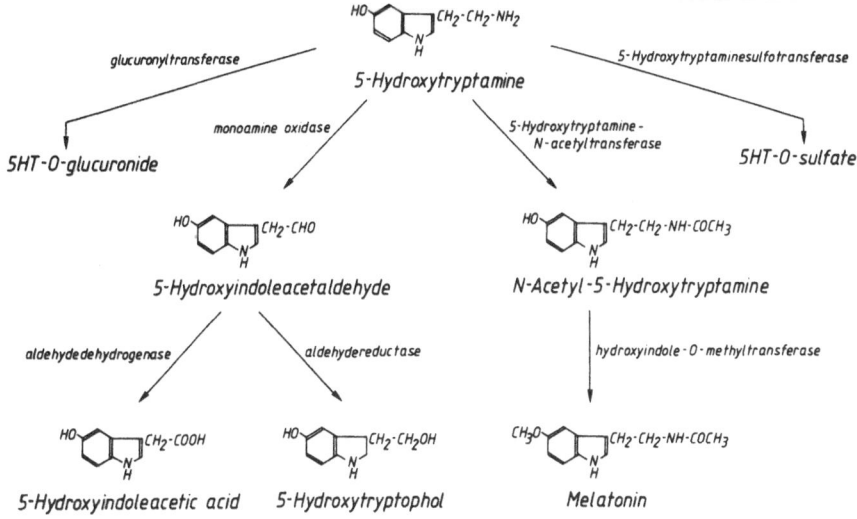

Figure 2. Metabolism of 5-hydroxytryptamine.

tion (Figure 2). In the pineal gland, N-acetylation of 5-HT followed by O-methylation of the N-acetyl-5-HT results in the formation of the hormone melatonin [6].

3. 5-HT in the cardiovascular system

Most of the 5-HT which reaches the cardiovascular system is believed to originate in the enterochromaffin cells of the gastrointestinal mucosa [7]. Part of the 5-HT released by the enterochromaffin cells overflows into the portal circulation where it is avidly taken up by the platelets; the 5-HT which escapes this uptake is metabolized in the liver or in the lungs [8]. The platelets are considered to be the most important source of 5-HT which interacts with the cardiovascular system. The interaction of 5-HT with the platelets will be discussed in Chapter 12.

Besides the 5-HT derived from the enterochromaffin cells, substantial amounts of the indoleamine have been detected in the heart and in the blood vessel wall of mammals, including humans [9—20]. In cerebral arteries of different species, including humans, and in human mesenteric arteries, 5-HT-like immunoreactivity has been detected in nerve fibres supplying these blood vessels [17, 21—25].

Despite the demonstration of the presence of 5-HT in the cardiac and blood vessel wall, information regarding its local biochemistry remains relatively sparse; the aim of this section is to briefly review our current knowledge on the local synthesis, storage, uptake, release and metabolism of 5-HT in the different compartments of the vasculature.

3.1. 5-HT in the heart

Hearts of mammals contain about 0.4 μg/g of 5-HT, a concentration which is about 6 times less than that of noradrenaline [9, 10, 12–14, 16]. Evidence for local synthesis of 5-HT in the heart has been presented by Sole et al. [14]; indeed, inhibition of tryptophan hydroxylase by α-propyldopacetamide resulted in a decreased cardiac 5-HT content in the hamster heart [14]. On the other hand, inhibition of monoamine oxidase causes an increased cardiac level of 5-HT and a decreased appearance of 5-HIAA illustrating the local metabolism of 5-HT in the heart [12, 14]. The exact location of the cardiac 5-HT remains to be determined; it has been demonstrated that the indoleamine levels in the heart were not associated with mast cells, platelets or 5-HT containing nerves [13, 14].

A physiological role for the cardiac 5-HT has not yet been described; it is well known, however, that the amine has profound effects on the mammalian heart and thus may be associated with the etiology of certain cardiac diseases [14].

3.2. 5-HT and the blood vessel wall

3.2.1. Introduction

Isolated blood vessels of different mammalian species including humans, contain 5-HT [12, 13, 15, 17–20]. In one paper, the local synthesis of 5-HT from its precursor L-tryptophan has been described for cultured endothelial cells of cerebral blood vessels [26]. Inhibition of monoamine oxidase causes an increased content of 5-HT and a decreased level of 5-HIAA in mesenteric arteries of rats, indicating that local metabolism of the indoleamine in these blood vessels can influence its tissue level [18]. Storage, release and metabolism of 5-HT appear to take place in the different cellular compartments of the vascular wall; thus interactions between 5-HT and endothelial cells, smooth muscle cells and sympathetic nerves have been described.

3.2.2. 5-HT and endothelial cells

Under normal conditions, most of the 5-HT present in the blood is stored in an inactive form in the dense granules of the platelets and hence the plasma levels of free 5-HT are too low (lower than 20 ng/ml) to produce significant cardiovascular effects. Any possible increase in the level of free 5-HT will be counteracted by two processes: enzymatic degradation by monoamine oxidase (especially in the liver) and removal of 5-HT by endothelial cells, particularly in the lungs [see 8]. Free 5-HT which escapes deamination in the liver will be rapidly cleared in the lung by uptake into the endothelial cells; this process is followed by inactivation of the amine by monoamine oxidase type A. This removal of 5-HT from the circulation, first observed by Starling and Verney in 1925, is considered to be one of the important non-ventilating functions of the lung [8, 27, 28].

Uptake of 5-HT by the endothelium is not restricted to the lung circulation; indeed, the endothelial cells of human umbilical veins, bovine and porcine aorta and porcine pulmonary artery [29, 30] have been shown to take up 5-HT by a process comparable to that described for the lung. Also brain capillaries can take up 5-HT by a mechanism similar to that described for the lung; this ability of the brain endothelium may be very important in regulating the passage of 5-HT from the blood to the brain [26, 31]. In a recent study Fukuda et al. [32] provided evidence that in the rat, little uptake of 5-HT takes place in the endothelium of the aorta while that of the mesenteric artery avidly accumulates the indoleamine; thus the functional role that the endothelial cells play by removing 5-HT from the circulation may vary in different vascular beds.

After uptake by the lung endothelial cells, 5-HT is rapidly degraded by monoamine oxidase of the A-type [8, 33]. The primary metabolite formed is 5-HIAA; however small amounts of 5-hydroxytryptophol have also been detected in the pulmonary effluent [34]. In brain capillaries, 5-HT is extensively degraded to 5-HIAA [26, 31]. In a recent study, we illustrated that intraluminal administration of [^{3}H]-5-HT to isolated perfused dog saphenous veins and coronary arteries resulted in a tissue accumulation of the indoleamine; the most likely storage site for the 5-HT are the sympathetic nerves [35, 36]. When the endothelium was removed from the perfused blood vessels, a marked augmentation of the accumulation of [^{3}H]-5-HT was observed (Figure 3) [36]. Whether the endothelial monoamine oxidase contributed significantly to the lower tissue accumulation of 5-HT in the blood vessels with endothelium remains to be determined; indeed, although treatment with pargyline resulted in an augmented tissue accumulation of 5-HT, this occurred both in the blood vessels with and in those without endothelium to a similar extent [36].

3.2.3. *5-HT and smooth muscle cells*

Besides the endothelial cells, the vascular smooth muscle cells have also been shown to take up and metabolize 5-HT. Thus, denervated blood vessels or vascular preparations, treated with inhibitors of the neuronal uptake mechanism for noradrenaline, accumulate significant amounts of [^{3}H]-5-HT [19, 35—38]. The extraneuronal uptake of 5-HT resembles that of catecholamines and possesses a corticoid-sensitive and a corticoid-resistant component [37]. In the rat aorta, a cocaine-sensitive extraneuronal uptake of 5-HT, which differs from that of noradrenaline, has been demonstrated; this uptake system appears to be located primarily in the smooth muscle layers adjacent to the lumen [32, 39]. After its uptake into the smooth muscle cells, 5-HT is rapidly metabolized mainly by monoamine oxidase of the A type [36, 37].

3.2.4. *5-HT and sympathetic nerves*

From experiments on non vascular tissues, it was known that 5-HT could be taken up by, be stored in and be released from sympathetic nerves [40, 41]. In the nerve vesicles of the sympathetic fibres supplying the pineal gland,

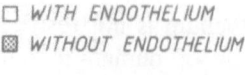

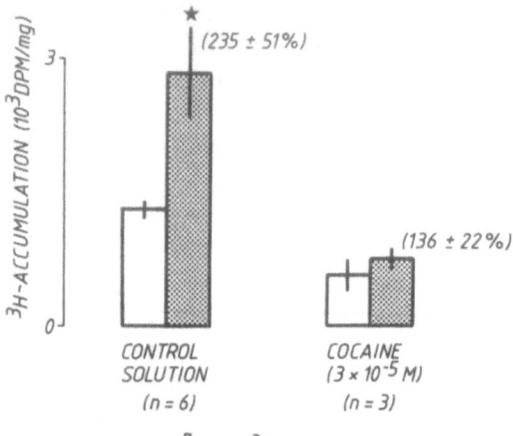

Figure 3. Accumulation of [³H]-5-HT in isolated perfused canine saphenous vein segments with or without endothelium. The tissues with endothelium accumulated significantly less 5-HT than the tissue without endothelium. Cocaine reduced the accumulation of [³H]-5-HT in both groups of tissues. (Data according to Verbeuren et al. [Ref 36] with permission).

5-HT appears to be co-stored with noradrenaline [6, 41, 42]; this observation probably was the first demonstration that nerve cells could contain more than one neurotransmitter.

In vascular tissues, indirect evidence suggests that 5-HT can enter the sympathetic nerve endings; indeed high concentrations of the indoleamine cause displacement of noradrenaline from its storage sites [43, 44]. The fact that the contractions caused by threshold concentrations of 5-HT are augmented by inhibitors of the neuronal uptake of noradrenaline [43, 45, 46] suggest that the entry of the indoleamine into the sympathetic nerves is not restricted to high concentrations.

Incubation of strips of canine saphenous veins and cerebral arteries with [³H]-5-HT causes a significant accumulation of the amine in the tissues. This accumulation is reduced by cocaine or by denervation with 6-hydroxydopamine suggesting that it occurs, for a large part, into the sympathetic nerves present in the vessel wall (Figure 4) [35]. These experiments have been confirmed in dog saphenous veins and basilar and coronary arteries, rabbit basilar arteries and in the rat mesenteric vasculature [19, 20, 36—38, 47—49]. In the dog saphenous vein, the cocaine sensitive accumulation of [³H]-5-HT was markedly potentiated by pargyline suggesting that rapid intra-neuronal deamination of the amine occurs [36].

5-HT derived from platelets can also enter the vessel wall and be incorporated into the sympathetic nerves; this transfer of platelet derived 5-HT to

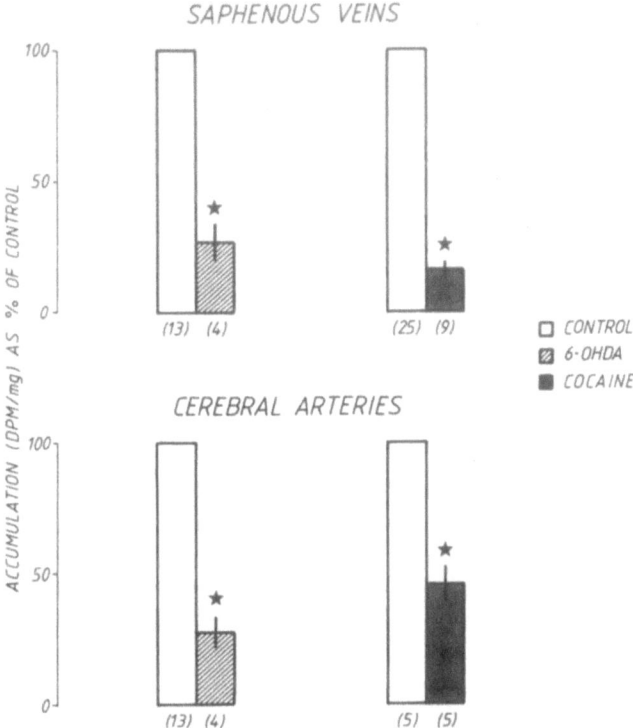

Figure 4. Effect of chemical denervation with 6- hydroxydopamine (6-OHDA) and of cocaine pretreatment on the accumulation of [³H]-5-HT in isolated saphenous veins and basilar arteries of dogs, incubated with 3×10^{-7} M of the [³H]-amine. Both denervation and inhibition of the uptake-system markedly decrease the accumulation of the [³H]-indoleamine but do not abolish it. (Data according to Verbeuren et al. [Ref 35]; with permission).

the nerve terminals is augmented after removal of the endothelium, both in vivo and in vitro [20, 36].

Evidence is available suggesting that cerebral arteries are innervated by 5-HT containing nerves (see above); the accumulation of [³H]-5-HT in dog and rabbit cerebral arteries appears to occur exclusively into the sympathetic nerves [19, 35, 49]. These experiments then seem to suggest that 5-HT and noradrenaline are co-localized in the nerves of the cerebral blood vessels, [35]; immunohistochemical data in support of this hypothesis have been presented for cerebral arteries of the guinea-pig, the rat and the monkey [23—25].

The [³H]-5-HT which accumulates into the sympathetic nerves of isolated arteries and veins spontaneously leaks from the storage sites; most of the amine detected in the basal [³H] efflux consists of [³H]-5-HIAA showing that the 5-HT which leaks from the intraneuronal sites is deaminated by monoamine oxidase before it reaches the synaptic cleft [35, 36, 38, 49]. The spontaneous 5-HT release depends upon the [³H] content of the tissues and is decreased by pretreatment of the blood vessels with cocaine or 6-hydroxy-dopamine [35, 36, 49]. Tyramine and rauwolscine have been shown to augment the basal [^{3}H]-5-HT release [35, 49].

Electrical stimulation of blood vessels labeled with [^{3}H]-5-HT releases the indoleamine [35—38, 47—49]; the pattern and the amount of the 5-HT released are similar to those of noradrenaline [49]. The release of 5-HT is frequency-dependent [35], blocked by tetrodotoxin, pretreatment with cocaine and 6-hydroxydopamine and by ommission of Ca^{2+} from the perfusion medium [35, 37, 38, 47]. The amine can also be released by elevation of the external K^+ concentration [35]. The stimulation-induced release of [^{3}H]-5-HT can be increased by alpha$_2$-adrenoceptor antagonists and be decreased by an alpha$_2$-adrenoceptor agonist; the 5-HT antagonists LY 53857 and methiothepin do not alter the release of 5-HT [35, 48, 49]. These results suggest that the release of [^{3}H]-5-HT is controlled by the presynaptic mechanisms which regulate the release of noradrenaline and thus reinforce the concept for a co-storage of the two amines [35].

Whether the accumulation of 5-HT and its subsequent release from sympathetic nerves contribute to its vascular activity in vivo remains to be determined. It was however described that 5-HT, previously incorporated into the rat mesenteric artery, can augment the constrictor response to nerve stimulation [47, 48], and in canine coronary arteries, 5-HT released from the sympathetic nerves converted the normal dilator response into a vasocon-strictor response [20, 38]. In perfused arteries and veins denuded of the endothelium, 5-HT penetrates the sympathetic nerves more easily than in control blood vessels [36]; this process also appears to occur in vivo [20]. These data then suggest that the interaction of 5-HT with the sympathetic nerves may contribute to the abnormal behaviour of the diseased blood vessel wall.

4. Conclusion

5-HT has been recognized as a neurotransmitter in the rat brain and as a precursor for melatonin in the pineal gland. Recent evidence strongly suggests that the indoleamine may be implicated in cardiovascular diseases such as hypertension or atherosclerosis. The observations that 5-HT can be synthesized, taken up, stored, released and metabolized in the various structures of the cardiovascular system certainly augments its potential role as a regulator of cardiovascular function in health and disease.

Acknowledgement

The author is grateful to Mrs Sophie Dumoulin for her excellent secretarial assistance.

References

1. Verbeuren TJ (1989): Synthesis, storage, release and metabolism of 5-HT in peripheral tissues, pp. 1—25 in: Fozard JR (ed), *Peripheral actions of 5-hydroxytryptamine*. Oxford University Press.
2. Tyce GM (1985): Biochemistry of serotonin, pp. 1—14 in: Vanhoutte PM (ed), *Serotonin and the cardiovascular system*. New York: Raven Press.
3. Johnston JP (1968): Some observations upon a new inhibitor of monoamine oxidase in brain tissue. *Biochem Pharmacol* 17: 1285—1297.
4. Knoll J, Magyar K (1972): Some puzzling pharmacological effects of monoamine oxidase inhibitors. *Adv Biochem Psychopharmacol* 5: 393—408.
5. Verbeuren TJ, Vanhoutte PM (1982): Deamination of released ^{3}H-norepinephrine in the canine saphenous vein. *Naunyn-Schmiedeberg's Arch Pharmacol* 318: 148—157.
6. Axelrod J (1974): The pineal gland: a neurochemical transducer. *Science* 184: 1341—1348.
7. Vanhoutte PM (1982): Does 5-hydroxytryptamine play a role in hypertension? *Trends Pharmacol Sci* 3: 370—373.
8. Gillis CN (1985): Peripheral metabolism of serotonin, pp. 27—36 in: Vanhoutte PM (ed), *Serotonin and the cardiovascular system*. New York: Raven Press.
9. Beauvallet M, Godefroy F, Weil-Fugazza J (1968): Modification de la teneur en 5-hydroxytryptamine du coeur au cours d'une surcharge de régime en chlorure de sodium. *CRS de la Soc de Biol Fil* (Paris) 162: 2085—2088.
10. Madan BR, Khanna NK, Godhwani JL, Pendse VK (1970): Changes in the 5-hydroxytryptamine content of the heart during ectopicventricular arrhythmias and consequent to its reversion by quinidine. *Ind J Med Res* 58: 130—134.
11. Votavova M, Boullin DJ, Costa E (1971): Specificity of action of 6-hydroxydopamine in peripheral cat tissues: depletion of noradrenaline without depletion of 5-hydroxytryptamine. *Life Sci* 10: 87—91.
12. Berkowitz BA, Lee CH, Spector S (1974): Disposition of serotonin in the rat blood vessels and heart. *Clin Exp Pharmacol Physiol* 1: 397—400.
13. Jarrott B, McQueen A, Graf L, Louis WJ (1975): Serotonin levels in vascular tissue and the effects of a serotonin synthesis inhibitor on blood pressure in hypertensive rats. *Clin Exp Pharmacol Physiol* (suppl) 2: 201—205.
14. Sole MJ, Shum A, Van Loon GR (1979): Serotonin: metabolism in the normal and failing heart. *Circ Res* 45: 629—634.
15. Kalsner S, Richards R (1984): Coronary arteries of cardiac patients are hyperreactive and contain stores of amines: a mechanism for coronary spasm. *Science* 223: 1435—1437.
16. Niwa M, Kunisada K, Himeno A, Kawaguchi A, Ozaki M (1984): 5-hydroxytryptamine content in the rat heart: quantitation by high-performance liquid chromatographic electrochemical detection. *Jap J Pharmacol* 34: 264—267.
17. Edvinsson L, Birath E, Uddman R, Lee TJF, Duverger D, MacKenzie ET, Scatton B (1984): Indoleaminergic mechanisms in brain vessels: localization, concentration, uptake and in vitro responses of 5-hydroxytryptamine. *Acta Physiol Scand* 121: 291—299.
18. Ozaki M, Himeno A, Uchida S, Ohta H, Niwa M (1986): Accelerated uptake of serotonin in mesenteric arteries of young spontaneously hypertensive rats. *J Hypertension* 4: S227—S228.
19. Levitt B, Duckles SP (1986): Evidence against serotonin as a vasoconstrictor neurotransmitter in the rabbit basilar artery. *J Pharmacol Exp Ther* 238: 880—885.
20. Cohen RA, Zitnay KM, Weisbrod RM (1987): Accumulation of 5-hydroxytryptamine leads to dysfunction of adrenergic nerves in canine coronary artery following intimal damage in vivo. *Circ Res* 61: 829—833.
21. Griffith SG, Lincoln J, Burnstock G (1982): Serotonin as a neurotransmitter in cerebral arteries. *Brain Res* 247: 388—392.

22. Griffith SG, Burnstock G (1983): Immunohistochemical demonstration of serotonin nerves supplying human cerebral and mesenteric blood vessels. *Lancet* 1983/1: 561–562.

23. Chang JY, Owman Ch (1986): Immunohistochemical and pharmacological studies on serotonergic nerves and receptors in brain vessels. *Acta Physiol Scand* 127 (suppl) 552: 49–53.

24. Chang JY, Hardebo JE, Owman Ch, Svendgaard Aa N (1987): Nerves containing serotonin, its interaction with noradrenaline, anc characterization of serotonin receptors in arteries of monkey. *J Auton Pharmac* 7: 317–329.

25. Jackowski A, Crockard A, Burnstock G (1988): Ultrastructure of serotonin-containing nerve fibres in the middle cerebral artery of the rat and evidence for its localisation within catecholamine-containing nerve fibres by immunoelectron microscopy. *Brain Res* 443: 159–165.

26. Maruki C, Spatz M, Ueki Y, Nagatsu I, Bembry J (1984): Cerebrovascular endothelial cell culture: metabolism and synthesis of 5-hydroxytryptamine. *J Neurochem* 43: 316–319.

27. Starling EH, Verney EG (1925): The secretion of urine as studied on the isolated kidney. *Proc Royal Soc London* 97: 321–363.

28. Junod AF (1975): Metabolism, production and release of hormones and mediators in the lung. *Am Rev Resp Dis* 112: 93–108.

29. Small R, Macarak E, Fisher AB (1976): Production of 5-hydroxyindoleacetic acid from serotonin by cultured endothelial cells. *J Cell Physiol* 90: 225–232.

30. Junod AF, Ody C (1977): Amine uptake and metabolism by endothelium of pig pulmonary artery and aorta. *Am J Physiol* 232: C88–C94.

31. Spatz M, Maruki C, Abe T, Rausch WD, Abe K, Merkel N (1981): The uptake and fate of the radiolabeled 5-hydroxytryptamine in isolated cerebral microvessels. *Brain Res* 220: 214–219.

32. Fukuda S, Su C, Lee TJ-F (1986): Extraneuronal serotonin accumulation in peripheral arteries of the rat. *Experientia* 42: 1244–1245.

33. Roth RA, Gillis CN (1975): Mutiple forms of amine oxidase in perfused rabbit lung. *J Pharmacol Exp Ther* 194: 537–544.

34. Crooks PA, Dreyer RN, Sulens CH, Gillis CN, Coward JK (1979): Deamination of 5-hydroxytryptamine metabolites in isolate perfused rabbit lung by high-performance liquid chromatography. *Anal Biochem* 93: 143–152.

35. Verbeuren TJ, Jordaens FH, Herman AG (1983): Accumulation and release of [³H]5-hydroxytryptamine in saphenous veins and cerebral arteries of the dog. *J Pharmacol Exp Ther* 226: 579–588.

36. Verbeuren TJ, Jordaens FH, Bult H, Herman AG (1988): The endothelium inhibits the penetration of serotonin and norepinephrine in the isolated canine saphenous vein. *J Pharmacol Exp Ther* 244: 276–282.

37. Paiva MQ, Caramona M, Osswald W (1984): Intra — and extraneuronal metabolism of 5-hydroxytryptamine in the isolated saphenous vein of the dog. *Naunyn-Schmiedeberg's Arch Pharmacol* 325: 62–68.

38. Cohen RA (1985): Platelet-induced neurogenic coronary contractions due to accumulation of the false neurotransmitter, 5-hydroxytryptamine. *J Clin Invest* 75: 286–292.

39. Fukuda S, Su C, Lee TJ-F (1986): Mechanisms of extraneuronal sertonin uptake in the rat aorta. *J Pharmacol Exp Ther* 239: 264–269.

40. Thoa NB, Eccleston D, Axelrod J (1969): The accumulation of C¹⁴-serotonin in the guinea-pig vas deferens. *J Pharmacol Exp Ther* 169: 68–73.

41. Jaim-Etcheverry G, Zieher LM (1971): Ultrastructural cytochemistry and pharmacology of 5-hydroxytryptamine in adrenergic nerve endings. III. Selective increase of norepinephrine in the rat pineal gland consecutive to depletion of neuronal 5-hydroxytryptamine. *J Pharmacol Exp Ther* 178: 42–48.

42. Owman C (1964): Sympathetic nerves probably storing two types of monoamines in the rat pineal gland. *Int J Neuropharmacol* 2: 105—112.
43. McGrath MA (1977): 5-hydroxytryptamine and neurotransmitter release in canine blood vessels. *Circ Res* 41: 428—435.
44. Starke K, and Weitzell R (1978): Is histamine involved in the sympathominetic effect of nicotine? *Naunyn-Schmiedeberg's Arch Pharmacol* 304: 237—248.
45. Curro FA, Greenberg S, Verbeuren TJ, and Vanhoutte PM (1978): Interaction between alpha-adrenergic and serotonergic activation of canine saphenous veins. *J Pharmacol Exp Ther* 207: 936—949.
46. Vanhoutte PM, Verbeuren TJ, Webb RC (1981): Local modulation of the adrenergic neuroeffector interaction in the blood vessel wall. *Physiol Rev* 61: 151—247.
47. Kawasaki H, Takasaki K (1984): Vasoconstrictor response induced by 5-hydroxytryptamine released from vascular adrenergic nerves by periarterial nerve stimulation. *J Pharmacol Exp Ther* 229: 816—822.
48. Kawasaki H, Takasaki K (1986): Pharmacological characterization of presynaptic alpha-adrenoceptors in the modulation of the 5-hydrotryptamine release from vascular adrenergic nerves in the rat. *Jap J Pharmacol* 42: 561—570.
49. Verbeuren TJ, Zonnekeyn LL, Jordaens FH, Herman AG (1986): Effects of iskedyl and its two constituents raubasine and dihydroergocristine on the release of [³H] noradrenaline and [³H] serotonin in canine basilar arteries. *Eur J Pharmacol* 125: 1—10.

II. 5-Hydroxytryptamine transport systems

DAVID GRAHAM and SALOMON Z. LANGER

1. Introduction

Studies on the uptake of radioactively-labelled 5-hydroxytryptamine (5-HT) have revealed the accumulation of this biogenic amine in a number of different tissues. In many instances this accumulation of 5-HT represents a temperature-dependent, saturable uptake process which can be inhibited by metabolic inhibitors and by certain selectively-acting compounds. These observations indicate the presence of specific carrier or transport systems involved in the active transport of 5-HT into specific tissue elements.

Active transport systems for 5-HT have an important physiological role in the homeostasis of this biogenic amine. In the central nervous system, for example, high-affinity transport systems associated with serotonergic nerve terminals serve to terminate 5-HT neurotransmission and maintain low levels of this transmitter in the synaptic cleft. As such, these uptake processes serve to conserve the neurotransmitter 5-HT molecules and reduce the need for their 'de novo' synthesis. Also, the vasoactive effects of 5-HT in the blood are inactivated principally by uptake and metabolism in the liver and the lung (particularly by the endothelium). In addition, the existence of specific transporters for the uptake and storage of 5-HT in platelets which do not possess the capability to synthetize this biogenic amine is indispensable for the subsequent role played by 5-HT released upon aggregation.

In active 5-HT transport systems, translocation of this biogenic amine is coupled to the movement of certain ions. Two main categories of active 5-HT transport have been identified: those that are coupled to sodium ions and those that are coupled to protons. In both platelets and serotonergic neurones, these two functionally-distinct transport systems or transporters are used sequentially in the uptake and storage of 5-HT (Figure 1). Both these transporters represent in effect secondary transport systems in that they are driven by primary ATP ion-pumps which generate ion gradients. Active 5-HT transport across the plasma membrane is effectuated by a sodium-coupled transporter which derives its energy from the co-transport of sodium

P.R. Saxena, D.I. Wallis, W. Wouters and P. Bevan (eds), Cardiovascular Pharmacology of 5-Hydroxytryptamine, pp. 15–30.
© 1990 Kluwer Academic Publishers, Dordrecht —

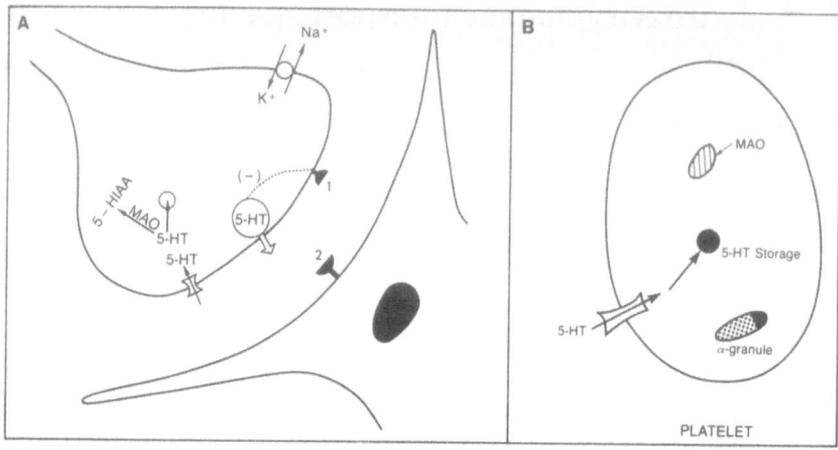

Figure 1. 5-HT Transport systems in serotonergic neurones and platelets. A. At serotonergic synapses exocytotically-released 5-HT crosses the synaptic cleft to activate postsynaptic receptor sites (2). The high synaptic cleft concentrations of 5-HT are subsequently reduced by active uptake of the biogenic amine across the presynaptic neuronal plasma membrane by the sodium-coupled 5-HT transporter. Intracellular 5-HT is then either degraded by MAO or taken up into storage vesicles by a proton-coupled transporter. In addition, the activation by 5-HT of the presynaptic autoreceptor (1) leads to a reduction in the amount of 5-HT released. B. The plasma membrane sodium-coupled 5-HT transporter and vesicular proton-coupled transporter associated with the uptake and storage of 5-HT in platelets.

ions moving down their electrochemical potential gradient. Uptake of 5-HT into storage vesicles is then mediated by a proton-coupled transporter in which the biogenic amine is translocated in exchange for H^+.

The scope of the present review is to describe the mechanistic and molecular properties of these principal 5-HT transport systems. The interactions of various drugs inhibiting 5-HT uptake are discussed together with the therapeutic potential of these drugs in certain disease states.

2. Proton-coupled 5-HT transport

Similarly to other biogenic amines, the bulk of 5-HT is localized intracellularly within specialized organelles or storage vesicles. These 5-HT storage systems present in platelets and in central and peripheral serotonergic neurones subserve a number of roles. Firstly, uptake of 5-HT into these vesicles not only limits intracellular metabolism of this biogenic amine by MAO but leads to the formation of a greater concentration gradient for 5-HT across the plasma membrane thus rendering more effective the overall process of 5-HT uptake into the cell. In addition, the acidic environment inside the storage vesicle helps to prevent degradation of stored indolealkylamine.

The uptake of 5-HT into the storage vesicles shows the properties expected of an active carrier-mediated process. Thus, transport of 5-HT across the vesicular membrane is not only temperature-dependent and saturable, but it is also energy-dependent with a requirement for ATP and Mg^{2+} ions [1, 2, 3]. Compounds such as reserpine [3, 4], tetrabenazine [5] and also ketanserin [6] interact with this vesicular monoamine transport process to inhibit vesicular uptake.

Current ideas on the energetics of this transport system are depicted in Figure 2. The uptake of 5-HT into the storage vesicle occurs by the operation of two sequential processes. First, a membrane-bound Mg^{2+}-dependent ATPase proton pump generates an electrochemical gradient across the vesicular membrane for H^+ (inside > outside). The subsequent coupling of protons to the 5-HT transporter then provides the energy for transport of the biogenic amine with the driving force coming from the movement of H^+ ions down their electrochemical potential gradient. This transporter functions therefore in an antiport configuration as 5-HT is taken up into the storage vesicle in exchange for H^+ ion extrusion.

The characteristics of vesicular 5-HT uptake processes shown by serotonergic neurones [5], platelets [3] and rat basophilic leukemic cells [7] are very similar to those exhibited by other monoamine vesicular storage systems e.g. adrenergic chromaffin granules of the adrenal medulla [8], noradrenergic synaptic vesicles in the heart [9] or dopaminergic and noradrenergic storage granules in the pheochromocytoma cell line PC 12 [10]. Each of these vesicular monoaminergic uptake systems is activated by ATP and Mg^{2+} ions

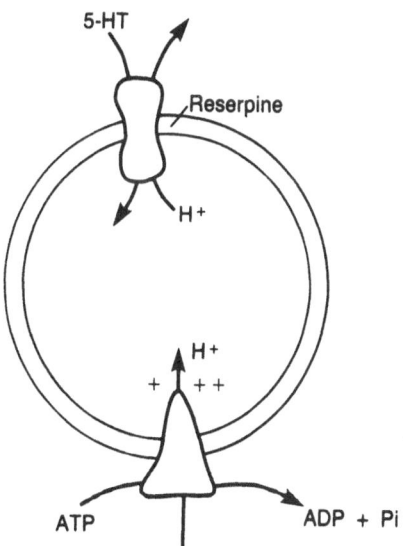

Figure 2. Energetics of proton-coupled vesicular 5-HT transport. The ATPase pump generates an electrochemical potential gradient for protons across the vesicular membrane which in turn drives the accumulation of 5-HT by the proton-coupled biogenic amine transporter.

and inhibited by reserpine and tetrabenazine. Moreover, the substrate specificity of the proton-coupled 5-HT transporters in these different monoaminergic tissues is rather broad. The chromaffin granule transporter for example can use not only adrenaline as substrate but also dopamine, noradrenaline and 5-HT [11]. Moreover, this chromaffin granule transporter was recently purified by affinity chromatography [58], and the purified transporter (a 45,000 polypeptide) photoaffinity-labelled by a radiolabelled derivative of 5-HT ([³H]4-azido-3-nitro-phenylazo-5-HT). The proton-coupled transporters studied using synaptic vesicle preparations from either dopaminergic, serotonergic or noradrenergic enriched brain regions exhibit similar turnover numbers (V_{max}/B_{max}) and affinities for 5-HT [5]. These findings therefore suggest that in different monoaminergic tissues a very similar or perhaps identical transporter species is involved in vesicular transport. As such, the biogenic amine content in storage organelles of different cell-types would be controlled by the substrate specificity of the plasma membrane transport systems and the synthetic machinery of the host cell.

3. Sodium-coupled 5-HT transport

3.1. *Location and properties of sodium-coupled 5-HT transport*

The requirement of sodium ions for the active transport of 5-HT across the plasma membrane is a feature common to 5-HT transport in a number of different tissue elements. In most instances this sodium-dependent process is mediated by a selective 5-HT transport system as defined by inhibition by specific blockers of sodium-dependent 5-HT uptake such as citalopram. The properties of these sodium-dependent 5-HT transporters have been studied principally in platelets [12, 13] and serotonergic neurones [14, 15, 16], although similar 5-HT transport systems have also been demonstrated in e.g. glial cells [17], astrocytes [18], mast cells [19] and lung endothelium [20, 21]. The principal characteristics of uptake by these sodium-coupled 5-HT transporters are shown in Table 1.

The many similarities between the sodium-coupled transport of 5-HT into platelets and brain serotonergic neurones have led to a widespread use of platelets as a simple and easily-accessible model for central serotonergic uptake processes [12, 22]. Nevertheless, differences do exist between these two 5-HT transporter entities. For example, whereas tryptamine is taken up by the platelet transporter [23], the nonhydroxylated indolealkylamine does not actively accumulate in the brain by a sodium-dependent process [24]. Also, the neurotoxin MPP⁺ is taken up by the sodium-dependent dopamine transporter and not the 5-HT transporter in the central nervous system, although this compound serves as a substrate for the platelet 5-HT transporter [25]. As such, the structural requirements for uptake by the neuronal

Table 1. Characteristics of uptake by the sodium-coupled 5-HT transporter.

Plasma membrane location
Sodium-dependent
Temperature-dependent
Saturable following Michaelis-Menten kinetics
$$K_m = 50-100 \text{ nM (synaptosomes)}$$
$= 600$ nM   (platelets)
Specific structural requirements for substrates
Inhibited by metabolic inhibitors and by ouabain
Inhibited by selective 5-HT uptake blockers e.g. citalopram, paroxetine,
SL 81.0385 and fluoxetine

5-HT transporter are more stringent compared to those of its platelet counterpart.

It should also be noted that sodium-coupled transport of 5-HT is not mediated exclusively by 5-HT transporter entities. Active accumulation of 5-HT in noradrenergic nerve endings has been reported to occur in tissues such as vas deferens [26], pancreatic β-cells [27], certain blood vessels [28] and the pineal [29]. In these instances, uptake is mediated by the sodium-coupled noradrenaline transporter.

3.2. *Energetics of the sodium-coupled 5-HT transporter*

The driving force for sodium-dependent 5-HT transport is provided by the electrochemical gradients generated across the plasma membrane for sodium and potassium ions (and indirectly chloride ions) by the enzyme Na^+/K^+ ATPase. Current ideas principally derived from studies with platelet plasma membrane vesicle preparations indicate that each of these ions actually participate in the translocation cycle of the sodium-dependent 5-HT transporter [30, 31]. In the first step of this process, 5-HT, sodium and chloride ions bind to the transporter on its exterior plasma membrane side (Figure 3). It has been suggested that the external sodium ions increase the affinity of the transporter for the biogenic amine [14, 32]. Subsequently, the biogenic amine together with the sodium and chloride ions are translocated to the cytoplasmic surface of the transporter where they dissociate (Figure 3). The binding of potassium to the cytoplasmic side of the transporter followed by the translocation of this monovalent ion then permits reorientation of the biogenic amine binding site so that the cycle can once again be initiated (Figure 3). Interestingly, protons to some extent are apparently capable of substituting the role played by potassium [33]. In this 5-HT transport cycle which has been estimated to occur with a turnover number of about 300 cycles per min in pig platelets [30], it is the translocation rather than the binding steps which are considered to be rate-limiting.

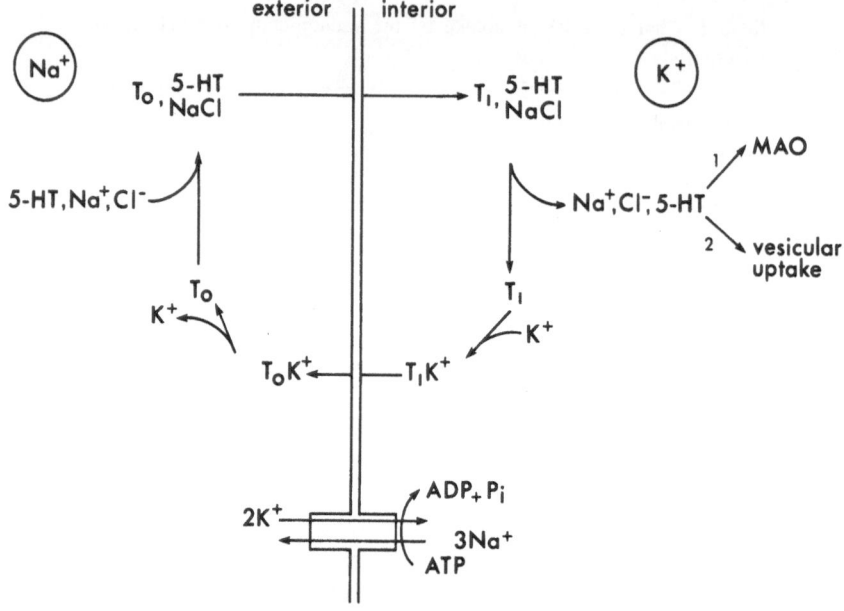

Figure 3. Model for the mechanism of sodium-coupled 5-HT transport across the plasma membrane. The Na^+/K^+ ATPase pump generates appropriate ion gradients across the plasma membrane which serve to power 5-HT translocation by the sodium-coupled 5-HT transporter. In the presence of Na^+ and Cl^-, 5-HT binds to the extracellular side of the transporter (To) to be co-transported together with these ions across the membrane. Upon dissociation of this complex at the cytoplasmic side of the membrane, the binding of K^+ to the transporter (Ti) serves to reorientate the 5-HT binding site to the extracellular membrane surface.

Controversy exists over whether or not the uptake of 5-HT by the sodium-coupled 5-HT transporter is an electrogenic or electroneutral event. Although the transport process in platelets has been claimed to be electroneutral [31], preliminary findings by another group have suggested that the 5-HT transporter of rat basophilic leukemic cells operates by an electrogenic mechanism [7]. Although one cannot totally discount that the platelet and leukemic cell 5-HT transporters could operate through different mechanisms, the discordancy noted in these studies might to some extent be explained by the use of membrane vesicle preparations which are known to be somewhat leaky. If net charge is indeed translocated by the sodium-coupled 5-HT transport system the possibility of using whole-cell recording techniques to demonstrate this could be considered. Such an approach has been used to characterize the electrogenic properties of the sodium-coupled alanine transporter in pancreatic acinar cells [34]. Interestingly, such whole-cell recording techniques have been used to elucidate the stoichiometry and order of binding of each of the components participating in electrogenic transporter function [35].

3.3. *5-HT uptake inhibitors*

Studies on the sodium-coupled 5-HT transport system have led to the identification of compounds such as the tricyclic antidepressant, imipramine, that inhibit uptake of 5-HT by interacting with the transporter macromolecule itself. Although imipramine is an equipotent inhibitor in vitro of both 5-HT and noradrenaline uptake, it is interesting to note that certain substitutions on the tricyclic dibenzazepine nucleus produce compounds which are much more potent inhibitors of 5-HT uptake in vitro compared to noradrenaline uptake e.g. chlorimipramine and cianopramine [36, 37].

During the past decade particular interest has been paid to the development of selective 5-HT uptake inhibitors chemically unrelated to the dibenzazepines. Novel chemical structures which have emerged include citalopram, paroxetine, SL 81.0385, indalpine, fluoxetine and fluvoxamine (Figure 4). Pharmacological studies with these nontricyclic drugs have revealed that they specifically inhibit the uptake of 5-HT compared to the

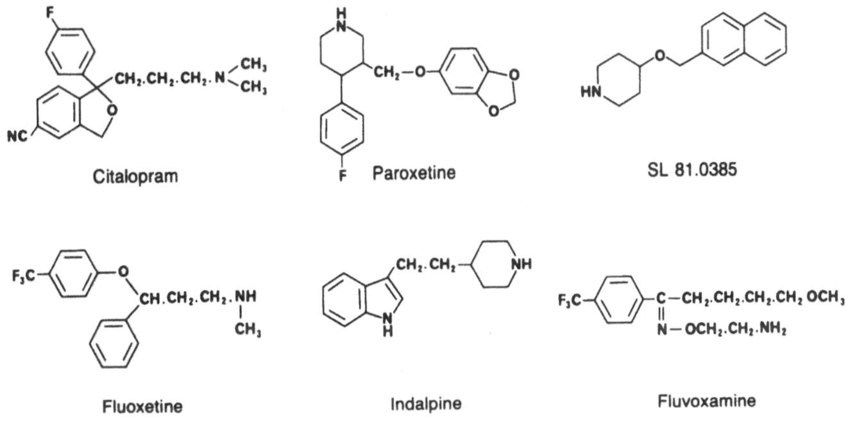

Figure 4.   Chemical structures of nontricyclic selective 5-HT uptake inhibitors.

uptake of other biogenic amines [36, 38—42]. Also, these compounds either do not interact with or show very low affinity for neurotransmitter receptors. The pronounced selectivity of these nontricyclic 5-HT uptake inhibitors thus makes these compounds suitable probes with which to characterize the sodium-coupled 5-HT transport system at a molecular level.

3.4. *[³H]Paroxetine binding*

Radiolabelled forms of 5-HT uptake inhibitors have been used extensively in in vitro membrane binding assays to study the sodium-coupled 5-HT transporter (for review see 43). In initial studies [³H]imipramine was used to label this transporter [44, 45]. However, over the past couple of years highly selective 5-HT uptake inhibitors such as [³H]paroxetine, [³H]citalopram and [³H]indalpine have been adopted for this purpose.

In our laboratory we have shown that [³H]paroxetine labels a single class of high-affinity binding sites in both platelet and cerebral cortical membrane preparations from several mammalian species [46, 47, unpublished observations]. Interestingly, although pretreatment of rats with 6-hydroxydopamine has no effect on the binding of [³H]paroxetine to cerebral cortical membranes, the binding of this radioligand and endogenous 5-HT levels are dramatically reduced upon 5,7-dihydroxytryptamine pretreatment of the animals. These lesioning data suggest that [³H]paroxetine binding sites in cerebral cortex are located on serotonergic neurones [46]. Moreover, the potencies of a number of compounds to inhibit [³H]paroxetine binding and [³H]5-HT uptake in both brain and platelets show an excellent correlation [46, 47]. These properties of [³H]paroxetine binding therefore indicate the suitability of this radioligand as a highly specific probe of the sodium-coupled 5-HT transporter.

Using the [³H]paroxetine binding assay we have recently examined the topographical arrangement of the 5-HT inhibitor binding sites on the neuronal sodium-coupled 5-HT transporter. In one series of experiments inhibition of [³H]paroxetine binding to rat cerebral cortical membranes by citalopram, imipramine and 5-HT was examined at different [³H]paroxetine concentrations. With each drug increases in the concentration of [³H]paroxetine used resulted in parallel shifts to the right of the sigmoidal inhibition curves with no reduction of I_{max} (Figure 5a, below). Moreover, "Schild plot type" analyses of the various curves produced by each drug revealed slopes close to unity (Figure 5b, p. 23). These data were highly suggestive of truly competitive interactions between citalopram, paroxetine, imipramine and

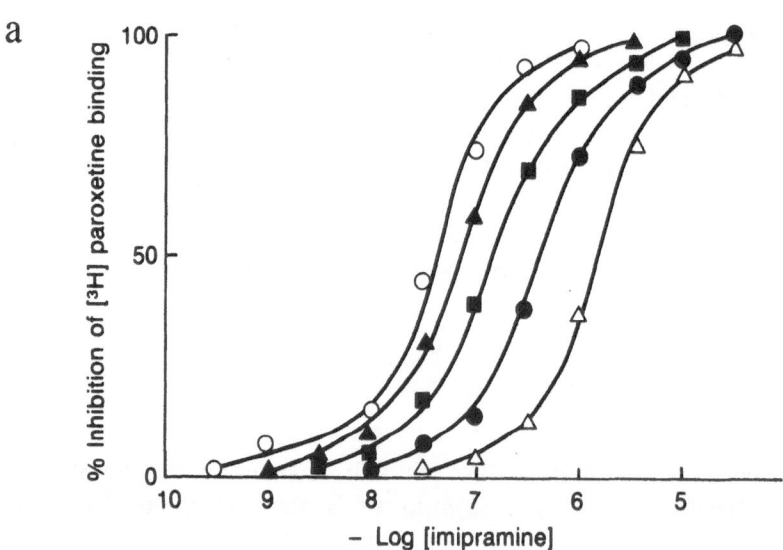

b

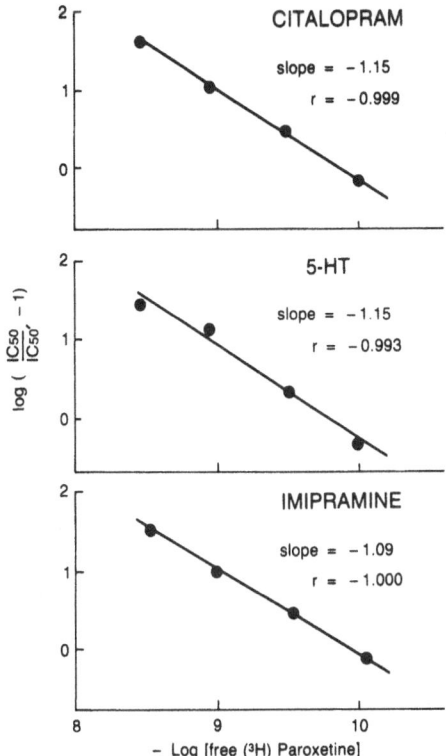

Figure 5a, b. Competitive inhibition of [³H]paroxetine binding by citalopram, imipramine and 5-HT. Competitive inhibition experiments were set up with at least 8 concentrations of citalopram, imipramine or 5-HT at different [³H]paroxetine concentrations (○—○, 0.05 nM; ▲—▲, 0.1 nM; ■—■, 0.3 nM; ●—●, 1.0 nM; △—△, 3.0 nM). A typical experiment for imipramine is shown in Figure 5a. The concentration of drug in each curve that inhibited specific [³H]paroxetine binding by 50% (IC_{50} value) was calculated using the non-linear regression analysis programme ALLFIT [63]. The various IC_{50} values obtained for each drug were then subjected to "Schild-type" analyses (Figure 5b) using the plot log $[(IC_{50}/IC_{50}^{1}) - 1]$ *V* log free [³H]paroxetine concentration, where IC_{50}^{1} represented the IC_{50} value for each drug obtained using 0.05 nM [³H]paroxetine.

5-HT. Consequently, a complementary study was performed in which we investigated the effects of several 5-HT uptake inhibitors and also 5-HT on the dissociation kinetics of [³H]paroxetine binding from equilibrium conditions. In these latter experiments imipramine, 5-HT and the nontricyclic 5-HT uptake inhibitors indalpine, paroxetine, SL 81.0385, fluoxetine and citalopram produced monophasic [³H]paroxetine binding dissociation curves with t 1/2 values similar to the rate of dissociation of [³H]paroxetine binding induced by dilution [unpublished observations]. We therefore interpret these findings as indicating that a common binding site (or at least overlapping binding domains) exists for the tricyclic and nontricyclic 5-HT uptake inhibitors which is located at the substrate recognition site of the neuronal sodium-dependent 5-HT transporter.

3.5. *Purification of the neuronal sodium-coupled 5-HT transporter*

In order to obtain further insight into the structure and functioning of the sodium-coupled 5-HT transporter we have started a programme to solubilize and purify this membrane-bound protein. Membrane preparations from rat cerebral cortex were solubilized using the non-ionic detergent, digitonin, and after ultracentrifugation, the binding of [³H]paroxetine to the supernatant detergent extracts examined [48]. Analysis of the equilibrium saturation isotherm of [³H]paroxetine binding to these digitonin-solubilized extracts revealed the presence of a single class of high-affinity binding sites for this radioligand with a K_d almost identical to the value obtained with the parent membrane preparation (Figure 6). In addition, the potency of a number of different drugs, including the 5-HT uptake inhibitors and 5-HT itself, to inhibit [³H]paroxetine binding to the solubilized and membrane preparations showed an excellent correlation [48]. Thus, the retention of substrate and inhibitor properties of [³H]paroxetine binding to these detergent extracts indicated that the solubilized neuronal sodium-dependent 5-HT transporter was maintained in a conformational state close to that of the native membrane-bound macromolecule.

The neuronal sodium-coupled 5-HT transporter was purified by means of an affinity chromatographic step using an agarose resin to which a derivative of the selective 5-HT uptake inhibitor, citalopram, had been covalently coupled. The digitonin extracts containing solubilized 5-HT transporter were passed over the resin and as a result 70-80% of the solubilized [³H]paroxe-

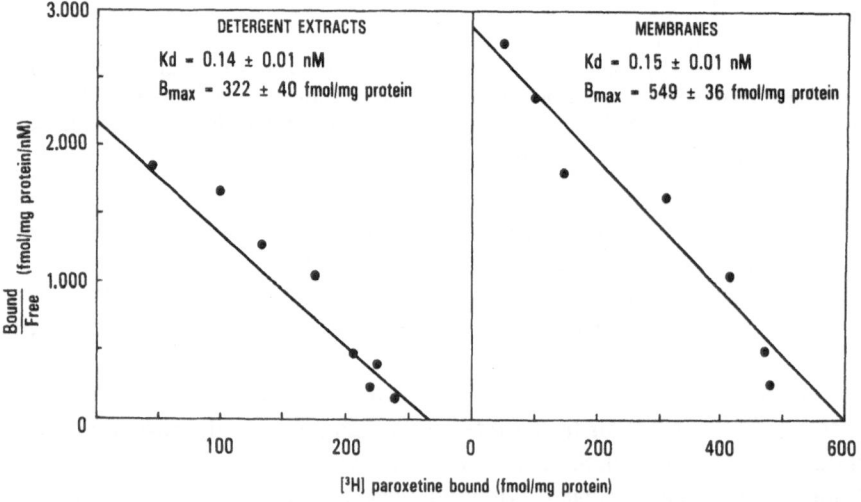

Figure 6. Scatchard transformation of equilibrium saturation [³H]paroxetine binding to digitonin-solubilized and membrane-bound forms of the neuronal sodium-dependent 5-HT transporter.

tine binding sites were adsorbed to the citalopram-resin. After extensive washing of the resin to remove non-specifically bound material, the transporter was biospecifically eluted with the selective 5-HT uptake inhibitor, SL 81.0385. Subsequently, the SL 81.0385 eluate was subjected to steric-exclusion HPLC to remove excess eluting ligand and then the various fractions obtained from the HPLC step analyzed for [³H]paroxetine binding activity. Equilibrium saturation analysis of [³H]paroxetine binding to the pooled active fractions revealed the presence of a single class of high-affinity binding sites with a K_d value of 0.71 nM (Figure 7). The B_{max} value of the binding sites was calculated to be > 1962 pmoles/mg protein (Figure 7) which indicated a purification of > 3,000-fold of [³H]paroxetine binding activity compared to that of the parent membrane preparation. The binding of [³H]paroxetine to this purified preparation was inhibited by citalopram, imipramine and 5-HT with K_i values of 19 nM, 123 nM and 3.5 μM, respectively. This profile therefore confirmed that purification of the neuronal sodium-coupled 5-HT transporter had indeed been obtained. SDS-polyacrylamide gel electrophoresis of the purified material under reducing conditions revealed a major polypeptide band of Mr = 110,000, suggesting that the transporter protein is probably comprised of this single polypeptide. Studies are currently underway to further characterize the purified transporter and it is hoped eventually to apply molecular biological techniques to gain more insight into the functioning of this macromolecule in sodium-coupled transport of 5-HT.

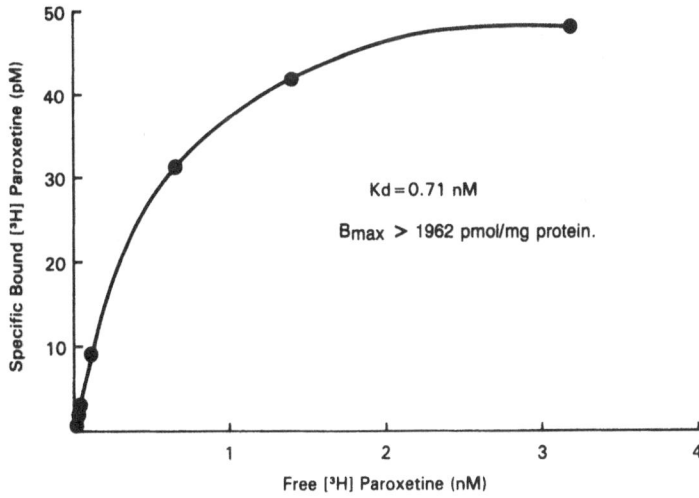

Figure 7. Equilibrium saturation of [³H]paroxetine binding to the purified neuronal sodium-dependent 5-HT transporter.

4. Selective 5-HT uptake inhibitors: therapeutic uses

The hypothesis that a deficit in serotonergic neurotransmission might be implicated in certain forms of depression [49, 50, 51] was the impetus that gave rise to the development of the selective 5-HT uptake inhibitors. Most of these compounds have been synthetized during the past decade and they are at various stages of evaluation as antidepressants (Table 2). In general, clinical studies with the selective 5-HT uptake inhibitors have revealed that

Table 2. Developmental status of selective 5-HT uptake inhibitors as antidepressants.

Launched	—	Fluoxetine, fluvoxamine
Pre-registration	—	Citalopram, femoxetine
Phase III Clinical Trials	—	Cianopramine, paroxetine, sertraline
Phase II Clinical Trials	—	SL 81.0385

they are as effective as the tricyclic antidepressants in the management of depression [52—54]. The principal advantage of these drugs is that they limit the appearance of a large number of the undesirable side-effects noted upon tricyclic antidepressant treatment. In particular, the highly selective pharmacological profile of these new antidepressants greatly reduces side-effects resulting from interactions at α-adrenergic, histaminergic and cholinergic receptors such as sedation, fatigue, orthostatic hypotension, dry mouth, constipation, blurred vision and urinary retention. In addition, these selective 5-HT uptake inhibitors do not produce arrhythmias, tachycardia or cardiac toxicity. Also, in spite of the peripheral effects of 5-HT on smooth muscle and the importance of platelets in the storage and release of this biogenic amine, treatment with these drugs has interestingly not revealed any particular cardiovascular complications for the patients.

Other possible applications for the selective 5-HT uptake inhibitors include their use in the treatment of obesity and alcoholism. Preliminary studies have indicated that zimelidine [55], femoxetine [56] and fluoxetine [57] lead to reductions in body weight in nondepressed obese human patients. Also, zimelidine and citalopram have been claimed to decrease alcohol consumption in nondepressed heavy drinkers [58, 59]. Finally, in view of the proposal of the role of 5-HT neurotransmission in memory, it is interesting to note that in certain animal models fluoxetine [60] and zimelidine [61] have been claimed to enhance memory processing.

5. Conclusions and perspectives

The general properties of sodium- and proton-coupled transport systems involved in the accumulation and/or removal of 5-HT are relatively-well characterized. Nonetheless, some pertinent questions regarding the role and functioning of these transporters have yet to be fully explored. For example, given the preliminary indications that stress and circadian rhythms exert an influence on 5-HT transport, what is the likehood and nature of regulatory mechanisms by which this transport could be controlled? In addition, since sodium-dependent 5-HT transporters have been reported to be associated with both serotonergic neurones and astrocytes in the brain, are there subtle differences in the properties of these transporter entities and do they exert different physiological roles? To address some of these issues, the availability of selective transporter ligands such as [³H]paroxetine for the sodium-coupled 5-HT transporter will no doubt prove useful.

A major direction for future research on 5-HT transport systems will be to elucidate the finer details of the functioning of the transporters during 5-HT translocation. The reported purification of these transporter entities now opens up the possibility to analyse the functional properties of transport at a structural level. The application of molecular biological techniques to elucidate the primary structure of these transporter macromolecules and studies of the effects of site-directed mutagenesis on transporter function should eventually provide detailed insights into the functioning of these transport systems.

Finally, the principle that selective 5-HT uptake inhibitors would prove to be effective antidepressants devoid of the anticholinergic and cardiovascular side-effects displayed by the tricyclic antidepressants has now been confirmed by clinical studies. Nevertheless, in view of the role of 5-HT in the cardiovascular system, it remains to be explored whether these drugs could find application in the treatment of certain cardiovascular disease states.

Acknowledgements

The authors thank Miss F. Péchoux for expert secretarial assistance in the preparation of this article.

References

1. Maron R, Kanner B, Schuldiner S (1979): The role of a transmembrane pH gradient in 5-hydroxytryptamine uptake by synaptic vesicles from rat brain. *FEBS Letts* 98: 237—240.
2. Wilkins JA, Greenawalt JW, Huang L (1978): Transport of 5-hydroxytryptamine by dense granules from porcine platelets. *J Biol Chem* 253: 6260—6265.
3. Rudnick G, Fishkes H, Nelson PJ, Schuldiner S (1980): Evidence for two distinct serotonin transport systems in platelets. *J Biol Chem* 255: 3638—3641.
4. Pletscher A, Da Prada M, Berneis KH, Tranzer JP (1971): New aspects on the storage of 5-hydroxytryptamine in blood platelets. *Experientia* 27: 993—1120.
5. Scherman D (1986): Dihydrotetrabenazine binding and monoamine uptake in mouse brain regions. *J Neurochem* 47: 331—339.

6. Darchen F, Scherman D, Laduron PM, Henry J-P (1988): Ketanserin binds to the monoamine transporter of chromaffin granules and of synaptic vesicles. *Mol Pharmacol* 33: 672 −677.

7. Kanner BI (1983): Bioenergetics of neurotransmitter transport. *Biochim Biophys Acta* 726: 293−316.

8. Njus D, Radda GK (1978): Bioenergetic processes in chromaffin granules: a new perspective on some old problems. *Biochim Biophys Acta* 463: 219−244.

9. Angelides KJ (1980): Transport of catecholamines by native and reconstituted rat heart synaptic vesicles. *J Neurochem* 35: 949−962.

10. Greene LA, Rein G (1977): Release, storage and uptake of catecholamines by a clonal cell line of nerve growth factor (NGF) responsive pheochromocytoma cells. *Brain Res* 129: 247−263.

11. Da Prada M, Obrist R, Pletscher A (1975): Discrimination of monoamine uptake by membranes of adrenal chromaffin granules. *Br J Pharmacol* 53: 257−265.

12. Sneddon JM (1973): Blood platelets as a model for monoamine-containing neurones. *Prog Neurobiol* 1: 151−198.

13. Stahl SM, Meltzer HY (1978): A kinetic and pharmacological analysis of 5-hydroxytryptamine transport by human platelets and platelet storage granules: comparison with central serotonergic neurons. *J Pharmacol Exp Ther* 205: 118−132.

14. Bogdanski DF, Tissari AH, Brodie BB (1970): Mechanism of transport and storage of biogenic amines. III. Effects of sodium and potassium on kinetics of 5-hydroxytryptamine and noradrenaline transport by rabbit synaptosomes. *Biochim Biophys Acta* 219: 189−199.

15. Shaskan EG, Snyder SH (1970): Kinetics of serotonin accumulation into slices from rat brain. Relationship to catecholamine uptake. *J Pharmacol Exp Ther* 175: 404−418.

16. Gershon MD, Jonakait GM (1979): Uptake and release of 5-hydroxytryptamine by enteric 5-hydroxytryptaminergic neurones: effects of fluoxetine (Lilly 110140) and chlorimipramine. *Br J Pharmacol* 66: 7−9.

17. Suddith RL, Hutchinson HT, Haber B (1978): Uptake of biogenic amines by glial cells in culture. 1. A neuronal-like transport of serotonin. *Life Sci* 22: 2179−2188.

18. Kimelberg HK (1986): Occurrence and functional significance of serotonin and catecholamine uptake by astrocytes. *Biochem Pharmacol* 35: 2273−2281.

19. Gripenberg J (1976): Inhibition by reserpine, guanethidine and imipramine of the uptake of 5-hydroxytryptamine by rat peritoneal mast cells in vivo. *Acta Physiol Scand* 96: 407−416.

20. Bosin TR, Lahr PD (1981): Mechanisms influencing the disposition of serotonin in mouse lung. *Biochem Pharmacol* 30: 3187−3193.

21. Raisman R, Langer SZ (1983): Specific high affinity [³H]imipramine binding sites in rat lung are related with a non-neuronal uptake site for serotonin. *Eur J Pharmacol* 94: 345−348.

22. Stahl SM (1977): The human platelet: a diagnostic and research tool for the study of biogenic amines in psychiatric and neurologic disorders. *Arch Gen Psychiat* 34: 509−516.

23. Segonzac A, Tateishi T, Langer SZ (1984): Saturable uptake of [³H]tryptamine in rabbit platelets is inhibited by 5-hydroxytryptamine uptake blockers. *Naunyn-Schmiedeberg's Arch Pharmacol* 328: 33−37.

24. Ross SB, Ask AL (1980): Structural requirements for uptake into serotonergic neurons. *Acta Pharmacol Toxicol* 46: 270−277.

25. Da Prada M, Cesura AM, Launay JM, Richards JG (1988): Platelets as a model for neurones. *Experientia* 44: 115−126.

26. Thoa NB, Ecclestone D, Axelrod J (1969): The accumulation of ¹⁴C-serotonin in the guinea-pig vas deferens. *J Pharmacol Exp Ther* 169: 68−73.

27. Lindström P, Sehlin J, Täljedal I-B (1980): Characteristics of 5-hydroxytryptamine transport in pancreatic islets. *Br J Pharmacol* 68: 773−778.

28. Verbeuren TJ, Jordaens FH, Herman AG (1983): Accumulation and release of [³H]5-hydroxytryptamine in saphenous veins and cerebral arteries of the dog. *J Pharmacol Exp Ther* 226: 579—588.

29. Ducis I, Di Stefano V (1980): Characterization of serotonin uptake in isolated pinealocyte suspensions. *Mol Pharmacol* 18: 447—454.

30. Talvenheimo J, Nelson PJ, Rudnick G (1979): Mechanism of imipramine inhibition of platelet 5-hydroxytryptamine transport. *J Biol Chem* 254: 4631—4635.

31. Nelson PJ, Rudnick G (1982): The role of chloride ion in platelet serotonin transport. *J Biol Chem* 257: 6151—6155.

32. Ross SB, Helder D (1977): Efflux of 5-hydroxytryptamine from synaptosomes of rat cerebral cortex. *Acta Physiol Scand* 99: 27—36.

33. Keyes SR, Rudnick G (1982): Coupling of transmembrane proton gradients to platelet serotonin transport. *J Biol Chem* 257: 1172—1176.

34. Jauch P, Läuger P (1986): Electrogenic properties of the sodium-alanine cotransporter in pancreatic acinar cells: II. Comparison with transport models. *J Memb Biol* 94: 117—127.

35. Jauch P, Läuger P (1988): Kinetics of the Na⁺/alanine cotransporter in pancreatic acinar cells. *Biochim Biophys Acta* 939: 179—188.

36. Hytell J (1982): Citalopram: pharmacological profile of a specific serotonin uptake inhibitor with antidepressant activity. *Prog Neuro-Psychopharmacol & Biol Psychiat* 6: 277—295.

37. Haefely W, Schaffner R, Burkard WP, Da Prada M, Kellar HH, Pole P, Richards JG (1978): Ro 11-2465, a potent and selective inhibitor of 5-hydroxytryptamine uptake. 11th C.I.N.P. Congress, Vienna, July abstracts p. 95.

38. Thomas DR, Nelson DR, Johnson AM (1987): Biochemical effects of the antidepressant paroxetine, a specific 5-hydroxytryptamine uptake inhibitor. *Psychopharmacology* 93: 193—200.

39. Scatton B, Claustre Y, Graham D, Dennis T, Serrano A, Arbilla S, Pimoule C, Schoemaker H, Bigg D, Langer SZ (1988): SL 81.0385: a novel selective and potent serotonin uptake inhibitor. *Drug Dev Res* 12: 29—40.

40. Le Fur G, Uzan A (1977): Effects of 4-(3-indolyl-alkyl)-piperidine derivatives on uptake and release of noradrenaline, dopamine and 5-hydroxytryptamine in rat brain synaptosomes, rat heart and human blood platelets. *Biochem Pharmacol* 26: 497—503.

41. Stark P, Fuller RW, Wong DT (1985): The pharmacologic profile of fluoxetine. *J Clin Psychiat* 46: 7—13.

42. Claassen V (1983): Review of the animal pharmacology and pharmacokinetics of fluvoxamine. *Br J Clin Pharmacol* 15: 349S—355S.

43. Graham D, Langer SZ (1988): The neuronal sodium-dependent serotonin transporter: studies with [³H]imipramine and [³H]paroxetine, pp. 367—391 in: Osborne NN, Hamon M (eds), *Neuronal Serotonin*. John Wiley and Sons Ltd.

44. Langer SZ, Moret C, Raisman R, Dubocovich ML, Briley MS (1980): High affinity [³H]imipramine binding in rat hypothalamus is associated with the uptake of serotonin but not norepinephrine. *Science* 210: 1133—1135.

45. Langer SZ, Briley M, Raisman R, Henry J-F, Morselli PL (1980): Specific [³H]imipramine binding in human platelets: influence of age and sex. *Naunyn-Schmiedeberg's Arch Pharmacol* 313: 189—194.

46. Habert E, Graham D, Tahraoui L, Claustre Y, Langer SZ (1985): Characterization of [³H]paroxetine binding to rat cortical membranes. *Eur J Pharmacol* 118: 107—114.

47. Segonzac A, Schoemaker H, Langer SZ (1987): Temperature-dependence of drug interaction with the platelet 5-HT transporter: a clue to the imipramine selectivity paradox. *J Neurochem* 48: 331—339.

48. Habert E, Graham D, Langer SZ (1986): Solubilization and characterization of the 5-hydroxytryptamine transporter complex from rat cerebral cortical membranes. *Eur J Pharmacol* 122: 197—204.

49. Goodwin FK, Post RM (1983): 5-hydroxytryptamine and depression: a model for the interaction of normal variance with pathology. *Br J Clin Pharmacol* 15: 393S—405S.
50. Shopsin B, Gershon S, Goldstein M, Friedman E, Wilk S (1975): The use of synthesis inhibitors in defining a role for biogenic amines during imipramine treatment in depressed patients. *Psychopharmacol Commun* 1: 239—249.
51. Shopsin B, Friedman E, Gershon S (1976): Parachlorophenylalanine reversal of trancypromine effects in depressed patients. *Arch Gen Psychiat* 33: 811—819.
52. Stark P, Hardison CD (1985): A review of multi-centered outpatient imipramine and placebo controlled studies of fluoxetine in the treatment of major depressive disorders. *J Clin Psychiatry* 46: 53—58.
53. Penfield P, Ward A (1986): Fluvoxamine. A review of its pharmacodynamic and pharmacokinetic properties, and therapeutic efficacy in depressive illness. *Drugs* 32: 313—334.
54. Anderson J, Bech P, Benjaminsen S et al. (1986): Citalopram: clinical effect profile in comparison with clomipramine. A controlled multicenter study. *Psychopharmacology* 90: 131—138.
55. Simpson RJ, Lawton DJ, Watt MH, Tiplady B (1981): Effect of zimelidine, a new antidepressant, on appetite and body weight. *Br J Clin Pharmacol* 11: 96—98.
56. Smedgegaard J, Christiansen P, Skrumsager B (1981): Treatment of obesity by femoxetine, a selective 5-HT uptake inhibitor. *Int J Obesity* 5: 377—378.
57. Ferguson JM (1986): Fluoxetine induced weight loss in non-depressed overweight humans. *Alimentazione Nutrizione Metabolismo* 7: (2) 19.
58. Naranjo CA, Sellers EM, Roach CA, Woodley DV, Sanchez-Craig M, Sykora K (1984): Zimelidine-induced variations in alcohol intake by nondepressed heavy drinkers. *Clin Pharmacol Ther* 35: 373—381.
59. Naranjo CA, Sellers EM, Sullivan JT, Woodley DV, Sanchez-Craig M, Sykora K (1987): The serotonin uptake inhibitor citalopram attenuates ethanol intake. *Clin Pharmacol Ther* 41: 266—274.
60. Flood JF, Cherkin A (1987): Fluoxetine enhances memory processing in mice. *Psychopharmacology* 93: 36—43.
61. Altman HJ, Nordy DA, Ögen SV (1984): Role of serotonin in memory: facilitation by alaproclate and zimelidine. *Psychopharmacology* 84: 496—502.
62. Gabizon R, Schuldiner S (1985): The amine transporter from bovine chromaffin granules. *J Biol Chem* 260: 3001—3005.
63. De Lean A, Munson PJ, Rodbard D (1978): Simultaneous analysis of families of sigmoidal curves: application to bioassay, radioligand assay and physiological dose-response curves. *Am J Physiol* 235: E97—E102.

III. Cloning of the choroid plexus 5-HT$_{1C}$ receptor

PAUL R. HARTIG

1. Molecular Biology of the G protein receptor family

In the limited time that molecular cloning techniques have been successfully applied to neurotransmitter receptors, we have learned of strong sequence homologies among one group of receptors, the G protein-coupled receptors, that unite these proteins into one structural family [1]. Members of this family include the muscarinic cholinoceptors, alpha- and beta-adrenoceptors, opsin and the Substance K receptor [1, 2]. All members of this family are single subunit proteins containing seven membrane-spanning domains with interconnecting extracellular and cytoplasmic sequences. The transmembrane domains exhibit strong sequence homologies among the family members, while the interconnecting water soluble domains are less well conserved. Recently, the 5-HT$_{1C}$ receptor became the first serotonergic member of this family of cloned G-protein-coupled receptors, and so became the first 5-hydroxytryptamine (5-HT) receptor subtype to be understood at the amino acid sequence level [3, 4]. The strategy used to clone the 5-HT$_{1C}$ receptor is a powerful new approach to molecular cloning, which will be broadly applicable to many receptor and ion channel proteins. The basics of this strategy will be reviewed in this chapter, along with information it has provided on the structure of the 5-HT$_{1C}$ receptor.

The most straightforward approach to molecular cloning is to purify the protein of interest, determine the 20 or so N-terminal amino acids of the protein (or of a peptide fragment derived from the protein), then translate the amino acid sequence into a nucleotide sequence. This nucleotide sequence is then synthesized in the laboratory and used to probe a cDNA or genomic library. Another strategy is to obtain antibodies to the protein of interest, then use these antibodies to screen an "expression library" in which bacteria or eukaryotic cells synthesize proteins which are encoded by a family of cDNA or genomic DNA clones. Alternatively, these antibodies can be used to precipitate polysomes containing mRNA for the corresponding protein. Unfortunately, these approaches are difficult to apply to the low-abundance

P.R. Saxena, D.I. Wallis, W. Wouters and P. Bevan (eds), Cardiovascular Pharmacology of 5-Hydroxytryptamine, pp. 31—39.
© 1990 *Kluwer Academic Publishers, Dordrecht* —

membrane proteins of interest to neurobiologists (receptors, transport proteins and ion channels), because these proteins are notoriously difficult to purify and very few antibodies are available for their study.

2. Use of oocytes in 5-HT receptor cloning

Recently, a new cloning strategy has been devised which utilizes Xenopus oocytes as a translation system for exogenous mRNA [3, 4]. These large (1 mm diameter) oocytes are poised for rapid development following sperm penetration, which makes them capable of efficiently translating foreign RNA injected into them. Injection of a few picograms of pure receptor RNA into oocytes leads to the expression of sufficient receptor molecules to provide a measurable current signal when the neurotransmitter agonist of choice is externally applied [4].

The first indication that the oocytes system could be useful to 5-HT researchers came in 1983, when Gundersen et al. [5] reported that injection of rat brain poly A^+ RNA into Xenopus oocytes led to the appearance of a large 5-HT-activated chloride conductance increase. Subsequently, Dascal et al. [6] and Lübbert et al. [7] characterized this response extensively, and determined that its pharmacological inhibition profile most closely resembled the binding properties of the choroid plexus 5-HT$_{1C}$ receptor. In addition, this response was G protein mediated, involving the release of intracellular calcium, and was most evident with RNA obtained from the choroid plexus, the tissue with the highest density of 5-HT$_{1C}$ receptors.

The electrophysiological response of oocytes to 5-HT appears to arise from the coupling of the 5-HT$_{1C}$ receptor (produced by translation of the injected RNA) to an endogenous oocyte G protein-phospholipase C system which is normally activated by a sperm receptor in the oocyte. This endogenous system releases IP$_3$ and intracellular calcium in response to fertilization, which leads to depolarization of the cell through calcium activation of a specific chloride channel, thereby blocking further sperm entry [2]. Fortunately, 5-HT$_{1C}$ receptor mRNA is efficiently translated by the oocyte and this receptor can efficiently couple to the oocyte's endogenous G protein pathway.

The ability of oocytes to serve as a sensitive assay system for 5-HT$_{1C}$ receptor mRNA was exploited in a scheme for the cloning of this receptor [3], which is outlined in Figure 1. The goals of this cloning strategy were: 1) to obtain receptor clones in the absence of amino acid sequence data or receptor-specific antibodies, 2) to be able to detect positive cDNA clones for a receptor even if the receptor contains multiple, functional subunits and the cDNA being tested contains only part of the coding sequence for one of the functional subunits, and 3) to obtain antisense hybridization probes (complementary to the coding strand) from single stranded plasmids, for use in hybridization to mRNA coding for the 5-HT$_{1C}$ receptor. A hybrid depletion approach was chosen for this cloning strategy, so that a cDNA clone would

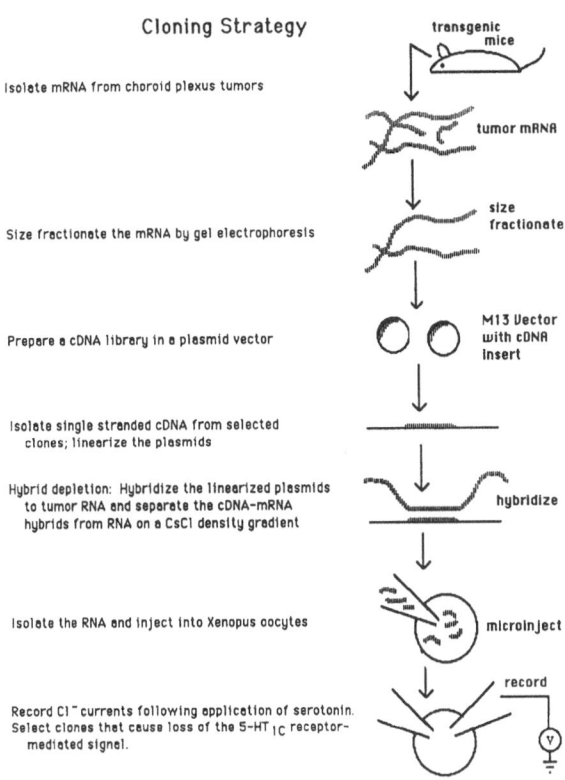

Cloning Strategy

Isolate mRNA from choroid plexus tumors

Size fractionate the mRNA by gel electrophoresis

Prepare a cDNA library in a plasmid vector

Isolate single stranded cDNA from selected clones; linearize the plasmids

Hybrid depletion: Hybridize the linearized plasmids to tumor RNA and separate the cDNA–mRNA hybrids from RNA on a CsCl density gradient

Isolate the RNA and inject into Xenopus oocytes

Record Cl⁻ currents following application of serotonin. Select clones that cause loss of the 5-HT$_{1C}$ receptor-mediated signal.

transgenic mice

tumor mRNA

size fractionate

M13 Vector with cDNA insert

hybridize

microinject

record

Figure 1. Initial scheme for cloning of the 5-HT$_{1C}$ receptor (from reference [3]). Poly A$^+$ RNA was isolated from mouse choroid plexus tumors, size fractionated on an agarose gel, and a cDNA library was constructed in the plasmid vector pUC119. Single-stranded DNA was isolated from groups of clones, linearized, and hybridized to choroid plexus tumor RNA. DNA-RNA hybrids were separated from unhybridized RNA on CsCl grandients, and the unhybridized RNA was injected into oocytes. Oocytes were later voltage-clamped and tested for the chloride conductance increase in response to 5-HT that is characteristic of the 5-HT$_{1C}$ receptor. Positive clones were identified by a loss of the 5-HT signal following hybrid depletion. After a partial clone for the 5-HT$_{1C}$ receptor was isolated by this method [3], the entire coding region was obtained by a variant of this procedure [4], as described in the text.

be detected even if it only coded for a portion of the functional receptor. In this approach, cDNA colonies were screened in groups for their ability to hybridize to mRNA for the 5-HT$_{1C}$ receptor (which was obtained from a mouse choroid plexus tumor [8]). cDNA-mRNA hybrids were formed in solution and separated from unhybridized RNA on a CsCl gradient containing guanidine hydrochloride. The hybrid-depleted RNA was harvested from the gradient and injected into oocytes. If the cDNA being tested contained part of the sequence of one functional subunit of the receptor, it would hybridize to the receptor mRNA, leading to depletion of this mRNA from the gradient RNA band. Thus, positive clones would cause a loss of the electrophysiological signal to 5-HT in oocytes injected with hybrid-depleted RNA. Additional refinements to the strategy included enrichment of the 5-HT$_{1C}$ receptor mRNA by size selection, prior to production of the cDNA library, and subtractive hybridization of the choroid plexus tumor cDNA library with kidney cDNA to remove clones (about 25% of the library) that were common to both tissues and thus could not code for the 5-HT_{1C} receptor.

This strategy was applied to a choroid plexus tumor cDNA library consisting of 35,000 individual clones [3]. These clones were screened in groups of 20, with each assay set requiring cDNA preparation, hybrid selection, injection, and electrophysiological assay of the oocytes. After 1,200 colonies had been screened, one positive clone (clone D9) was identified which contained a 1.9 kb cDNA insert. Later work showed that this clone consisted entirely of 3' untranslated sequence for the 5-HT_{1C} receptor [9]. The presence of a long stretch of 3' untranslated region, which does not code for protein, is quite common in mammalian mRNA, and the length of both 3' and 5' untranslated regions is longer for brain-specific mRNA than for other mRNA [10]. Little is known about the function of these untranslated regions, although they probably play a role in regulating translation initiation and stability of the mRNA [10].

Clone D9 was then used as a hybridization probe to screen the entire cDNA library for other clones which contained a portion of the same nucleotide sequence (homology screening). The longest clones picked from this library were 4 kb in length, lacking 1 kb of sequence from the 5' end of the mRNA from which they were derived. Unfortunately, these clones terminated within the coding region of the 5-HT_{1C} receptor, so that the entire amino acid sequence of the receptor could not be determined [9]. This failure to obtain a full length cDNA is not an uncommon problem in the cloning of brain proteins, since the unusual length of brain-specific messenger RNA's puts great demands on the reverse transcriptase enzyme, and on second strand cDNA synthesis, to transcribe faithfully several thousand bases without premature termination.

The full coding region of the 5-HT_{1C} receptor was first obtained by a different research group (at Columbia University) who devised a variation of the oocyte strategy described above [4]. This group constructed their cDNA library in a bacteriophage expression vector, Lambda-ZAP, which contains promoters for T3 and T7 RNA polymerase flanking the region of the cDNA insert. These promoters allow the cDNA insert to be transcribed in vitro into a cRNA which can be capped with Gppp and injected into oocytes. This strategy provides a direct assay for full length cDNA, since the oocytes will only provide a signal if the cDNA spans the entire coding region of the receptor. Since the oocyte was able to detect extremely low levels of 5-HT_{1C} receptor cDNA amid many negative clones, a sib selection procedure was utilized in which 5 pools of clones (each pool containing 10^5 separate clones) were transcribed in vitro and tested in oocytes, producing a relatively weak (20 to 50 nA) electrophysiological signal in one pool. This pool was divided into 5 pools of 20,000 clones each and further subdivided for four more rounds of screening, until a single positive clone was selected from a total library of 1.2×10^6 independent clones.

The strategy developed by the Columbia University group requires a very high quality cDNA library, so that the entire protein coding region will be contained in at least one clone in the library. This strategy is therefore an "all or none" approach which can quickly produce the full length coding sequence, while the approach of Lübbert et al. [3] will produce positive oocyte signals from clones containing even a fragment of the mRNA sequence (coding or noncoding region). The Columbia strategy has the advantage of immediately focussing on the most useful region of the cDNA clone, the protein coding region, while the approach of Lübbert et al. [3] requires only that a partial fragment of the receptor clone be present in the cDNA library. Since a partial clone can be used either as a hybridization probe to isolate the missing sequence from a cDNA or genomic library, or as a specific primer to direct synthesis of the missing sequence from an impure RNA mixture, the approach of Lübbert et al. [3] should eventually succeed once an initial fragment has been isolated. Also, it should be noted that the Columbia strategy is a powerful and rapid approach for single subunit receptors while the hybrid depletion strategy of Lübbert et al. [3] can be applied to both multiple and single subunit receptors.

3. Structure of the 5-HT$_{1C}$ receptor

The 5-HT$_{1C}$ clone obtained by the Columbia group is a 3 kb coding region fragment derived from the 5 kb mRNA for this receptor. This clone is missing most of the 3' untranslated sequence for this mRNA, even though it was obtained from a cDNA library primed by oligo dT. This primer would be expected to produced cDNA extending all the way to the poly A tail at the 3' terminus of the mRNA. It is possible that part of the 3' untranslated region may have been lost during the construction and screening of this cDNA library or that priming of the cDNA synthesis occurred at an internal site rich in adenine. The Columbia clone contains a single open reading frame encoding a protein of 460 amino acids with a molecular weight of 52,000 daltons. Hydrophobicity analysis of this amino acid sequence suggests the presence of seven membrane spanning domains, in agreement with other G protein-coupled receptors [4].

Figure 2 shows the predicted membrane topology of this receptor, starting with a long extracellular amino terminal end and terminating with an intracellular COOH terminal segment joined to transmembrane region 7. The amino acid sequence and predicted secondary structure of the 5-HT$_{1C}$ receptor are homologous to other G protein-coupled receptors, such as the human beta-adrenoceptor, hamster beta$_2$-adrenoceptor, bovine substance K, rat muscarinic M1 and M3, pig muscarinic, and human alpha$_2$-adrenoceptors [4]. Regions of highest homology are in the transmembrane domains, as is found among other members of this receptor family [1, 4].

This conservation of transmembrane domains would be expected, since recent work has demonstrated the importance of these transmembrane segments for ligand binding in other members of this receptor family. Dixon et al. [11, 12] have constructed deletion mutants of the beta-adrenoceptor which show that the hydrophilic sequences (cytoplasmic and extracellular) of this receptor are not important for ligand binding. The cytoplasmic segments do, however, play an important role in second messenger signalling. In particular, the cytoplasmic loop between transmembrane segments 5 and 6 has been implicated as part of the G-protein binding site of the beta-adrenoceptor [13]. Since the G-protein receptor family appears to interact with a diverse family of different G-proteins, it is not surprising that the cytoplasmic loop between transmembrane segments 5 and 6 shows large variations in length and in amino acid sequence between members of the G-protein receptor family [1].

Certain individual amino acids which are thought to be critical to adrenoceptor function are conserved in the same topological positions in the 5-HT$_{1C}$ receptor. Strader, Dixon and co-workers [11, 12, 14] have determined that Aspartate 79 in transmembrane segment 2, Aspartate 113 in transmembrane segment 3, and Asparagine 318 in transmembrane segment 7 of the hamster beta-adrenoceptor are all important for ligand binding (positions 79 and 318 for agonist binding, and position 113 for antagonist binding). The recent construction of chimeric adrenoceptors by Kobilka et al. [13] has also pointed to the importance of transmembrane segment 7 in ligand binding. In the 5-HT$_{1C}$ receptor, the same two aspartic acid residues and one asparagine residue are present in the same positions as seen for the beta-adrenoceptor (note the inverse coloured amino acids in Figure 2. This fact is consistent with the theory that they play the same critical role in the binding of the monoamine ligand for all of these receptors (possibly via a salt bridge to the amino group of the neurotransmitter).

Another interesting amino acid conservation involves cysteine residues in the extracellular segments. The beta-adrenoceptor has two key cysteine residues, one on the loop between transmembrane segments 2 and 3 and the other on the loop between transmembrane segments 4 and 5. Dixon and Strader have hypothesized that these cysteines form a disulphide bridge between these segments [12]. The same cysteines are conserved at the same positions in the 5-HT$_{1C}$ receptor and thus may play the same role in this protein. Site directed mutation and deletion mutation analysis of the 5-HT$_{1C}$ receptor clone should help verify these ideas and will allow identification of the 5-HT binding and G protein interaction domains of this receptor.

4. New Directions in the 5-HT Receptor Field

The successful cloning of the 5-HT$_{1C}$ receptor and elucidation of its amino acid sequence has provided a gateway for the cloning of other 5-HT receptor subtypes in the near future. We can expect that G protein-coupled 5-HT

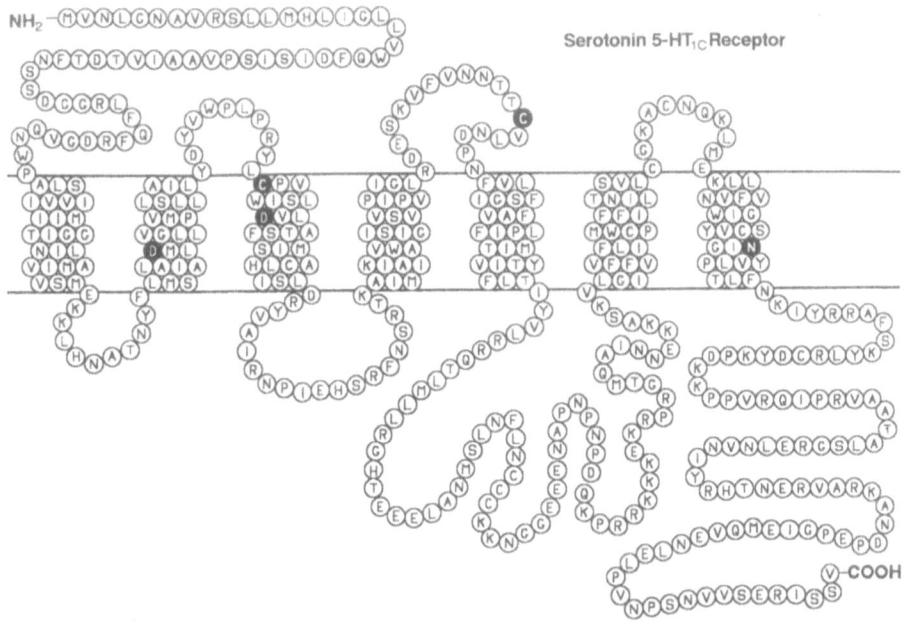

Figure 2. Amino acid sequence and predicted membrane topology of the rat choroid plexus 5-HT$_{1C}$ receptor. The diagram shows the predicted distribution of the 5-HT$_{1C}$ receptor sequence between transmembrane domains and cytoplasmic or extracellular domains, assuming that the amino terminal end lies on the extracellular face of the membrane (sequence data from reference [4]). The five amino acid residues highlighted in reverse text are believed to be important for ligand binding in other members of the G-protein receptor family, and are found in the same topological positions as in the 5-HT$_{1C}$ receptor.

receptors (which now appear to include the 5-HT$_2$, 5-HT$_{1A}$, 5-HT$_{1B}$, 5-HT$_{1P}$ and 5-HT$_{1D}$ receptors) will all prove to be single subunit proteins with seven transmembrane domains and some similarities in amino acid sequence. This information, along with the availability of the 5-HT$_{1C}$ clone, should lead to cloning of all these G protein-coupled 5-HT receptor subtypes in the near future. Other 5-HT receptor subtypes, such as the 5-HT$_3$ receptor, may be multisubunit proteins which are directly coupled to an ion channel [15]. Such multi-subunit ion channels would require a different cloning approach.

The availability of the gene and amino acid structures of this increasingly important receptor family should help settle long-standing controversies on the number and diversity of 5-HT receptor subtypes. At the current time, at least six distinct 5-HT receptor subtypes have been named [16] and several more appear poised to join this list. Inherent limitations in binding and response assays have triggered frequent, often spirited debates over various receptor classification schemes. The ultimate resolution of these continuing controversies will only come with the cloning and sequencing of genes coding for these receptors. Elucidation of the primary amino acid sequences of these receptors will reveal enough about their structures and diversity to provide a truly molecular basis for 5-HT receptor classification [17]. Unfortunately, we may have to absorb an increase rather than a decrease in the number of 5-HT receptor subtypes during this process, if the experience with other monoamine receptor families provides any indication of the future [2]. Molecular pharmacologists should not, however, be timid in demanding proof that the receptor proteins predicted from nucleic acid data are indeed expressed and functional in native biological systems before accepting claims that yet another 5-HT receptor subtype must be reckoned with.

In the field of cardiovascular and periperal 5-HT receptors, in particular, molecular biology may well bring about a revolution in our understanding of 5-HT receptor action. Many of the benefits of receptor binding technology have bypassed this field because of the low density of 5-HT receptors in these tissues and the subsequent difficulty in studying them by radioligand binding. Molecular biology provides new approaches (Northern blot analysis, 'in situ' hybridization) that can, in difficult systems, be much more sensitive and selective than current receptor binding assays. Molecular cloning techniques give us the power to isolate cDNA clones for very low abundance mRNA species (encoding 0.01% or less of the cellular protein), then produce large amounts of these rare proteins by transfecting these clones into appropriate cell lines. This technology should enable the study of very rare receptor subtypes present at extremely low density in the central and peripheral nervous systems. Discovery of additional receptor subtypes, and rapid progress in our understanding of the molecular basis of 5-HT receptor pharmacology, can confidently be expected to follow from these new initiatives in molecular biology.

References

1. Dohlman HG, Caron MG, Lefkowitz RJ (1987): A family of receptors coupled to guanine nucleotide regulatory proteins, *Biochemistry* 26: 2657–2664.
2. Lester HA (1988): Heterologous expression of excitability proteins: route to more specific drugs? *Science* 241: 1057–1063.
3. Lübbert H, Hoffman BJ, Snutch TP, van Dyke T, Levine AJ, Hartig PR, Lester HA, Davidson N (1987): cDNA cloning of a serotonin 5-HT$_{1C}$ receptor by using electrophysiological assays of mRNA-injected Xenopus oocytes. *Proc Natl Acad Sci USA* 84: 4332–4336.
4. Julius D, MacDermott AB, Axel R, Jessell TM (1988): Molecular characterization of a functional cDNA encoding the serotonin 5-HT$_{1C}$ receptor. *Science* 241: 558–564.
5. Gundersen CB, Miledi R, Parker I (1983): Serotonin receptors induced by exogenous messenger RNA in Xenopus oocytes. *Proc Royal Soc London* B219: 103–109.
6. Dascal N, Ifune C, Hopkins R, Snutch TP, Lübbert H, Davidson N, Simon MI, Lester HA (1986): Involvement of a GTP-binding protein in mediation of serotonin and acetylcholine responses in Xenopus oocytes injected with rat brain messenger RNA *Mol Brain Res* 1: 201–209.
7. Lübbert H, Snutch TP, Dascal N, Lester HA, Davidson N (1987): Rat brain 5-HT$_{1C}$ receptors are encoded by a 5-6 kbase mRNA size class and are functionally expressed in injected Xenopus oocytes. *J Neurosci* 7: 1159–1165.

8. Yagaloff KA, Lozano G, van Dyke T, Levine AJ, Hartig PR (1986): Serotonin 5-HT$_{1C}$ receptors are expressed at high density on choroid plexus tumors from transgenic mice. *Brain Res* 385: 389—394.

9. Hoffman BJ (1988): Molecular pharmacology of serotonin receptors: radioligand development, mechanisms of signal transduction, and cloning of a receptor gene. Doctoral thesis, Johns Hopkins University.

10. Sutcliffe JG (1988): mRNA in the mammalian central nervous system. *Ann Rev Neurosci* 11: 157—198.

11. Dixon RAF, Sigal IS, Rands E, Register RB, Candelore MR, Blake AD, Strader CD (1987): Ligand binding to the beta-adrenergic receptor involves its rhodopsin-like core, *Nature* 326: 73—77.

12. Dixon RAF, Sigal IS, Candelore MR, Register RB, Scattergood W, Rands E, Strader CD (1987): Structural features required for ligand binding to the beta-adrenergic receptor, *EMBO Journal* 6: 3269—3275.

13. Kobilka BK, Kobilka TS, Daniel K, Regan JW, Caron MG, Lefkowitz RJ (1988): Chimeric alpha$_2$-, beta$_2$-adrenergic receptors: delineation of domains involved in effector coupling and ligand binding specificity, *Science* 240: 1310—1316.

14. Strader CD, Sigal IS, Register RB, Candelore MR, Rands E, Dixon RAF (1987): Identification of residues required for ligand binding to the beta-adrenergic receptor, *Proc Natl Acad Sci USA* 84: 4384—4388.

15. Hoyer D (1988): Moleuclar pharmacology and biology of 5-HT$_{1C}$ receptors, *Trends Pharm Sci* 9: 89—94.

16. Peroutka SJ (1988): 5-Hydroxytryptamine Receptor Subtypes, *Ann Rev Neurosci* 11: 45—60.

17. Hartig PR (1989): Molecular biology of 5-HT receptors. *Trends Pharm Sci* 10: 64—69.

IV. Regional differences in the transduction mechanisms of 5-hydroxytryptamine receptors in the mammalian brain

M. HAMON, M. B. EMERIT, S. EL MESTIKAWY,
M. C. GALLISSOT, and H. GOZLAN

1. Introduction

During the last ten years, binding studies with selective radioligands have contributed to the present knowledge of central 5-hydroxytryptamine (5-HT) receptors, leading to the identification of membrane-bound specific sites with pharmacological properties expected for such receptors. Three main classes of 5-HT binding sites designated 5-HT_1, 5-HT_2 and 5-HT_3 have been identified so far [1]. Apparently a single homogeneous population of sites corresponds to each of the two latter classes (at least in the CNS), but clearcut evidence of heterogeneity of 5-HT_1 sites has been reported [2]. Thus it could be established that 5-HT_1 sites are a mixture of 4 distinct classes of high affinity sites for $[^3H]5\text{-HT}$ called 5-HT_{1A}, 5-HT_{1B}, 5-HT_{1C} and 5-HT_{1D}, whose proportions are extremely variable from one brain area to another, and also from one species to another.

Binding studies are useful for identification of specific binding sites, but tell nothing regarding their correspondence to authentic receptors. Pharmacological, electrophysiological and biochemical investigations have to be carried out to demonstrate this. In particular, at the cellular level, the binding of 5-HT and related agonists to these sites should trigger a biological response with measurable biochemical and electrophysiological correlates. Receptors for monoamines, notably catecholamines, function with second messengers such as cyclic AMP (cAMP) and the breakdown products of phosphatidylinositol bisphosphate (i.e. mainly diacylglycerol-DAG and inositol trisphosphate IP_3); the possible effects of 5-HT on such compounds in target cells have been explored. In 1975 Von Hungen et al. [3] reported stimulation of adenylate cyclase (AC) activity in brain by 5-HT. However, identification of the 5-HT receptors responsible for this effect could not then be achieved because of poor knowledge of 5-HT binding sites, and of the limited number of 5-HT agonists and antagonists available to define the pharmacological profile of the 5-HT-evoked response. Recently, the development of numerous new drugs with marked selectivity for the various classes of 5-HT

P.R. Saxena, D.I. Wallis, W. Wouters and P. Bevan (eds), Cardiovascular Pharmacology of 5-Hydroxytryptamine, pp. 41–59.
© 1990 *Kluwer Academic Publishers, Dordrecht* —

binding sites allowed investigations on the possible coupling of these sites to second messenger systems. Thus it could be demonstrated that 5-HT_{1A}, 5-HT_{1B} and 5-HT_{1D} are coupled with AC whereas 5-HT_{1C} and 5-HT_2 control phosphoinositide (PI) turnover in brain [see 4, 5 for reviews].

The present article recalls the main experimental facts which led to these conclusions. However, evidence for coupling of 5-HT receptors to other transducing mechanisms also exists, and will be discussed in relation to the marked regional differences in the functions and modulations of 5-HT receptors in brain.

2. Indirect evidence of the coupling of central 5-HT binding sites with AC and PI turnover

The coupling of a neurotransmitter binding subunit with the enzyme synthesizing the second messengers, i.e. AC for cAMP and phosphoinositide-specific phospholipase C (PLC) for DAG and inositolphosphates from phosphatidylinositol-bisphosphate, is not direct but involves specific proteins having the capacity of binding guanine nucleotides, and designated G proteins [6]. Several families of these proteins have been identified, depending on their role in the functional coupling between the receptor subunit (R) and the enzyme synthesizing the second messengers; e.g. Gs for those ensuring AC stimulation upon binding of an agonist to R, Gi for those implicated in AC inhibition after the same molecular event, Gp (still poorly identified) for PLC modulation in the case of receptors controlling PI turnover.

Extensive studies on receptors coupled to AC have demonstrated that G proteins not only control the enzyme activity but also the receptor subunit R. Indeed a receptor exhibits a high affinity for agonists when it is physically associated (RG) with the G protein in membranes, whereas the free form R has a markedly lower affinity for agonists [6]. In contrast, the affinity of R for antagonists is not, or poorly, affected by its association with the G protein. It can be predicted whether R functions with or without a G protein from exploring its binding capacity towards agonists in the presence or absence of GTP (or an active analogue, for instance GppNHp). Indeed in the presence of an agonist, GTP has the capacity to dissociate the complex RG, and therefore to reduce the affinity of R for the agonist. In contrast, for R not coupled to G, the nucleotide will not affect its affinity for any ligand, agonist or antagonist.

Soon after the identification of 5-HT binding sites in brain, Peroutka et al. [7] reported that GTP affects the binding of agonists to 5-HT_1 sites specifically labelled by [^{3}H]5-HT, but not to 5-HT_2 sites specifically labelled by [^{3}H]spiperone. Extensive studies then demonstrated that only the first part of this statement was correct, as numerous groups [8—12] including ours [8, 9], clearly showed that the binding of agonists to 5-HT_2 sites is also modulated by GTP as expected from the coupling of 5-HT_2 receptors to G proteins. More recent investigations, using appropriate ligands for the specific labelling of the various classes of 5-HT_1 binding sites, confirmed the coupling with G proteins of 5-HT_{1A} [13, 14], 5-HT_{1B} [14] and 5-HT_{1D} [15] binding subunits. In contrast, no evidence of such coupling has yet been reported for 5-HT_{1C} sites, since the only study devoted to this question mentioned that the binding of 5-HT to 5-HT_{1C} sites was unaffected by the stable GTP analogue GppNHp [16]. This finding is surprising as the recent sequencing of the 5-HT_{1C}-R molecule (see Chapter III) revealed that it belongs to the family of G protein-coupled receptors, which are thought to traverse the cytoplasmic membrane seven times [17]. Furthermore, the 5-HT_{1A}-R, for which clearcut evidence of coupling with G protein has been reported [13, 14], exhibits the same molecular organization (the sequence of the human 5-HT_{1A}-R is in fact that of the G21 protein [18, M. G. Caron, personal communication]). In contrast, guanine nucleotides have been shown to be inactive upon central 5-HT_3 receptors [19] suggesting that the latter do not function with G proteins in brain membranes.

3. Coupling of central 5-HT receptors with adenylate cyclase

3.1 *Positive coupling*

As previously observed for other monoamine receptors (β-adrenoceptors, D_1) coupled to G proteins, a positive interaction between 5-HT receptors and AC is observed in the brain of various mammalian species [3, 20, 21]. As shown in Figure 1, a concentration-dependent stimulatory effect of 5-HT on cAMP production from ATP by brain tissue homogenates can be found in adult as well as in new born rats. Indeed, this effect is more pronounced during early life, which led Enjalbert et al. [22, 23] to explore the characteristics of the corresponding receptor in young animals. This 5-HT receptor was found to be postsynaptically located, with a regional distribution more or less related to that of 5-HT_1 sites, but with pharmacological properties completely different from those of 5-HT_1 subtypes. For instance, RU 24969, an agonist in the nM range at 5-HT_{1A}, 5-HT_{1B} and 5-HT_{1D} receptors, does not stimulate 5-HT-sensitive AC [24], and the potent 5-HT_1 antagonists propranolol and alprenolol [25] do not prevent the increased enzyme activity due to 5-HT [20, 26]. Furthermore, 5-HT exerts no effect on AC activity in the choroid plexus where 5-HT_{1C} sites are highly concentrated [16]. Therefore, it is unlikely (but see [27]) that any of the 5-HT_1 subtypes corresponds to the 5-HT receptor positively coupled to AC in the rat brain. In addition, the latter receptor is not 5-HT_2 since ketanserin does not prevent AC stimulation by 5-HT in rat hippocampal membranes [26].

Recently Dumuis et al. [28] proposed that the 5-HT receptor positively coupled to AC in rat colliculi might correspond to the 5-HT_3 type since ICS

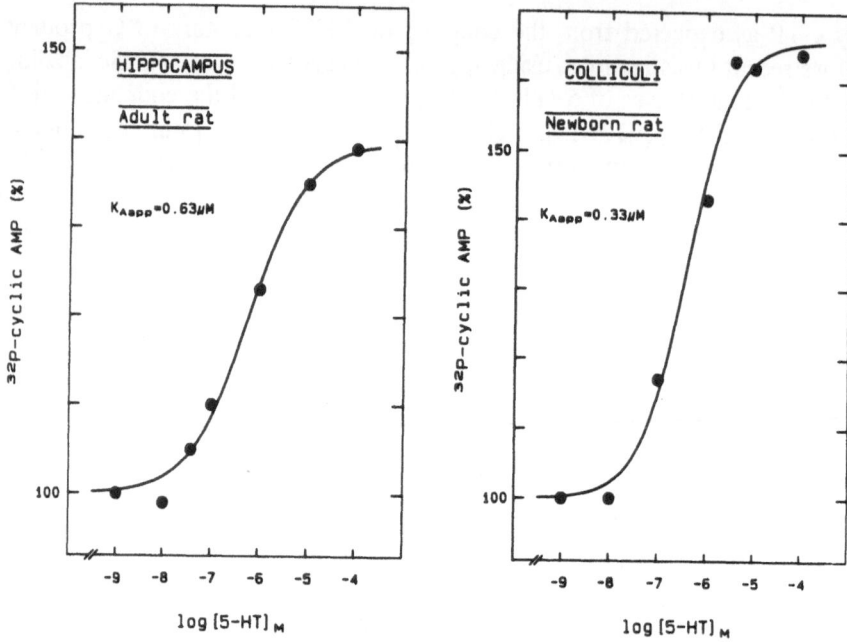

Figure 1. Concentration-dependent stimulation by 5-HT of basal adenylate cyclase activity in homogenates from the hippocampus of adult rats and the colliculi of new born rats.

Adenylate cyclase was assayed with 0.5 mM [^{32}P]ATP [22]. Adult rats were 3 month-old and new born rats were 4 day-old. 5-HT-induced increase in [^{32}P]cAMP production is expressed as percentage over basal AC activity (100%). Each point is the mean of triplicate determinations in two separate experiments. K_{Aapp}: 5-HT concentration producing half-maximal stimulation of adenylate cyclase activity.

205-930, a selective 5-HT$_3$ antagonist, was found to prevent the stimulatory effect of 5-HT upon cAMP production. However, in colliculi homogenates from new born rats, ICS 205-930 (1 μM) did not affect AC stimulation (+47%) by 5 μM 5-HT [unpublished observations]. Indeed this postulated coupling is surprising since the 5-HT$_3$ receptor does not function with a G protein (see above).

In conclusion, the 5-HT receptor positively coupled to AC in rat brain at least (particularly in adult hippocampus) cannot be included in the classification generally accepted in most laboratories [1]. Its function regarding 5-HT neurotransmission is still puzzling, as its postnatal development is completely different from that of serotoninergic fibres and terminals invading progressively various brain structures. It might be involved in the trophic effect of 5-HT during brain maturation [29], but further investigations should be performed to assess this point. In addition, it cannot be excluded that the 5-HT receptor positively coupled to AC in the rat does not extend to other species, since part of the stimulatory effect of 5-HT upon AC activity in guinea pig hippocampal membranes involves 5-HT$_{1A}$ receptors [see 30].

3.2 *Negative coupling*

Using the assay conditions devised by De Vivo and Maayani [31] which consist of measuring AC activity in the presence of its direct activator, forskolin, a negative effect of 5-HT upon this enzyme could be found in various brain areas (Table 1). The inhibitory effect was maximum in hippocampus, and then decreased in the following order: substantia nigra, cerebral cortex, septum, raphe area, hypothalamus. No significant effect of 5-HT was detected on forskolin-stimulated AC activity in striatum and cerebellum (Table 1). Since this regional distribution was markedly different from that of any of the 5-HT binding sites [see 1], it could be proposed that the 5-HT effect involves either another unidentified 5-HT receptor type, or a "mixture" of these receptors. Indeed the second hypothesis proved to be the right one.

Table 1. Inhibitory effect of 5-HT and 8-OH-DPAT on forskolin-stimulated adenylate cyclase activity in various regions of the rat brain.

Brain region	[^{32}P]cyclic AMP (nmoles/mg prot)		
	None	+1 μM 5-HT	+0.1 μM 8-OH-DPAT
Raphe area	2.35 ± 0.08	2.04 ± 0.06* (−13%)	2.07 ± 0.05* (−12%)
Hippocampus	2.97 ± 0.09	2.13 ± 0.07* (−28%)	2.09 ± 0.06* (−30%)
Hypothalamus	3.36 ± 0.11	2.99 ± 0.09* (−11%)	3.03 ± 0.10 (−10%)
Substantia nigra	4.12 ± 0.21	3.04 ± 0.09* (−26%)	3.98 ± 0.14 (−3%)
Cerebellum	4.14 ± 0.24	3.81 ± 0.14 (−8%)	4.05 ± 0.18 (−2%)
Cerebral cortex	4.92 ± 0.18	4.00 ± 0.20* (−19%)	4.12 ± 0.21* (−16%)
Septum	5.97 ± 0.24	5.00 ± 0.21* (−16%)	4.95 ± 0.19* (−17%)
Striatum	20.87 ± 0.84	19.62 ± 0.79 (−6%)	19.93 ± 1.01 (−5%)

Adenylate cyclase assays were performed in the presence of 0.5 mM [^{32}P]ATP, 0.1 M NaCl, 10 μM GTP and 10 μM forskolin, plus 1 μM 5-HT or 0.1 μM 8-OH-DPAT as indicated. The enzyme activity is expressed in nmoles [^{32}P]cyclic AMP synthesized per mg protein and per 20 min at 30 °C. Each value is the mean ± S.E.M. of 3 separate determinations. The percent reduction due to 5-HT or 8-OH-DPAT is indicated in parentheses.
* P < 0.05 when compared to respective control value, in the absence of 5-HT or 8-OH-DPAT.

As shown in Table 1, the 5-HT$_{1A}$ selective agonist, 8-OH-DPAT, also exerted a significant inhibitory effect on forskolin-stimulated AC activity in hippocampus, septum, cerebral cortex and raphe area, where 5-HT$_{1A}$ binding sites are concentrated in adult rats [32].

Surprisingly, an inhibitory effect of 5-HT and 8-OH-DPAT on the forskolin-stimulated enzyme was also found in cerebellum homogenates from new born rats (Table 2), whereas, as expected from the lack of 5-HT$_{1A}$ binding sites [32], both agonists were inactive in the cerebellum of adults. However further investigations on 5-HT$_{1A}$ binding sites during development revealed that these sites exist in the rat cerebellum for the first two weeks after birth only [33]. Therefore, in young as in adult animals, a close correlation exists between the regional distribution of 8-OH-DPAT-induced inhibition of forskolin-stimulated AC activity and that of 5-HT$_{1A}$ sites. Extensive pharmacological investigations on 5-HT-induced inhibition of the forskolin-stimulated enzyme in the adult rat hippocampus also led to the conclusion that this effect involves 5-HT$_{1A}$ receptors. In addition to 8-OH-DPAT, other selective 5-HT$_{1A}$ agonists such as ipsapirone, buspirone (Table 2) and gepirone mimicked (at least partially) the 5-HT effect, whereas 5-HT$_{1A}$ antagonists prevented it [31, 34—36].

Table 2. Effects of various 5-HT$_{1A}$ agonists on forskolin-stimulated adenylate cyclase activity in homogenates from adult rat hippocampus or new born rat cerebellum.

Addition	Hippocampus Adult rat	Cerebellum New born rat
	[^{32}P]cyclic AMP (nmol/mg prot)	
None	3.29 ± 0.15	0.72 ± 0.04
5-HT (1 μM)	2.42 ± 0.09* (−26%)	0.59 ± 0.05* (−18%)
8-OH-DPAT (1 μM)	2.38 ± 0.08* (−28%)	0.59 ± 0.03* (−18%)
Ipsapirone (1 μM)	2.46 ± 0.11* (−25%)	0.60 ± 0.04* (−17%)
Buspirone (1 μM)	2.81 ± 0.07* (−15%)	0.63 ± 0.04* (−13%)

Adenylate cyclase was assayed with 0.5 mM [^{32}P]ATP in the presence of 10 μM forskolin, 10 μM GTP and 0.1 M NaCl, plus 1 μM of various 5-HT$_{1A}$ agonists at indicated. Each value (in nmoles [^{32}P]cyclic AMP synthesized per mg protein and per 20 min at 30 °C) is the mean ± S.E.M. of 3 independent determinations. The percent reduction due to each agonist is indicated in parentheses.
* P < 0.05 when compared to respective control values.

In contrast to hippocampus, 8-OH-DPAT did not mimic the inhibitory effect of 5-HT on forskolin-stimulated AC activity in the rat substantia nigra (Table 1). Conversely, agonists acting on 5-HT_{1B} sites such as RU 24969 and CGS 12066B did (Figure 2). Furthermore, 5-HT_{1B} antagonists such as cyanopindolol and propranolol, but not the 5-HT_{1A} (and 5-HT_2) antagonist spiperone, the 5-HT_{1C} antagonist mesulergine and the 5-HT_2 antagonist ketanserin, prevented the 5-HT-induced inhibition of the nigral enzyme [37]. Accordingly, it can be concluded that 5-HT_{1B} sites are negatively coupled to AC in the substantia nigra, where they are highly concentrated in the adult rat [32].

Several reports suggest that 5-HT_{1B} sites correspond to presynaptic autoreceptors which control 5-HT release from nerve endings [38], but binding studies revealed that most (if not all) of these sites are postsynaptically located [32]. Similarly, we found that selective lesion of serotoninergic projections to substantia nigra by 5,7-dihydroxytryptamine treatment did not significantly alter the 5-HT-induced inhibition of forskolin-stimulated nigral

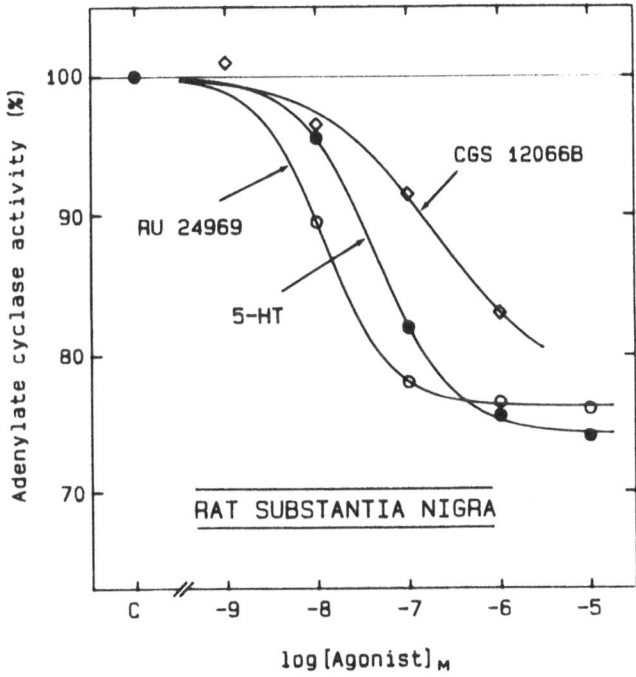

Figure 2. Concentration-dependent inhibition of forskolin-stimulated adenylate cyclase activity by 5-HT, RU 24969 and CGS 12066B in substantia nigra homogenates from adult rats.

Adenylate cyclase was assayed with 0.5 mM [^{32}P]ATP in the presence of 10 μM forskolin, 10 μM GTP and 0.1 M NaCl [31], plus various concentrations of each agonist as indicated on the abscissa. The enzyme activity is expressed as percentage of the control value (C), without drugs. Each point is the mean of triplicate determinations.

AC activity in rats (Figure 3), indicating that, like 5-HT$_{1B}$ sites, the coupled receptors are postsynaptic. In line with these observations, it has recently been established that presynaptic autoreceptors controlling 5-HT release do not function through a coupling with AC [39].

On the basis of their identical pharmacological properties and common location at the synaptic level, it can be inferred that postsynaptic 5-HT$_{1B}$ sites are the 5-HT receptors negatively coupled to AC in the rat substantia nigra. Although much less has been done on the possible transduction mechanism

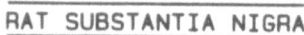

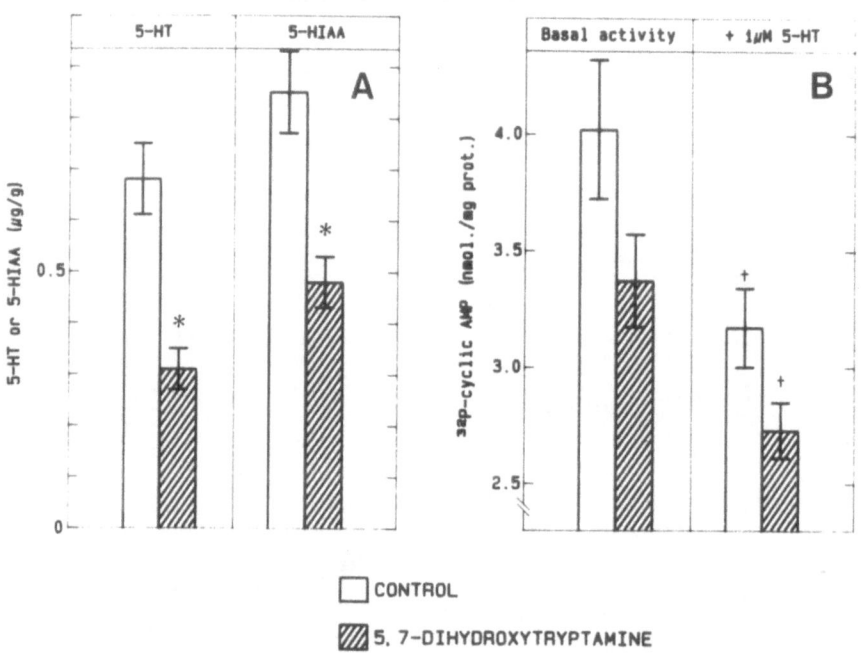

Figure 3. 5-HT and 5-HIAA levels (A) and 5-HT-sensitive adenylate cyclase activity (B) in the rat substantia nigra after 5,7-DHT lesion.

5,7-DHT (8 μg/4 μl) was injected intracerebrally [13] and adult rats were sacrificed three weeks later. 5-HT and 5-HIAA levels were measured by HPLC coupled to electrochemical detection [36], and adenylate cyclase was assayed with 0.5 mM [^{32}P]ATP in the presence of 10 μM forskolin, 10 μM GTP and 0.1 M NaCl plus or minus 1 μM 5-HT as indicated. Each bar represents the mean ± S.E.M. of 6 independent determinations.

* P < 0.05 when compared to respective values in control rats.

† P < 0.05 when compared to "basal" adenylate cyclase activity, in the absence of 5-HT.

Although some reduction in adenylate cyclase activity was found in 5,7-DHT-lesioned rats compared to controls, the absolute decrease due to 5-HT was not significantly different in the two groups of animals (controls: 0.83 ± 0.12 nmol [^{32}P]cAMP/mg prot/20 min at 30 °C; lesioned: 0.64 ± 0.15 nmol/mg prot/20 min).

of 5-HT$_{1D}$ sites, recent evidence reports a negative coupling of these sites with AC in calf substantia nigra [40], suggesting that 5-HT$_{1D}$ sites are probably equivalent to 5-HT$_{1B}$ sites in species (including man [41]) where the latter are absent.

In conclusion, convincing evidence exists for the negative coupling of 5-HT$_{1A}$, 5-HT$_{1B}$ and 5-HT$_{1D}$ binding sites with AC in selected brain regions. Conversely, clearcut pharmacological data demonstrate that AC does not participate in the transduction mechanisms of 5-HT$_{1C}$, 5-HT$_2$ and 5-HT$_3$ receptors.

4. Coupling of central 5-HT receptors with PLC

In the rat choroid plexus, 5-HT stimulates PI turnover and this effect can be mimicked by agonists and prevented by antagonists acting preferentially on 5-HT$_{1C}$ sites [42]. Indeed, a significant correlation exists between the pharmacological profile of the 5-HT-evoked response and that of 5-HT$_{1C}$ binding sites labelled by [^{125}I]LSD [42—44], demonstrating that these sites are functionally coupled to PLC.

A stimulatory effect of 5-HT upon PI turnover also occurs in various brain regions, but the relative efficacies of a series of agonists to mimic, and of antagonists to prevent, the 5-HT-induced effect are markedly different from those noted in the choroid plexus [42—44]. The pharmacological profile of the 5-HT-evoked response in the cerebral cortex showed a significant correlation with that of 5-HT$_2$ binding sites, strongly suggesting that the latter are functionally coupled to PI turnover [45, 46]. Confirmation comes from studies on in vivo modulations of 5-HT$_2$ sites. A good parallelism is observed between changes in 5-HT-induced stimulation of PI turnover and in the density of 5-HT$_2$ binding sites in the cerebral cortex after various pharmacological treatments [46, 47].

The cell types with 5-HT$_2$ receptors functionally coupled to PLC in the cerebral cortex have not been clearly identified, but recent evidence suggests that they might in part be astrocytes [48]. Interestingly, the other receptor type coupled to PLC, i.e. the 5-HT$_{1C}$, is also located on non-neuronal cells (i.e. epithelial cells) in the choroid plexus [49]. Therefore, in marked contrast with 5-HT$_1$ receptors coupled to AC which appear to be exclusively located on neurones in brain [48, 50], the 5-HT receptors controlling PI turnover are — at least partly — located on other cell types.

5. Functional 5-HT receptors uncoupled to AC or PLC

Electrophysiological recording from pyramidal cells in hippocampal slices has shown that 5-HT causes a large hyperpolarization due to a selective increase in K$^+$ conductance. This effect is probably mediated through

5-HT$_{1A}$ receptors, since it can be reproduced (partially) by 8-OH-DPAT and prevented by spiperone [51]. Furthermore, 5-HT-evoked responses were most prominent in the stratum radiatum where 5-HT$_{1A}$ sites are the most abundant [51]. Nevertheless, these receptors do not seem to correspond to the 5-HT$_{1A}$ type coupled to AC, since neither bath application of the membrane-soluble cAMP analogue, 8-bromo-cyclic AMP, nor the intracellular injection of the cyclic nucleotide itself, reduced the response to 5-HT. This is in contrast to what would be expected if the latter was triggered by the negative influence of the amine upon cAMP production [52]. The involvement of second messengers derived from PI turnover could also be ruled out, since activation of protein kinase C (normally by DAG) fails to mimic the 5-HT-evoked response. Furthermore, the latter is independent of intracellular Ca^{2+}, in contrast to the effects mediated by IP$_3$, the other main second messenger derived from PI hydrolysis.

Nevertheless, as expected from the involvement of an authentic 5-HT$_{1A}$ receptor, that mediating the hyperpolarization of hippocampal pyramidal cells by 5-HT is functionally coupled to a Gi (or Go) protein, since inactivation of the latter by Pertussis toxin completely prevented the 5-HT-evoked response. Conversely, direct activation of G proteins by GTPγS mimicked the effect of the indoleamine [52]. These observations led to the conclusion that at least some 5-HT$_{1A}$ receptors in rat hippocampus may be physically associated with a Gi or Go protein for controlling a K^+channel [52]. According to this view, 5-HT$_{1A}$ receptors should be considered functionally equivalent to GABA B and adenosine receptors, since coupling of the two latter to the same K^+-channel via a Pertussis toxin-sensitive G protein has been recently demonstrated [53].

In addition to the hippocampus, where the most complete and elegant studies have been performed [51—53], other brain areas rich in 5-HT$_{1A}$ receptors such as the septum [54] and the dorsal raphe nucleus [55] probably function in the same way regarding 5-HT synaptic transduction mechanisms. 5-HT$_{1A}$ agonists also trigger hyperpolarization by opening a K^+channel in septal and raphe cells.

6. Regional differences in the functioning of central 5-HT receptors

On account of marked differences in the regional distributions of various classes of 5-HT receptors functionally coupled to distinct transducing mechanisms (Table 3), variable effects of 5-HT will be observed from one area to another depending on the relative proportions of these receptors in each area. But in addition to these expected differences, others have been noted which demonstrate that 5-HT receptors of apparently the same type may not be perfectly equivalent in various brain areas. Clearcut evidence of such heterogeneity has been reported for 5-HT$_{1A}$ and 5-HT$_2$ "related" receptors.

Table 3. Main locations and cellular transduction mechanisms of central 5-HT receptors.

Receptor type	Main location	Coupling mechanism	Second messengers
5-HT$_{1A}$	Hippocampus	-negative (Gi) with adenylate cyclase	cyclic AMP ↘
		-K$^+$ channel (via Gi or Go)	none
5-HT$_{1B}$	Substantia nigra (rat)	-negative (Gi) with adenylate cyclase	cyclic AMP ↘
5-HT$_{1D}$	Substantia nigra (calf)	-negative (Gi) with adenylate cyclase	cyclic AMP ↘
5-HT$_{1C}$	Choroid plexus	-positive, phosphatidylinositol turnover	-inositol ↗ trisphosphate -diacylgly- ↗ cerol
5-HT$_2$	Frontal cortex	-positive, phosphatidylinositol turnover	-inositol ↗ trisphosphate -diacylgly- ↗ cerol
5-HT$_3$	Entorhinal cortex area postrema	cation channels	none

6.1 *5-HT$_{1A}$-related receptors*

5-HT$_{1A}$ receptors are heterogeneous in their cellular location, since lesion studies have demonstrated that those within the dorsal and median raphe nuclei are located presynaptically on the soma and dendrites of serotoninergic neurones [32, 56, 57], whereas in other brain areas these receptors are located postsynaptically [32]. Apparently, such differential locations are associated with different pharmacological properties since several behavioural [58—60] and metabolic [36] effects of 5-HT$_{1A}$ agonists are compatible with a preferential action on the presynaptic sites located in the raphe nuclei. The same effects could be evoked either by systemic administration or intra raphe injection of these drugs. In contrast, other pharmacological effects of 5-HT$_{1A}$ agonists seem to depend on the preferential stimulation of postsynaptic sites [61].

    In an attempt to understand why *either* the pre- *or* postsynaptic 5-HT$_{1A}$ receptors apparently mediate the effects of a given 5-HT$_{1A}$ agonist, we compared the pharmacological properties of corresponding binding sites in the dorsal raphe nucleus where they are presynaptic and in the dentate gyrus where they are exclusively postsynaptic. As shown in Figure 4, no real difference was noted in these two regions, indicating that 5-HT$_{1A}$ binding

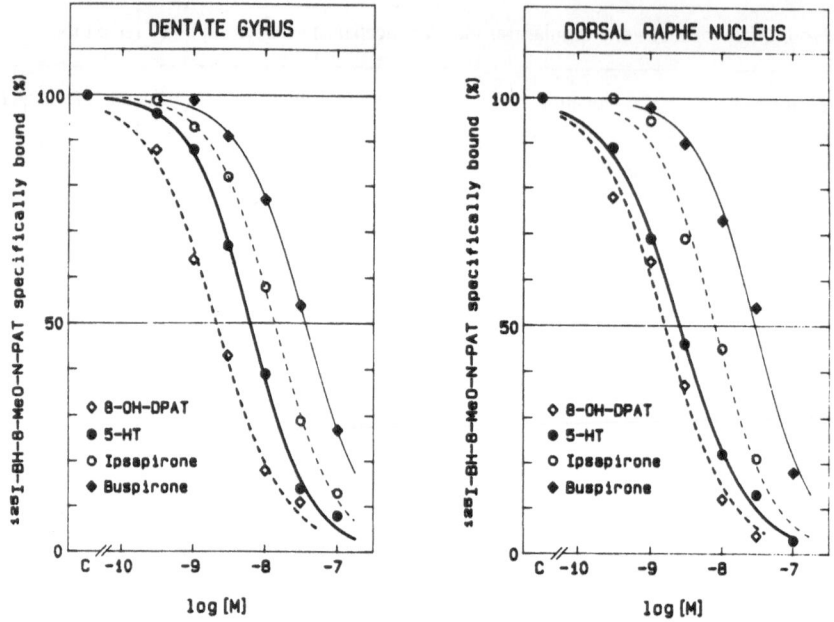

Figure 4. Concentration-dependent inhibition by various agonists of the specific binding of [^{125}I]BH-8-MeO-N-PAT to 5-HT$_{1A}$ sites in the dentate gyrus and the dorsal raphe nucleus of adult rats.

Brain sections (16 μm thick) were incubated with 80 pM [^{125}I]BH-8-MeO-N-PAT and various concentrations of each agonist (8-OH-DPAT, 5-HT, ipsapirone, buspirone) as indicated, and then processed for quantitative autoradiography as described [32]. Optical density in both regions was converted into fmol. of [^{125}I]BH-8-MeO-N-PAT specifically bound (i.e. minus that measured on films from sections incubated with 10 μM 5-HT), and expressed in percent of that found with sections incubated with the radioligand alone (C on the abscissa). Each point is the mean of 14—18 measurements in two independent experiments. Only minor differences were noted between these agonists in inhibiting [^{125}I]BH-8-MeO-N-PAT binding to *presynaptic* 5-HT$_{1A}$ sites in dorsal raphe nucleus and to *postsynaptic* 5-HT$_{1A}$ sites in dentate gyrus.

sites exhibit the same pharmacological profile whether they are pre- or post-synaptically located. Another possible explanation of the preferential involvement of pre-synaptic 5-HT$_{1A}$ receptors in the effects of 5-HT$_{1A}$ agonists in vivo (at least in some circumstances) would be that the efficiency of 5-HT$_{1A}$ receptor coupling to transducing mechanisms is higher at pre- than at post-synaptic sites. Indirect estimate of coupling efficiency can be inferred from guanine nucleotide-induced modulations of agonist binding, since they depend on functional interactions between receptor and G protein. However, in this case too, no difference was found between pre- and post-synaptic 5-HT$_{1A}$ sites; the GTP analogue, GppNHp, similarly reduced the binding of [^{125}I]BH-8-MeO-N-PAT to 5-HT$_{1A}$ sites in the dorsal raphe nucleus and in the hippocampus (dentate gyrus and CA1, Figure 5).

In contrast to binding studies, electrophysiological recording of 5-HT$_{1A}$-evoked pre- and post-synaptic responses was more successful in explaining

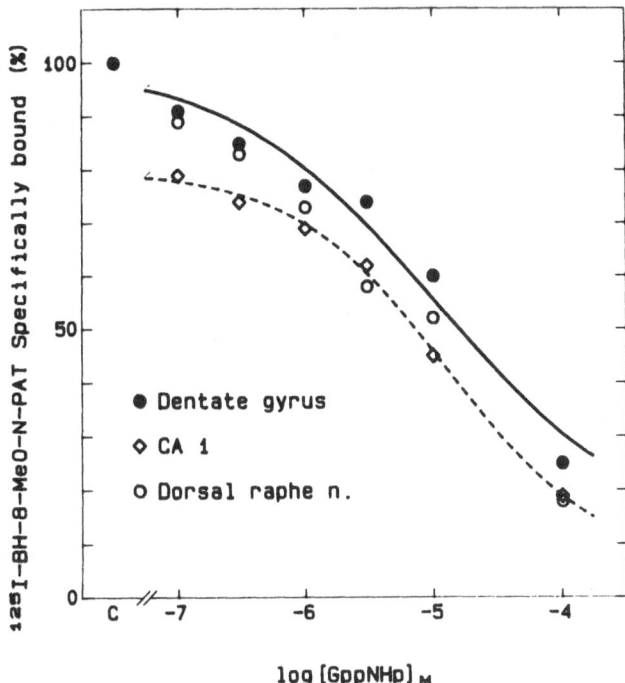

Figure 5. Concentration-dependent inhibition by GppNHp of the specific binding of [^{125}I]BH-8-MeO-N-PAT to 5-HT$_{1A}$ sites in the dentate gyrus and CA1 area of the hippocampus, and in the dorsal raphe nucleus of adult rat.

The same protocol as that described in the legend to Figure 4 was used except that the GTP analogue, GppNHp, was added instead of 5-HT$_{1A}$ agonists to the incubating medium of brain sections. Each point is the mean of 14—18 measurements in two independent experiments. In hippocampal areas where 5-HT$_{1A}$ sites are *postsynaptic* as in the dorsal raphe nucleus where these sites are *presynaptic*, the IC50 of GppNHp is around 10 μM.

— at least partly — why 5-HT$_{1A}$ agonist-induced effects in vivo seem to depend on stimulation of pre- but not post-synaptic receptors. Within the dorsal raphe nucleus, 5-HT$_{1A}$ agonists, such as 8-OH-DPAT, ipsapirone, buspirone and LY 165163, are *full* agonists and can even hyperpolarize serotoninergic cells to a greater extent than 5-HT itself [62]. In contrast, on post-synaptic target cells in the hippocampus, the same drugs are only *partial* agonists, partly mimicking the hyperpolarizing effect of 5-HT through 5-HT$_{1A}$ receptors [63, 64]. One group even reported that 8-OH-DPAT may be a 5-HT antagonist in the rat hippocampus [65]. Behavioural data also support the notion that some 5-HT$_{1A}$ agonists at the presynaptic raphe level are antagonists at post-synaptic sites, e.g., buspirone and ipsapirone prevent several components of the "5-HT behavioural syndrome" due to 5-methoxy-N,N-dimethyltryptamine in rats [66].

Altogether these observations explain why — at least some — 5-HT$_{1A}$ agonists induce behaviour typical of blockade of 5-HT transmission; activation of presynaptic autoreceptors triggers inhibitory control of the electrical and metabolic activity of serotoninergic neurones [36, 62] and, concomitantly, these drugs block the postsynaptic action of 5-HT.

Other examples of 5-HT$_{1A}$ agonists acting as full agonists in a given brain region, but as partial agonists and even antagonists in other regions, have also been reported for 5-HT$_{1A}$ receptors which are exclusively post-synaptic. Thus, Dumuis et al. [67] recently demonstrated that ipsapirone and buspirone are potent agonists of 5-HT$_{1A}$ receptors negatively coupled to AC in hippocampal neurones, but behave as competitive antagonists of the same receptors in cortical neurones. Similarly, spiroxatrine is a potent antagonist of 5-HT$_{1A}$ receptors on (canine) cerebral vessels [68], but an agonist of these receptors in hippocampus [69] and dorsal raphe nucleus [unpublished observations]. The new 5-HT$_{1A}$ ligand, MDL 72832, has also been shown to act as an antagonist on peripheral 5-HT$_{1A}$ receptors but as an agonist on central 5-HT$_{1A}$ receptors [70, unpublished observations].

Such differential effects of selective 5-HT$_{1A}$ ligands in various areas might also explain why these receptors are not regulated in the same way in one brain region compared to another. In particular, the full agonist properties of these drugs in the dorsal raphe nucleus, and their partial agonist or antagonist properties in hippocampus and cerebral cortex, might well account for their efficiency in desensitizing pre-synaptic 5-HT$_{1A}$ receptors on raphe cells without altering post-synaptic 5-HT$_{1A}$ receptors in vivo [71, 72]. Since the same receptor modulations can be triggered by some antidepressants [73], such changes may well account for the antidepressant action of 5-HT$_{1A}$ agonists [72].

6.2   *5-HT$_2$-related receptors*

Although it is well established that 5-HT$_2$ receptors are functionally coupled to PLC in cerebral cortex, the situation is largely unsolved for other brain regions. For instance in the hippocampus, where 5-HT$_2$ binding sites are abundant, 5-HT also evokes a marked increase in PI turnover but the pharmacological profile of this effect does not fit with that of 5-HT$_2$ sites [45, 74]. More generally, there is no correlation between the regional distribution of 5-HT$_2$ sites labelled by [^{3}H]ketanserin and that of 5-HT-induced stimulation of PI turnover [45]. Accordingly, this effect may be mediated by various 5-HT receptor types. Alternatively, several subtypes of 5-HT$_2$ receptor with different pharmacological properties might exist throughout the brain.

7. Conclusions and future trends

Studies on transduction mechanisms at the cellular level have been of crucial importance in demonstrating that the various recognition sites for 5-HT identified in binding studies are authentic 5-HT receptors in brain. It is now well established that 5-HT$_{1A}$, 5-HT$_{1B}$ and 5-HT$_{1D}$ receptors are negatively coupled to AC, whereas $5\text{-}HT_{1C}$ and $5\text{-}HT_2$ are positively coupled to PLC. However this view is an oversimplification, since the same category of binding sites can be coupled to several transduction mechanisms. This is particularly true of $5\text{-}HT_{1A}$ binding sites for which cellular transduction mechanisms involve not only AC but also K^+ channels, and even PI turnover. Indeed, Claustre et al. [75] recently described a negative influence of $5\text{-}HT_{1A}$ receptor stimulation on carbachol-induced increase in PI turnover in rat hippocampus, but not striatum and cerebral cortex. This finding further illustrates the marked differences observed in the effects of 5-HT ligands on a given class of 5-HT receptor from one brain region to another. Such regional differences not only depend on the transduction mechanism coupled to the binding site, but also on the varying efficiency of this coupling throughout the brain.

Variations in the nature and efficiency of coupling might explain why a ligand is a full agonist within the dorsal raphe nucleus, for instance, but only a partial agonist in the hippocampus. Preliminary results in our laboratory have shown no change in $5\text{-}HT_{1A}$-dependent AC activity in hippocampus at a time when the local density of $5\text{-}HT_{1A}$ sites has been reduced by 70% as a result of an electrolytic lesion of the septum [unpublished observations]. This observation further supports the view that not all $5\text{-}HT_{1A}$ binding sites are coupled to AC, and even suggests that non-functional $5\text{-}HT_{1A}$ sites to which agonists may bind in vivo may exist at the hippocampal level. Whether the relative proportions of functional and non-functional $5\text{-}HT_{1A}$ binding sites are variable from one area to another deserves further investigation.

Studies on adrenergic receptors have shown that agonist and antagonist binding do not depend on exactly the same parts of the receptor molecule [76]. This concept could also apply to the agonist properties of a 5-HT receptor ligand in a given brain region, and the antagonist properties of the same drug on the same receptor type in other areas (or tissues). Whether discrete changes in the molecular structure of this receptor actually exist, depending on its environment, should also be considered in future studies. Finally, little is known yet about the transduction mechanisms of $5\text{-}HT_3$ receptors; research in this field should be strongly supported in the light of the potential clinical interest of $5\text{-}HT_3$ ligands [1].

Acknowledgements

Original data reported in this review have been obtained thanks to grants by INSERM and BAYER-PHARMA.

References

1. Bradley PB, Engel G, Feniuk W, Fozard JR, Humphrey PPA, Middlemiss DN, Mylecharane EJ, Richardson BP, Saxena PR (1986): Proposals for the classification and

nomenclature of functional receptors for 5-hydroxytryptamine. *Neuropharmacology* 25: 563—575.

2. Pedigo NW, Yamamura HI, Nelson DL (1981): Discrimination of multiple [³H]5-hydroxytryptamine binding sites by the neuroleptic spiperone in rat brain. *J. Neurochem* 36: 220—226.

3. Von Hungen K, Roberts S, Hill DF (1975): Serotonin-sensitive adenylate cyclase activity in immature rat brain. *Brain Research* 84: 257—267.

4. Roth BL, Chuang DM (1987): Multiple mechanisms of serotonergic signal transduction. *Life Sci* 41: 1051—1064.

5. Hamon M, Gozlan H, EI Mestikawy S, Emerit MB, Cossery JM, Lutz O. (1988): Biochemical properties of central serotonin receptors, pp. 393—422 in: Osborne NN, Hamon M (eds), *Neuronal Serotonin*. Chichester: John Wiley & Sons Ltd.

6. Neer EJ, Clapham DE (1988): Roles of G protein subunits in transmembrane signalling. *Nature (Lond)* 333: 129—134.

7. Peroutka SJ, Lebovitz RM, Snyder SH (1979): Serotonin receptor binding sites affected differentially by guanine nucleotides. *Mol Pharmacol* 16: 700—708.

8. Hamon M, Nelson DL, Herbet A, Glowinski J (1980): Multiple receptors for serotonin in the rat brain, pp. 223—233 in: Pepeu G, Kuhar MJ, Enna SJ (eds), *Receptors for Neurotransmitters and Peptide Hormones*. N.Y.: Raven Press.

9. Hamon M, Goetz C, Gozlan H (1983): Reciprocal modulations of central 5-HT receptors by GTP and cations, pp. 349—359 in: Mandel P, de Feudis FV (eds), *CNS receptors — from molecular pharmacology to behavior*. N.Y.: Raven Press.

10. Kendall DA, Nahorski SR (1983): Temperature-dependent 5-hydroxytryptamine (5-HT)-sensitive [³H]spiperone binding to rat cortical membranes: regulation by guanine nucleotide and antidepressant treatment. *J Pharmacol Exp Ther* 227: 429—434.

11. Battaglia G, Shannon M, Titeler M (1984): Guanyl nucleotide and divalent cation regulation of cortical S_2 serotonin receptors. *J Neurochem* 43: 1213—1219.

12. Shearman MS, Strange PG (1988): Guanine nucleotide effects on agonist binding to serotonin 5-HT_2 receptors in rat frontal cortex. *Biochem Pharmacol* 37: 3097—3102.

13. Gozlan H, El Mestikawy S, Pichat L, Glowinski J, Hamon M (1983): Identification of presynaptic serotonin autoreceptors using a new ligand: ³H-PAT. *Nature (Lond)* 305: 140—142.

14. Hall MD, Gozlan H, Emerit MB, El Mestikawy S, Pichat L, Hamon M (1986): Differentiation of pre- and post-synaptic high affinity serotonin receptor binding sites using physico-chemical parameters and modifying agents. *Neurochem Res* 11: 891—912.

15. Heuring RE, Peroutka SJ (1987): Characterization of a novel ³H-5-hydroxytryptamine binding site subtype in bovine brain membranes. *J Neurosci* 7: 894—903.

16. Palacios JM, Markstein R, Pazos A (1986): Serotonin-1C sites in the choroid plexus are not linked in a stimulatory or inhibitory way to adenylate cyclase. *Brain Research* 380: 151—154.

17. Julius D, Mac Dermott AB, Axel R, Jessell TM (1988): Molecular characterization of a functional cDNA encoding the serotonin 1C receptor. *Science* 241: 558—564.

18. Kobilka BK, Frielle T, Collins S, Yang-Feng T, Kobilka TS, Francke U, Lefkowitz RJ, Caron MG (1987): An intronless gene encoding a potential member of the family of receptors coupled to guanine nucleotide regulatory proteins. *Nature (Lond)* 329: 75—79.

19. Kilpatrick GJ, Jones BJ, Tyers MB (1987): Identification and distribution of 5-HT_3 receptors in rat brain using radioligand binding. *Nature (Lond)* 330: 746—748.

20. Tsang D, Lal S (1977): Effect of monoamine receptor agonists and antagonists on cyclic AMP accumulation in human cerebral cortex slices. *Can. J. Physiol Pharmacol* 55: 1263—1269.

21. Ahn HS, Makman MH (1978): Stimulation of adenylate cyclase activity in monkey anterior limbic cortex by serotonin. *Brain Research* 153: 636—640.

22. Enjalbert A, Bourgoin S, Hamon M, Adrien J, Bockaert J (1978): Postsynaptic serotonin-

sensitive adenylate cyclase in the central nervous system. I. Development and distribution of serotonin- and dopamine-sensitive adenylate cyclases in rat and guinea pig brain. *Mol Pharmacol* 14: 2—10.

23. Enjalbert A, Hamon M, Bourgoin S, Bockaert J (1978): Postsynaptic serotonin-sensitive adenylate cyclase in the central nervous system. II. Comparison with dopamine- and isoproterenol-sensitive adenylate cyclases in rat brain. *Mol Pharmacol* 14: 11—23.

24. Euvrard C, Boissier JR (1980): Biochemical assessment of the central 5-HT agonist activity of RU 24969 (a piperidinyl indole). *Europ J Pharmacol* 63: 65—72.

25. Middlemiss DN, Blakeborough L, Leather SR (1977): Direct evidence for an interaction of β-adrenergic blockers with the 5-HT receptor. *Nature (Lond)* 267: 289—290.

26. Barbaccia ML, Brunello N, Chuang DM, Costa E (1983): Serotonin-elicited amplification of adenylate cyclase activity in hippocampal membranes from adult rat. *J Neurochem* 40: 1671—1679.

27. Markstein R, Hoyer D, Engel G (1986): 5-HT$_{1A}$-receptors mediate stimulation of adenylate cyclase in rat hippocampus. *Naunyn-Schmiedeberg's Arch Pharmacol* 333: 335—341.

28. Dumuis A, Bouhelal R, Sebben M, Bockaert J (1988): A 5-HT receptor in the central nervous system, positively coupled with adenylate cyclase, is antagonized by ICS 205 930. *Europ J Pharmacol* 146: 187—188.

29. Hamon M, Bourgoin S (1982): Characteristics of 5-HT metabolism and function in the developing brain, pp. 197—220 in: Osborne NN (ed), *Biology of serotonergic transmission*. Chichester: John Wiley & Sons Ltd.

30. Shenker A, Maayani S, Weinstein H, Green JP (1987): Pharmacological characterization of two 5-hydroxytryptamine receptors coupled to adenylate cyclase in guinea pig hippocampal membranes. *Mol Pharmacol* 31: 357—367.

31. De Vivo M, Maayani S (1986): Characterization of the 5-hydroxytryptamine$_{1A}$ receptor-mediated inhibition of forskolin-stimulated adenylate cyclase activity in guinea pig and rat hippocampal membranes. *J Pharmacol Exp Ther* 238: 248—253.

32. Vergé D, Daval G, Marcinkiewicz M, Patey A, El Mestikawy S, Gozlan H, Hamon M (1986): Quantitative autoradiography of multiple 5-HT$_1$ receptor subtypes in the brain of control or 5,7-dihydroxytryptamine treated rats. *J Neurosci* 6: 3474—3482.

33. Daval G, Vergé, D, Becerril A, Gozlan H, Spampinato U, Hamon M (1987): Transient expression of 5-HT$_{1A}$ receptor binding sites in some areas of the rat CNS during postnatal development. *Int J Devl Neurosci* 5: 171—180.

34. Bockaert J, Dumuis A, Bouhelal R, Sebben M, Cory RN (1987): Piperazine derivatives including the putative anxiolytic drugs, buspirone and ipsapirone, are agonists at 5-HT$_{1A}$ receptors negatively coupled with adenylate cyclase in hippocampal neurons. *Naunyn-Schmiedeberg's Arch Pharmacol* 335: 588—592.

35. Hamon M (1987): Second messenger systems linked to different serotonin (5-HT) receptors, pp. 281—284 in: Rand MJ, Raper C (eds), *Pharmacology*. Elsevier Sci. Publ.

36. Hamon M, Fattaccini CM, Adrien J, Gallissot MC, Martin P, Gozlan H (1988): Alterations of central serotonin and dopamine turnover in rats treated with ipsapirone and other 5-HT$_{1A}$ agonists with potential anxiolytic properties. *J Pharmacol Exp Ther* 246: 745—752.

37. Bouhelal R, Smounya L, Bockaert J (1988): 5-HT$_{1B}$ receptors are negatively coupled with adenylate cyclase in rat substantia nigra. *Europ J Pharmacol* 151: 189—196.

38. Engel G, Göthert M, Hoyer D, Schlicker E, Hillenbrand, K (1986): Identity of inhibitory presynaptic 5-hydroxytryptamine (5-HT) autoreceptors in the rat brain cortex with 5-HT$_{1B}$ binding sites. *Naunyn-Schmiedeberg's Arch Pharmacol* 332: 1—7.

39. Schlicker E, Fink K, Classen K, Göthert M (1987): Facilitation of serotonin (5-HT) release in the rat brain cortex by cAMP and probable inhibition of adenylate cyclase in 5-HT nerve terminals by presynaptic α_2-adrenoceptors. *Naunyn-Schmiedeberg's Arch Pharmacol* 336: 251—256.

40. Hoyer D, Schoeffter P (1988): 5-HT$_{1D}$ receptor-mediated inhibition of forskolin-stimulated adenylate cyclase activity in calf substantia nigra. *Europ J Pharmacol* 147: 145—147.

41. Hamblin MW, Ariani K, Adriaenssens PI, Ciaranello RD (1987): [^{3}H]-Dihydroergotamine as a high affinity, slowly dissociating radioligand for 5-HT$_{1B}$ binding sites in rat brain membranes: evidence for guanine nucleotide regulation of agonist affinity states. *J Pharmacol Exp Ther* 243: 989—1001.

42. Conn PJ, Sanders-Bush E, Hoffman BJ, Hartig PR (1986): A unique serotonin receptor in choroid plexus is linked to phosphatidyl-inositol turnover. *Proc Natl Acad Sci USA* 83: 4086—4088.

43. Conn PJ, Sanders-Bush E (1986): Agonist-induced phosphoinositide hydrolysis in choroid plexus. *J Neurochem* 47: 1754—1760.

44. Conn PJ, Sanders-Bush E (1987): Relative efficacies of piperazines at the phosphoinositide hydrolysis-linked serotonergic (5-HT$_2$ and 5-HT$_{1C}$) receptors. *J Pharmacol Exp Ther* 242: 552—557.

45. Conn PJ, Sanders-Bush E (1985): Serotonin-stimulated phosphoinositide turnover: mediation by the S$_2$ binding site in rat cerebral cortex but not in subcortical regions. *J Pharmacol Exp Ther* 234: 195—203.

46. Kendall DA, Nahorski SR (1985): 5-hydroxytryptamine-stimulated inositol phospholipid hydrolysis in rat cerebral cortex slices: pharmacological characterization and effects of antidepressants. *J Pharmacol Exp Ther* 233: 473—479.

47. Conn PJ, Sanders-Bush E (1986): Regulation of serotonin-stimulated phosphoinositide hydrolysis: relation to the serotonin 5-HT$_2$ binding site. *J Neurosci* 6: 3669—3675.

48. Hansson, E, Simonsson P, Alling C (1987): 5-hydroxytryptamine stimulated the formation of inositol phosphate in astrocytes from different regions of the brain. *Neuropharmacology* 26: 1377—1382.

49. Yagaloff KA, Hartig PR (1985): [^{125}I]-LSD binds to a novel serotonergic site on rat choroid plexus epithelial cells. *J Neurosci* 5: 3178—3183.

50. Bockaert J, Premont J, Tassin JP, Hamon M, Deterre P, Ebersolt C, Prochiantz A (1982): Pharmacological characteristics and neuronal localization of dopamine- and serotonin-sensitive adenylate cyclases in rat brain and snail neurones, pp. 155—166 in: Dumont JE, Nunez J, Schultz G (eds), *Hormones and Cell Regulation* 6. Elsevier Biomed Press.

51. Andrade R, Nicoll RA (1987): Pharmacologically distinct actions of serotonin on single pyramidal neurones of the rat hippocampus recorded in vitro. *J Physiol (Lond)* 394: 99—124.

52. Andrade R, Malenka RC, Nicoll RA (1986): A G protein couples serotonin and GABA$_B$ receptors to the same channels in hippocampus. *Science* 234: 1261—1265.

53. Nicoll RA (1988): The coupling of neurotransmitter receptors to ion channels in the brain. *Science* 241: 545—551.

54. Joëls M, Shinnick-Gallagher P, Gallagher JP (1987): Effect of serotonin and serotonin analogues on passive membrane properties of lateral septal neurons in vitro. *Brain Research* 417: 99—107.

55. Aghajanian GK, Lakoski JM (1984): Hyperpolarization of serotonergic neurons by serotonin and LSD: studies in brain slices showing increased K$^+$-conductance. *Brain Research* 305: 181—185.

56. Vergé D, Daval G, Patey A, Gozlan H, El Mestikawy S, Hamon M (1985): Presynaptic 5-HT autoreceptors on serotonergic cell bodies and/or dendrites but not terminals are of the 5-HT$_{1A}$ subtype. *Europ J Pharmacol* 113: 463—464.

57. Weissmann-Nanopoulos D, Mach E, Magre J, Demassey Y, Pujol JF (1985): Evidence for the localization of 5-HT$_{1A}$ binding sites on serotonin containing neurons in the raphe dorsalis and raphe centralis nuclei of the rat brain. *Neurochem Int* 7: 1061—1072.

58. Hutson PH, Dourish CT, Curzon G (1986): Neurochemical and behavioural evidence for mediation of the hyperphagic action of 8-OH-DPAT by 5-HT cell body autoreceptors. *Europ J Pharmacol* 129: 347—352.

59. Carli M, Samanin R (1988): Potential anxiolytic properties of 8-hydroxy-2-(di-n-propylamino) tetralin, a selective serotonin$_{1A}$ receptor agonist. *Psychopharmacology* 94: 84—91.
60. Invernizzi RW, Cervo L, Samanin R (1988): 8-hydroxy-2-(di-n-propylamino) tetralin, a selective serotonin$_{1A}$ receptor agonist, blocks haloperidol-induced catalepsy by an action on raphe nuclei medianus and dorsalis. *Neuropharmacology* 27: 515—518.
61. Hutson PH, Donohoe TP, Curzon G (1987): Hypothermia induced by the putative 5-HT$_{1A}$ agonists LY 165163 and 8-OH-DPAT is not prevented by 5-HT depletion. *Europ J Pharmacol* 143: 221—228.
62. Sprouse JS, Aghajanian GK (1987): Electrophysiological responses of serotoninergic dorsal raphe neurons to 5-HT$_{1A}$ and 5-HT$_{1B}$ agonists. *Synapse* 1: 3—9.
63. Martin KF, Mason R (1987): Isapirone is a partial agonist at 5-hydroxytryptamine$_{1A}$ (5-HT$_{1A}$) receptors in the rat hippocampus: electrophysiological evidence. *Europ J Pharmacol* 141: 479—483.
64. Andrade R, Nicoll RA (1987): Novel anxiolytics discriminate between postsynaptic serotonin receptors mediating different physiological responses on single neurons of the rat hippocampus. *Naunyn-Schmiedeberg's Arch Pharmacol* 336: 5—10.
65. Colino A, Halliwell JV (1986): 8-OH-DPAT is a strong antagonist of 5-HT action in rat hippocampus. *Europ J Pharmacol* 130: 151—152.
66. Smith LM, Peroutka SJ (1986): Differential effects of 5-hydroxytryptamine$_{1A}$ selective drugs on the 5-HT behavioral syndrome. *Pharmacol Biochem Behav* 24: 1513—1519.
67. Dumuis A, Sebben M, Bockaert J (1988): Pharmacology of 5-hydroxtryptamine$_{1A}$ receptors which inhibit cAMP production in hippocampal and cortical neurons in primary culture. *Mol Pharmacol* 33: 178—186.
68. Nelson DL, Taylor EW (1986): Spiroxatrine: a selective serotonin$_{1A}$ receptor antagonist. *Europ J Pharmacol* 124: 207—208.
69. Herrick-Davis K, Titeler M (1988): [^{3}H]spiroxatrine: a 5-HT$_{1A}$ radioligand with agonist binding properties. *J Neurochem* 50: 528—533.
70. Mir AK, Hibert M, Tricklebank MD, Middlemiss DN, Kidd EJ, Fozard JR (1988): MDL 72832: a potent and stereoselective ligand at central and peripheral 5-HT$_{1A}$ receptors. *Europ J Pharmacol* 149: 107—120.
71. Blier P, De Montigny C (1987): Modification of 5-HT neuron properties by sustained administration of the 5-HT$_{1A}$ agonist gepirone: electrophysiological studies in the rat brain. *Synapse* 1: 470—480.
72. Kennett, GA, Marcou M, Dourish CT, Curzon G (1987): Single administration of 5-HT$_{1A}$ agonists decreases 5-HT$_{1A}$ presynaptic, but not postsynaptic receptor-mediated responses: relationship to antidepressant-like action. *Europ J Pharmacol* 138: 53—60.
73. Blier P, De Montigny C (1983): Electrophysiological investigations on the effect of repeated zimelidine administration on serotonergic neurotransmission in the rat. *J Neurosci* 3: 1270—1278.
74. Claustre Y, Rouquier L, Scatton B (1988): Pharmacological characterization of serotonin-stimulated phosphoinositide turnover in brain regions of the immature rat. *J Pharmacol Exp Ther* 244: 1051—1056.
75. Claustre Y, Bénavides J, Scatton B (1988): 5-HT$_{1A}$ receptor agonists inhibit carbachol-induced stimulation of phosphoinositide turnover in the rat hippocampus. *Europ J Pharmacol* 149: 149—153.
76. Kobilka BK, Kobilka TS, Daniel K, Regan JW, Caron MG, Lefkowitz RJ (1988): Chimeric α_2-, β_2-adrenergic receptors: delineation of domains involved in effector coupling and ligand binding specificity. *Science* 240: 1310—1316.

V. Reduction of a distinct pool of monoamines by ketanserin in peripheral tissues

J. E. LEYSEN, J. WYNANTS, A. EENS and P. A. J. JANSSEN

1. Introduction

Ketanserin is a prototype of a 5-HT$_2$ antagonist which also has moderate α_1-adrenoceptor blocking properties. These properties are thought to underly its demonstrated antithrombotic and antivasoconstrictive activities (for reviews see [1, 2]).

[^{3}H]ketanserin is the most widely used ligand to label 5-HT$_2$ receptors [3]. However, in brain tissue and platelets [^{3}H]ketanserin also labels non-serotonergic, saturable binding sites which were recently identified. Ketanserin and the monoamine depleting agent, tetrabenazine [4], bind with nanomolar affinity and reversibly to these sites; reserpine interacts with them in a non-reversible way. The drugs trigger the release of catecholamines, 5-HT and their acid metabolites from brain slices and platelets, with potencies corresponding to their binding affinities [5, 6] suggesting a role of the binding sites in the release process.

In view of these recently discovered in vitro properties of ketanserin, which it has in common with tetrabenazine, we have now investigated the effects of these drugs on the levels of monoamines and metabolites in the brain and in peripheral tissues of young, senescent and spontaneously hypertensive rats.

2. Experimental procedures

Young male Wistar rats (200 g), senescent male Wistar rats (6—11 months old) and spontaneously hypertensive male Okamota rats (200 g), were acutely or repeatedly treated i.p. with ketanserin or tetrabenazine (see below). Control rats received saline injections. The animals were killed by decapitation two hours after the last injection. Brain and peripheral tissues were rapidly dissected, immediately weighed, frozen in liquid nitrogen and lyophilized. The tissue content of monoamines: noradrenaline (NA), dopa-

P.R. Saxena, D.I. Wallis, W. Wouters and P. Bevan (eds), Cardiovascular Pharmacology of 5-Hydroxytryptamine, pp. 61—66.

mine (DA), 5-hydroxytryptamine (5-HT) and of monoamine metabolites 3,4 dihydroxybenzene acetic acid (DOPAC), homovanillic acid (HVA), 3-methoxytyramine (3-MT) and 5-hydroxy indole acetic acid (5-HIAA) was determined on high performance liquid chromatography (HPLC) as previously described [7]. Ketanserin-tartaric acid salt (R 49 945, Janssen Research Foundation, Beerse, Belgium) and tetrabenazine (Holffmann-La Roche, Basle, Switzerland) were dissolved in saline.

3. Results

Young male Wistar rats were acutely treated with 5 or 20 mg/kg ketanserin and tetrabenazine, control animals received saline. Two hours later the frontal cortex, striatum, vas deferens, spleen, left ventricle, caudal artery and portal vein were dissected and prepared for HPLC analysis. The data on the content of the biogenic amines and their metabolites are presented in Table 1. At a dose of 20 mg/kg, ketanserin caused an average reduction by about 20% of the monoamine levels in the brain, whereas the levels in the cardiovascular tissues and in the spleen were reduced by more than 40%. In the vas deferens the NA levels were reduced by 34% but the DA levels by 85%. Ketanserin did not markedly affect the monoamine metabolites in the brain. 5 mg/kg ketanserin had little effect on brain monoamine levels and on NA and 5-HT levels in the peripheral tissues, however, the DA levels in the vas deferens were still reduced by 62%.

Tetrabenazine, at a dose of 20 mg/kg caused a total depletion of brain monoamine and 3-MT levels, concomitant with a large increase of the acid metabolites (DOPAC, HVA and 5-HIAA). In contrast, peripheral 5-HT and NA levels were less reduced (−54% for 5-HT, −70% for NA). However, DA levels in the vas deferens were nearly totally depleted. 5 mg/kg tetrabenazine still caused substantial reductions of the monoamine levels in central and peripheral tissues.

After repeated treatment of the rats with 2 × 10 mg/kg. day of ketanserin or tetrabenazine for 6, 13 and 20 days, similar reductions in monoamine levels, measured in the brain and in the vas deferens, were seen as after acute treatment. Investigations in old male Wister rats and in spontaneously hypertensive Okamota rats revealed that in the control animals of these series, central DA and 5-HT levels were significantly increased by about 20% as compared to the levels in young Wistar rats. In the vas deferens of these animals, the NA levels were about 30% lower, but the DA levels were 300% and 500% higher in the old Wistar and the Okamota rats respectively. The effects of acute (20 mg/kg) and 6 days (2 × 10 mg/kg.day) treatment with ketanserin or tetrabenazine on the monoamine and metabolite levels in the brain tissues and in the vas deferens, were the same as those observed in the young male Wistar rats (data not shown).

Table 1. Biogenic amine and metabolite levels in tissues of young male Wistar rats, 2 hours after treatment (i.p.) with ketanserin or tetrabenazine.

Tissue	Compound	Control values (pmoles/mg dry weight)	Per cent of matched controls (mean values ± SD, n)			
			Ketanserin		Tetrabenazine	
			5 mg/kg	20 mg/kg	5 mg/kg	20 mg/kg
Frontal cortex	NA	7.7 ± 2.0 (32)	85 ± 17 (8)*	63 ± 11 (5)***	31 ± 14 (8)***	0 (5)***
	DA	1.6 ± 0.5 (34)	113 ± 27 (7)	71 ± 21 (5)***	60 ± 24 (6)**	0 (5)***
	DOPAC	0.39 ± 0.23 (34)	123 ± 31 (4)	83 ± 61 (5)	147 ± 28 (4)*	283 ± 55 (5)***
	5-HT	11.5 ± 1.7 (34)	86 ± 8 (8)***	80 ± 9 (5)***	46 ± 18 (6)***	12 ± 3 (5)***
	5-HIAA	5.6 ± 0.9 (35)	95 ± 12 (8)	104 ± 14 (5)	138 ± 19 (8)***	169 ± 24 (5)***
Striatum	DA	311 ± 46 (35)	96 ± 13 (8)	78 ± 12 (6)***	15 ± 6 (8)***	4 ± 1 (6)***
	DOPAC	32.1 ± 5.3 (33)	94 ± 9 (8)	103 ± 25 (6)	198 ± 21 (8)***	216 ± 22 (6)***
	HVA	20.0 ± 4.8 (35)	78 ± 15 (8)**	134 ± 19 (6)***	265 ± 36 (8)***	434 ± 79 (6)***
	3-MT	9.9 ± 2.9 (35)	73 ± 29 (8)*	95 ± 44 (6)	21 ± 15 (7)***	0 (6)***
	5-HT	8.4 ± 1.4 (36)	94 ± 21 (8)	88 ± 17 (6)	50 ± 11 (7)***	17 ± 6 (6)***
	5-HIAA	10.1 ± 1.5 (35)	91 ± 23 (8)	107 ± 24 (6)	140 ± 20 (8)	188 ± 49 (6)***
Vas deferens	NA	322 ± 74 (35)	89 ± 10 (7)**	69 ± 15 (6)***	73 ± 7 (7)***	33 ± 10 (6)***
	DA	8.6 ± 3.4 (34)	38 ± 12 (7)***	15 ± 4 (6)***	20 ± 5 (8)***	7 ± 3 (6)***
Spleen	NA	17.6 ± 6.5 (17)	93 ± 26 (8)	34 ± 22 (8)***	43 ± 9 (7)***	8 ± 4 (8)***
	5-HT	41.5 ± 10.2 (16)	95 ± 15 (7)	71 ± 20 (8)***	53 ± 14 (8)***	46 ± 11 (8)***
Left ventricle	NA	16.1 ± 4.9 (24)	90 ± 22 (8)	57 ± 10 (8)***	62 ± 14 (8)***	38 ± 19 (8)***
Caudal artery	NA	76.7 ± 36.4 (23)	124 ± 40 (8)	61 ± 6 (8)***	62 ± 37 (8)**	22 ± 5 (8)***
Portal vein	NA	76.6 ± 19.0 (23)	72 ± 12 (4)**	56 ± 8 (8)***	40 ± 6 (4)***	11 ± 6 (8)***

Statistic analysis was according to the Student's t-test (two-tailed).
Significance of difference from controls, ***$p \leq 0.001$; **$p \leq 0.005$; *$p \leq 0.05$; no indication $p > 0.05$.
NA, noradrenaline; DA, dopamine; DOPAC, 3,4 dihydroxybenzene acetic acid; 5-HIAA, 5-hydroxy indole acetic acid; 3-MT, 3-methyoxytryramine.

4. Discussion

In this study, we showed that ketanserin at a dose of 20 mg/kg, produced a partial reduction of monoamine levels, which was more pronounced in peripheral tissues than in the brain. In contrast, tetrabenazine produced complete depletion of brain monoamines and was less active in peripheral tissues. As a result, the effect of ketanserin and tetrabenazine differed less in some peripheral tissues; a similar extensive decrease of DA levels in the vas deferens was noted. An accumulative effect of the drugs during prolonged treatment was not observed.

The presently described findings have implications for the interpretation of the mechanism of the monoamine depleting action of the drugs and for interpreting the ketanserin effects on cardiovascular pathologies in humans.

Based on the findings in this study, we suggest that at least two mechanisms are involved in the depletion of the monoamines. Tetrabenazine acts via both mechanisms, ketanserin seems to act only on one system in vivo. The first mechanism, insensitive to ketanserin in vivo, probably is the classically proposed inhibition of the uptake of the monoamines in the storage vesicles. This mechanism, apparently is predominant in the brain and is responsible for the large depletion of central monoamines by tetrabenazine, an effect which is not obtained with ketanserin. The second mechanism is release of the monoamines from a ketanserin-sensitive pool. This pool appears to be relatively more important in peripheral tissues. A distinction in sensitivity of the various amines is noted (DA > NA > 5-HT) and for a given amine the relative size of the pool varies with tissues. The differential effect of ketanserin on the DA and the NA levels in the vas deferens, which are totally and only 30% reduced respectively, is highly suggestive of the existence of two distinct pools. Based on our studies in vitro (see above) it can be suggested that the release of the content of the ketanserin-sensitive monoamine pool is triggered by interaction of the drugs with the release evoking ketanserin binding sites, presumably localized on the plasma membranes. It is at present not yet clear, whether a similar type of binding site would be associated with the monoamine transporter on the storage vesicles as suggested by Darchen et al. [8]). The possibility remains, that the latter intracellular sites are not sufficiently reached by ketanserin in vivo.

Ketanserin is known to have potent antithrombotic and antivasoconstrictive activities due to concomitant blockade of $5-HT_2$ receptors and α-adrenoceptors on platelets and vessel walls (see above). These properties are thought to underly the beneficial effects of ketanserin in cardiovascular pathologies, but they could not explain its entire profile of activities [2]. The presently described, partial monoamine depleting effects, may provide an additional explanation for certain actions of ketanserin. The partial monoamine depleting activity of ketanserin has been confirmed in studies in humans, in which a reduction by about 20% of platelet-bound 5-HT has been observed following ketanserin treatment at therapeutic dosages (De Clerck et al., personal communication). Our results in laboratory animals show that the ketanserin-sensitive monoamine pool is larger in hypertensive and in old animals. This could be related to the clinical observation that ketanserin is particularly effective in elderly patients with essential hypertension [9]. The demonstrated preferential activity in peripheral tissues on a particular ketanserin-sensitive monoamine pool, distinguishes the action of ketanserin from that of tetrabenazine- and reserpine-like drugs and make noxious side effects, known for the latter unlikely.

5. Conclusions

The differential effects of ketanserin and tetrabenazine on monoamine depletion suggest that two different mechanisms may be involved: (i) inhibition of uptake of monoamines in the storage vesicles; a property of tetrabenazine not shared by ketanserin in vivo, (ii) release of monoamines from a ketanserin-sensitive pool, triggered by both, ketanserin and tetrabenazine, a phenomenon which is relatively more important in peripheral tissues than in the brain.

Acknowledgements

The technical assistance of Boris Petrov is highly appreciated. Chris Verellen is thanked for typing the manuscript.

References

1. Van Nueten JM, Janssen , 'AJ, Symoens J, Janssens WJ, Heykants J, De Clerck F, Leysen JE, Vancauteren H, Vanhoutte PM (1987): Ketanserin, pp. 1—56 in: Scriabine A (ed), *New Cardiovascular Drugs*. New York: Raven Press.
2. Vanhoutte PM, Ball SG, Berdeaux A, Cohen ML, Hedner T, McCall R, Ramage A, Reimann IH, Richer C, Saxena PR, Schalekamp MADH, Struyker-Boudier HAJ, Symoens J, Van Nueten JM, Van Zwieten PA (1986): Mechanism of action of ketanserin in hypertension. *Trends Pharmacol Sci* 7: 58—59.
3. Leysen JE, Niemegeers CJE, Van Nueten JM, Laduron PM (1982): [³H]Ketanserin (R 41 468), a selective ³H-ligand for serotonin₂ receptor binding sites. *Mol Pharmacol* 21: 301—314.
4. Pletscher A, Brossi A, Gey KF (1962): Benzoquinolizine derivates: a new class of monoamine decreasing drugs with psychotropic action. *Int Rev Neurobiol* 4: 275—306.
5. Leysen JE, Eens A, Gommeren W, Van Gompel P, Wynants J, Janssen PAJ (1987): Non-serotonergic [³H]ketanserin binding sites in striatal membranes are associated with a dopac release system on dopaminergic nerve endings. *Eur J Pharmacol* 134: 373—375.
6. Leysen JE, Eens A, Gommeren W, Van Gompel P, Wynants J, Janssen PAJ (1988): Identification of nonserotonergic [³H]ketanserin binding sites associated with nerve terminals in rat brain and with platelets; relation with release of biogenic amine metabolites induced by ketanserin- and tetrabenazine-like drugs. *J Pharmacol Exp Ther* 244: 310—321.
7. Leysen JE, Gommeren W, Van Gompel P, Wynants J, Janssen PFM, Laduron PM

(1985): Receptor-binding properties in vitro and in vivo of ritanserin. A very potent and long acting serotonin-S_2 antagonist. *Mol Pharmacol* 27: 600—611.

8. Darchen F, Scherman D, Laduron PM, Henry J-P (1988): Ketanserin binds to the monoamine transporter of chromaffin granules and of synaptic vesicles. *Mol Pharmacol* 33: 672—677.

9. De Cree J, Leempoels J, Geukens H, De Cock W, Verhaegen H (1981): The antihypertensive effects of ketanserin (R 41 468), a novel 5-hydroxytryptamine-blocking agent, in patients with essential hypertension. *Clin Sci* 61: 473s—476s.

Receptors

VI. Putative agonists and antagonists at 5-HT$_1$-like receptors

WASYL FENIUK and PATRICK P. A. HUMPHREY

1. Introduction

There is little doubt that the classification of 5-hydroxytryptamine (5-HT) receptors has gone through a major transition over the last few years. Indeed it has been argued [1] that even the recent classification of Bradley and colleagues [2] is now outmoded. This need for change has largely arisen from some major advances from radioligand binding studies. However the acceptability and credibility of any receptor classification will be clearly dependent upon the selectivity and specificity of the agonists and antagonists which are used to define such receptor sites. It is perhaps worth emphasising, even at this early stage, that few selective and specific agonists and *no specific antagonists* are available in the area of 5-HT$_1$ receptor research. Consequently the classification of 5-HT$_1$ receptors, which has been so markedly influenced by the data generated from ligand binding studies, has on occasion, been met with scepticism [3]. Not withstanding such a criticism, certain new drug tools particularly agonists showing high degrees of selectivity [4] have recently become available. These may help unify a classification which seems in part to be based on ligand binding studies and in part on functional studies [1, 2].

The aim of this article is to outline some of the characteristics of the 5-HT$_1$ recognition sites and where possible to equate such sites with functional correlates. It is also our intention to outline the pharmacological properties of certain receptor types termed '5-HT$_1$-like' [2] which bear certain similarities to the 5-HT$_1$ recognition site but are not identical to any of the known sub-groups of such a recognition site [see 5].

2. 5-HT$_1$ "receptors" — a classification on the basis of ligand binding studies

On the basis of ligand binding studies in brain tissue, Peroutka and Snyder

P.R. Saxena, D.I. Wallis, W. Wouters and P. Bevan (eds), Cardiovascular Pharmacology of 5-Hydroxytryptamine, pp. 69—80.

[6] proposed the existence of two types of 5-HT "receptor" in the central nervous system. Namely, they identified a 5-HT$_1$ "receptor" which can be labelled with a high (nM) affinity by [^{3}H]5-HT and a 5-HT$_2$ "receptor" at which 5-HT has a low (μM) affinity but which can be labelled with high affinity by a variety of 5-HT receptor blocking drugs such as spiperone and ketanserin [7]. It must be emphasised that the characterisation of 5-HT receptor sites on the basis of agonist affinity alone is a considerable handicap since, on the basis of ligand binding studies, 5-HT itself is a selective 5-HT$_1$ receptor agonist while in functional studies it clearly is not. Hence other claims of agonist selectivity on the basis of ligand binding experiments must be viewed with the utmost caution. Indeed several agents which are commonly used as selective 5-HT$_1$ receptor agonists such as RU24969 and a variety of halogenated phenylpiperazines [8–11] have all been shown to have marked functional activity in isolated tissues containing 5-HT$_2$ receptors [12–14].

3. Subdivision of 5-HT$_1$ receptors

As has already been mentioned, the 5-HT$_1$ "receptor" was clearly defined [6] as having a high affinity for 5-HT. However Pedigo et al. [15] using spiperone to displace [^{3}H]5-HT from its binding site demonstrated that the 5-HT$_1$ site was heterogeneous and should be subdivided. The terms '5-HT$_{1A}$' to differentiate the high affinity site for spiperone and '5-HT$_{1B}$' for the low affinity sub-site were consequently introduced. The identification of more selective ligands such as 8-OH-DPAT [16, 17] from binding studies certainly supported this differentiation. Indeed numerous subsequent studies have shown that 8-OH-DPAT is the archetypal agonist with which to identify not only binding sites but also functional responses mediated via the activation of 5-HT$_{1A}$ receptors (see below). However, one should be wary of attributing all the actions of 8-OH-DPAT as being mediated via 5-HT$_{1A}$ receptor activation since the compound has clear pharmacological actions at receptors other than 5-HT receptors [18]. More recently 5-HT$_1$ recognition sites have been further subdivided into 5-HT$_{1C}$ and 5-HT$_{1D}$ subtypes with the identification of other 'apparently' selective ligands [5, 19]. The subdivisions of 5-HT$_1$ binding sites and their characteristics are summarised in Table 1. It is particularly noteworthy, that although each of the subtypes of the 5-HT$_1$ binding site can be identified by the unique binding profile of particular ligands, certain agents such as 5-carboxamidotryptamine (5-CT) and methiothepin exhibit varying degrees of affinity across all of the subtypes and both agents are also fundamental to the definition of functional 5-HT$_1$-like receptor as defined by Bradley and colleagues [2] (see below).

Table 1. Characteristics of 5-HT$_1$ binding sites (modified from Heuring and Peroutka [5]).

	5-HT$_{1A}$	5-HT$_{1B}$	5-HT$_{1C}$	5-HT$_{1D}$
Radiolabelled by	[³H]5-HT [³H]8-OH-DPAT	[³H]5-HT [¹²⁵I]cyanopindol	[³H]5-HT [³H]mesulergine	[³H]5-HT
High density	Raphé nuclei Hippocampus	Substantia nigra Globus pallidus	choroid plexus	caudate nucleus basal ganglia substantia nigra
Putative agonists	5-CT Dipropyl 5-CT 8-OH-DPAT	5-CT RU24969	5-CT (lower affinity) RU24969 (lower affinity)	5-CT RU24949
Putative antagonists	Spiperone Methiothepin Cyanopindolol Pindolol BMY 7378 MDL 72832 Metergoline	Methiothepin Cyanopindolol Pindolol Metergoline	Mesulergine Methiothepin Ketanserin Mianserin Metergoline	Methiothepin Metergoline
Functional Responses	see Table 2	Terminal autoreceptors Potentiation of neurogenic contractions in mouse bladder [Rodent specific receptor site]	Stimulation of Phosphoinositide turnover	Inhibition of adenylate cyclase

3.1 5-HT$_{1A}$ receptors

There now seems little doubt that 5-HT$_{1A}$ receptors, identified by the ability of spiperone to displace [^{3}H]5-HT binding curves in a biphasic manner [15] and the selective binding profile of 8-OH-DPAT [16], mediate certain functional responses (see Table 2). These have largely been characterised on the basis of the agonist properties of 8-OH-DPAT and antagonism by

Table 2. Proposed Pharmacological consequences following 5-HT$_{1A}$ receptor activation in vitro and in vivo.

Response	Species/Preparation	Reference
Hypotension by a central action	Dog, Rat, Cat	[20—22]
Hyperpolarisation	Rat hippocampal neurones	[23, 24]
Inhibition of acetylcholine release	guinea-pig enteric neurones	[25]
Stimulation of adenylate cyclase	Rat hippocampus	[26]
Inhibition of adenylate cyclase	Rat hippocampus guinea-pig hippocampus	[27, 28]
Stimulation of ACTH secretion	Rat	[29]
Hyperglycaemia/ Hypoinsulinemia	Rat	[30]
Inhibition of 5-HT release	Rat somatodendritic terminals	[16]

compounds possessing amongst other actions, a high affinity at 5-HT$_{1A}$ binding sites such as pindolol, spiperone and methiothepin [1]. In view of the fact that the binding profile of the 5-HT$_{1A}$ recognition site correlates with the pharmacology of 8-OH-DPAT in a variety of functional test systems, the use of the term "receptor" to define such recognition sites does not seem inappropriate [3]. In more recent years a variety of compounds possessing varying degress of efficacy at 5-HT$_{1A}$ receptors has been identified. Of particular interest amongst these are buspirone and ipsapirone which appear to be partial agonists [31, 32] at 5-HT$_{1A}$ receptors and have anxiolytic activity in man. In addition flesinoxan, which possess marked hypotensive activity in laboratory animals, is currently being developed as a novel anti-hypertensive agent [33]. However the potential impact that such compounds may have in the treatment of central nervous system disorders and hypertension still remains to be determined and is outside the scope of this article.

Although compounds such as 8-OH-DPAT, 5-CT, dipropyl 5-CT and flesinoxan may all be used as 5-HT_{1A} agonists [27], to our knowledge no compound behaves as a selective *and* specific 5-HT_{1A} receptor antagonist. However a recently identified buspirone analogue, BMY 7378 (8-[2-[4-(2-methoxyphenyl)-1-piperazinlyl]ethyl]-8-azapirol [4.5]-decane-7,9-dione dihydrochloride]), appears to produce a selective antagonism of 5-CT, 5-HT and 8-OH-DPAT-induced inhibition of forskolin stimulated adenylate cyclase [34]. In addition MDL 72832 whose enantiomers show some degree of stereoselectivity at the 5-HT_{1A} recognition site [35] may prove to be useful antagonists for defining functional responses mediated via 5-HT_{1A} receptor activation. However their antagonist activities in a *range* of functional test systems (Table 2) remain to be determined. Such studies are clearly of importance in determining whether all such responses are mediated via one and the same receptor type. Indeed recent studies in the guinea-pig ileum provide some evidence which suggests that 5-HT_{1A} receptors may be heterogeneous [36].

3.2 *5-HT₁B receptors*

In contrast to the situation for 5-HT_{1A} receptors, there are no specific or selective agonists or antagonists for the 5-HT_{1B} receptor. Thus the characterisation of functional responses which appear to be mediated via the activation of 5-HT_{1B} receptors has largely been carried out by the exclusion of other receptor mechanisms. For example, the central 5-HT terminal autoreceptor in rat cortex has been characterised as being a 5-HT_{1B} receptor on the basis of the antagonist potency of such drugs as cyanopindolol, pindolol and methiothepin [37] and the high agonistic potency of such drugs as 5-CT. Although all of these agents also have a high affinity at 5-HT_{1A} sites [37], an action at 5-HT_{1A} receptors can be excluded on the basis of a lack of agonist activity of 8-OH-DPAT and lack of antagonist activity of such drugs as spiperone. Other functional responses which appear to be mediated via the activation of 5-HT_{1B} receptors include enhancement of neurogenically mediated contraction in the mouse bladder [38], inhibition of sympathetic neurotransmission in the rat vena cava [39] and inhibition of adenylate cyclase in rat substantia nigra [40]. It is however important to note that 5-HT_{1B} receptors appear to be entirely confined to rodent species and appear to be absent in human brain [41].

3.3 5-HT$_{1C}$ and 5-HT$_{1D}$ receptors

More recently 5-HT$_1$ binding sites have been further subdivided into 5-HT$_{1C}$ and 5-HT$_{1D}$ sites [42, 5]. Although the distribution of 5-HT$_{1C}$ sites is quite different to the distribution of 5-HT$_2$ receptors, there is a remarkable similarity in the affinities of a variety of agonists and antagonists between the two sites [see 42]. Even 5-CT, which has a high affinity for 5-HT$_{1A}$, $_{1B}$ and $_{1D}$ sites and is a potent agonist at 5-HT$_1$-like receptors [2], has a lower affinity for 5-HT$_{1C}$ sites and is also a weak agonist at 5-HT$_2$ receptors mediating contraction of the rabbit aorta [43]. No specific agonists or antagonists at 5-HT$_{1C}$ or 5-HT$_{1D}$ receptors have so far been described and the functional consequences of the activation of such sites at the cellular level seems obscure. However at the intracellular level it has been shown that 5-HT$_{1C}$ receptor activation in rat choroid plexus leads to inositol phospholipid metabolism [42] whilst 5-HT$_{1D}$ receptor activation causes an inhibition of forskolin-stimulated adenylate cyclase [47]. The ligands commonly used to identify 5-HT$_{1C}$ and 5-HT$_{1D}$ recognition sites are listed in Table 1, but none of these drug probes can be considered to be sufficiently specific and selective enough to properly 'fingerprint' these sites.

3.4 5-HT$_1$-like receptors

Although most 5-HT$_1$ receptors (5-HT$_{1A}$, $_{1B}$ and $_{1D}$) and the responses mediated via the activation of such sites can at least in part be characterised by the high affinities and/or agonist potencies of such drugs as methiothepin and 5-CT, each of the subtypes can be differentiated on the basis of the differing actions of other various ligands e.g. 8-OH-DPAT, cyanopindolol, mesulergine, etc. There are however numerous examples of functional responses in isolated peripheral tissues (Table 3), that are mediated through the activation of specific 5-HT receptors, which are neither 5-HT$_2$- nor 5-HT$_3$-mediated and which have subsequently been classified as 5-HT$_1$-like [2]. All these responses can be characterised by the high agonist potency of 5-CT and their succeptibility to antagonism by methiothepin. Yet none of these responses can be equated with any of the known 5-HT$_1$ binding sites and hence the appellation 5-HT$_1$-like. Thus in studies by our group in a variety of preparations containing functional 5-HT$_1$-like receptors compounds such as 8-OH-DPAT, cyanopindolol, mesulergine and metergoline are virtually inactive as either agonists or antagonists (e.g. see [4]).

Although there is no doubt that 5-CT remains an important probe with which to characterise and explore the pharmacology of 5-HT$_1$-like receptors in vitro and in vivo [43—48], we have recently identified a novel agonist, GR43175 (3-2[dimethylamino]ethyl-N-methyl-1H-indole-5-methane sulphonamide) which is an even more selective 5-HT$_1$-like agonist than 5-CT and which provides evidence on the basis of functional studies that 5-HT$_1$-

Table 3. A comparison of the pharmacological activity of 5-carboxamidotryptamine (5-CT) and GR43175 in a range of preparations containing different 5-HT receptor types.

Receptor	Preparation	Response	Equi-effective molar potency ratio (5-HT = 1)*		Reference
			5-CT	GR43175	
5-HT$_1$-like	Dog saphenous v.	Contraction	0.4	4.6	[4, 43]
5-HT$_1$-like	Dog saphenous v.	Neuronal inhibition	0.3	4.2	[4, 51]
5-HT$_1$-like	Dog basilar a.	Contraction	0.9	8.8	[49]
5-HT$_1$-like	Human basilar a.	Contraction	1.4	6.4	[50]
5-HT$_1$-like	Cat saphenous v.	Relaxation	0.03	INACTIVE	[4, 52]
5-HT$_1$-like	Pig vena cava	Relaxation	0.01	INACTIVE	[53, 54]
5-HT$_1$-like	Pig vena cava	Adenylate cyclase activation	0.01	INACTIVE	[53–55]
5-HT$_1$-like	Anaesthetised cat	Tachycardia	0.02	INACTIVE	[45, 48, unpublished observations]
5-HT$_2$	Rabbit aorta	Contraction	26	INACTIVE	[4, 43]
5-HT$_3$	Rat vagus nerve	Depolarisation	INACTIVE	INACTIVE	[4, unpublished observations]

* Values less than unity indicate a greater potency than that for 5-HT.

like receptors are heterogeneous [4]. The high agonist potency of 5-CT in a range of preparations containing different 5-HT receptors is shown in Table 3. Also shown but often ignored is the weak agonist activity of 5-CT at 5-HT$_2$ receptors. It is clear that the agonist potency of 5-CT in a wide range of preparations containing 5-HT$_1$-like receptors falls into two distinct categories. In some preparations, predominantly those where 5-CT mediates contraction of some vascular smooth muscle or where 5-CT inhibits sympathetically mediated contraction of the dog isolated saphenous vein, 5-CT is approximately equipotent with 5-HT. In other preparations where 5-CT mediates relaxation of vascular smooth muscle, tachycardia or stimulation of adenylate cyclase, 5-CT is 30—100 times more potent than 5-HT. Although such a difference in the relative potencies of 5-CT can hardly be considered as unequivocal evidence for receptor heterogeneity, the agonist activities of GR43175 provide us with more definitive evidence for such a claim. In those preparations where 5-CT is approximately equipotent with 5-HT, GR43175 is a potent agonist being approximately 5—10 times weaker that 5-HT [4, 43, 49—51]. In contrast in those preparations where 5-CT is much more potent than 5-HT, GR43175 is devoid of both agonist and antagonist activity [4, 48, 52—55].

Although GR43175 is structurally related to 5-HT [4] it is reasonable to question whether evidence exists that GR43175 activates a specific 5-HT receptor. Experiments in the dog saphenous vein using methiothepin (Figure 1) clearly show that methiothepin antagonises the contractile response to 5-HT and GR43175 equally whilst having no effect on the contractile response to the thromboxane A$_2$ mimetic, U46619. Similar results have recently been obtained in both human and primate cerebral blood vessels [49, 50]. There therefore seems little doubt on the basis of such studies that GR43175 is a highly selective 5-HT$_1$-like receptor agonist, being even more selective than 5-CT and should provide a tool for the further characterisation

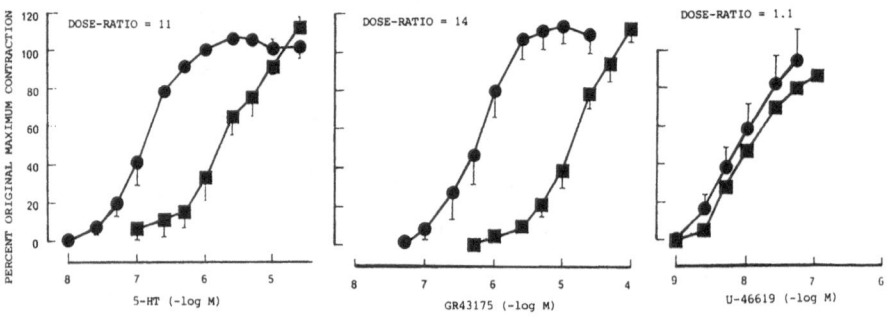

Figure 1. Antagonist effects of methiothepin (0.1 μM) against 5-HT and GR43175, but not U-46619 in dog isolated saphenous vein. Control agonist concentration response curves (●), concentration response curves in presence of methiothepin (■).

of the 5-HT$_1$-like receptor sub-type for which it appears selective. Other studies in vitro with GR43175 have now provided evidence that the GR43175-sensitive 5-HT$_1$-like receptor is confined largely to cranial blood vessels. Indeed recent studies have shown that GR43175 causes a selective vasoconstriction in the cranial circulation of anaesthetised dogs by an agonist action specifically mediated by the 5-HT$_1$-like receptor like that found in the dog saphenous vein and isolated cranial vessels [56]. The same receptor may also function as the autoreceptor on serotoninergic nerves in the mammalian brain [57]. It therefore seems only a matter of time before an equivalent 5-HT$_1$ binding sub-site is found in brain.

Undoubtedly major advances in our understanding of 5-HT receptor function both in the central nervous system and periphery have been and will be brought about with the advent of such drugs as 5-CT, 8-OH-DPAT, and GR43175. Although such agonists are useful probes to study the distribution of 5-HT$_1$ and 5-HT$_1$-like receptors, the physiological and pathological importance of these receptors will only be determined by the use of specific and selective blocking drugs. To date, none have been described but let us hope that our wait for such drugs will not be too long. Recent studies [58] have shown that GR43175 has a high affinity for the 5-HT$_{1D}$ binding site. However, this site appears to be heterogeneous [59].

References

1. Fozard JR (1987): 5-HT: The enigma variations. *Trends in Pharmacol Sci* 100: 501—506.
2. Bradley PB, Engel G, Feniuk W, Fozard JR, Humphrey PPA, Middlemiss DN, Mylecharane EJ, Richardson BP, Saxena PR (1986): Proposals for the classification and nomenclature of functional receptors for 5-hydroxytryptamine. *Neuropharmacol* 25: 563—576.
3. Leff P, Martin GR (1988): The classification of 5-hydroxytryptamine receptors. *Med Res Rev* 8: 187—202.
4. Humphrey PPA, Feniuk W, Perren MJ, Connor HE, Oxford AW, Coates IH, Butina D (1988): GR43175 a selective agonist for the 5-HT$_1$-like receptor in dog isolated saphenous vein. *Br J Pharmacol* 94: 1123—1132.
5. Heuring RE, Peroutka SJ (1987): Characterisation of a novel ³H-5-hydroxytryptamine binding site in bovine brain membranes. *J Neuroscience* 7: 894—903.
6. Peroutka SJ, Snyder SH (1979): Multiple serotonin receptors: Differential binding of [³H]-5-hydroxytryptamine, [³H] by lysergic acid diethylamide and [³H]-spiroperidol. *Mol Pharmacol* 16: 687—699.
7. Leysen JE, Awouters F, Kennis L, Laduron PM, Vandenberk J, Janssen PAJ (1981): Receptor binding profile of R41468, a novel antagonist at 5-HT$_2$ receptors. *Life Sci* 28: 1015—1022.
8. Hunt P, Oberlander C (1981): The interaction of indole derivatives with the serotonin receptor and non-dopaminergic circling behaviour. *Adv Exp Med Biol* 133: 547—562.
9. Middlemiss DN (1985): The putative 5-HT$_1$ receptor agonist RU24969 inhibits the efflux of 5-hydroxytryptamine from rat frontal cortex slices by stimulation of the 5-HT autoreceptor. *J Pharm Pharmac* 37: 434—437.
10. Sills M, Wolfe BB, Frazer A (1984): Determination of selective and non selective

compounds for the 5-HT$_{1A}$ and 5-HT$_{1B}$ receptor subtypes in rat frontal cortex. *J Pharm Exp Ther* 231: 480—487.

11. Martin LL, Sanders-Bush E (1982): Comparison of the pharmacological characteristics of 5-HT$_1$ binding sites with those of serotonin autoreceptors which modulate serotonin release. *Naunyn-Schmiedeberg's Arch Pharmacol* 321: 165—170.

12. Cohen ML, Mason N, Wiley, KS, Fuller RW (1983): Further evidence that vascular serotonin receptors are of the 5-HT$_2$ type. *Biochem Pharmacol* 32: 567—570.

13. Alper RH, Snider JM (1987): Activation of serotonin$_2$ (5-HT$_2$) receptors by quipazine increases arterial pressure and renin secretion in conscious rats. *J Pharmacol Exp Ther* 243: 829—833.

14. Feniuk W, Humphrey PPA (1989): Mechanisms of 5-hydroxytryptamine-induced vaso-constriction, in: Fozard JR (ed), *The Peripheral Actions of 5-Hydroxytryptamine*. Oxford University Press.

15. Pedigo NW, Yamamura HI, Nelson DL (1981): Discrimination of multiple [^{3}H]-5-hydroxytryptamine binding sites by the neuroleptic spiperone in rat brain. *J Neurochem* 36: 220—226.

16. Gozlan H, El-Mestikawy S, Picket L, Glowinsky J, Hammon M (1983): Identification of presynaptic serotonin autoreceptors using a new ligand: ^{3}H-PAT. *Nature (Lond)* 305: 140—142.

17. Middlemiss DN, Fozard JR (1983): 8-Hydroxy-2-(di-n-propylamino)-tetralin discriminates between subtypes of the 5-HT$_1$-recognition site. *Eur J Pharmacol* 90: 151—153.

18. Crist J, Suprenant A (1987): Evidence that 8-Hydroxy-2-(n-propylamino)-tetralin (8-OH-DPAT) is a selective α_2-adrenoceptor antagonist on guinea-pig submucous neurones. *Br J Pharmacol* 92: 341—347.

19. Pazos A, Hoyer D, Palacios JM (1984): The binding of serotonergic ligands to the porcine choroid plexus: Characterisation of a new type of serotonin recognition site. *Eur J Pharmacol* 106: 539—546.

20. Fozard JR, Mir AK, Middlemiss DN (1987): Cardiovascular response to 8-Hydroxy-2-(di-n-propylamino) tetralin (8-OHDPAT) in the rat: Site of action and pharmacological analysis. *J Cardiovasc Pharmacol* 9: 328—347.

21. Di Francesco GF, Petty AM, Fozard JR (1988): Antihypertensive effects of 8-hydroxy-2-(di-n-propylamino) tetralin (8-OH-DPAT) in conscious dogs. *Eur J Pharmacol* 147: 287—290.

22. Ramage AG, Fozard JR (1987): Evidence that the putative 5-HT$_{1A}$ receptor agonists, 8-OH-DPAT and ipsapirone have a central hypotensive action that differs from that of clonidine in anaesthetised cats. *Eur J Pharmacol* 138: 179—191.

23. Martin KF, Mason R (1987): Isapirone is a partial agonist at 5-hydroxytryptamine$_{1A}$ (5-HT$_{1A}$) receptors in the rat hippocampus: electrophysiological evidence. *Eur J Pharmacol* 141: 479—483.

24. Colino A, Halliwell JV (1986): 8-OHDPAT is a strong antagonist of 5-HT actions in rat hippocampus. *Eur J Pharmacol* 130: 151—152.

25. Fozard JR, Kilbinger H (1985): 8-OH-DPAT inhibits transmitter release from guinea-pig enteric cholinergic neurones by activating 5-HT$_{1A}$ receptors. *Br J Pharmacol* 86: 601P.

26. Markstein R, Hoyer D, Engel G (1986): 5-HT$_{1A}$ receptors mediate stimulation of adenylate cyclase in rat hippocampus. Naunyn-Schmiedebergs Arch Pharmacol 333: 335—341.

27. Schoeffter P, Hoyer D (1988): Centrally acting hypotensive agents with affinity for 5-HT$_{1A}$ binding sites inhibit forskolin-stimulated adenylate cyclase activity in calf hippocampus. *Br J Pharmacol* 95: 975—985.

28. De Vivo M, Maayani S (1986): Characterisation of the 5-hydroxytryptamine$_{1A}$ receptor-mediated inhibition of forskolin-stimulated adenylate cyclase activity in guinea-pig and rat hippocampus membranes. *J Pharmacol Exp Ther* 238: 248—253.

29. Gilbert F, Brazell C, Tricklebank MD, Stahl S (1988): Activation of the 5-HT$_{1A}$ receptor subtype increases rat plasma ACTH concentration. *Eur J Pharmacol* 147: 431—439.

30. Chauloff F, Jeanrenaud B (1987): 5-HT$_{1A}$ and alpha-2 adrenergic receptors mediate the hyperglycemic and hypoinsulinemic effects of 8-Hydroxy-2-(di-n-propylamino) tetralin in the conscious rat. *J Pharmacol Exp Ther* 243: 1159—1166.

31. Bockaert J, Dumuis A, Bouhelal R, Sebben M, Cory RN (1987): Piperazine derivatives including the putative anxiolytic drugs buspirone and ipsapirone, are agonists at 5-HT$_{1A}$ receptors negatively coupled with adenylate cyclase in hippocampal neurones. *Naunyn-Schmiedebergs Arch Pharmacol* 335: 588-592.

32. Goldberg HL, Finnesty RJ (1979): The comparitive efficacy of buspirone and diazepam in the treatment of anxiety. *Am J Psychiatry* 136: 1184—1187.

33. Wouters W, Tulp MThM, Bevan P (1988): Flesinoxan lowers blood pressure and heart rate in cats via 5-HT$_{1A}$ receptors. *Eur J Pharmacol* 149: 213—223.

34. Yocca FD, Hyslop DK, Smith DW, Maayani S (1987): BMY 7378, a buspirone analog with high affinity, selectivity and low intrinsic activity at the 5-HT$_{1A}$ receptor in rat and guinea-pig hippocampal membranes. *Eur J Pharmacol* 137: 293—294.

35. Fozard JR, Hilbert M, Kidd EJ, Middlemiss DN, Mir AK, Tricklebank MD (1987): MDL 72832: a potent, selective and stereospecific ligand for 5-HT$_{1A}$ receptors. *Br J Pharmacol* 90: 273P.

36. Wouters W, Rademaker B (1988): Discrepancies between 5-HT$_{1A}$ binding sites in the rat CNS and the guinea-pig ileum. *Proc Cardiovascular Pharmacology of 5-HT Symposium.* Amsterdam P62.

37. Engel G, Göthert M, Hoyer D, Schliker E, Hillenbrand K (1986): Identity of inhibitory presynaptic 5-hydroxytryptamine (5-HT) autoreceptors in the rat brain cortex with 5-HT$_{1B}$ binding sites. *Naunyn Schmiedebergs Arch Pharmacol* 332: 1—7.

38. Holt SE, Cooper M, Wyllie JH (1986): On the nature of the receptor mediating the action of 5-hydroxytryptamine in potentiating responses of the mouse urinary bladder to electrical stimulation. *Naunyn Schmiedebergs Arch Pharmacol* 334: 333—340.

39. Moldering GJ, Fink K, Schliker E, Göthert M (1987): Inhibition of noradrenaline release via presynaptic 5-HT$_{1B}$ receptors of the rat vena cava. *Naunyn Schmiedebergs Arch Pharmacol* 336: 245—250.

40. Bouhelal R, Smounya L, Bockaert J (1988): 5-HT$_{1B}$ receptors are negatively coupled with adenylate cyclase in rat substantia nigra. *Eur J Pharmacol* 151: 189—196.

41. Hoyer D, Pazos A, Probst A, Palacios JM (1986): Serotonin receptors in human brain. 1. Characterisation and autoradiographic localisation of 5-HT$_{1A}$ recognition sites. Apparent absence of 5-HT$_{1B}$ recognition sites. *Brain Res* 376: 85—96.

42. Hoyer D (1988): Molecular pharmacology and biology of 5-HT$_{1C}$ receptors. *Trends in Pharmacol Sci* 9: 89—94.

43. Feniuk W, Humphrey PPA, Perren MJ, Watts AD (1985): A comparison of 5-hydroxytryptamine receptors mediating contraction in rabbit aorta and dog saphenous vein: evidence for different receptor types obtained by use of selective agonists and antagonists. *Br J Pharmacol* 86: 697—704.

44. Saxena PR, Lawang A (1985): A comparison of cardiovascular and smooth muscle effects of 5-hydroxytryptamine and 5-carboxamidotryptamine, a compound with selectivity for 5-HT$_1$ binding sites. *Arch Int Pharmacodyn* 277: 235—252.

45. Saxena PR, Mylecharane EJ, Heiligers J (1985): Analysis of the heart rate effects of 5-hydroxytryptamine in the cat; Mediation of tachycardia by 5-HT$_1$-like receptors. *Naunyn Schmiedebergs Arch Pharmacol* 330: 121—129.

46. Saxena PR, Verdouw PD (1985): 5-Carboxamide tryptamine, a compound with high affinity for 5-HT$_1$ binding sites, dilates arterioles and constricts arteriovenous anastomoses. *Br J Pharmacol* 84: 533—544.

47. Schoeffter P, Waeber C, Palacios JM, Hoyer D (1988): The 5-hydroxytryptamine 5-HT$_{1D}$

receptor subtype is negatively coupled to adenylate cyclase in calf susbtantia nigra. *Naunyn-Schmiederbergs Arch. Pharmacol* 337: 602—607.

48. Connor HE, Feniuk W, Humphrey PPA, Perren MJ (1986): 5-carboxamidotryptamine is a selective agonist at 5-hydroxytryptamine receptors mediating vasodilatation and tachycardia in anaesthetised cats. *Br J Pharmacol* 87: 417—426.
49. Connor HE, Feniuk W, Humphrey PPA (1989): Characterisation of 5-HT receptors mediating contraction of canine and primate basilar artery using GR43175, a selective 5-HT$_1$-like receptor agonist. *Br J Pharmacol* 96: 379—387.
50. Parson AA, Whalley ET, Feniuk W, Connor HE, Humphrey PPA (1989): 5-HT$_1$-like receptors mediate 5-hydroxytryptamine induced contraction of human isolated basilar artery. *Br J Pharmacol* 96: 434—449.
51. Feniuk W, Humphrey PPA, Watts AD (1981): Further characterisation of pre- and post-junctional receptors for 5-hydroxytryptamine in isolated vasculature. *Br J Pharmacol* 73: 191—192P.
52. Feniuk W, Humphrey PPA, Watts AD (1984): 5-Carboxamidotryptamine — a potent agonist at 5-hydroxytryptamine receptors mediating relaxation. *Br J Pharmac* 82: 209P.
53. Trevethick MA, Feniuk W, Humphrey PPA (1986): 5-Carboxamidotryptamine: A potent agonist mediating relaxation and elevation of cyclic AMP in the isolated neonatal porcine vena cava. *Life Sci* 38: 1521—1528.
54. Sumner MJ, Humphrey PPA, Feniuk W (1987): Characterisation of the 5-HT$_1$-like receptor mediating relaxation of porcine vena cava. *Br J Pharmacol* 92: 574P.
55. Sumner MJ, Feniuk W, Humphrey PPA (1989): Further characterisation of the 5-HT receptor mediating vascular relaxation and elevation of cyclic AMP in isolated porcine vena cava. *Br J Pharmac* (In press).
56. Feniuk W, Humphrey PPA, Perren MJ (1989): The selective carotid arterial vaso-constrictor action of GR43175 in anaesthetised dogs. *Br J Pharmacol* 96: 83—90.
57. Middlemiss DN, Bremer ME, Smith SM (1988): A pharmacological analysis of the 5-HT receptors mediating inhibition of 5-HT release in the guinea-pig frontal cortex. *Eur J Pharmacol* 157: 101—108.
58. Peroutka SJ, McCarthy BG (1989): Sumatriptan (GR43175) interacts selectively with 5-HT$_{1B}$ and 5-HT$_{1D}$ binding sites. *Eur J Pharmacol* 163: 133—136.
59. Sumner MJ, Humphrey PPA (1989): 5-HT$_{1D}$ binding sites in porcine brain can be sub-divided by GR43175. *Br J Pharmacol* 98: 29—31.

VII. Agonists and antagonists of 5-HT$_2$ receptors

E. J. MYLECHARANE

1. Introduction

In the context of an update on new drugs used in the characterization of functional receptors for 5-hydroxytryptamine (5-HT), a review such as this on 5-HT$_2$ receptor agonists and antagonists needs to address the criteria currently used to classify these receptors, and to consider the validity of these criteria in the light of the relevant data available on functional actions. In particular, any evidence suggesting heterogeneity within this functional receptor classification needs to be evaluated, thus quantitative functional data obtained in vitro for several 5-HT$_2$ receptor antagonists in a range of tissues containing 5-HT$_2$ receptors have been considered in some detail. Comparisons have also been made with data obtained in ligand binding studies. The question of specificity has also been briefly considered, and some recently developed 5-HT$_2$ receptor agonists and antagonists have been discussed.

2. Criteria for defining functional 5-HT$_2$ receptors

The criteria now generally used to define functional 5-HT$_2$ receptors are those proposed recently by Bradley et al. [1]. For classification as a 5-HT$_2$ receptor-mediated response, the effect of 5-HT must be blocked by ketanserin, cyproheptadine, methysergide, or related agents such as methiothepin, spiperone or pizotifen. While most of these antagonists are highly selective for 5-HT$_2$ receptors as opposed to 5-HT$_1$-like and 5-HT$_3$ receptors, methysergide and methiothepin also have appreciable affinities for 5-HT$_1$ binding sites (7—38-fold less than those for 5-HT$_2$ sites [2, 3]). The pA$_2$ or pK$_B$ values for ketanserin, cyproheptadine and methysergide should be of the order of 8.9, 8.8 and 8.7, respectively. 5-HT$_3$ receptor antagonists such as (−)-cocaine, MDL 72222 and ICS 205-930 must be ineffective. The availability of selective antagonists has pre-empted the necessity to specify selective agonists in the criteria defining this group of functional receptors.

P.R. Saxena, D.I. Wallis, W. Wouters and P. Bevan (eds), Cardiovascular Pharmacology of
5-Hydroxytryptamine, pp. 81—100.
© 1990 *Kluwer Academic Publishers, Dordrecht* —

In accordance with these criteria, 5-HT$_2$ receptors were identified by Bradley et al. [1] as being responsible for vascular smooth muscle contraction in a variety of preparations; contraction of uterine, bronchial, gastro-intestinal and bladder smooth muscle; platelet aggregation; increased capillary permeability; and some behavioural syndromes in rodents such as head twitch and wet-dog shakes. Other effects mediated by 5-HT$_2$ receptors include the release of adrenaline from the dog adrenal medulla [4], and the discriminative stimulus properties of 5-hydroxytryptophan and hallucinogens such as lysergic acid diethylamide (LSD) and 1-(2,5-dimethoxy-4-methyl-phenyl)-2-aminopropane (DOM) in rodents [5—7], although the lack of efficacy of ritanserin (a more specific 5-HT$_2$ receptor antagonist) in the latter model raises the possibility of involvement of catecholaminergic pathways in discriminative stimulus activity [8].

Recent electrophysiological studies have shown that the excitatory effects of 5-HT on rat brainstem neurons satisfy the criteria for mediation by a 5-HT$_2$ receptor [9]. 5-HT-induced depolarization of guinea-pig cortical pyramidal neurons also appears to be mediated by 5-HT$_2$ receptors [10], but other central neuroexcitatory effects of 5-HT are not, for example in rat spinal neurons [9] and hippocampal CA$_1$ neurons [11]. Inhibition of glutamate release from rat cerebellum slices involves both 5-HT$_1$-like and 5-HT$_2$ receptors [12]. Evidence is also emerging that 5-HT$_2$ receptors are involved in hypothalamic-anterior pituitary neuroendocrine function. 5-HT$_2$ receptors contribute substantially to β-endorphin and corticosterone secretion in rats [13], and also interact with opiate pathways to produce marked augmentation of luteinizing hormone release in ovariectomized rats [14], despite the fact that 5-HT systems yield only a modest stimulatory effect and opiates result in inhibition when these pathways are activated separately. 5-HT$_2$ receptors make little or no contribution to prolactin or growth hormone secretion in rats [15—17], but do appear to be involved in prolactin (but not growth hormone or corticosteroid) release in rhesus monkeys [18].

3. Comparisons of the effects of antagonists on functional 5-HT$_2$ receptors

Bradley et al. [1] noted that strict measurements of K$_B$ values for 5-HT$_2$ receptor antagonists were not able to be determined for all responses classified as 5-HT$_2$ receptor-mediated, and some anomalies existed; however, it was considered that the available data did not yet warrant the conclusion that 5-HT$_2$ receptors were heterogeneous. Leff and Martin [19] drew attention to the instances of non-surmountable antagonism with ketanserin and methysergide and the "inordinately large range" of K$_B$ estimates for ketanserin and spiperone in smooth muscle preparations. Differences in experimental conditions and analytical methods were recognized as possible sources of these discrepancies [1, 19], but Leff and Martin [19] also argued that either genuine heterogeneity in these receptors could exist or that the antagonists used were unreliable.

Detailed comparisons of the effects of several 5-HT$_2$ receptor antagonists have therefore been made over a range of functional 5-HT$_2$ receptor-mediated responses in peripheral tissue preparations. Table 1 lists pA$_2$ values (or equivalent pK$_B$ values) against 5-HT for the principal antagonists presently used to characterize functional 5-HT$_2$ receptors [1], as well as data for trazodone and LY53857, in vascular and other smooth muscle preparations in which the contractile responses to 5-HT have been accepted as being mediated by 5-HT$_2$ receptors. The data included have been confined to values where the antagonism was competitive. In most instances, evidence of simple competition is based on analysis using the established criteria of Schild plots [20] or the equivalent, but in some cases the evidence provided is limited to parallel rightward shifts in the 5-HT log concentration-effect curves in the presence of antagonist, and fully surmountable antagonism (e.g. [37]). Data described as pA$_2$ or pK$_B$ values have not been included where the antagonism clearly does not involve simple competition. Tissues have been included in Table 1 only when at least two of the antagonists have been evaluated in that tissue, to try to ensure that any pattern of apparent heterogeneity is not due to a particular antagonist. In some instances, there are literature reports of non-competitive as well as competitive antagonism for a particular antagonist-tissue combination; these instances have been identified in Table 1.

Overall, the differences between the lower and upper limits of the values for each antagonist vary between 0.58 log units (pizotifen) and 2.45 log units (methysergide). Differences in experimental conditions and methods of analysis could well contribute to these relatively large ranges. It is impossible to define a set of "standard" conditions and analysis from the studies included in Table 1; the small but numerous differences in methodology from various laboratories doubtless bear testament to the individuality of pharmacologists. Nevertheless, the data reported do suggest that genuine differences may be present in the various antagonist-receptor interactions studied.

The values listed in Table 1 for ketanserin (which have an overall mean of 8.92) can be divided into two distinct groupings. One subgroup is confined to several (but not all) preparations from rats. The mean of the values in rat caudal artery, femoral artery, jugular vein and uterus preparations is 9.31 ± 0.22 (n = 8), while that in the remaining preparations is 8.66 ± 0.14 (n = 12). Thus although there is an overall difference of 2.31 log units between the lowest and highest values in all preparations, the ranges reduce to 8.42–10.41 (difference 1.99 log units) in the rat preparation subgroup, and 8.10–9.93 (difference 1.83 log units) in the remaining subgroup. The latter difference has been inflated by almost 1 log unit because of a single high value in the rat portal vein.

It has been suggested on the basis of findings with trazodone that the 5-HT$_2$ receptor in the rabbit aorta may differ from those in other tissues, and the possibility of heterogeneity has been raised [1, 19]. As can be seen in Table 1, however, almost all the data for trazodone is in the rat preparation subgroup; values in the remaining subgroup have only been obtained in

Table 1. pA$_2$ and pK$_B$ values of 5-HT$_2$ receptor antagonists for contractile responses to 5-HT in smooth muscle tissue preparations.

Tissue	Ketanserin	Cyproheptadine	Methysergide	Spiperone	Pizotifen	Trazodone	LY53857
Rat:							
aorta	8.40 [21]	8.76 [38] a[21]	7.97 [38] a[21]	9.72 [43]	—	—	—
caudal a.	8.80 [21] 9.08 [22] 9.23 [23] 8.42 [98] a[19, 24, 25]	8.70 [21]	9.11 [23] a[19, 21, 22, 24]	9.63 [19]	—	8.32 [19]	—
femoral a.	10.41 [26]	—	10.42 [26]	—	—	—	—
jugular v.	9.05 [19] 9.70 [27]	—	—	9.66 [19] 10.00 [27] 10.13 [43]	—	8.02 [19] 8.70 [27]	10.35 [48]
portal v.	8.20 [28] 9.93 [100] a[29]	—	—	9.90 [28]	—	7.70 [28]	8.40 [28]
uterus	9.80 [30] a[33, 34]	—	—	—	—	8.49 [47]	10.10 [30]
Rabbit:							
aorta	8.56 [19] 8.72 [31] 8.67 [32]	8.73 [39] 8.88 [40]	8.25 [19] 8.49 [39] 8.25 [42]	9.28 [19] 8.92 [31] 8.64 [32] 9.26 [44] 9.21 [45]	9.42 [39]	7.23 [19] 7.22 [42]	—

Table 1 (Continued)

Tissue	Ketanserin	Cyproheptadine	Methysergide	Spiperone	Pizotifen	Trazodone	LY53857
common carotid a.	8.49 [33]	9.19[b]	8.80[b]	—	9.20 |46|	—	—
femoral a.	8.27 [35]	—	—	—	8.84 |46|	—	—
Dog:							
femoral a.	8.10 [36]	8.55 [41]	8.52 |41|	—	—	—	—
gastro-splenic v.	8.88 [22]	—	8.56 [22]	—	—	—	—
Guinea-pig:							
trachea	9.00 [30] 8.73 [33] a[37]	—	—	—	—	—	9.30 [30]
Means ± s.e.:	8.92 ± 0.14	8.80±0.09	8.71 ± 0.24	9.49 ± 0.14	9.15±0.17	7.95±0.22	9.54 ± 0.44
Range:	8.10—10.41 (2.31)	8.44—9.19 (0.64)	7.97—10.42 (2.45)	8.64—10.13 (1.49)	8.84—9.42 (0.58)	7.22—8.70 (1.48)	8.40—10.35 (1.95)

Literature values are shown, together with references in square parentheses. For each antagonist, the mean ± s.e. of all pA_2 (or pK_B) values is listed, together with the range of the values expressed as lower and upper limits and as the difference between the limits (in log units, in parentheses). Abbreviations: a. = artery; v. = vein.

[a] potent antagonism, not competitive.
[b] (E. J. Mylecharane, M. C. Pye, J. K. Markus and C. A. Phillips, unpublished).

rabbit aorta and rat portal vein. As with ketanserin, values are consistently higher in the rat subgroup, but studies in other tissues in the remaining subgroup need to be conducted before concluding that trazodone identifies the same subgroups as are apparently identified by ketanserin. Like ketanserin and trazodone, values for spiperone are higher in the rat subgroup and lower in rabbit aorta, but the values are also high in rat aorta and portal vein. Spiperone has not been tested in other tissues in the remaining subgroup. There are extensive data for methysergide in the remaining subgroup, with values ranging between 7.97 and 8.80, but only two values have been determined in tissues from the rat subgroup. Although these are higher (by 0.31 and 1.62 log units, respectively), more data are needed to establish if a pattern similar to that with ketanserin can be obtained. Of the other antagonists, both cyproheptadine and pizotifen give consistent values in the remaining subgroup; the sole value in the rat subgroup (for cyproheptadine, in rat caudal artery) is similar. The limited data for LY53587 show similar high values in the rat subgroup, and lower (but widely differing) values in guinea-pig trachea and rat portal vein.

Thus the pattern of two distinct subgroups apparent with ketanserin is also suggested by the data with trazodone, methysergide and LY53587, although there are insufficient data available to allow firm conclusions to be drawn. Spiperone also yields two apparent subgroups, but the composition of these subgroups does not correspond exactly with those for ketanserin; again, more data are needed. The limited data available for cyproheptadine suggest that it may not be able to discriminate 5-HT$_2$ receptor subgroups.

Apart from the need to obtain more data before concluding that there are two functional 5-HT$_2$ receptor subgroups, some other aspects of antagonism in these tissues make it necessary to draw any such conclusions with caution. These aspects are characterized by the occurrence of an end result of blockade which does not fulfil the criteria for simple competition; a meaningful identification of receptor subtypes depends on an equilibrium model of competitive interaction between agonist, antagonist and receptor. Table 1 shows several instances of reports of antagonism with ketanserin, cyproheptadine and methysergide which is potent but not competitive (i.e. occurring at concentrations similar to those producing competitive blockade), for tissue/antagonist combinations where competitive antagonism has been reported in other studies. There are also uniform reports of potent but not competitive antagonism in several of the tissues included in Table 1: cyproheptadine in rat portal vein [29] and guinea-pig trachea (E. J. Mylecharane, M. C. Pye, J. K. Markus and C. A. Phillips, unpublished); methysergide in rat jugular vein [19], rat portal vein [29], rat uterus [34, 47] and guinea-pig trachea [37]; spiperone in the rat uterus [34]; and pizotifen in the guinea-pig trachea (E. J. Mylecharane, M. C. Pye, J. K. Markus and C. A. Phillips, unpublished).

The mechanisms underlying the propensity of many of the 5-HT$_2$ receptor antagonists to produce blockade which does not fulfil the criteria for simple competitive antagonism have not been clarified. The nature of the blockade produced by each of these agents is variable: usually non-surmountable, with parallel or non-parallel rightward shifts, but occasionally non-surmountable with no shifts, or surmountable with variable shifts. No particular tissue- or antagonist-related pattern is discernable. Uptake and metabolism of 5-HT have been controlled in some studies and not in others, but direct comparisons have seldom been made. These factors are important when tryptamine is used as an agonist, but antagonism of 5-HT does not appear to be greatly influenced, at least in rat caudal artery preparations [23], and $uptake_1$ does not appear to be a variable influence in rabbit common carotid artery [46]. Variable degrees of desensitization of 5-HT responses (independent of uptake or metabolism) might also influence functional agonist-antagonist interactions; guinea-pig trachea has a rapid desensitization rate relative to that in rabbit aorta preparations [49]. The possibility of activation of mixed receptors influencing agonist-antagonist interactions has likewise not yet been systematically addressed, as evidenced for example by the availability of data with $5-HT_3$ antagonists in rabbit aorta and rat uterus preparations but its absence in rat caudal artery, dog gastrosplenic vein and guinea-pig trachea when Bradley at al. [1] recently classified 5-HT receptors. The $5-HT_3$ receptor antagonists MDL 72222 and ICS 205-930 have since been shown to have no effect on responses to 5-HT in guinea-pig trachea [50]. Possible involvement of $5-HT_1$-like receptors in the responses being monitored is difficult to assess at present because of the lack of selective $5-HT_1$-like receptor antagonists. Given the experimental techniques usually adopted in preparing the vascular tissues investigated, an endothelium-derived relaxing factor component in the response, mediated by $5-HT_1$-like receptors [51], is unlikely, but its possible influence has not been systematically assessed or controlled. One way to minimize the complications of mixed receptor responses would be to use selective $5-HT_2$ receptor agonists instead of 5-HT as the agonist in functional studies with antagonists. This approach has not yet been adopted, perhaps because of the emphasis which has been placed on the availability of selective $5-HT_2$ receptor antagonists. Some of the more recently developed selective agonists (see section 6) may be useful in this regard.

In some other tissues (not included in Table 1), pA_2 values against 5-HT have been evaluated for only a single $5-HT_2$ receptor antagonist. Any pattern suggestive of heterogeneity is therefore unable to be verified with other antagonists as yet, but further information will doubtless emerge. The data obtained in some of these studies, however, are of relevance to the previously outlined problems associated with production of antagonism which does not fulfil the criteria of simple competition.

Ketanserin has been reported to have pK_B values of 9.51 in calf trachea [37], 9.18 and 9.45 in calf coronary artery [52, 53], and 9.38 in calf pulmonary artery [53]; methysergide produces potent but non-surmountable blockade in these tissues [37, 54]. Kaumann and his colleagues [37, 54] have suggested that the non-surmountable effect of methysergide in these calf preparations, and also in guinea-pig trachea, involves binding to an allosteric site on the $5\text{-}HT_2$ receptor, which induces a conformational change such that 5-HT can only elicit a "residual" response (presumably because the changes in the receptor alter the post-receptor events). This residual response to 5-HT is resistant to antagonism by ketanserin and methysergide, indicating that the conformational change in the $5\text{-}HT_2$ receptor may also result in a decrease in affinity for $5\text{-}HT_2$ receptor antagonists. Ketanserin also appears to act in this way on the allosteric site in guinea-pig trachea (but not in the other tissues), thereby producing non-surmountable antagonism in that tissue. In all four tissues, however, ketanserin was also able to restore the methyser-gide-reduced maximal response to 5-HT. It was concluded that ketanserin is able to act as a competitive antagonist at the allosteric site, thereby reversing the action of methysergide and the consequent conformational changes in the receptor. Allosteric regulation of $5\text{-}HT_2$ receptors may therefore contribute to the non-surmountable antagonism produced by these and other $5\text{-}HT_2$ receptor antagonists in other tissues.

In other tissues purported to contain $5\text{-}HT_2$ receptors, pA_2 or pK_B values for antagonists have not been determined. Ketanserin and methysergide, for example, have been shown to be potent antagonists of 5-HT-induced contraction in longitudinal muscle strips prepared from the distal ileum of juvenile guinea-pig [55], but pA_2 values were not established.

Several human vascular preparations have been studied, but $5\text{-}HT_1$-like receptors also appear to be involved in the contractile response, and non-surmountable antagonism frequently occurs. Ketanserin is a potent but not competitive antagonist of 5-HT in gastric and colonic arteries and veins [56]. In human saphenous veins, a relatively weak non-competitive antagonism has been obtained with ketanserin, cyproheptadine, methysergide and pizotifen [56—58], and a $5\text{-}HT_2$ receptor-mediated component has been suggested. Competitive blockade with yohimbine was demonstrated [58], but the pA_2 value obtained was approximately 1.5 log units less than those for $5\text{-}HT_2$ receptor-mediated contraction in calf coronary and pulmonary arteries [52, 53], and approximately 2.5 log units less than that in the rat stomach fundus [59], where a $5\text{-}HT_1$-like receptor appears to be responsible for 5-HT-induced contraction [1].

The effects of ketanserin and methysergide in human umbilical artery preparations vary with O_2 tension. At low pO_2 levels (equivalent to the normal physiological level), methysergide was a potent competitive antago-nist of the contractile response to 5-HT, but ketanserin, despite being very potent, resulted in blockade which was not competitive [60, 61]. When pO_2 was increased (to levels normally present in the systemic arterial circulation), the potency of 5-HT increased, both methysergide and ketanserin produced biphasic shifts in the 5-HT concentration-response curve, methysergide behaved as a partial agonist, and the selective $5\text{-}HT_1$-like receptor agonist

5-carboxamidotryptamine displayed much greater contractile activity [61, 62], suggesting that elevation of pO$_2$ activates a 5-HT$_1$-like receptor-mediated component in the vasoconstrictor response. In another investigation in which relatively high pO$_2$ levels were used, ketanserin acted as a competitive antagonist against 5-HT in human umbilical artery and vein preparations, but the pA$_2$ values obtained were substantially less than that expected for 5-HT$_2$ receptor-mediated actions [63].

There are conflicting reports concerning the nature of the receptor mediating the contractile response to 5-HT in dog coronary arteries. Brazenor and Angus [64, 65] found that ketanserin, cyproheptadine and pizotifen were potent but non-surmountable antagonists of 5-HT; methysergide behaved either as a partial agonist [64] or as a potent non-surmountable antagonist [Porquet et al., 66] and trazodone was a relatively weak non-surmountable antagonist [65]. Frenken and Kaumann [67], however, subsequently reported that ketanserin at a concentration of 0.1 μM unmasked a ketanserin-resistant component in the 5-HT response, but a partly surmountable blocking component was also present; at 1 μM, the first component was much less pronounced, and a substantial partly surmountable antagonism was again observed. In contrast, Cohen [36] found that ketanserin and cyproheptadine acted as non-surmountable antagonists in endothelium-denuded dog coronary artery preparations, but these agents were much less potent than previously reported; the effects of 1 μM ketanserin in these experiments, for example, were comparable with those produced by 0.01 μM ketanserin in the experiments described by Brazenor and Angus [65]. Houston and Vanhoutte [68] described an even weaker blocking effect with 1 μM ketanserin in endothelium-denuded preparations. Methiothepin was a competitive antagonist of the contractile response to 5-HT, with pA$_2$ values of 8.00 [36] and 8.78 [68] being reported. There is little other data available on pA$_2$ values for methiothepin. Estimates range from 6.99 to 7.71 for blockade of 5-HT-induced pre-synaptic inhibition of neurotransmitter release from tryptaminergic, cholinergic and noradrenergic neuronal terminals [69–71], actions which are all mediated by 5-HT$_1$-like receptors [1]. In tissues where the contractile response to 5-HT is mediated by 5-HT$_2$ receptors, the only pA$_2$ value for methiothepin is 8.80, in the dog femoral artery [36]; in the rabbit common carotid artery, methiothepin (0.01–0.3 nM) produces surmountable (but not competitive) antagonism, and at concentrations of 0.01–300 nM, it acts as a non-surmountable antagonist in guinea-pig trachea (E. J. Mylecharane, I. Fong, J. D. Nicol and C. A. Phillips, unpublished). Presumably, both 5-HT$_1$-like and 5-HT$_2$ receptors contribute to the contractile response to 5-HT in the dog coronary artery, which may be further complicated (at least in the earlier investigations) by an endothelium-mediated relaxant component.

Similarly, the nature of the receptor mediating the contractile response to 5-HT in the dog basilar artery is disputed. Van Nueten et al. [22] reported

Table 2. pK$_i$ values of 5-HT$_2$ receptor antagonists for inhibition of binding at 5-HT$_2$ sites in membrane preparations.

Tissue and ligand	Ketanserin	Cyproheptadine	Methysergide	Spiperone	Pizotifen	Trazodone	LY53857
Rat cortex:							
[3H]spiperone	8.68 [3]	8.70[2]	8.59 [2]	9.29 [2]	8.19 [3]	7.65 [27]a	7.65 [28]a
	8.95 [27]a	8.19 [3]	7.92 [3]	8.92 [3]	8.34 [7]a	7.80 [28]a	
	8.75 [28]a	8.07 [7]a	8.10 [7]a	9.40 [27]a	8.66 [81]		
	8.70 [82]a	8.62 [79]	8.51 [79]	9.35 [28]a			
		8.45 [81]	8.36 [81]	8.58 [81]			
[3H]ketanserin	8.86 [55]	9.36 [80]	8.62 [55]	9.28 [80]	9.55 [80]	—	8.17 [59]
	9.37 [59]	8.90 [83]	8.77 [59]	8.80 [83]			
	9.41 [80]	8.46 [84]	9.03 [80]	8.76 [84]			
	8.90 [83]		8.60 [83]				
[3H]LSD (plus 0.3 μM 5-HT)	—	8.77 [2]	8.55 [2]	9.12 [2]	—	—	—
[125I]LSD	8.80 [72]	8.38 [72]	8.65 [72]	8.64 [72]	8.83 [72]	—	—
[3H]mesulergine	9.00 [83; 73%]	8.30 [83]	8.90 [83; 79%]	8.40 [83]	—	—	—
	7.10 [83; 27%]		6.70 [83; 21%]				
Pig cortex:							
[3H]ketanserin	8.40 [83]	—	7.70 [83; 44%]	8.10 [83]	—	—	—
			5.30 [83; 56%]				
[3H]mesulergine	7.00 [83]	—	8.70 [83]	5.90 [83]	—	—	—

Table 2 (Continued)

Tissue and ligand	Ketanserin	Cyproheptadine	Methysergide	Spiperone	Pizotifen	Trazodone	LY53857
Human cortex:							
[³H]ketanserin	8.64 [85]	—	7.10 [83; 64%] 5.60 [83; 36%] 8.28 [85]	8.60 [83] 9.04 [85]	—	—	—
[³H]spiperone	8.22 [86]	—	—	—	—	—	—
Rat striatum:							
[³H]ketanserin	9.24 [87]	9.00 [87]	8.64 [87]	9.35 [87]	—	—	—
Cat platelets:							
[³H]ketanserin	9.22 [87]	8.70 [87]	8.15 [87]	8.96 [87]	—	—	—
Human platelets:							
[³H]spiperone	7.30 [86]	—	—	—	—	—	—
Rat uterus:							
[³H]ketanserin	6.84 [88]	—	6.82 [88]	6.87 [88]	—	—	—
Means ± s.e.:	8.49±0.19	8.61±0.10	7.98±0.22	8.63±0.21	8.71±0.24	7.73	7.91
Range:	6.48—9.41	8.07—9.36	5.30—9.03	5.90—9.40	8.19—9.55	7.65—7.80	7.65—8.17
	(2.93)	(1.29)	(3.73)	(3.50)	(1.36)	(0.15)	(0.52)

Literature values are shown, together with references in square parentheses. For each antagonist, the mean ± s.e. of all pK$_i$ values is listed, together with the range of the values expressed as lower and upper limits and as the difference between the limits (in log units, in parentheses). Abbreviations: LSD = lysergic acid diethylamide.

^{a}—log IC$_{50}$ values; insufficient data to calculate pK$_i$ values.

potent but non-surmountable antagonism with ketanserin, but methysergide-induced blockade was competitive (pA_2 = 8.43); Müller-Schweinitzer and Engel [72] found that various antagonists, including ketanserin, cyproheptadine, methysergide, spiperone and pizotifen, produced potent non-surmountable blockade. In contrast, Peroutka et al. [73—75] concluded that 5-HT$_2$ receptors made little or no contribution to the response (based largely on functional studies with ketanserin, cyproheptadine, methysergide and spiperone, and on autoradiographic binding studies with 5-HT, spiperone and LSD), and presented evidence for involvement of a receptor which resembles the 5-HT$_{1A}$ binding site. Cohen and Colbert [76] likewise reported only minimal shifts in 5-HT concentration-response curves with ketanserin (0.1 μM) and spiperone (0.01 μM), and also with LY53587 (0.01 μM), but found a correlation between antagonist potencies in the dog basilar artery and the rat stomach fundus. Taylor et al. [77] concluded from agonist studies that the receptor mediating contraction to 5-HT resembled the 5-HT$_{1A}$ binding site. An involvement of both 5-HT$_2$ and non-5-HT$_2$ receptors was suggested by Frenken and Kaumann [78]; evidence was obtained for potent and partly surmountable antagonism with ketanserin, and a ketanserin-resistant component in the response, similar to the effects observed in the dog coronary artery [67].

4. Affinities of antagonists for 5-HT$_2$ binding sites

The 5-HT$_2$ binding site affinities of the antagonists discussed in detail in section 3 have been compared in a similar manner. Table 2 lists a range of literature K_i values for inhibition by these agents of radiolabelled ligand binding in several membrane preparations. For ease of comparison with the functional values in Table 1, the K_i values have all been expressed as pK_i values (i.e. $-\log K_i$).

As in the functional studies, there is some variability in the data for each antagonist. There are some obvious discrepancies for rat uterus and human platelet data; the relatively low values reported may reflect inherent difficulties in determining values when receptor density is low. However, the data in cat platelets seem to be very similar to those obtained in the various brain membrane preparations. Other discrepancies appear when [^{3}H]mesulergine is the ligand; Pazos et al. [83] reported that in rat cortex, [^{3}H]mesulergine and [^{3}H]ketanserin labelled similar sites (based on pK_i values for ketanserin, cyproheptadine, methysergide and spiperone), but in pig cortex, clear differences were seen, with the pK_i values for [^{3}H]-mesulergine binding being lower than those for [^{3}H]ketanserin binding in the case of ketanserin and spiperone, and higher in the case of methysergide (cyproheptadine was not tested). Pazos et al. [83] were unable to determine pK_i values in human cortex for [^{3}H]mesulergine binding, because of the very low level of specific binding with this ligand. Species differences may well account for these discrepancies; biphasic inhibition profiles were also obtained in several instances, which complicates analysis (in such cases, pK_i values for both the high and low affinity components are included in Table 2, together with the % proportions of binding at each site).

If these clearly discrepant data are excluded (i.e. rat uterus and human platelet data, [³H]mesulergine data in pig cortex, and low affinity site pK_i data), the ranges between the lowest and highest values decrease to 1.19 log units (ketanserin), 1.93 log units (methysergide) and 1.30 log units (spiperone). No particular pattern of variability in the remaining values is discernible, however. In general, the mean pK_i values in Table 2 correspond well to the overall mean pA_2 values in Table 1; exclusion of the above discrepant data from Table 2 increases the means for ketanserin, methysergide and spiperone, giving a better correspondence with the functional data. The only exception is LY53857; the limited binding inhibition data give a mean value which is 1.63 log units less than the overall mean in the functional studies (which are also few in number).

5. Specificity of 5-HT₂ receptor antagonists

As noted previously, most 5-HT₂ receptor antagonists have little or no affinity for 5-HT₁ binding sites or 5-HT₁-like receptors, the exceptions being methysergide and methiothepin amongst the antagonists discussed in detail in the previous sections. There are considerable data available for comparing 5-HT₁ and 5-HT₂ binding site affinities [for example, see references 2, 3, 27, 28, 79, 84]; comparisons with functional actions mediated by 5-HT₁-like receptors have also been made in many investigations [for example, see references 1, 30, 47, 59, 69—71, 82, 84]. These aspects are covered in more detail in other contributions in this volume.

The actions of the 5-HT₂ receptor antagonists at other receptors and binding sites are also well-documented. Comparisons of actions at α-adrenoceptors are particularly important, because many of the responses to 5-HT are mimicked by α-adrenoceptor agonists. Ketanserin acts as an antagonist at α-adrenoceptors in vascular preparations at concentration of the order of 10-fold higher than those effective at 5-HT₂ receptors [for example 1, 22, 25, 32, 33, 65], as does spiperone [32]; methiothepin has a high affinity for α_1-adrenergic binding sites [3]. Little is known of the activity of trazodone at α-adrenoceptors, although it has been reported to have antagonist activity in dog coronary artery [65]. The other 5-HT₂ receptor antagonists have considerably less α-adrenoceptor affinity [3, 22, 38, 39, 41, 46, 48], except in the dog coronary artery where pizotifen appeared to be a potent antagonist of noradrenaline-induced contraction [65].

6. Recently developed 5-HT$_2$ receptor agonists and antagonists

A noteworthy aspect is the increasing interest in developing selective 5-HT$_2$ receptor agonists. As noted previously, selective agonists may prove to be of value in characterizing functional 5-HT$_2$ receptors, particularly where mixed 5-HT receptors may influence the response being monitored.

Non-tryptamine agonists such as quipazine and MK-212 (6-chloro-2-[1-piperazinyl]-pyrazine) have been available for some time, but these agents have appreciable affinity for other 5-HT receptors. Selective 5-HT$_2$ receptor agonist activity has been found, however, in a series of phenylisopropyla-mines, such as the hallucinogen DOM, and its bromo and iodo congeners 1-(2,5-dimethoxy-4-bromophenyl)-2-aminopropane (DOB) and 1-(2,5-dime-thoxy-4-iodophenyl)-2-aminopropane (DOI). These agents have a high selectivity for 5-HT$_2$ binding sites [89—91]; in addition to hallucinogenic actions, DOI has recently been reported to produce 5-HT$_2$ receptor-mediated actions such as anorexia in rats [92], inhibition of glutamate release from the rat cerebellum [12], and increases in spontaneous discharge in cat cardiac sympathetic nerves following i.v. administration [93]. [^{3}H]DOB and [^{125}I]DOI have been developed as 5-HT$_2$ receptor ligands [94].

Nelson et al. [95] found that tetrahydropyridylindole derivatives of the selective 5-HT$_1$-like receptor agonist RU 24969 with a benzyl substitution in the C-1 position were almost devoid of 5-HT$_{1A}$ binding site affinity, but affinity for 5-HT$_2$ sites was markedly enhanced. These agents acted as 5-HT$_2$ receptor agonists in the rabbit femoral artery and as antagonists in the rat aorta.

Relatively little has been reported on new 5-HT$_2$ receptor antagonists. A benzoxathiepin analog, CV-5197, has been shown to be a highly specific 5-HT$_2$ receptor antagonist in rat caudal and pig coronary arteries, although it did not alter the head twitch response to 5-HT; it was highly selective for 5-HT$_2$ binding sites in rat brain [96]. The recently developed antagonist ICI 169,369 is a specific blocker of several actions of 5-HT mediated by 5-HT$_2$ receptors and is selective for 5-HT$_2$ binding sites [97, 98], but it is a potent antagonist of the contractile responses to 5-HT in rat stomach fundus, rabbit basilar artery and human basilar artery [98, 99], which are classified as 5-HT$_1$-like receptor-mediated actions [1].

7. Conclusion

The quantitative data available for functional actions of several 5-HT$_2$ receptor antagonists in smooth muscle preparations suggest the possibility that two subgroups of the functional 5-HT$_2$ receptor might exist. A subgroup of rat preparations (caudal artery, femoral artery, jugular vein and uterus) have consistently higher pA$_2$ values for ketanserin compared with the remaining subgroup (rat aorta and portal vein; rabbit aorta, common carotid artery and femoral artery; dog femoral artery and gastrosplenic vein; and guinea-pig trachea). The pattern of blockade with methysergide, trazodone and LY53857 is consistent with this, although there are insufficient data available to confirm this possibility. Although more data are needed, spiperone also appears to identify two similar but not identical subgroups, but cyproheptadine does not seem to discriminate any subgroups. A limiting factor in comparisons of this kind is the propensity of many of the antagonists to produce blockade which does not fulfil the criteria for simple competitive inhibition; differences in experimental conditions and analysis methods also pose problems. Any real differences in the data may reflect a genuine heterogeneity in 5-HT$_2$ receptors, but the differences could equally be inherent in the diverse chemical natures of the antagonists used. Nevertheless, consistent patterns of blockade with antagonists are still useful in characterizing the nature of receptors mediating particular responses. The use of selective 5-HT$_2$ receptor agonists may prove to be helpful in clarifying these possibilities. 5-HT$_2$ binding data show some discrepancies, usually related to use of a particular ligand ([^{3}H]mesulergine) or tissue (rat uterus; human platelet). In general, the binding data correlate well with functional data. The clinical and therapeutic implications of heterogeneity in functional 5-HT$_2$ receptors remain to be established.

Acknowledgements

Investigations conducted in the author's laboratory were supported in part by the National Health and Medical Research Council of Australia, and Janssen Pharmaceutica (Australia).

References

1. Bradley PB, Engel G, Feniuk W, Fozard JR, Humphrey PPA, Middlemiss DN, Mylecharane EJ, Richardson BP, Saxena PR (1986): Proposals for the classification and nomenclature of functional receptors for 5-hydroxytryptamine. *Neuropharmacology* 25: 563—576.
2. Peroutka SJ, Snyder SH (1979): Multiple serotonin receptors: differential binding of [^{3}H]5-hydroxytryptamine, [^{3}H]lysergic acid diethylamide and [^{3}H]spiroperidol. *Mol Pharmacol* 16: 687—699.
3. Leysen JE, Awouters F, Kennis L, Laduron PM, Vandenberk J, Janssen PAJ (1981): Receptor binding profile of R 41 468, a novel antagonist at 5-HT$_2$ receptors. *Life Sciences* 28: 1015—1022.
4. Feniuk W, Hare J, Humphrey PPA (1981): An analysis of the mechanism of 5-hydroxytryptamine-induced vasopressor responses in ganglion-blocked anaesthetized dogs. *J Pharm Pharmacol* 33: 155—160.
5. Colpaert FC, Niemegeers CJE, Janssen PAJ (1982): A drug discrimination analysis of lysergic acid diethylamide (LSD): in vivo agonist and antagonist effects of purported 5-hydroxytryptamine antagonists and of pirenperone, a LSD-antagonist. *J Pharmacol Exp Ther* 221: 206—214.
6. Glennon RA, Young R, Rosecrans JA (1983): Antagonism of the effects of the hallucinogen DOM and the purported 5-HT agonist quipazine by 5-HT$_2$ antagonists. *Eur J Pharmacol* 91: 189—196.

7. Friedman RL, Barrett RJ, Sanders-Bush E (1984): Discriminative stimulus properties of quipazine: mediation by serotonin$_2$ binding sites. *J Pharmacol Exp Ther* 228: 628—635.

8. Tricklebank MD (1985): The behavioural response to 5-HT receptor agonists and subtypes of the central 5-HT receptor. *Trends Pharmacol Sci* 6: 403—407.

9. Roberts MHT, Davies M (1989): In vivo electrophysiology of receptor subtypes mediating the central nervous system actions of 5-hydroxytryptamine, pp. 70—76 in: Mylecharane EJ, Angus JA, de la Lande IS, Humphrey PPA (eds), *Serotonin: Actions, Receptors, Pathophysiology. Proceedings of Satellite Symposium of the IUPHAR 10th International Congress of Pharmacology, Heron Island, 4—6 September 1987.* London: Macmillan.

10. Davies MF, Deisz RA, Prince DA, Peroutka SJ (1987): Physiological and pharmacological characterization of the response of guinea pig neocortical neurons to serotonin. *Soc Neurosci Abstracts* 13: 801.

11. Gurevich N, Wu PH, Carlen PL (1987): Complexities of serotonin and serotonin antagonist interactions measured intracellularly in hippocampal CA$_1$ neurons. *Soc Neurosci Abstracts* 13: 1650.

12. Maura G, Roccatagliata E, Ulivi M, Raiteri M (1988): Serotonin-glutamate interaction in rat cerebellum: involvement of 5-HT$_1$ and 5-HT$_2$ receptors. *Eur J Pharmacol* 145: 31—38.

13. Koenig JI, Gudelsky GA, Meltzer HY (1987): Stimulation of corticosterone and β-endorphin secretion in the rat by selective 5-HT receptor subtype activation. *Eur J Pharmacol* 137: 1—8.

14. Lenahan SE, Seibel HR, Johnson JH (1987): Opiate-serotonin synergism stimulating luteinizing hormone release in estrogen-progesterone-primed ovariectomized rats: mediation by serotonin$_2$ receptors. *Endocrinology* 120: 1498—1502.

15. Meltzer HY, Simonovic M, Gudelsky GA (1983): Effects of pirenperone and ketanserin on rat prolactin secretion in vivo and in vitro. *Eur J Pharmacol* 92: 83—89.

16. Willoughby JO, Menadue MF, Liebelt H (1987): Activation of serotonin receptors in the medial basal hypothalamus stimulates growth hormone secretion in the unanaesthetized rat. *Brain Res* 404: 319—322.

17. Willoughby JO, Menadue MF, Liebelt H (1988): Activation of 5-HT 1 serotonin receptors in the medial basal hypothalamus stimulates prolactin secretion in the unanaesthetized rat. *Neuroendocrinology* 47: 83—87.

18. Heninger GR, Charney DS, Smith A (1987): Effects of serotonin receptor agonists and antagonists on neuroendocrine function in rhesus monkeys. *Soc Neurosci Abstracts* 13: 801.

19. Leff P, Martin GR (1986): Peripheral 5-HT$_2$-like receptors. Can they be classified with the available antagonists? *Br J Pharmacol* 88: 585—593.

20. Arunlakshana O, Schild HO (1959): Some quantitative uses of drug antagonists. *Br J Pharmacol* 14: 48—58.

21. Bradley PB, Humphrey PPA, Williams RH (1983): Are vascular 'D' and '5-HT$_2$' receptors for 5-hydroxytryptamine the same? *Br J Pharmacol* 79: 295P.

22. Van Nueten JM, Janssen PAJ, Van Beek J, Xhonneux R, Verbeuren TJ, Vanhoutte PM (1981): Vascular effects of ketanserin (R 41 468), a novel antagonist of 5-HT$_2$ serotonergic receptors. *J Pharmacol Exp Ther* 218: 217—230.

23. Bradley PB, Humphrey PPA, Williams RH (1985): Tryptamine-induced vasoconstriction responses in rat caudal arteries are mediated predominantly via 5-hydroxytryptamine receptors. *Br J Pharmacol* 84: 919—925.

24. Hicks PE, Langer SZ (1983): Antagonism by tetrahydro-β-carboline of the vasoconstrictor responses to tryptamine in rat tail arteries. *Eur J Pharmacol* 96: 145—149.

25. Marwood JF, Stokes GS (1983): Vascular smooth muscle serotonin and α-adrenoceptors. *Clin Exp Pharmacol Physiol* 10: 265—267.

26. Mecca TE, Webb RC (1984): Vascular responses to serotonin in steroid hypertensive rats. *Hypertension* 6: 887—892.

27. Cohen ML, Mason N, Wiley KS, Fuller RW (1983): Further evidence that vascular serotonin receptors are of the 5HT$_2$ type. *Biochem Pharmacol* 32: 567—570.

28. Lemberger HF, Mason N, Cohen ML (1984): 5HT$_2$ receptors in the rat portal vein: desensitization following cumulative serotonin addition. *Life Sci* 35: 71—77.

29. Doggrell SA (1987): The effects of drugs on the contractile responses of the rat portal vein to phenylephrine and 5-hydroxytryptamine. *Clin Exp Pharmacol Physiol* Suppl. 10: 34—35.

30. Cohen ML, Schenck KW, Colbert W, Wittenauer L (1985): Role of 5-HT$_2$ receptors in serotonin-induced contractions of nonvascular smooth muscle. *J Pharmacol Exp Ther* 232: 770—774.

31. Humphrey PPA, Feniuk W, Watts AD (1982): Ketanserin — a novel antihypertensive drug? *J Pharm Pharmacol* 34: 541.

32. Feniuk W, Humphrey PPA, Perren MJ, Watts AD (1985): A comparison of 5-hydroxytryptamine receptors mediating contraction in rabbit aorta and dog saphenous vein: evidence for different receptor types obtained by use of selective agonists and antagonists. *Br J Pharmacol* 86: 697—704.

33. Sutherland RMcD, Fishburn PA, Phillips CA, Mylecharane EJ (1989): The actions of ketanserin in smooth muscle preparations (in preparation).

34. Ichida S, Hayashi T, Terao M (1983): Selective inhibition by ketanserin and spiroperidol of 5-HT-induced myometrial contraction *Eur J Pharmacol* 96: 155—158.

35. Van Nueten JM, Janssen PAJ, De Ridder W, Vanhoutte PM (1982): Interaction between 5-hydroxytryptamine and other vasoconstrictor substances in the isolated femoral artery of the rabbit; effect of ketanserin (R 41 468). *Eur J Pharmacol* 77: 281—287.

36. Cohen RA (1986): Contractions of isolated canine coronary arteries resistant to S$_2$-serotonergic blockade. *J Pharmacol Exp Ther* 237: 548—552.

37. Lemoine H, Kaumann AJ (1986): Allosteric properties of 5-HT$_2$ receptors in tracheal smooth muscle. *Naunyn-Schmiedebergs Arch Pharmacol* 333: 91—97.

38. Forster C, Whalley ET (1982): Analysis of the 5-hydroxytryptamine induced contraction of the human basilar arterial strip compared with the rat aortic strip in vitro. *Naunyn-Schmiedebergs Arch Pharmacol* 319: 12—17.

39. Apperley E, Humphrey PPA, Levy GP (1976): Receptors for 5-hydroxytryptamine and noradrenaline in rabbit isolated ear artery and aorta. *Br J Pharmacol* 58: 211—221.

40. Stollak JS, Furchgott RF (1983): Use of selective antagonists for determining the types of receptors mediating the actions of 5-hydroxytryptamine and tryptamine in the isolated rabbit aorta. *J Pharmacol Exp Ther* 224: 215—221.

41. Apperley E, Feniuk W, Humphrey PPA, Levy GP (1980): Evidence for two types of excitatory receptor for 5-hydroxytryptamine in dog isolated vasculature. *Br J Pharmacol* 68: 215—224.

42. Black JW, Brazenor RM, Gerskowitch VP, Leff P (1983): The problem of insurmountable antagonism in 5-hydroxytryptamine receptor classification *Br J Pharmacol* 80: 607P.

43. Cohen ML, Fuller RW, Wiley KS (1981): Evidence for 5-HT$_2$ receptors mediating contraction in vascular smooth muscle. *J Pharmacol Exp Ther* 218: 421—425.

44. Maayani S, Wilkinson CW, Stollak JS (1984): 5-hydroxytryptamine receptor in rabbit aorta: characterization by butyrophenone analogs. *J Pharmacol Exp Ther* 229: 346—350.

45. Clancy BM, Maayani S (1985): 5-hydroxytryptamine receptor in isolated rabbit aorta: characterization with tryptamine analogs. *J Pharmacol Exp Ther* 233: 761—769.

46. Black JL, French RJ, Mylecharane EJ (1981): Receptor mechanisms for 5-hydroxytryptamine in rabbit arteries. *Br J Pharmacol* 74: 619—626.

47. Wrigglesworth SJ (1983): Heterogeneity of 5-hydroxytryptamine receptors in the rat uterus and stomach strip. *Br J Pharmacol* 80: 691—697.

48. Cohen ML, Fuller RW, Kurz KD (1983): LY53857, a selective and potent serotonergic (5-HT$_2$) receptor antagonist, does not lower blood pressure in the spontaneously hypertensive rat. *J Pharmacol Exp Ther* 227: 327—332.

49. Ben-Harari RR, Dalton B, Kaplan J, Maayani S (1987): Kinetic characterization of the response to 5-hydroxytryptamine in airway and vascular tissues. *Soc Neurosci Abstracts* 13: 343.

50. Fong I, Philips CA, Mylecharane EJ (1987). 5-Hydroxytryptamine receptor subtypes in rabbit common carotid artery, guinea-pig trachea and rat stomach fundus preparations. *Clin Exp Pharmacol Physiol* Suppl. 11: 189.

51. Leff P, Martin GR, Morse JM (1987): Differential classification of vascular smooth muscle and endothelial cell 5-HT receptors by use of tryptamine analogues. *Br J Pharmacol* 91: 321—331.

52. Kaumann AJ (1983): Yohimbine and rauwolscine inhibit 5-hydroxytryptamine-induced contraction of large coronary arteries of calf through blockade of 5-HT$_2$ receptors. *Naunyn-Schmiedebergs Arch Pharmacol* 323: 149—154.

53. Frenken M, Kaumann AJ (1984): Interaction of ketanserin and its metabolite ketanserinol with 5-HT$_2$ receptors in pulmonary and coronary arteries of calf. *Naunyn-Schmiedebergs Arch Pharmacol* 326: 334—339.

54. Kaumann AJ, Frenken M (1985). A paradox: the 5-HT$_2$-receptor antagonist ketanserin restores the 5-HT-induced contraction depressed by methysergide in large coronary arteries of calf. Allosteric regulation of 5-HT$_2$-receptors. *Naunyn-Schmiedebergs Arch Pharmacol* 328: 295—300.

55. Engel G, Hoyer D, Kalkman H, Wick MB (1985): Pharmacological similarity between the 5-HT-D-receptor on the guinea-pig ileum and the 5-HT$_2$ binding site. *Br J Pharmacol* 84: 106P.

56. Eccles NK, Grimmer AJ, Leathard HL (1981): Action of ketanserin, a new 5-hydroxytryptamine antagonist, on human isolated blood vessels. *Br J Pharmacol* 74: 831P—832P.

57. Müller-Schweinitzer E (1984): Alpha-adrenoceptors, 5-hydroxytryptamine receptors and the action of dihydroergotamine in human venous preparations obtained during saphenectomy procedures for varicose veins. *Naunyn-Schmiedebergs Arch Pharmacol* 327: 299—303.

58. Docherty JR, Hyland L (1986): An examination of 5-hydroxytryptamine receptors in human saphenous vein. *Br J Pharmacol* 89: 77—81.

59. Clineschmidt BV, Reiss DD, Pettibone DJ, Robinson JL (1985): Characterization of 5-hydroxytryptamine receptors in rat stomach fundus. *J Pharmacol Exp Ther* 235: 696—708.

60. McGrath JC, MacLennan SJ, Stuart-Smith K (1985): Characterization of the receptor mediating contraction of human umbilical artery by 5-hydroxytryptamine. *Br J Pharmacol* 84: 199—202.

61. McGrath JC, MacLennan SJ (1986): Oxygen modifies the potency of 5-HT, and of 5-HT antagonists, in human umbilical artery (HUA). *Br J Pharmacol* 88: 320P.

62. MacLennan SJ, McGrath JC (1986): Evidence for "5-HT$_1$-like" receptors in human umbilical artery (HUA). *Br J Pharmacol* 89: 587P.

63. Tuncer M, Dogan N, Oktay S, Kayaalp SO (1985): Receptor mechanisms for 5-hydroxytryptamine in isolated human umbilical artery and vein. *Arch Int Pharmacodyn Ther* 276: 17—27.

64. Brazenor RM, Angus JA (1981): Ergometrine contracts isolated coronary arteries by a serotonergic mechanism: no role for alpha adrenoceptors. *J Pharmacol Exp Ther* 218: 530—536.

65. Brazenor RM, Angus JA (1982): Actions of serotonin antagonists on dog coronary artery. *Eur J Pharmacol* 81: 569—576.

66. Porquet M-F, Pourrias B, Santamaria R (1982): Effects of 5-hydroxytryptamine on canine isolated coronary arteries. *Br J Pharmacol* 75: 305—310.

67. Frenken M, Kaumann AJ (1985): Ketanserin causes surmountable antagonism of 5-hydroxytryptamine-induced contractions of large coronary arteries of dog. *Naunyn-Schmiedebergs Arch Pharmacol* 328: 301—303.

68. Houston DS, Vanhoutte PM (1988): Comparison of serotonergic receptor subtypes on the smooth muscle and endothelium of the canine coronary artery. *J Pharmacol Exp Ther* 244: 1—10.

69. Engel G, Göthert M, Müller-Schweinitzer E, Schlicker E, Sistonen L, Stadler PA (1983): Evidence for common pharmacological properties of [³H]-5-hydroxytryptamine binding sites, presynaptic 5-hydroxytryptamine autoreceptors in CNS and inhibitory presynaptic 5-hydroxytryptamine receptors on sympathetic nerves. *Naunyn-Schmiedebergs Arch Pharmacol* 324: 116—124.

70. Kilbinger H, Pfeuffer-Friedrich I (1985): Two types of receptors for 5-hydroxytryptamine on the cholinergic nerves of the guinea-pig myenteric plexus. *Br J Pharmacol* 85: 529—539.

71. Molderings GJ, Fink K, Schlicker E, Göthert M (1987): Inhibition of noradrenaline release via presynaptic 5-HT$_{1B}$ receptors of the rat vena cava. *Naunyn-Schmiedebergs Arch Pharmacol* 336: 245—250.

72. Müller-Schweinitzer E, Engel G (1983): Evidence for mediation by 5-HT₂ receptors of 5-hydroxytryptamine-induced contraction of canine basilar artery. *Naunyn-Schmiedebergs Arch Pharmacol* 324: 287—292.

73. Peroutka SJ, Noguchi M, Tolner DJ, Allen GS (1983): Serotonin-induced contraction of canine basilar artery: mediation by 5-HT₁ receptors. *Brain Res* 259: 327—330.

74. Peroutka SJ, Kuhar MJ (1984): Autoradiographic localization of 5-HT₁ receptors to human and canine basilar arteries. *Brain Res* 310: 193—196.

75. Peroutka SJ, Huang S, Allen GS (1986): Canine basilar artery contractions mediated by 5-hydroxytryptamine$_{1A}$ receptors. *J Pharmacol Exp Ther* 237: 901—906.

76. Cohen ML, Colbert WE (1986): Relationship between receptors mediating serotonin (5-HT) contractions in the canine basilar artery to 5-HT₁, 5-HT₂ and rat stomach fundus 5-HT receptors. *J Pharmacol Exp Ther* 237: 713—718.

77. Taylor EW, Duckles SP, Nelson DL (1986): Dissociation constants of serotonin agonists in the canine basilar artery correlate to K_i values at the 5-HT$_{1A}$ binding site. *J Pharmacol Exp Ther* 236: 118—125.

78. Frenken M, Kaumann AJ (1986): Surmountable antagonism by ketanserin of 5-hydroxytryptamine-induced contractions in dog basilar artery. *Br J Pharmacol* 89: 550P.

79. Peroutka SJ, Lebovitz RM, Snyder SH (1981): Two distinct central serotonin receptors with different physiological functions. *Science* 212: 827—829.

80. Leysen JE, Niemegeers CJE, Van Nueten JM, Laduron PM (1982): [³H]Ketanserin (R 41 468), a selective ³H-ligand for serotonin₂ receptor binding sites: binding properties, brain distribution, and functional role. *Mol Pharmacol* 21: 301—314.

81. Martin LL, Sanders-Bush E (1982): Comparison of the pharmacological characteristics of 5HT₁ and 5HT₂ binding sites with those of serotonin autoreceptors which modulate serotonin release. *Naunyn-Schmiedebergs Arch Pharmacol* 321: 165—170.

82. Cohen ML, Wittenauer LA (1985): Relationship between serotonin and tryptamine receptors in the rat stomach fundus. *J Pharmacol Exp Ther* 233: 75—79.

83. Pazos A, Hoyer D, Palacios JM (1985): Mesulergine, a selective serotonin-2 ligand in the rat cortex, does not label these receptors in porcine and human cortex: evidence for species differences in brain serotonin-2 receptors. *Eur J Pharmacol* 106: 531—538.

84. Engel G, Göthert M, Hoyer D, Schlicker E, Hillenbrand K (1986): Identity of inhibitory presynaptic 5-hydroxytryptamine (5-HT) autoreceptors in the rat brain cortex with 5-HT$_{1B}$ binding sites. *Naunyn-Schmiedebergs Arch Pharmacol* 332: 1—7.

85. Schotte A, Maloteaux JM, Laduron PM (1983): Characterization and regional distribution of serotonin S₂-receptors in human brain. *Brain Res* 276: 231—235.

86. McBride PA, Mann JJ, McEwen B, Biegon A (1983): Characterization of serotonin binding sites on human platelets. *Life Sci* 33: 2033—2041.

87. Leysen JE, de Chaffoy de Courcelles D, De Clerck F, Niemegeers CJE, Van Nueten

JM (1984): Serotonin-S_2 receptor binding sites and functional correlates. *Neuropharmacology* 23: 1493—1501.

88. Ichida S, Hayashi T, Kita T, Murakami T (1985): Estradiol-induced increase of specific [^{3}H]ketanserin binding sites on rat uterine membranes. *Eur J Pharmacol* 108: 257—264.

89. Shannon, M, Battaglia G, Glennon RA, Titeler M (1984): 5-HT_1 and 5-HT_2 binding properties of the hallucinogen 1-(2,5-dimethoxyphenyl)-2-aminopropane (2,5-DMA). *Eur J Pharmacol* 102: 23—29.

90. Lyon RA, Titeler M, Glennon RA (1987): LSD and phenylisopropylamine hallucinogen interactions with multiple radiolabelled brain serotonin receptors. *Soc Neurosci Abstracts* 13: 1183.

91. Wang SS, Peroutka SJ (1987): 2,5-Dimethoxy-4-bromoamphetamine (DOB) interactions with 5-HT receptor subtypes. *Soc Neurosci Abstracts* 13: 1237.

92. Schechter LE, Simansky KJ (1987): 1-(2,5-Dimethoxy-4-iodophenyl)-2-aminopropane HCl (DOI), a selective 5-HT_2 agonist, exerts an anorexic action in rats that is prevented by LY53857, a selective 5-HT_2 antagonist. *Soc Neurosci Abstracts* 13: 1339.

93. McCall RB, Harris LT (1988): 5-HT_2 receptor agonists increase spontaneous sympathetic nerve discharge. *Eur J Pharmacol* 151: 113—116.

94. Glennon RA, Seggel MR, Soine WH, Davis KH, Lyon RA, Titeler M (1987): [^{125}DOI]: a new radiolabel for 5-HT_2 serotonin sites. *Soc. Neurosci Abstracts* 13: 1181.

95. Nelson DL, Killam AL, Lambert G, Nikam SS, Weck B, Martin AR (1987): Structure-activity relationships of a series of tetrahydropyridylindoles at serotonin$_{1A}$ and serotonin$_2$ receptors. *Soc Neurosci Abstracts* 13: 1236.

96. Hirata M, Imamoto T, Shibouta Y, Kurihara Y, Kito G, Sugihara H (1986): A selective S_2-serotonin blocker, CV-5197, a benzoxathiepin analog. *Blood Vessels* 23: 76.

97. Blackburn TP, Cox B, Pearce RJ, Thornber CW (1987): In vivo pharmacology of ICI 169,369 — a new 5-HT_2 antagonist. *Br J Pharmacol* 90: 256P.

98. Blackburn TP, Thornber CW, Pearce RJ, Cox B (1988): In vitro studies with ICI 169,369, a chemically novel 5-HT antagonist. *Eur J Pharmacol* 150: 247—256.

99. Blackburn TP, Cox B, Grant TL, Growcott JW (1987): ICI 169369 is an antagonist of 5-HT in tissues claimed to contain 5-HT_{1A} and 5-HT_{1C} receptors. *Soc Neurosci Abstracts* 13: 801.

100. Cummings SA, Groszmann RJ, Kaumann AJ (1986): Hypersensitivity of mesenteric veins to 5-hydroxytryptamine- and ketanserin-induced reduction of portal pressure in portal hypertensive rats. *Br J Pharmacol* 89: 501—513.

VIII. Agonists and antagonists of 5-HT$_3$ receptors

JOHN R. FOZARD

1. Introduction

There can be little doubt that the basis of the recent remarkable advances in
our understanding of the physiological and pathophysiological roles of 5-HT
has been the identification and development of compounds with selectivity
for 5-HT receptor subtypes [1—4]. Among these, none has been more
spectacular nor of potentially greater therapeutic significance than the advent
of ligands with potency and selectivity for the 5-HT$_3$ receptor subtype. The
purpose of this article is to describe these compounds and their use as tools
to identify 5-HT$_3$ receptors and their properties. Both selective agonists and
antagonists will be considered as well as a number of their radiolabelled
counterparts. The historical development of these compounds will *not* be
dealt with since it has been the subject of recent comprehensive review
[5—8].

2. Agonist ligands useful for discriminating 5-HT$_3$ receptors

Three compounds are chosen for inclusion under this heading: 5-methoxy-
tryptamine, 2-methyl-5-HT and phenylbiguanide. Their formulae are given in
Figure 1; their properties are summarized in Table 1 and discussed in detail
in the sections which follow.

2.1 *5-Methoxytryptamine*

Paradoxically, perhaps, the value of 5-methoxytryptamine as a tool to
discriminate responses mediated through 5-HT$_3$ receptors stems from its
complete *lack* of affinity for these sites. This was first clearly demonstrated in
studies by Fozard and Mobarok Ali [9] who compared the agonist properties
of a number of tryptamine analogues at the 5-HT$_3$ receptor of the terminal

P.R. Saxena, D.I. Wallis, W. Wouters and P. Bevan (eds), Cardiovascular Pharmacology of
5-Hydroxytryptamine, pp. 101—115.
© 1990 *Kluwer Academic Publishers, Dordrecht —*

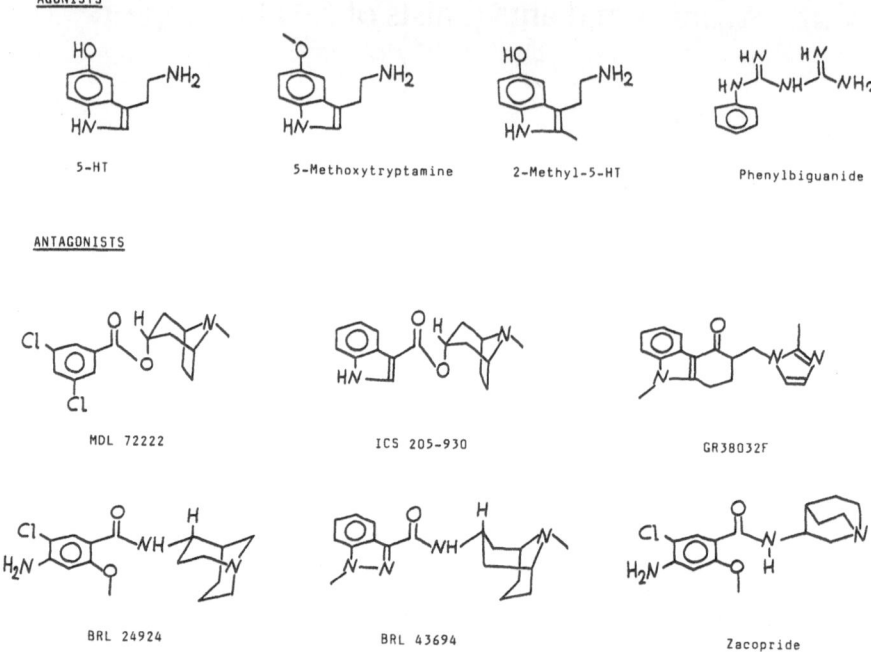

Figure 1. Formulae of 5-HT$_3$ receptor discriminatory agonists and antagonists.

sympathetic fibres of the rabbit heart with their potencies at the D (5-HT$_2$) and M (*not* 5-HT$_3$ — see below) receptors [10] of the guinea-pig ileum. 5-Methoxytryptamine proved a powerful stimulant of the 5-HT$_2$ and M receptors yet was devoid of either agonist or antagonist activity at the 5-HT$_3$ receptor of the heart [9; Figure 2]. The remarkable loss of activity when the

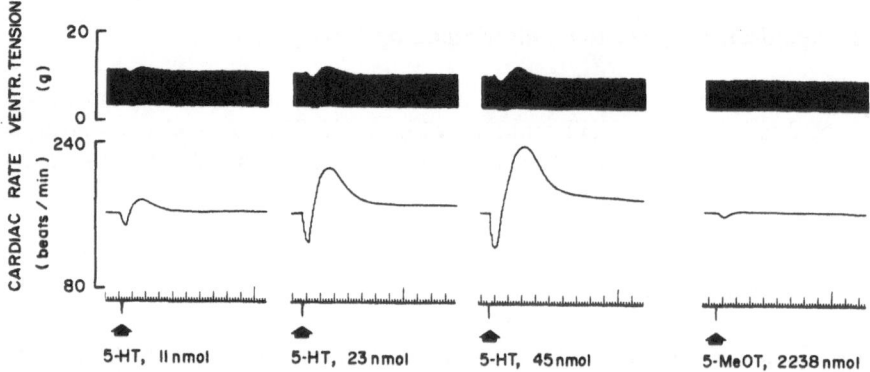

Figure 2. Comparison between 5-HT and 5-methoxytryptamine (5-MeOT) on the rabbit isolated heart. Hearts were perfused by the Langendorff technique with modified Tyrode solution as described in detail previously [9, 31]. Bolus injections of 5-HT (arrows) induce biphasic (inhibition followed by stimulation) effects on ventricular tension development and cardiac rate due to the release of acetylcholine and noradrenaline from the cardiac parasympathetic and sympathetic nerves, respectively [12, 56]. 5-Methoxytryptamine was essentially inactive.

hydroxyl group in 5-HT is substituted by methoxy has now been demonstrated for the 5-HT_3 receptors present on peripheral sympathetic [11], parasympathetic [12; Figure 2] and afferent [13] neurones. Moreover, 5-methoxytryptamine has been repeatedly shown to have activity approaching that of 5-HT at each of the other major 5-HT receptor subtypes [14—16; see Table 1]. Thus, failure to mimic an effect of 5-HT with 5-methoxytryptamine would point strongly to the response being 5-HT_3 receptor mediated.

Table 1. Properties of agonist ligands useful for discriminating 5-HT_3 receptors.

		5-HT	5-methoxy-tryptamine	2-methyl-5-HT	Phenyl-biguanide
5-HT₃ receptors					
Functional					
afferent (rabbit[a] [rat][b] vagus)	pD_2	6.0 [6.2]	<4	5.7 [5.6]	[6.1]
autonomic (rabbit heart[a,c,d])	EC_{50} (nmol)	11	>2200	18	170
enteric (guinea-pig ileum[a,d])	pD_2	5.9	<4	5.4	<4
Binding					
[³H]ICS 205-930 (mouse N1E cells[e])	pK_D	6.4	4.5	5.9	6.1
[³H]GR65630 (rat cortex[f])	pK_I	6.9	no data	7.1	no data
Other 5-HT receptor subtypes					
Functional					
M receptor (guinea-pig ileum[d,g])	pD_2	7.2	6.7	<4	<4
Binding					
5-HT_{1A} (pig cortex[h])	pK_D	8.5	8.0	5.6	<4
5-HT_{1B} (rat cortex[h])	pK_D	7.6	6.4	4.4	<4
5-HT_{1C} (pig choroid plexus[h])	pK_D	7.5	7.6	5.9	4.5
5-HT_{1D} (calf caudate)	pK_D	8.4	8.4	6.4	4.1
5-HT_2 (rat cortex[h])	pK_D	5.5	5.5	5.0	4.2

Data sources: [a] Richardson and Buchheit, 1988 [7]; Richardson, B. P. unpublished data; [b] Ireland and Tyers, 1987 [21]; [c] Fozard and Mobarok Ali, 1978 [9]; Fig. 1; [d] Buchheit, K. H. unpublished data; [e] Hoyer and Neijt, 1988 [43]; [f] Kilpatrick et al., 1987 [42]; [g] Buchheit et al., 1985 [18]; Fig. 3; [h] Hoyer, 1989 [51]; Hoyer, D. unpublished observations.

A good example of where the discriminatory properties of 5-methoxy-tryptamine have been of particular value is in differentiating the twin components of the indirect (neuronally mediated) stimulant response to 5-HT in guinea-pig ileum. The dose-response curve for the indirect effects of 5-HT is clearly biphasic [17; see also Figure 3]; only the "low affinity" component, thought to be substance P mediated [17, 18], can be blocked by $5-HT_3$ receptor antagonists [18, 19]. The "high affinity" component is cholinergic [18; see also Figure 3], resistant to $5-HT_3$ receptor blockade [18, 19] and corresponds to the M receptor of Gaddum and Picarelli [10]. As can be seen in Figure 3, unlike 5-HT, 5-methoxytryptamine does not show a biphasic dose-response relationship on guinea-pig ileum treated with methysergide. Moreover, although in agreement with the literature, responses to high doses of 5-HT are resistant to blockade with atropine, responses to 5-methoxytryptamine can be abolished by low concentrations of this agent (Figure 3). In tissues desensitized with an excess of 5-methoxytryptamine,

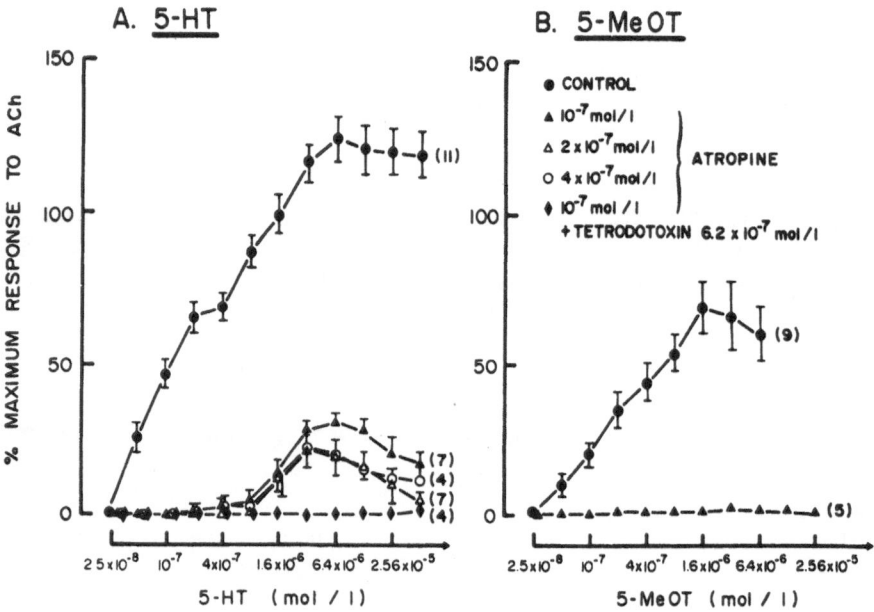

Figure 3. Comparison between 5-HT (A) and 5-methoxytryptamine (5-MeOT; B) on guinea-pig ileum: effects of atropine or atropine plus tetrodotoxin. Segments of guinea-pig ileum were set up in modified Tyrode solution containing methysergide, 10^{-7} M, as previously described [9, 31]. Agonist dose-response curves were generated non-cumulatively; antagonists at the concentrations indicated or vehicle were included in the Tyrode solution 15 min prior to establishing the curves. Points represent mean values ($\pm$ SEM) from the number of individual experiments shown in parentheses. Responses to 5-methoxytryptamine and *low* ($< 4 \times 10^{-7}$ M) concentration of 5-HT were abolished by atropine. The residual response to 5-HT in the presence of atropine was abolished by tetrodotoxin confirming its indirect (neuronal stimulant) basis. For further details, see text.

only the first phase of the dose-response curve to 5-HT is inhibited (Figure 4); in contrast, desensitization with 5-HT leads to elimination of responses both to 5-methoxytryptamine and to 5-HT (Figure 5). The data clearly indicate differences between the receptors mediating the "high" and "low affinity" components of the enteric neuronal stimulant response to 5-HT in guinea-pig ileum. Further, to conclude, based on the lack of response to 5-methoxytryptamine, that the "low affinity" site is the 5-HT_3 receptor would be in complete accord with the conclusion drawn from the analysis of the response using antagonists [18—20].

2.2   *2-Methyl-5-HT*

During a systematic structure-activity relationship study with methyl substituted derivatives of 5-HT, Richardson et al. [20] observed that 2-methyl-5-HT was a substantially more potent agonist (expressed relative to 5-HT) at autonomic, afferent and enteric neuronal 5-HT_3 receptors than at the non-5-HT_3 receptors present in rat uterus or rat cerebral cortex membranes. That 2-methyl-5-HT stimulates 5-HT_3 receptors with a potency slightly less than that of 5-HT has been amply confirmed [19, 21, 22]; however, on both rat vagus nerve and rabbit cervical sympathetic trunk preparations, 2-methyl-5-HT appeared to be a partial agonist with $60 - 70\%$ of the efficacy of 5-HT [21, 22].

Unfortunately, apart from those referred to above, there are few data from functional tests with which to assess the selectivity of action of 2-methyl-5-HT. In the guinea-pig ileum, 2-methyl-5-HT does not activate the "high affinity" M receptor [19]. However, from radioligand binding studies (see Table 1) the compound has highest affinity at 5-HT_{1D} sites and shows relatively little selectivity for 5-HT_3 receptors vis à vis 5-HT_{1A} or 5-HT_{1C} sites. Thus, whilst 2-methyl-5-HT is indeed useful as a 5-HT_3 receptor probe, it remains less than ideal due to limited selectivity and the possibility of response variability due to differences in receptor reserve.

2.3   *Phenylbiguanide*

Phenylbiguanide has been recognized for many years to mimic selectively many of the neuronal stimulant effects of 5-HT both in vivo and in vitro [23—27]. More recently direct evidence has been obtained both from functional studies [19, 21, 28, 29] and radioligand binding assays (Table 1) that these actions of phenylbiguanide are mediated through 5-HT_3 receptors. Phenylbiguanide is equipotent with 5-HT in depolarizing rat superior cervical ganglia [27] and only slightly less active than 5-HT in depolarizing rat vagus nerve [21] and in a 5-HT_3 receptor radioligand binding assay (Table 1); the

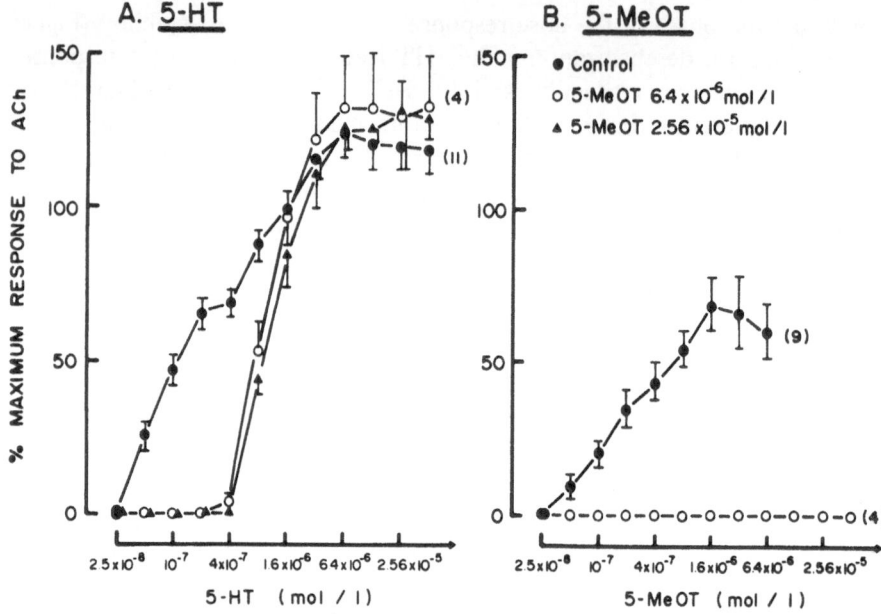

Figure 4. Effects of continuous incubation with high concentrations of 5-methoxytryptamine (5-MeOT) on responses of guinea-pig ileum to 5-HT (A) and 5-methoxytryptamine (B). Experimental details as in legend to Figure 3.

Incubation with a high concentration (6.4×10^{-6} M) of 5-hydroxytryptamine desensitized the tissue to 5-methoxytryptamine (B) and responses to the lower concentrations of 5-HT were abolished (A). Contractile effects to the higher concentrations of 5-HT were unaffected by an increase in the desensitizing concentration of 5-methoxytryptamine to 2.56×10^{-5} M (A). For further details, see text.

maximum depolarization of rat superior cervical ganglion was similar to that of 5-HT but amounted to only 80% of that of 5-HT on the vagus nerve [21]. Of significance is the fact that phenylbiguanide does not appear to stimulate either the enteric neuronal 5-HT$_3$ receptor or the M receptor (Table 1).

Phenylbiguanide appears to interact highly selectively with the 5-HT$_3$ receptors of autonomic and afferent neurones. Thus, it has no direct contractile effects on smooth muscle of rat blood vessels, stomach fundus or mouse duodenum in vitro [24, 26]. Moreover in radioligand binding assays, phenylbiguanide has negligible affinity for all 5-HT receptor subtypes with the exception of 5-HT$_3$ (Table 1).

2.4 Conclusion

The use of small molecule agonists with close structural resemblance to the endogenous ligand is considered an important approach to the definition of 5-HT receptor subtypes [30]. In such an approach, compounds like 5-methoxytryptamine, which has no affinity for 5-HT$_3$ receptors but mimics

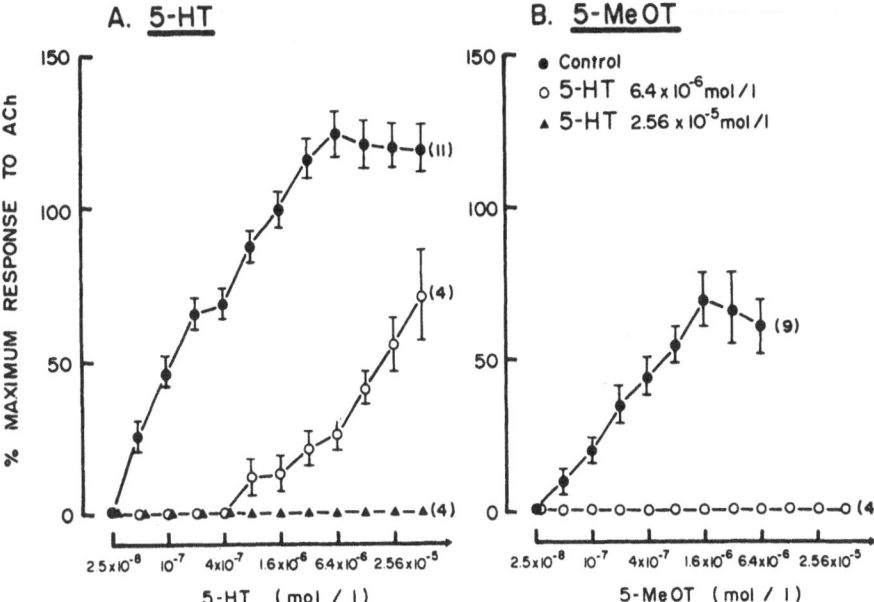

Figure 5. Effects of continuous incubation with high concentrations of 5-HT on responses of guinea-pig ileum to 5-HT (A) and 5-methoxytryptamine (5-MeOT; B). Experimental details as in legend to Figure 3.

Incubation with a high concentration of 5-HT (6.4×10^{-6} M) desensitized the tissue to 5-methoxytryptamine (B) and responses to 5-HT up to 4×10^{-7} M were abolished (A). Increasing the incubation concentration of 5-HT to 2.56×10^{-5} M desensitized completely the ileum to 5-HT. For further details, see text.

5-HT closely at other sites, and phenylbiguanide, which shows marked selectivity for autonomic and afferent 5-HT₃ receptors, are of inestimable value. 2-Methyl-5-HT is also of value although its only advantage over phenylbiguanide may be its capacity to stimulate the enteric neuronal 5-HT₃ receptor; its relative lack of selectivity can be considered a significant disadvantage.

3. Antagonist ligands useful for discriminating 5-HT₃ receptors

3.1 *General*

Since 1984 when the properties of the first potent and highly selective 5-HT₃ receptor antagonist MDL 72222, were described [31], a number of such compounds has become available. The formulae of the principal selective 5-HT₃ receptor antagonists and their properties on representative afferent, autonomic and enteric neurones and in radioligand binding assays from both peripheral (N1E mouse neuroblastoma cells) and central (rat entorhinal cortex) tissues are shown in Figure 1 and Table 2.

Table 2. Properties of antagonist ligands useful for discriminating 5-HT$_3$ receptors.

	Afferent (rabbit vagus) pA$_2$	Autonomic (rabbit heart) pA$_2$	Enteric (guinea-pig ileum) pA$_2$	[³H] ICS 205-930[i] (mouse N1E cells) pK$_D$	[³H] GR65630[j] (rat cortex) pK$_I$
MDL 72222	7.9[a]	9.3[b]	<6[b]	8.2	7.3
ICS 205-930	10.2[c]	10.6[c]	7.9[c]	9.1	8.5
BRL 24924	8.5[d]	8.9[e]	7.6[e]	8.5	no data
BRL 43694	9.9[d]	10.7[f]	8.1[f]	8.9	9.2
GR38032F	9.4[g]	10.1[d]	7.3[g]	7.9	8.5
Zacopride	10.1[h]	no data	8.5[h]	9.7	8.7*

Data sources: [a] Donatsch et al., 1984 [52]; [b] Fozard, 1984 [31]; [c] Richardson et al., 1985 [20]; [d] Buchheit, K. H. and Richardson, B. P., unpublished data; [e] Sanger, 1987 [32]; [f] Fake et al., 1987 [53]; [g] Butler et al., 1988 [19]; [h] Smith et al., 1988 [54]; [i] Hoyer and Neijt, 1988 [46], Hoyer, D. unpublished observations; [j] Kilpatrick et al., 1987 [42]; * Measured against [³H] zacopride binding, Barnes et al., 1988 [55].

A number of general points can be made concerning the 5-HT$_3$ receptor antagonists. First, compounds such as MDL 72222, ICS 205-930, GR38032F and BRL 43694 are impressively *selective* as 5-HT$_3$ receptor antagonists; no meaningful activity other than 5-HT$_3$ receptor blockade has been reported for any of these agents at concentrations below micromolar; BRL 24924 and zacopride, by contrast, appear to have agonist/partial agonist activity at the "high" affinity M receptor of the guinea-pig ileum [32, 33], a phenomenon well known to occur with the related substituted benzamide, metoclopramide [34]. Second, each compound is 1.5–2 log units more active at the 5-HT$_3$ receptors on afferent and autonomic neurones than on the enteric neurones of the guinea-pig ileum; this has been taken as evidence for the existence of at least two subtypes of the 5-HT$_3$ recognition site [35, 36]. Finally there is an excellent correlation between effects in functional tests and affinities in the several radioligand binding assays now available (Table 3); the use of the latter thus provides a straightforward and reliable approach to detecting agents with affinity at these sites (see section 3.3 below).

3.2   *The question of non-surmountability of antagonism*

For drugs to be optimally useful in receptor characterization, evidence that they interact competitively and reversibly with the receptor should be available. In fact, for several of the 5-HT$_3$ receptor antagonists, evidence *inconsistent* with simple reversible competition has been obtained. This is the case for MDL 72222 on rabbit heart [31], rabbit superior cervical and nodose ganglia [37, 38] and rat vagus nerve [21], for ICS 205-930 on rabbit superior cervical and nodose ganglia [30] and rat vagus nerve [21] and for GR38032F on rabbit heart and rabbit vagus nerve [19]. That this may be more a reflection of the tissue and/or experimental conditions used rather than an intrinsic property of the antagonist is suggested by the fact that *low* concentrations (< 0.1 μM) of MDL 72222 and ICS 205-930 cause parallel shifts of 5-HT dose-response curves to the right on rabbit heart and superior cervical and nodose ganglia [31, 37–39]. Moreover, on guinea-pig ileum (ICS 205-930) and rabbit preganglionic cervical sympathetic nerves (MDL 72222 and ICS 205-930), these antagonists show apparently competitive kinetics over a wide concentration range [20, 22]. Interestingly, on isolated rabbit heart, whether the antagonism of 5-HT by GR38032F appears competitive depends on the initial sensitivity of the preparation to the agonist [19]!

There can be many reasons why changes in dose-response curves may appear inconsistent with a simple competitive interaction between agonist and antagonist at the receptor site [40]. With respect to 5-HT$_3$ receptors, a particularly significant factor may be the rapid desensitization which is a consistent feature of the depolarization generated in neurones by 5-HT$_3$

Table 3. Radioligands identifying 5-HT$_3$ recognition sites.

	[³H] GR65630[a]	[³H] Zacopride[b]	[³H] Quipazine[c]	[³H] Q-ICS 205-930[d]	[³H] GR67330[e]
Tissue (rat)	Entorhinal cortex	Entorhinal cortex	Cortex	Cortex	Entorhinal cortex
K_D (nM)	0.4	0.8	1.2	1	0.04
B_{max} (fmol/mg protein)	32	78	[3.0]*	75	23
Non-specific binding (%)	30—40	40	30—50	ca 25	ca 30
	K_i (nM)	K_i (nM)	K_i (nM)	K_i (nM)	K_i (nM)
ICS 205-930	3	2	0.6	0.6	0.9
GR38032F	3	5	no data	0.6	2
MDL 72222	55	no data	9	14	no data
BRL 43694	0.6	3	1	no data	1
Quipazine	1	no data	1	2	0.2
Metoclopramide	360	326	190	100	no data

Data sources: [a] Kilpatrick et al., 1987 [42]; [b] Barnes et al., 1988 [55]; [c] Peroutka and Hamik, 1988 [50]; Peroutka, 1988 [45]; [d] Watling et al., 1988 [57]; [e] Kilpatrick et al., 1989 [58]. * pmol/g tissue wet weight. Data with [³H] ICS 205-930 appears in Tables 1 and 2.

receptor activation [41]. It bears emphasis that in 5-HT$_3$ receptor binding assays competitive kinetics are usually observed; thus, displacement of the radioligand by 5-HT$_3$ antagonists is invariably monophasic and Hill slopes close to unity are normally obtained [42, 43].

3.3 Radioligands for identifying 5-HT$_3$ receptors

The availability of potent and selective antagonists for 5-HT$_3$ receptors provided the means to develop radioligands for use in binding assays. Attempts to label 5-HT$_3$ receptors with [^{3}H] MDL 72222 foundered due to unacceptably high non-specific binding [44, 45]. [^{3}H] ICS 205-930 has been used successfully to label 5-HT$_3$ receptors in membranes prepared from cells in culture [43, 46; see Tables 1 and 2] and intact tisuses [47]. Recently, five additional radioligands have been described which appear to be satisfactory for labelling 5-HT$_3$ receptors in a number of tissues. These are [^{3}H] GR65630, [^{3}H] zacopride, [^{3}H] quipazine, [^{3}H] quaternary-ICS 205-930 and [^{3}H] GR67330; a summary of the major features of these ligands and details of the displacing effects of a number of antagonists is given in Table 3.

Certain generalizations can again be made. First, binding in all cases is to a single saturable site of high ($<$ nM) affinity. Second, compounds with high affinity for 5-HT$_1$ and 5-HT$_2$ sites or other neurotransmitter receptors have minimal displacing activity [48]; conversely, selective 5-HT$_3$ receptor antagonists and agonists inhibit the binding with high affinities which correlate reasonably well with their activities defined in functional tests (compare Tables 1–3). Finally, there appear to be marked differences between species with respect to 5-HT$_3$ receptor densities. For instance, using [^{3}H] GR65630, markedly higher levels of specific binding were seen in a variety of brain areas of rat and mouse than in ferret, rabbit or cynomolgus monkey brains [49]; using [^{3}H]quipazine, specific binding of the radioligand could be detected in both rat and pig cortical membranes but not in membranes prepared from human, cow, dog, turtle, mouse, guinea-pig, chicken or rabbit brains [50]. However, the area postrema seems to be enriched in 5-HT$_3$ receptors irrespective of species [49].

3.4 Conclusion

The rapid developments in the field of 5-HT$_3$ receptor antagonists allows the prospective user the luxury of choice. For historical reasons the largest "data base" exists for MDL 72222 and ICS 205-930 and used sensibly these compounds are perfectly satisfactory tools for defining 5-HT$_3$ receptor function. MDL 72222 may indeed have a particular advantage over the other compounds in that it has minimal activity at the 5-HT$_3$ receptor in guinea-pig ileum [31; Table 2]; since sub-types of 5-HT$_3$ receptors are likely [7, 20, 35, 36], such selectivity could have practical significance.

The several radioligands which have evolved from the 5-HT$_3$ receptor antagonists are suitable for use in binding essays or for autoradiography. For the present, there seems to be little to choose between the compounds available. What does appear to be crucial is the choice of tissue since in several species many brain areas do not contain sufficient 5-HT$_3$ receptors for quantitative evaluation.

4. General conclusions

This account of 5-HT$_3$ receptor agonists and antagonists reveals a particularly healthy state of affairs. Highly potent and selective antagonists from different chemical structural classes and agonists with intriguing selectivities are now available. These agonists and antagonists allow responses mediated through 5-HT$_3$ receptors to be convincingly discriminated from those initiated by other 5-HT$_3$ receptor subtypes. Radioligands based on the antagonists enable affinities at 5-HT$_3$ receptors to be easily and rapidly determined and, by autoradiography, their tissue distribution to be defined. These tools have provided data which hint strongly at the existence of 5-HT$_3$ receptor subtypes; that they do not allow their definitive characterization indicates that, despite impressive developments, progress remains to be made.

Acknowledgements

I am grateful to Drs. K. H. Buchheit, D. Hoyer and B. P. Richardson for permission to include their unpublished results.

References

1. Bradley PB, Engel G, Feniuk W, Fozard JR, Humphrey PPA, Middlemiss DN, Mylecharane EJ, Richardson BP, Saxena PR (1986): Proposals for the classification and nomenclature of functional receptors for 5-hydroxytryptamine. *Neuropharmacology* 25: 563—576.
2. Fozard JR (1987): 5-HT: The enigma variations. *Trends Pharmacol Sci* 8: 501—506.
3. Glennon RA (1987): Central serotonin receptors as targets for drug research. *J Med Chem* 30: 1—12.
4. Peroutka SJ (1988): 5-Hydroxytryptamine receptor subtypes: molecular, biochemical and physiological characterization. *Trends Neurosci* 11: 496—500.
5. Costall B, Naylor RJ, Tyers MB (1988): Recent advances in the neuropharmacology of 5-HT$_3$ agonists and antagonists. *Reviews Neurosci* 2: 41—65.
6. Sanger GJ, King FD (1988): From metoclopramide to selective gut motility stimulants and 5-HT$_3$ receptor antagonists. *Drug Design and Delivery* 3: 273—295.

7. Richardson BP, Buchheit KH (1988): The pharmacology, distribution and function of 5-HT₃ receptors, pp. 465—507 in: Osborne NN, Hamon M (eds), *Neuronal Serotonin.* Chichester: John Wiley and Sons, Ltd.

8. Fozard JR (1989): The development and early clinical evaluation of selective 5-HT₃ receptor antagonists, pp. 354—376 in: Fozard JR (ed), *The Peripheral Actions of 5-Hydroxytryptamine.* Oxford: Oxford University Press.

9. Fozard JR, Mobarok Ali ATM (1978): Blockade of neuronal tryptamine receptors by metoclopramide. *Europ J Pharmacol* 49: 109—112.

10. Gaddum JH, Picarelli ZP (1957): Two kinds of tryptamine receptor. *Brit J Pharmacol Chemother* 12: 323—328.

11. Wallis D, Nash H (1981): Relative activities of substances related to 5-hydroxytryptamine as depolarizing agents of superior cervical ganglion cells. *Europ J Pharmacol* 70: 381—392.

12. Fozard JR (1984): Characteristics of the excitatory 5-HT receptor on the cholinergic nerves of the rabbit heart, 1189P, *Proceedings of the 9th International Congress of Pharmacology.* London: Macmillan Press Ltd.

13. Fozard JR (1983): Failure of 5-methoxytryptamine to evoke the Bezold-Jarisch effect supports homology of excitatory 5-HT receptors on vagal afferents and postganglionic sympathetic neurones. *Europ J Pharmacol* 95: 331—332.

14. Vane JR (1959): The relative potencies of some tryptamine analogues on the isolated rat stomach strip preparation. *Brit J Pharmacol* 14: 97—98.

15. Bertaccini G, Zamboni P (1961): The relative potency of 5-hydroxytryptamine-like substances. *Arch Int Pharmacody Ther* 133: 138—156.

16. Schoeffter P, Waeber C, Palacios JM, Hoyer D (1988): The 5-hydroxytryptamine 5-HT₁D receptor subtype is negatively coupled to adenylate cyclase in calf substantia nigra. *Naunyn-Schmiedeberg's Arch Pharmacol* 337: 602—608.

17. Chahl LA (1983): Substance P mediates atropine-sensitive responses of guinea-pig ileum to serotonin. *Europ J Pharmacol* 87: 485—489.

18. Buchheit KH, Engel G, Mutschler E, Richardson BP (1985): Study of the contractile effect of 5-hydroxytryptamine (5-HT) in the isolated longitudinal muscle strip from the guinea-pig ileum. *Naunyn-Schmiedeberg's Arch Pharmacol* 329: 36—41.

19. Butler A, Hill JM, Ireland SJ, Jordan CC, Tyers MB (1988): Pharmacological properties of GR38032F, a novel antagonist at 5-HT₃ receptors. *Brit J Pharmacol* 94: 397—412.

20. Richardson BP, Engel G, Donatsch P, Stadler PA (1985): Identification of serotonin receptor subtypes and their specific blockade by a new class of drugs. *Nature* 316: 126—131.

21. Ireland SJ, Tyers MB (1987): Pharmacological characterization of 5-hydroxytryptamine-induced depolarization of the rat isolated vague nerve. *Brit J Pharmacol* 90: 229—238.

22. Elliott P, Wallis DI (1988): The depolarizing action of 5-hydroxytryptamine in rabbit isolated preganglionic cervical sympathetic neurones. *Naunyn-Schmiedeberg's Arch Pharmacol,* in press.

23. Paintal AS (1955): Impulses in vagal afferent fibres from specific pulmonary deflation receptors. The response of these receptors to phenyl diguanide, potato starch, 5-hydroxytryptamine and nicotine and their role in respiratory and cardiovascular reflexes. *Quart J Exp Physiol* 40: 348—363.

24. Fastier FN, McDowall MA, Waal H (1959): Pharmacological properties of phenyl-diguanide and other amidine derivatives in relation to those of 5-hydroxytryptamine. *Brit J Pharmacol* 14: 527—535.

25. Gyermek L (1964): Action of guanidine derivatives on autonomic ganglia. *Arch Int Pharmacodyn Ther* 150: 570—581.

26. Drakontides AB, Gershon MD (1968). 5-Hydroxytryptamine receptors in the mouse duodenum. *Brit J Pharmacol* 33: 480—492.

27. Fortune DH, Ireland SJ, Tyers MB (1983): Phenylbiguanide mimics the effects of 5-

hydroxytryptamine on the rat isolated vagus nerve and superior cervical ganglion. *Brit J Pharmacol* 79: 298P.

28. Ravi K, Dev NB (1988): Metoclopramide blocks the phenyl diguanide and 5-hydroxy-tryptamine induced cardio-respiratory reflexes in cats and dogs. *Can J Physiol Pharmacol* 66: 776—782.

29. Armstrong DJ, Kay IS (1985): MDL 72222 (a 5-HT antagonist) antagonizes the pulmonary depressor and respiratory chemoreflexes evoked by phenylbiguanide in anaesthetized rabbits. *J Physiol (Lond)* 365: 104P.

30. Leff P, Martin GR (1988): The classification of 5-hydroxytryptamine receptors. *Med Res Rev* 8: 187—202.

31. Fozard JR (1984): MDL 72222: a potent and highly selective antagonist at neuronal 5-hydroxytryptamine receptors. *Naunyn-Schmiedeberg's Arch Pharmacol* 326: 36—44.

32. Sanger GJ (1987): Increased gut cholinergic activity and antagonism of 5-hydroxy-tryptamine M-receptors by BRL 24924: Potential clinical importance of BRL 24924. *Brit J Pharmacol* 91: 77—87.

33. Alphin RS, Smith WL, Jackson CB, Droppleman DA, Sancilio LF (1986): Zacopride (AHR 11190B): a unique and potent gastrointestinal prokinetic and antiemetic agent in laboratory animals. *Dig Dis Sci* 31: 4825.

34. Sanger GJ (1987): Activation of a myenteric 5-hydroxytryptamine-like receptor by metoclopramide. *J Pharm Pharmacol* 39: 449—453.

35. Fozard JR (1985): Peripheral neuronal 5-hydroxytryptamine receptors and their bio-logical significance, pp. 37—56 in: Lambert RW (ed), *Proceedings of the third SCI/RSC Medicinal Chemistry Symposium*. London: The Royal Society of Chemistry.

36. Richardson BP, Engel G (1986): The pharmacology and functions of 5-HT$_3$ receptors. *Trends Neurosci* 7: 424—428.

37. Azami J, Fozard JR, Round AA, Wallis DI (1985): The depolarizing action of 5-hydroxytryptamine on rabbit vagal primary afferent and sympathetic neurones and its selective blockade by MDL 72222. *Naunyn-Schmiedeberg's Arch Pharmacol* 328: 423—429.

38. Round A, Wallis DI (1987): Further studies on the blockade of 5-HT depolarizations of rabbit vagal afferent and sympathetic ganglion cells by MDL 72222 and other antago-nists. *Neuropharmacology* 26: 39—48.

39. Round A, Wallis DI (1986): The depolarising action of 5-hydroxytryptamine on rabbit vagal afferent and sympathetic neurones in vitro and its selective blockade by ICS 205-930. *Brit J Pharmacol* 88: 485—494.

40. Kenakin TP (1984): The classification of drugs and drug receptors in isolated tissues. *Pharmacol Rev* 36: 165—222.

41. Wallis DI (1989): Interaction of 5-hydroxytryptamine with autonomic and sensory neurones, pp. 220—246 in: Fozard JR (ed), *The Peripheral Actions of 5-hydroxytrypta-mine*. Oxford: Oxford University Press.

42. Kilpatrick GJ, Jones BJ, Tyers MB (1987): Identification and distribution of 5-HT$_3$ receptors in rat brain using radioligand binding. *Nature* 330: 746—748.

43. Hoyer D, Neijt HC (1988): Identification of serotonin 5-HT$_3$ recognition sites in membranes of N1E-115 neuroblastoma cells by radioligand binding. *Mol Pharmacol* 33: 303—309.

44. Middlemiss DN, Fozard JR, unpublished observations.

45. Peroutka SJ (1988): Species variations in 5-HT$_3$ recognition sites labeled by ^{3}H-quipazine in the central nervous system. *Naunyn-Schmiedeberg's Arch Pharmacol* 338: 472—475.

46. Neijt HC, Karpf A, Schoeffter P, Engel G, Hoyer D (1988): Characterisation of 5-HT$_3$ recognition sites in membranes of NG 108—15 neuroblastoma-glioma cells with [^{3}H] ICS 205-930. *Naunyn-Schmiedeberg's Arch Pharmacol* 337: 493—499.

47. Waeber C, Dixon K, Hoyer D, Palacios JM (1988): Localisation by autoradiography of neuronal 5-HT$_3$ receptors in the mouse CNS. *Europ J Pharmacol* 151: 351—352.

48. Watling KJ (1988): Radioligand binding studies identify 5-HT₃ recognition sites in neuroblastoma cell lines and mammalian CNS. *Trends Pharmacol Sci* 9: 227—229.

49. Kilpatrick GJ, Jones BJ, Tyers MB (1988): Binding of the 5-HT₃ ligand [³H] GR65630, to rat area postrema, vagus nerve and the brains of several species. *Europ J Pharmacol* 159: 157—164.

50. Peroutka SJ, Hamik A (1988): [³H] Quipazine labels 5-HT₃ recognition sites in rat cortical membranes. *Europ J Pharmacol* 148: 297—299.

51. Hoyer D (1989): 5-Hydroxytryptamine receptors and effector coupling mechanisms in peripheral tissues, pp. 72—99 in: Fozard JR (ed), *The Peripheral Actions of 5-hydroxy-tryptamine*. Oxford: Oxford University Press.

52. Donatsch P, Engel G, Richardson BP, Stadler PA (1984): Subtypes of neuronal 5-hydroxytryptamine (5-HT) receptors as identified by competitive antagonists. *Brit J Pharmacol* 81: 33P.

53. Fake CS, King FD, Sanger GJ (1987): BRL 43694: A potent and novel 5-HT₃ receptor antagonist. *Brit J Pharmacol* 91: 335P.

54. Smith WW, Sancilio LF, Owera-atepo JB, Naylor RJ, Lambert I (1988): Zacopride, a potent 5-HT₃ antagonist. *J Pharm Pharmacol* 40: 301—302.

55. Barnes NM, Costall B, Naylor RJ (1988): [³H] Zacopride: Ligand for the identification of 5-HT₃ recognition sites. *J Pharm Pharmacol* 40: 548—551.

56. Fozard JR, Mwaluko GMP (1976): Mechanism of the indirect sympathomometic effect of 5-hydroxytryptamine on the isolated heart of the rabbit. *Brit J Pharmacol* 57: 115—125.

57. Watling KJ, Aspley S, Swain CJ, Saunders J (1988): [³H] Quaternised ICS 205-930 labels 5-HT₃ receptor binding sites in rat brain. *Europ J Pharmacol* 149: 397—398.

58. Kilpatrick GJ, Jones BJ, Tyers MB (1989): [³H] GR67330, a very high affinity ligand for central 5-HT₃ receptor. *Brit J Pharmacol* 96: 8P.

IX. The continuing story of 5-hydroxytryptamine receptors: a 5-HT$_3$ receptor modulates dopamine release from rat striatal slice

PATRIZIO BLANDINA, JOSEPH GOLDFARB and
JACK PETER GREEN

1. The plethora of 5-hydroxytryptamine (5-HT) receptors

To the large number of 5-HT receptors that have been catalogued [1—4] can now be added the 5-HT$_{1D}$ receptor, first described as a binding site [5] and recently shown to be negatively coupled to adenylyl cyclase in the calf substantia nigra [6]. Yet additional 5-HT receptors exist, not only in mammalian smooth muscles and other peripheral tissues [1, 3] but in brain as well. For example, the hippocampus has binding sites (and probably the homologous receptors) for all known 5-HT receptors [5, 7—10]. But some 5-HT-induced excitatory responses in the hippocampus cannot be attributed to any of these receptors. These include a slow depolarization of pyramidal cells which has been attributed to a decrease in a K$^+$ current [11, 12]; a decrease in the calcium-dependent K$^+$ current responsible for the slow after-spike hyperpolarization in pyramidal cells [11, 12]; and a transient increase in population spike amplitude [13].

Hippocampal membranes have a receptor with low affinity for 5-HT that stimulates adenylyl cyclase activity [14, 15]. This receptor (in adult hippocampus) may be the same receptor as found in infant rat colliculi, and it has not been classified [15].

As noted before [3], the large number of receptors for 5-HT compared with the number of receptors for other endogenous ligands may be more apparent than real. The 5-HT receptors appear to be more readily manifest than many others, in part perhaps because of the rush of syntheses of antagonists and agonists designed to explore 5-HT receptors. In contrast, for example, it was commonly believed for decades that only one muscarinic receptor exists, an opinion that was first corrected with the advent of pirenzepine, after which cloning revealed four muscarinic receptors [16], and yet more are being revealed. A similar progression of events revealed the multiplicity of receptors for other transmitters [17]. Availability of new antagonists and agonists and increased application of the techniques of molecular biology may well reveal yet additional 5-HT receptors.

P.R. Saxena, D.I. Wallis, W. Wouters and P. Bevan (eds), Cardiovascular Pharmacology of 5-Hydroxytryptamine, pp. 117—126.
© 1990 *Kluwer Academic Publishers, Dordrecht —*

2. The risks of too quickly associating a receptor with a specific transducing mechanism: the 5-HT$_{1A}$ receptor as an example

One of the 5-HT receptors linked to *stimulation* of adenylyl cyclase activity in guinea pig and rat hippocampal membranes was shown to be the 5-HT$_{1A}$ receptor [15]. The same receptor in the same tissue was shown to be linked to *inhibition* of adenylyl cyclase activity [18]. Table 1 compares the responses to stimulation and inhibition. The agonists and the antagonist that were tested did not distinguish the receptor linked to the two effects. Availability and testing of other agonists and antagonists may reveal that stimulation and inhibition are, in fact, mediated by distinct receptors.

Table 1. Comparative responses of 5-HT stimulation of adenylyl cyclase activity (by R$_H$, the high-affinity receptor) [15] with 5-HT inhibition of forskolin-stimulated adenylyl cyclase activity in guinea pig hippocampal membranes [18]. Each value is the geometric mean ± standard error.

Substance	Stimulation (R$_H$) EC$_{50}$(nM)	Inhibition EC$_{50}$(nM)
5-HT	43 ± 6	53 ± 4
5-methoxytryptamine	51 ± 12	49 ± 5
5-carboxamidotryptamine	6 ± 1	5 ± 0.2
8-hydroxy-2-(di-*n*-propylamino)tetralin	29 ± 1	18 ± 1
	K$_D$(nM)	K$_D$(nM)
Spiperone	24 ± 3	26 ± 1

Alternatively, the dual effects may rest on the capacity of a stimulated receptor, specifically the 5-HT$_{1A}$ receptor, to react with different guanine nucleotide-binding proteins, a G$_s$ protein to stimulate adenylyl cyclase and a G$_i$ to inhibit adenylyl cyclase. As pointed out before, it has been shown that a β-adrenoceptor agonist binds to membranes from cells lacking G$_s$ but possessing G$_i$, and the binding is sensitive to GTP [19]. Incorporation of the β-adrenoceptor and G$_i$ into phospholipid vesicles resulted in vesicles that responded to β-adrenoceptor agonists as measured by high-affinity binding of a guanine nucleotide and in stimulation of GTPase activity; these responses were no different from those in vesicles containing G$_s$ and the β-adrenoceptor [20]. Similarly, the μ opioid receptor can couple to different guanine nucleotide binding proteins [21]. It is therefore plausible that in homogenized hippocampal cells, the 5-HT$_{1A}$ receptor can bind to both G$_s$ and G$_i$. Which interaction is favored may be determined by the media in which the assays are conducted. For example, it is known that Na$^+$ influences both G$_s$- and G$_i$-mediated effects on adenylyl cyclase [22, 23].

The electrophysiological responses to stimulation of the 5-HT$_{1A}$ receptor cannot be presumed to be related to either stimulation or inhibition of adenylyl cyclase activity. In the rat hippocampal slice in vitro, activation of the 5-HT$_{1A}$ receptor decreases CA1 population spike amplitude [13], probably as a consequence of hyperpolarization of pyramidal cells by a 5-HT$_{1A}$ activated K$^+$ conductance [12]. Treating the rat with pertussis toxin, which ADP-ribosylates some G-proteins, blocks the effects of 5-HT$_{1A}$ stimulation on the hyperpolarization [24], the decrease in population spike amplitude [25], and its effect on adenylyl cyclase [25]. The magnitude of the effects of pertussis toxin on the 5-HT$_{1A}$ effects on population spike amplitude and adenylyl cyclase were correlated [25]. These observations might imply that the 5-HT$_{1A}$ coupled adenylyl cyclase accounts for the electrophysiologi-cal effects. However, since neither application of 8-bromo-cAMP to the bath nor intracellular injection of cAMP reduces the hyperpolarization, the 5-HT$_{1A}$ receptor activated G protein appears to be linked directly to the K$^+$ channel [24]. Whatever linkage the 5-HT$_{1A}$ receptor has to adenylyl cyclase appears unrelated to these electrophysiological effects. G proteins are known to function directly in other receptor regulated ion channels [26, 27].

3. 5-HT and dopamine (DA) interactions

DA release has been shown to be influenced by many endogenous sub-stances, including 5-HT [28]. Interactions between the serotonergic and dopaminergic systems have been described for over a decade [29, 30]. Paradoxical findings have accumulated, but they have hope of being resolved with the advent of specific agonists and antagonists. Some experiments show that 5-HT inhibits DA release from striatum. A concentration-related inhibition of K$^+$-evoked [^{3}H]DA release was produced by 5-HT over the concentration range 10^{-7} to 10^{-5} M; methiothepin, methysergide, cyprohept-adine, and mianserin antagonized this effect of 5-HT [31]. Others confirmed the inhibitory action of 5-HT on the K$^+$-evoked release of exogenous, labeled DA from striatal slices and, on the basis of blockade by ketanserin, suggested that the effect was mediated by the 5-HT$_2$ receptor [32]. Since ketanserin and structural analogues increase exogenous [^{3}H]DA release [33], the assignment is not certain. Behavioural experiments show that 5-HT injections into the nucleus accumbens inhibit the hyperactivity produced by injections of amphetamine or DA into this same nucleus [34]. Evidence has been presented that cell firing in the striatum is inhibited by stimulation of the dorsal raphe nucleus [35] and by the iontophoretic application of 5-HT in the striatum [36]. Methysergide antagonized both effects.

However, Bevan et al., [37] reported that iontophoresis of 5-HT pro-duced mainly excitation. Analogously, in vivo electrical stimulation of the dorsal raphe increased the striatal extracellular DOPAC, measured by means of implanted carbon fibre electrodes [38]. Other studies have shown that 5-HT enhances DA release. Addition of 5-HT, at a concentration of 5 × 10^{-5} M to a bath containing rat striatal slices previously incubated with

[3H]tyrosine, increased the release of [3H]DA [39]. 5-HT also stimulated [14C]DA release from striatal synaptosomes preincubated with the labeled amine and potentiated the release induced by 56 mM K+, but high con-centrations, i.e., 2×10^{-5} M 5-HT and greater were required; neither methysergide nor cyproheptadine antagonized this effect of 5-HT [40]. Others have shown that 5-HT reduced the K+-induced release of exogenous [3H]DA from the nucleus accumbens but enhanced the basal release, and both effects were eliminated by nomifensine [41]. Treatment of rats with p-chloroamphetamine, which releases 5-HT, caused a pronounced release of DA from the striatum [42]. Inhibitors of 5-HT uptake increased striatal concentrations of DA metabolites [43]. Injections of a 5-HT$_3$ antagonist, GR38032F, into the nucleus accumbens inhibited the hyperactivity produced by injections of DA or amphetamine into the same nucleus; interestingly, this antagonist did not affect striatal DA related behaviours [34]. GR38032F also inhibited the hyperactivity and the increased DA turnover in the nucleus accumbens produced by a neurokinin agonist injected into the ventral tegmental area [44]. 5-HT agonists enhanced DA turnover in the striatum, hypothalamus and cerebral cortex of rats [45]. The correlation between the levels of 5-hydroxindoleacetic acid and homovanillic acid in human cere-brospinal fluid fostered the suggestion that 5-HT facilitates DA turnover [46].

4. Evidence that stimulation of a 5-HT$_3$ receptor in the rat striatum releases DA

5-HT$_3$ receptors have been extensively characterized in guinea pig ileum, rabbit vagus nerve, and rabbit heart [1, 47]. 5-HT$_3$ high-affinity binding sites have been shown in brain [9, 48—52]. DA-rich areas such as the nucleus accumbens, tuberculum olfactorium, and striatum were among the regions showing high density of 5-HT$_3$ receptors [9]. Although, as noted above, a linkage between 5-HT$_3$ receptors and the dopaminergic systems has been shown, the discrete mechanisms remain to be elucidated. The role of the 5-HT$_3$ receptor in contributing to the modulation of DA release was therefore investigated.

4.1 Methods

Male Sprague-Dawley rats (250—300 g) were allowed free access to food pellets and water and were housed in a temperature controlled room (22—24 °C) which was lit from 7 a.m. to 8 p.m.

After decapitation the brains were removed and placed on ice. The striatum was dissected and cut sagitally into 400 μ sections with a manually operated McIlwain tissue slicer. The slices were removed from the blade with a fine sable brush, placed in chilled medium and six to nine of them immediately transferred to a plastic chamber the volume of which was 300 μl. They were superfused in an overflow manner at a rate of 0.5 ml/min at 37 °C with the medium which was prewarmed and continously gassed with 95% O_2 and 5% CO_2. The composition (mM) of the medium was: NaCl, 113; $NaHCO_3$ 25; KCl, 4.75; NaH_2PO_4. 1.18; $CaCl_2$, 2.52; $MgSO_4$, 1.19; glucose, 10; tyrosine, 0.050; nomifensine, 0.01; and pargyline, 0.01. After equilibration for 60 min, 1.5 ml (3 min periods) fractions were collected into tubes containing 166 μl of a solution of lN $HClO_4$ and 10 μM ascorbic acid, and 2.5 pg epinine as an internal standard. At selected times, slices were exposed to the substances under investigation by transferring the chamber inflow tubing to reservoirs containing the medium of appropriate composition. Samples were kept on ice during the collection period and stored at −20 °C until assayed. DA was measured by high-performance liquid chromatography-electrochemical detection (HPLC-ECD) (Waters, Milford MA, USA). After extraction with alumina [53], 25 μl aliquots of extracts were injected onto a reverse-phase column (Altex Ultrasphere Ion Pair, 5 μm, 150 × 4.6 mm) at room temperature. The mobile phase had the following composition (mM): chloroacetic acid, 222; NaOH, 116; Na_2EDTA 2; sodium octyl sulfate 2.5; methanol to 9% (pH 2.8). The potential of the glassy carbon electrode was set at 0.7 V against the reference electrode. The flow rate was 0.8 ml/min. The peaks were first identified by comparison of their retention times with those of the standards. Addition of authentic substances to the samples increased areas of specific compounds, and varying the pH of the mobile phase failed to reveal other substances coeluting with the compounds under investigation.

The amount of DA in the superfusate was calculated by comparing the sample peak area with the external standard peak area, both corrected by the internal standard peak area and expressed as pmol/mg protein/3 min. Results are given as percent increase in basal release, calculated as the mean of three observations. The peak area of DA divided by the peak area of the internal standard versus the amounts of DA was linear between 40 and at least 400 fmol ($r^2 = 0.99$), embracing the amounts measured. Protein was measured by the method of Lowry et al. [54].

The substances used in this study included, DA.HCl, epinine.HCl, 5-HT.HCl, pargyline.HCl and 1-tyrosine (all from Sigma); ICS 205−930 and 2-methyl-5-HT (2-Me-5-HT) (from Sandoz Ltd, Basel); nomifensine maleate (from Hoechst-Roussel, Sommerville, NJ); octyl sodium sulfate (from Eastman Kodak, Rochester, NY); sodium chloride ultrapure (from Alpha Products, Danvers, MA). All other reagents and solvents were of HPLC grade or the highest grade available (from Fisher or Sigma).

4.2 Results and discussion

Table 2 shows that superfusion with 1 μM and 6 μM 5-HT increased DA released by 70% and 109%, respectively. 6 μM and 10 μM 2-methyl-5-HT,

Table 2. The release of DA from rat striatal slices. The basal release of DA was 0.35 ± 0.03 pmol/mg protein/3 min (n = 20). Each value is the mean $\pm$ standard error.

Substance	Conc.	DA, % increase	n
5-HT	$1 \mu M$	70 ± 7	3
5-HT	$6 \mu M$	109 ± 15	3
2-Me-5-HT	$6 \mu M$	45 ± 3	3
2-Me-5-HT	$10 \mu M$	110 ± 19	3
5-HT	$6 \mu M$		
+ ICS 205-930	0.4 nM	42 ± 11	4
5-HT	$6 \mu M$		
+ ICS 205-930	0.9 nM	6 ± 2	4

which is a highly selective 5-HT_3 agonist [47], produced similar increases, 45% and 110%, respectively. In the presence of 2 mM EGTA and the absence of Ca^{2+}, 6 μM 5—HT had very slight effect on DA release. DOI ((2,5-dimethoxy-4-iodophenyl)-2-amino-propane), the selective 5-HT_2 agonist, at a concentration of 10 μM had insignificant effect on DA release as did 5-carboxamidotryptamine (1 μM), the selective 5-HT_1-like receptor agonist.

Concentration-response curves showed that 5-HT had an EC_{50} value of 0.79 μM, 2-Me-5-HT of 3.9 μM. The relative EC_{50} values of 5-HT and 2-Me-5-HT could favour attribution of the effect to either the 5-HT_{3A} or 5-HT_{3C} receptor [47].

The effect on DA release of 10 μM of 5-HT was not blocked by 1 μM methysergide.

0.4 nM ICS 205-930 ((3α-tropanyl) 1H-indole-3-carboxylic acid ester) reduced the effect of 6 μM 5-HT, and 0.9 nM ICS 205-930 almost completely blocked that effect (Table 2). At these concentrations, ICS 205-930 is an antagonist selective for 5-HT_3 receptors [47]. Our concentration-response curves for the effects of 5-HT and 2-Me-5-HT in releasing DA from striatal slices in the presence of ICS 205-930 suggest that the antagonist had K_B values of 0.032 nM ($pK_B = 10.5$) and 0.039 nM ($pK_B = 10.4$), respectively. These values of ICS 205-930 are similar to those on the 5-HT_{3A} ($pA_2 = 10.2$) 5-HT_{3B} ($pA_2 = 10.6$) receptors and much different from the pA_2 value of 7.9 on the 5-HT_{3C} receptor [47]. Indeed, the effect of 6 μM 5-HT in reducing the C-fibre action potential in desheathed rabbit vagus nerve, which rests on the 5-HT_{3A} receptor [47], is diminished by 50% in the presence of 0.5 nM ICS 205-930 and abolished in the presence of 2 nM ICS 205-930 [55]. Hence, from the EC_{50} values of the two agonists and the K_B of ICS 205-930, the 5-HT_{3A} receptor is probably implicated in DA release from the striatal slice. Further experiments are needed to probe this suggestion.

The modulation of striatal DA release by 5-HT_3 receptor(s) may offer an approach to therapy of dyskinesias. Of additional interest is to learn which

5-HT$_3$ receptor influences DA release in other parts of the brain, notably in the mesolimbic system. The 5-HT$_3$ receptor may offer opportunities for pharmacotherapy in addition to those as antiemetics [56] and anxiolytics [57]. Recently, both ICS 205-930 and another 5-HT$_3$ antagonist, MDL 72222, were shown to reduce the rewarding properties in rats of morphine and nicotine but not of amphetamine [58]. Work reported in abstract-form described experiments showing that GR 38032F, a 5-HT$_3$ antagonist, decreased ethanol consumption in rats [59]. Another abstract states that ICS 205-930, after systemic administration to rats or injection into the ventral tegmental area, prevented the increase in DA release from the nucleus accumbens that followed subcutaneous injections of morphine, nicotine or ethanol [60].

Acknowledgments

This work was supported by research grant DA 01875 from the National Institute on Drug Abuse. We thank G. Engel of Sandoz, Ltd. for gifts of 2-Me-5-HT and ICS 205-930, G. Cohen and S. Maayani for helpful comments, B. Royal and D. A. Jaeger for technical assistance.

References

1. Bradley PB, Engel G, Feniuk W, Fozard JR, Humphrey PPA, Middlemiss DN, Mylecharane EJ, Richardson BP, Saxena PR (1986): Proposals for the classification, and nomenclature of functional receptors for 5-hydroxytryptamine. *Neuropharmacology* 25: 563—576.
2. Arvidsson L-E, Hacksell U, Glennon RA (1986): Recent advances in central 5-hydroxytryptamine receptor agonists and antagonists. *Prog Drug Res* 30: 365—471.
3. Green JP, Maayani S (1987): Nomenclature, classification, and notation of receptors: 5-hydroxytryptamine receptors and binding sites as examples pp. 237—267 in: Black JW. Jenkinson DH Gerskowitch VP (eds), *Perspectives on receptor classification*, Liss: New York.
4. Peroutka SJ (1988): 5-Hydroxytryptamine receptor subtypes *Ann Rev Neurosci* 11: 45—60.
5. Heuring RE, Peroutka SJ (1987): Characterization of a novel ^{3}H-5-HT binding site subtype in bovine brain membrane. *J Neurosci* 7: 894—903.
6. Schoeffter P, Waeber C, Palacios JM, Hoyer D (1988): The 5-hydroxytryptamine 5-HT$_{1D}$ receptor subtype is negatively coupled to adenylate cyclase in calf substantia nigra *Naunyn-Schmiedeberg's Arch Pharmacol* 337: 602—608.
7. Pazos A, Cortes I, Palacios JM (1985): Quantitative autoradiographic mapping of serotonin receptors in the rat brain. I. Serotonin-2 receptors. *Brain Res* 346: 231—249.
8. Pazos A, Palacios JM (1985): Quantitative autoradiographic mapping of serotonin receptors in the rat brain. II. Serotonin-1 receptors. *Brain Res* 346: 205—230.
9. Kilpatrick GJ, Jones BJ, Tyers MB (1987): The identification and distribution of the 5-HT$_3$ receptors in rat brain using radioligand binding. *Nature* 330: 746—748.
10. Herrick-Davis K, Titeler M (1988): Detection and characterization of the serotonin 5-HT$_{1D}$ receptor in rat and human brain. *J Neurochem* 50: 1624—1631.

11. Colino A, Halliwell JV (1987): Differential modulation of three separate K^+-conductances in hippocampal CA1 neurons by serotonin. *Nature* 328: 73—77.
12. Andrade R, Nicoll RA (1987): Pharmacologically distinct actions of serotonin on single pyramidal neurones of the rat hippocampus recorded in vitro. *J Physiol (Lond.)* 394: 99—124.
13. Beck SG, Clarke WP, Goldfarb J (1985): Spiperone differentiates multiple 5-hydroxytryptamine responses in rat hippocampal slices in vitro. *Europ J Pharmacol* 116: 195—197.
14. Shenker A, Maayani S, Weinstein H, Green JP (1985): Two 5-HT receptors linked to adenylate cyclase in guinea pig hippocampus are discriminated by 5-carboxamidotryptamine and spiperone. *Eur J Pharmacol* 109: 427—429.
15. Shenker A, Maayani S, Weinstein H, Green, JP (1987): Pharmacological characterization of two 5-hydroxytryptamine receptors coupled to adenylate cyclase in guinea pig hippocampal membranes. *Mol Pharmacol* 31: 357—367.
16. Bonner TI, Buckley NJ, Young AC, Brann MR (1987): Identification of a family of muscarinic acetylcholine receptor genes. *Science* 237: 527—532.
17. Green JP (1987): Polypharmic antagonists — a class of their own. *Trends Pharmacol Sci* 8: 377—379.
18. De Vivo M, Maayani S (1986): Characterization of the 5-hydroxytryptamine$_{1A}$ receptor mediated inhibition of forskolin-stimulated adenylate cyclase activity in guinea pig and rat hippocampal membranes. *J Pharmacol Exp Ther* 238: 248—253.
19. Abramson SN, Molinoff PB (1985): Properties of beta-adrenergic receptors of cultured mammalian cells: interaction of receptors with a guanine nucleotide-binding protein in membranes prepared from L6 myoblast and from wild-type and cyc-S49 lymphoma calls. *J Biol Chem* 260: 14580—14588.
20. Asano T, Katada T, Gilman AG, Ross, EM (1984): Activation of the inhibitory GTP-binding protein of adenylate cyclase, G_i by beta-adrenergic receptors in reconstituted phospholipid vesicles, *J Biol Chem* 259: 9351—9354.
21. Ueda H, Harada H, Nozaki M, Katada T, Ui M, Satoh M, Takagi H (1988): Reconstitution of rat brain μ opioid receptors with purified guanine nucleotide-binding regulatory proteins, G_i and G_o. *Proc Natl Acad Sci USA* 85: 7013—7017.
22. Cooper DMF, Londos C, Rodbell M (1980): Adenosine receptor-mediated inhibition of rat cerebrat cortical adenylate cyclase by a GTP-dependent process. *Mol Pharmacol* 18: 598—601.
23. Jacobs KH, Aktories K, Minuth M, Schultz G (1985): Inhibition of adenylate cyclase vol. 19 pp. 137—150, in: Cooper DMF, Seamon KB (eds), *Advances in cyclic nucleotide and protein phosphorylation research*, Raven Press: New York.
24. Andrade R, Malenka RC, Nicoll RA (1986): A G protein couples serotonin and GABA-B receptors to the same channels in hippocampus. *Science* 234: 1261—1265.
25. Clarke WP, DeVivo M, Beck SG, Maayani S, Goldfarb J (1987): Serotonin decreases population spike amplitude in hippocampal cells through a pertussis toxin substrate. *Brain Res* 410: 357—361.
26. Gilman AG (1987): G proteins: transducers of receptor-generated signals. *Ann Rev Biochem* 56: 615—649.
27. Iyengar R, Birnbaumer L (1987): Signal transduction by G-proteins. ISI Atlas of Science: *Pharmacol* 213—221.
28. Glowinski J, Cheramy A, Romo R, Barbeito L (1988): Presynaptic regulation of dopaminergic transmission in the striatum. *Cell Mol Neurobiol* 8: 7—17.
29. Costall B, Naylor RJ (1974): Stereotyped and circling behavior induced by dopaminergic agonists after lesions of the midbrain raphe nuclei. *Eur J Pharmacol* 29: 206—212.
30. Samanin R, Quattrone A, Consolo S, Ladinsky H, Algeri S (1978): Biochemical and pharmacological evidence for the interaction of serotonin with other aminergic systems in the brain pp. 383—399 in: Garattini S, Pujol JF, Samanin R (eds), *Interactions between putative neurotransmitters in the brain*, Raven Press: New York.

31. Ennis C, Kemp JD, Cox B (1981): Characterization of inhibitory 5-hydroxytryptamine receptors that modulate dopamine release in the striatum. *J Neurochem* 36: 1515—1520.

32. Muramutsu M, Tamahi-Ohashi J, Usuki C, Araki H, Chaky S, Aihara H (1988): 5-HT$_2$ antagonists and minaprine block the 5-HT-induced inhibition of dopamine release from rat brain striatal slices. *Eur J Pharmacol* 153: 89—95.

33. Leysen JE, Eens A, Gommeren W, van Gompel P, Wynants J, Jansen PAJ (1988): Identification of nonserotonergic ^{3}H-ketanserin binding sites associated with nerve terminals in rat brain and with platelets; relation with release of biogenic amine metabolites induced by ketanserin- and terabenazine-like drugs. *J Pharmacol Exp Ther* 244: 310—321.

34. Costall B, Domeney AM, Naylor RJ, Tyers MB (1987): Effects of the 5-HT$_3$ receptor antagonist, GR38032F, on raised dopaminergic activity in the mesolimbic system of the rat and marmoset brain. *Br J Pharmacol* 92: 881—894.

35. Miller JJ, Richardson TL, Fibiger HC, Mc Lennan H (1975): Anatomical and electrophysiological identification of a projection from the mesencephalic raphe to the caudate putamen in the rat brain. *Brain Res* 97: 133—138.

36. Davies J, Tongroach P. (1978): Neuropharmacological studies on the nigro-striatal and raphe-striatal system in the rat. *Eur J Pharmacol* 51: 91—100.

37. Bevan P, Bradshaw CM, Szabaldi E (1975): Effects of desipramine on neuronal responses to dopamine, noradrenaline, 5-hydroxytryptamine and acetylcholine in the caudate nucleus of the rat. *Br J Pharmacol* 54: 285—293.

38. De Simoni MG, Dal Toso G, Fodritto F, Sokola A, Algeri S (1987): Modulation of striatal dopamine metabolism by the activity of dorsal raphe serotonergic afferents. *Brain Res* 411: 81—88.

39. Besson MJ, Cheramy A, Feltz P, Glowinski J (1969): Release of newly synthesized dopamine from dopamine-containing terminals in the striatum of the rat. *Proc Nat Acad Sci U.S.A.* 62: 741—748.

40. de Belleroche J, Bradford H (1980): Presynaptic control of the synthesis and release of dopamine from striatal synaptosomes: a comparison between the effects of 5-hydroxytryptamine, acetylcholine and glutamate. *J Neurochem* 35: 1227—1234.

41. Nurse B, Russel VA, Taljaard JJF (1988): Characterization of the effects of serotonin on the release of ^{3}H-Dopamine from rat nucleus accumbens and striatal slices. *Neurochem Res* 13: 403—407.

42. Sharp T, Zetterstrom T, Christmanson L, Ungerstedt U (1986): p-Chloroamphetamine releases both serotonin and dopamine into brain dialysates in vivo. *Neurosci Lett* 72: 320—324.

43. Waldmeier PC, Delini-Stula AA (1979): Serotonin-dopamine interactions in the nigrostriatal system. *Eur J Pharmacol* 55: 363—373.

44. Hagan RM, Butler A, Hill JM, Jordan CC, Ireland SJ, Tyers MB (1987): Effect of the 5-HT$_3$ receptor antagonist, GR38032F, on responses to injection of a neurokinin agonist into the ventral tegmental area of the rat brain. *Eur J Pharmacol* 138: 303—305.

45. Hamon M, Fattaccini C-M, Adrien J, Gallissot M-C, Martin P, Gozlan H (1988): Alteration of central serotonin and dopamine turnover in rats treated with ipsapirone and other 5-hydroxytryptamine$_{1A}$ agonists with potential anxiolytic properties. *J Pharmacol Exp Ther* 246: 745—752.

46. Agren H, Mefford IN, Rudorfer MV, Linnoila M, Potter WZ (1986): Interacting neurotransmitter systems. A non-experimental approach to the 5HIAA-HVA correlation in human CSF. *J Phychiat Res* 20: 175—193.

47. Richardson BP, Buchheit KH (1988): The pharmacology, distribution and function of 5-HT$_3$ receptors pp. 465—506, in: Osborne NN, Hamon M (eds), *Neuronal Serotonin, John Wiley &Sons* New York.

48. Hoyer D, Neijt HC (1987): Identification of serotonin 5-HT$_3$ recognition sites by radioligand binding in NG 108-15 neuroblastoma-glioma cells. *Eur J Pharmacol* 143: 291—292.

49. Barnes NM, Costall B, Naylor RJ (1988): [^{3}H]-Zacopride identifies 5-HT$_3$ binding sites in rat entorhinal cortex. *Br J Pharmacol* 94: 391 P.

50. Peroutka SJ, Hamik A (1988): [^{3}H]Quipazine labels 5-HT$_3$ recognition sites in rat cortical membranes. *Eur J Pharmacol* 148: 297—299.

51. Waeber C, Dixon K, Hoyer D, Palacios JM (1988): Localisation by autoradiography of neuronal 5-HT$_3$ receptors in the mouse CNS. *Eur J Pharmacol* 151: 351—352.

52. Watling KJ (1988): Radioligand binding studies identify 5-HT$_3$ recognition sites in neuroblastoma cell lines and mammalian CNS. *Trends Pharmacol Sci* 9: 227—229.

53. Misu Y, Goshima Y, Ueda H, Kubo T (1985): Presynaptic inhibitory dopamine receptors on noradrenergic nerve terminals: analysis of biphasic actions of dopamine and apomorphine on the release of endogenous norepinephrine in rat hypothalamic slices. *J Pharmacol Exp Ther* 235: 771—777.

54. Lowry OH, Rosebrough NJ, Farr AL, Randall RJ (1951): Protein measurement with the Folin phenol reagent. *J Biol Chem* 193: 265—273.

55. Richardson BP, Engel G, Donatsch P, Stadler PA (1985): Identification of serotonin M-receptor subtypes and their specific blockade by a new class of drugs. *Nature* 316: 126—131.

56. Andrews PLR, Rapeport WG, Sanger GJ (1988): Neuropharmacology of emesis induced by anti-cancer therapy. *Trends Pharmacol Sci* 9: 334—341.

57. Jones BJ, Costall B, Domeney AM, Kelly ME, Naylor RJ, Oakley NR, Tyers MB (1988): The potential anxiolytic activity of GR38032F, a 5-HT$_3$-receptor antagonist. *Br J Pharmacol* 93: 985—993.

58. Carboni E, Acquas E, Leone P, Perezzani L, Di Chiara G (1988): 5-HT$_3$ receptor antagonists block morphine- and nicotine-induced place-preference conditioning. *Eur J Pharmacol* 151, 159—160.

59. Sellers EM, Kaplan HL, Lawrin MO, Somer G, Naranjo CA, Frecker RC (1988): The 5-HT$_3$ antagonist GR38032F decreases alcohol consumption in rats. *Soc Neurosci Abstr* 14: 41.

60. Imperato A, Angelucci L (1988): 5-HT$_3$ receptors control dopamine release in the limbic system of freely-moving rats. *Soc Neurosci Abstr* 14: 611.

X. Allosteric modulation of arterial 5-HT$_2$ receptors

A. J. KAUMANN and A. M. BROWN

1. Introduction

Interaction of arterial 5-HT$_2$ receptors with their ligands are variable and complex. Some produce a surmountable, apparently competitive inhibition of the effects of 5-hydroxytryptamine (5-HT), causing a simple rightward shift of the concentration-effect curve for 5-HT. Other antagonists cause a rightward shift of the concentration-effect curve and a depression of maximum responses to 5-HT which cannot be surmounted by increased concentrations of 5-HT. However, in some cases, the unsurmountable action of one antagonist can be prevented or reversed by exposure to another, surmountable antagonist.

Kaumann and Frenken [1] proposed an allosteric receptor model to explain these results. It was proposed that the 5-HT$_2$ receptor can exist in two states, one on which 5-HT is highly active and the other on which 5-HT exerts low activity. The highly active state mediates fast contractions by 5-HT and the low active state mediates slow contractions. Agents modulate the interconversion between the two states by an action at an allosteric site. We describe here a formalisation of such a scheme which provides a good theoretical fit to experimental data obtained with several ligands interacting with two animal vascular tissues. We also provide evidence, for the first time, that pathological changes may alter the receptor type which predominates in human coronary artery.

2. 5-HT receptors involved in arterial contraction

5-HT causes contraction of arterial smooth muscle through 5-HT$_2$ receptors and other 5-HT receptors. 5-HT$_2$ receptors have by definition a relatively low affinity for 5-HT [2]. Equilibrium dissociation constants (i.e. reciprocal affinities) around 200 nM ($K_{5\text{-HT}}$) have been estimated by receptor occlusion with phenoxybenzamine for 5-HT$_2$ receptors of rabbit and calf arteries [3, 4].

P.R. Saxena, D.I. Wallis, W. Wouters and P. Bevan (eds), Cardiovascular Pharmacology of 5-Hydroxytryptamine, pp. 127–142.
© 1990 *Kluwer Academic Publishers, Dordrecht* −

Concentrations of 5-HT causing half maximum contractions of these arterial preparations are moderately lower (EC_{50} values 40—100 nM, Table 1) than the corresponding K_{5-HT} values suggesting the existence of some 5-HT$_2$ receptor reserve.

The introduction of high affinity antagonists has greatly stimulated research with 5-HT$_2$ receptors. Ketanserin, introduced by van Nueten et al. [5], has a subnanomolar equilibrium dissociation constant (K_B) for smooth muscle 5-HT$_2$ receptors (Table 1), as estimated from competitive antagonism

Table 1. 5-HT$_2$ receptor activators.

Tissue	5-HT $-\log EC_{50}(M)$	Ligand	$-\log K_B(M)^b$	Reference
Calf coronary artery	7.0	ICI 169,369[a]	9.1	[12]
Rat tail artery	7.2	ICI 169,369	8.8	[12]
Guinea-pig trachea	7.3	ICI 169,369	9.0	[14]
Calf coronary artery	7.3	Ketanserin	9.4	[1]
Calf trachea	7.4	Ketanserin	9.5	[13]
Rat tail artery	7.3	Ketanserin	9.4	[15]
Calf pulmonary artery	7.2	Ketanserin	9.5	[4, 28]
Calf coronary artery	7.0	Phentolamine	7.4	[22]
Rat tail artery	7.3	ICI 170,809[c]	10.0	[17]

[a] ICI 169,369 = 2-(2-dimethylaminoethylthio)-3-phenylquinoline
[b] K_B = equilibrium dissociation constant, estimated from competitive antagonism
[c] ICI 170,809 = 2-2(dimethylamino-2-methylpropylthio)-3-phenylquinoline [16]

on rat and calf arteries. In these arteries 5-HT acts mostly through 5-HT$_2$ receptors. On the other hand, in human coronary artery the use of ketanserin as a tool revealed that not only 5-HT$_2$ receptors but also non-5-HT$_2$ receptors are involved in the mediation of contractile responses to 5-HT. Furthermore, unlike arteries from healthy rats and calves, there even appear to exist regional differences between the relative contribution of 5-HT$_2$ receptors and non-5-HT$_2$ receptors in mediating contractions caused by 5-HT in a diseased human artery. The circumflex coronary artery, obtained from a patient with terminal ischaemic heart disease, undergoing heart transplant, presented a thrombotic occlusion but was patent on either side of the occlusion. The prestenotic but not poststenotic segment presented atheromatous plaques. Four arterial helicoids were prepared as described [6] from each of the prestenotic and poststenotic segments. The results are shown on Figure 1. The sensitivity to 5-HT of the prestenotic and poststenotic segments was similar. However, the effects of ketanserin were quite different in the 2 segments. Ketanserin blocked most of the 5-HT-induced contractions in the poststenotic segments and only a small (less than 20% of

Human Circumflex Coronary Artery

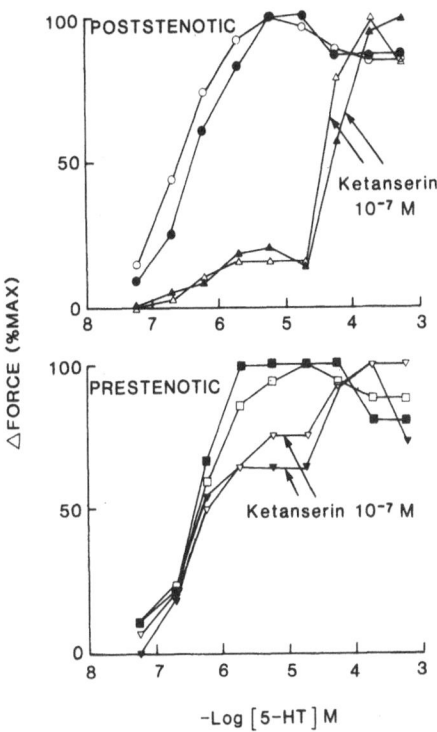

Figure 1. Differential blockade of the effects of 5-HT by ketanserin on helicoids dissected from a coronary artery of a patient (♀ 45 years) with terminal ischaemic heart disease. Experiment carried out at 37 °C as described [6]. Only a single concentration-effect curve for 5-HT was determined on each helicoid. Ketanserin was incubated 90 minutes before starting the cumulative administration of 5-HT. For further details see text.

maximum) component of the responses to low 5-HT concentrations were resistant to blockade. On the other hand, in prestenotic segments ketanserin was unable to block a large (up to 70% of maximum) portion of the responses to low 5-HT concentrations and only blocked the responses to high 5-HT concentrations. The experiments suggest that at least 2 distinct 5-HT receptors mediate 5-HT-induced contractions in human coronary artery, one ketanserin-resistant (non-5-HT$_2$), the other ketanserin-sensitive (i.e. 5-HT$_2$). 5-HT$_2$ receptors appear to predominate in arterial smooth muscle devoid of plaques whilst non-5-HT$_2$ receptors are perhaps located in newly formed smooth muscle that surrounds the atheromatous plaque. Our finding of a ketanserin-resistant component of 5-HT-induced contraction agrees with the lack of effect of ketanserin in coronary spasm [7] but does not rule out the participation of 5-HT. The coparticipation of 5-HT$_2$ receptors and non-5-HT$_2$ receptors in the mediation of 5-HT-induced contractions has also been described in canine coronary artery [8] and basilar artery [9].

3. The allosteric 5-HT₂ receptor system

5-HT-induced contractions of vascular smooth muscle can be blocked by antagonists in a manner that is surmountable or unsurmountable with 5-HT [1, 10, 11]. Surmountable antagonists (e.g. ketanserin, ICI 169, 369) usually cause competitive antagonism [1, 12], but the same drug can, in other tissues, also exhibit a non-competitive component (guinea-pig trachea [13, 14]). Unsurmountable antagonists (e.g. methysergide can either cause reversible blockade [1, 15]) or irreversible blockade [4]. Reversible unsurmountable antagonists cause non-competitive antagonism but often a component of competitive antagonism can also be shown for these drugs (ICI 170,809 [16] in calf coronary artery Figure 2 [17]; methysergide in rat tail artery Figure 3 [15]). Surmountable antagonists can prevent or reverse the depression of responses to 5-HT caused by reversible unsurmountable antagonists (Figures 2, 3).

Unsurmountable antagonists often uncover contractions with high 5-HT concentrations that are considerably slower than contractions observed with low 5-HT concentrations (for representative tracings see [1, 11, 15]). These experimental results, taken together, suggest the existence of the 5-HT₂ receptor in two interconvertible states R ⇌ R'. R mediates fast contractions and R' slow contractions. Drugs that favour R and R' are called activators and deactivators respectively [11, 18]. Drugs that cause both partially unsurmountable and competitive antagonism are called partial deactivators. A partial deactivator can also partially prevent the depression of the response to 5-HT depressed by a deactivator (Figure 2). A plausible analysis of a possible mechanism for the R ⇌ R' interconversion is given below.

The ability of a ligand to stabilise the R-state is not necessarily related to its affinity for the 5-HT₂ receptor. The rank order of some ligands in stabilising the R-state is ICI 169,369 > ketanserin > ICI 170,809 > (+)-LSD > LY 53857* > methysergide > ritanserin. (For data on LY 53857 and (+)-LSD see [11], for ritanserin data see [11, 15]). On the other hand, the rank order of the affinity for the 5-HT₂ receptor, estimated from competitive antagonism ($-\log M$ K_B values between parentheses; see also Table 1) is ICI 170,809 (10.0 $-$ 10.4) > ketanserin (9.4 $-$ 9.5) > ICI 169,369 (8.8 $-$ 9.1) > methysergide (8.3, [20]).

The rank order for depressing maximum responses to 5-HT in calf coronary artery and rat tail artery is ritanserin > methysergide > LY 53857 > (+)-LSD > ICI 170,809 > ketanserin (Table 2). High 5-HT concentrations (> 10 μM) cause slow contractions in the presence of ritanserin, methysergide or LY 53857.

Tryptamine [21] and (+)-LSD [11] have both agonistic and deactivating properties in calf coronary artery. Tryptamine causes both fast and slow contractions and depresses the maximum response to 5-HT.

---

* LY 53857 is (4-isopropyl-7-methyl-9-hydroxy-1-methylpropoxycarboxyl) 4,6,6A,7,8,9, 10,10A-octahydroindole-(4,3-FG) quinoline [19]

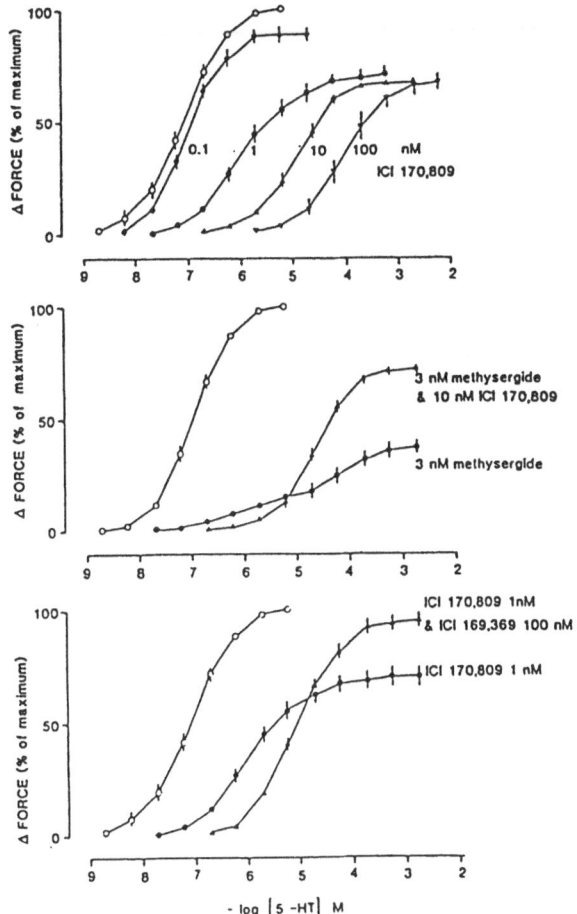

Figure 2. Interactions of 5-HT, the deactivators ICI 170,809 and methysergide, and the activator ICI 169,369 with the 5-HT₂ receptor system for calf coronary artery (adapted from [17]). The antagonists were incubated at least for 2 h before starting a concentration-effect curve for 5-HT.

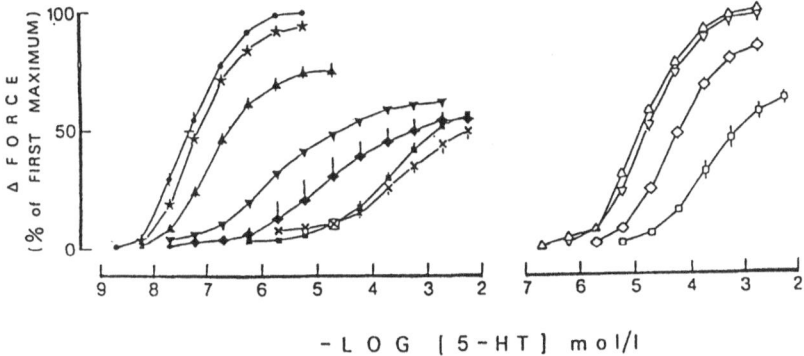

Figure 3. Unsurmountable antagonism by methysergide (left panel). Prevention by ketanserin 100 nM of methysergide-induced depression of the response to 5-HT (right panel). Experiments on rat tail artery [15]. Methysergide (nM): ★0.1, ▲△1, ▼▽10, ◆◇100, ■□1000, × 10000. Open symbols are in the presence of 100 nM ketanserin.

Table 2. 5-HT$_2$ receptor deactivators.

Tissue	Ligand	max %[a]	−log IC$_{50}$ (M)[b]	−log K$_B$ (M)[c]	Reference
Calf coronary artery	Ritanserin	> 85	8.9	d	[15]
Rat tail artery	Ritanserin	70	9.3	d	[15]
Calf coronary artery	Methysergide	70	9.8	d	[1]
Rat tail artery	Methysergide	40	9.0	> 8.0[e]	[15]
Guinea-pig trachea	Methysergide	80	> 9.0	d	[13]
Guinea-pig trachea	Ketanserin	40	~ 9.5	9.6	[13]
Calf coronary artery	ICI 170,809	35	~ 9.5	10.4	[17]

[a]   − Maximum depression of the maximum response to 5-HT
[b]   IC$_{50}$ = Concentration of deactivator that causes half maximum depression of the maximum response to 5-HT
[c]   K$_B$ = Equilibrium dissociation constant, estimated from competitive antagonism
[d]   − A component of competitive antagonism was not detected
[e]   − Competitive antagonism between $10^{-8} - 10^{-6}$ M but not at 10^{-5} M methysergide

Whether the 5-HT$_2$ component of the 5-HT-induced contractions in human coronary artery is also allosterically modulated has yet to be established.

4. Analysis of a formal model for allosteric modulation of 5-HT$_2$ receptors

Kaumann and Frenken [1, 12] have proposed that the 5-HT$_2$ receptor of various arterial tissues can exist and interact with 5-HT in two interconvertible forms, one highly active (R-form) and the other a low active (R' form). The R-state mediates fast contractions of 5-HT and the R'-state mediates slow contractions at high 5-HT concentrations. They proposed that agents can modulate the interconversion of the receptor between these two forms, agents classed as deactivators favouring the R' form and activators favouring the R form [4, 11, 15, 18, 21, 22].

To assess whether the experimental data could be consistent with this proposal we have carried out a formal kinetic analysis of a simple reaction scheme embodying the main features of this proposal. This scheme, shown in figure 4, has two reaction sites. One (shown in panel (i)) is the 5-HT receptor itself existing in two interconvertible forms, R and R'. Each of these is assumed to mediate force generation when 5-HT (shown as S in Figure 4) binds, with the dissociation constant K$_1$ to the R form and K$_2$ to the R' form. Deactivators (shown as D) and activators (shown as A) are known to compete with 5-HT with dissociation constants (K$_4$ and K$_5$ respectively in panel (i)) for which values have been determined experimentally (K$_B$ values in Tables 1, 2). For simplicity, these interactions are assumed to occur only

(i) 5 – HT – binding site (R,R^I)

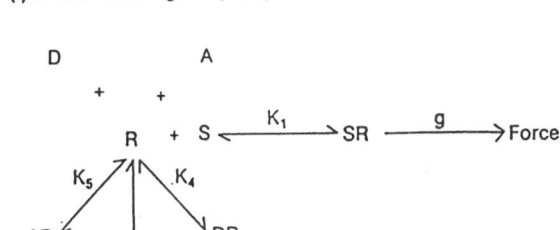

·(ii) Allosteric site (E)

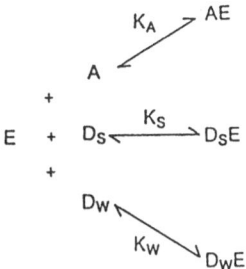

Figure 4. A two-state model for the 5-HT$_2$ receptor system.

with the R form of the receptor. In the absence of an added deactivator or activator it is assumed that the receptor is almost entirely in the R form and for this condition endogenous rate constants have been assigned for k_{-3} and k_{+3} respectively, giving an endogenous dissociation constant for the R to R′ interconversion (K_3) of 10000. This interconversion is assumed to be fully reversible. The mechanism by which activators and deactivators modulate the interconversion between R and R′ is assumed to occur through interactions of these agents with another (allosteric) site (designated E) associated with the 5-HT receptor, altering the value of the rate constant k_{+3}. These interactions are defined in panel (ii) of Figure 4. Interactions involving weak (shown as D_w) and strong (D_s) deactivators as well as an activator (A) are shown separately. k_{+3} is assumed to be proportional to the concentrations [ED$_w$] and [ED$_s$] with proportionality constants, f_w and f_s respectively having a value of 1 for a full deactivator and between 0 and 1 for a weak deactivator. An example of a strong deactivator is methysergide in calf coronary artery [1]; a weak deactivator is ketanserin in guinea-pig trachea [13, 14]. In this model, activators have been assumed simply to compete with deactivators at site E, to produce an inactive complex [AE] and to have no effect on the conversion in the R′ to R direction via changes in k_{-3}. These assumptions were made since there is no evidence that activators can increase 5-HT-induced contractions in the absence of a deactivator.

Considering panel (i), the total amount of the R receptor, $[R^{tot}]$, is given by the expression:

$$[R^{tot}] = [R] + [R'] + [SR] + [SR'] + [AR] + [DR] \tag{1}$$

$[R']$, $[SR]$, $[SR']$, $[AR]$ and $[DR]$ can each be expressed in terms of $[R]$ and the appropriate dissociation constant so that equation (1), on rearrangement, can be rewritten as:

$$[R] = [R^{tot}]/L \tag{2}$$

where L is $(1 + 1/K_3 + [S]/K_1 + [S]/K_2K_3 + [D]/K_4 + [A]/K_5)$

Force generation is given by the expression:

$$\text{Force} = g.[SR] + g'[SR'] \tag{3}$$

where g and g' are transduction functions. Combining equations (2) and (3), the expression for force is given by:

$$\text{Force} = [R^{tot}] (g.[S]/K_1 + g'[S]/K_2K_3)/L \tag{4}$$

A similar analysis of the scheme in panel (ii) yields the following expression for k_{+3}:

$$k_{+3} = N + P(f_s[D_s]/K_s + f_w[D_w]/K_w)/M \tag{5}$$

where M is $(1 + [A]/K_A + [D_w]/K_w + [D_s]/K_s)$, N is the endogenous rate constant for conversion of R to R' and P is a constant of proportionality. K_3 is then given by dividing k_{-3}, the endogenous rate constant for conversion of R' to R, by the expression in equation (5). We have assumed that during an experiment the system remains constant except for changes described by the model.

Attempts to simulate experimental data with this model were carried out using a Tandon computer with a program written in BASIC. In order to do this, values had to be assigned to the constants in these equations. Some of these had been determined experimentally, e.g. K_1, K_4, K_5. Most of the others were chosen to produce the best fit to all the data available. In most cases, only a small range of values yielded a reasonable fit, being constrained by data in more than one experiment and using more than one modulating agent. The choice of transduction functions g and g' was also determined empirically. However, choice was constrained somewhat by the rather surprising result that whatever affinities were assigned to the R and R' forms, the two forms have identical *overall* affinities when the whole scheme is considered, i.e. for both R and R' the concentration of 5-HT giving half maximal receptor occupancy is:

$$5\text{-HT}_{0.5} = K_1.K_2.(1 + K_3)/(K_1 + K_2.K_3). \tag{6}$$

This meant that with simple proportionality constants for g and g', the model was unable to generate force-5HT response curves showing the combination of high and low affinity responses observed in experiments. g' was therefore chosen to depend on 5-HT concentration in a Michaelis-Menten type dependency, i.e.

$$g' = G.[S]/([S] + K_g) \qquad (7)$$

where the values of K_g and G were determined empirically to give the best fit to the data. In view of the results in equation (6), K_1 and K_2 were assigned the same value in the simulation process. The values for the scheme constants giving the best fit of the model to the experimental data for rat tail artery and calf coronary artery are summarised in Table 3.

Table 3. Constants used in simulations (model shown in Figure 4).

		Calf coronary artery	Rat tail artery
Constants for 5-HT site:			
K_1	(nM)	100	100
K_2	(nM)	100	100
K_4	Methysergide (nM)	0.4	0.4
	Ketanserin (nM)	—	0.398
	ICI 170,809 (nM)	0.0398	—
K_5	ICI 169,369 (nM)	1.0	—
Constants for allosteric site:			
K_S	Methysergide (nM)	0.6	4.0
f_S	Methysergide	1	0.17
K_W	Ketanserin (nM)	—	0.7
f_W	Ketanserin	—	0.005
K_W	ICI 170,809 (nM)	0.1	—
f_W	ICI 170,809	0.075	—
K_A	ICI 169,369 (nM)	0.5	—
Other constants:			
R^{tot}		100	100
N		1	1
P		100,000	100,000
k_{-3}		10,000	10,000
g		1	1
G		0.25	0.25
k_g		10,000	20,000

Figures 5—9 compare experimental results and simulations.

The results with the partial deactivator ICI 170,809 on calf coronary artery (Figure 2, top panel) are simulated in Figure 5. The simulated concentration-effect curves for 5-HT in the presence of 1, 10 and 100 nM ICI 170,809 reasonably reproduced the experimental curves. The simulated curve for 5-HT in the presence of 0.1 nM ICI 170,809 showed a slightly greater rightward shift than the experimental curve. A possible reason for

Contractile force vs 5–HT concentration

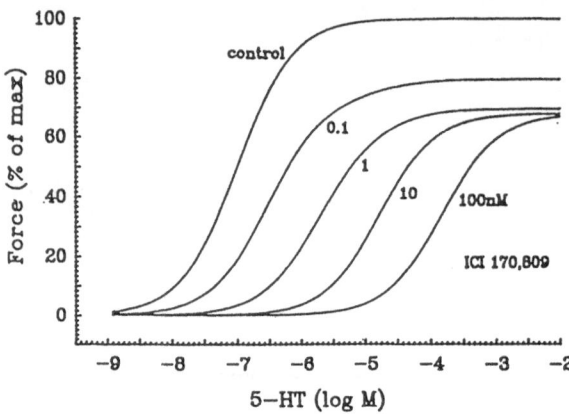

Figure 5. Simulation of the experiments of Figure 2 (top panel).

Contractile force vs 5–HT concentration

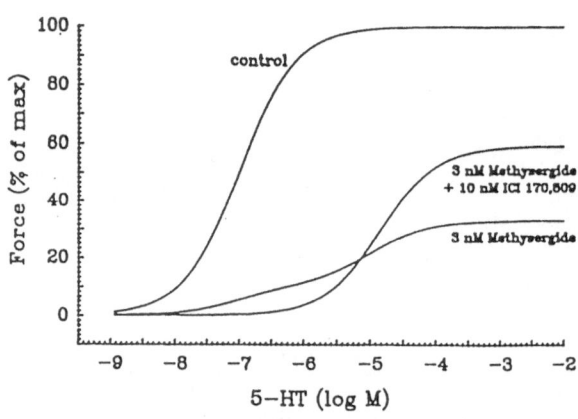

Figure 6. Simulation of the experiment of Figure 2 (middle panel).

this discrepancy is that at this low concentration, ICI 170,809 may not have been at equilibrium despite the long incubation time (150 minutes).

ICI 170,809 is a partial activator with respect to the deactivator methysergide because it partially prevents the depression of the maximum response to 5-HT (Figure 2 middle panel). The activator ICI 169,369 prevents the depression caused by ICI 170,809 (Figure 2 bottom panel). These two situations, observed in calf coronary artery, were satisfactorily simulated in Figures 6 and 7.

The results with the deactivator methysergide on rat tail artery (Figure 3, left panel) are reasonably well simulated with the exception of the effect of 10,000 nM methysergide which caused less blockade than predicted by the

Contractile force vs 5-HT concentration

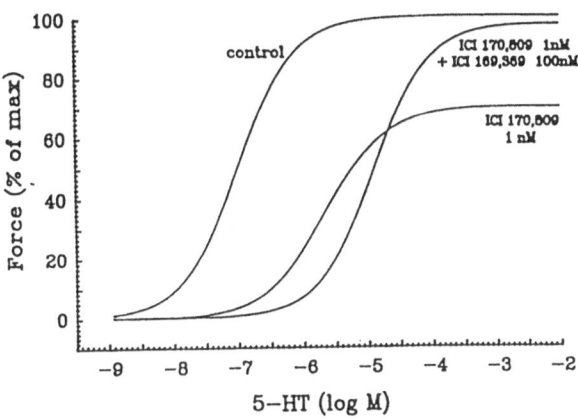

Figure 7. Simulation of the experiment of Figure 2 (bottom panel).

Contractile force vs 5-HT concentration

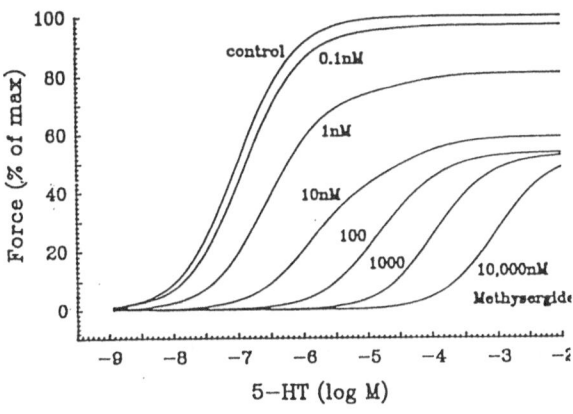

Figure 8. Simulation of the experiment of Figure 3 (left panel)

model (Figure 8). A plausible reason for this discrepancy could be that high 5-HT concentrations cause an effect not mediated through 5-HT$_2$ receptors (i.e. not blockable by methysergide). Instead, the methysergide-resistant effect of 5-HT could be mediated through α_1-adrenoceptors (see [6, 22] for references). The experiments of Figure 3 (right panel), showing that 100 nM ketanserin prevents the depression of the 5-HT responses caused by 1 and 10 nM methysergide, are reasonably well simulated in Figure 9.

The constants used in the simulations are shown in Table 3. A K$_1$ = K$_2$ value of 100 nM for 5-HT was chosen for convenience because it avoids the need to incorporate the modest spare receptor reserve into the model. In order to generate responses with a low apparent affinity for 5-HT, the model

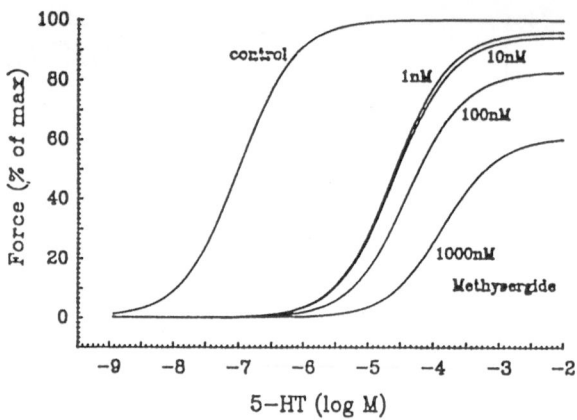

Figure 9. Simulation of the experiment of Figure 3 (right panel plus control curve for 5-HT).

assumes a difference in the transduction functions for R and R'. Thus, while contractile effects of 5-HT are merely proportional to receptor occupancy of R, R' is causing slow responses via the transduction function of equation (7). The biochemical implications would be that either R' is partially uncoupled from the biochemical cascade leading to contractile force compared to R or, alternatively, biochemical events caused by the 2 states are qualitatively different. There is circumstantial evidence consistent with a role of inositol 1,4,5 triphosphate in the 5-HT_2 receptor-mediated effects of 5-HT through the R-state in smooth muscle [23, 24]. The slow response to 5-HT resembles that produced by phorbol esters in arterial muscle [25] suggesting that protein kinase C could also be involved [11].

The experimental dissociation constants of ICI 170,809 and ICI 169,369 for the R-state resemble the corresponding constants for the allosteric site obtained from the model, suggesting that the allosteric site resembles the 5-HT receptor. The affinity estimates for methysergide also match for the R-state and allosteric site in calf coronary artery. However there is a 10-fold discrepancy in rat tail artery, which somewhat weakens the above suggestion. It should be pointed out, however, that the model is insensitive to the value of K_4 for methysergide in calf coronary and that more experiments and simulations are needed to understand the mode of action of methysergide.

Methysergide at low concentrations has a 36-fold greater ability to interconvert the receptor into the R'-state on calf coronary than on rat tail artery due to a greater value of f_s and lower K_s (see Table 3). Thus, the R $\rightleftharpoons$ R' interconversion could be species or tissue-dependent. (Preliminary experiments also suggest that it may be temperature dependent).

Lemoine and Teng [26] have recently reported experiments on the effects of methysergide and ICI 169,369 on rat tail artery in the presence of prazosin to block α-adrenoceptors. These essentially confirmed the findings by Frenken and Kaumann [15]. Lemoine and Teng also analysed their data with an allosteric model whose basic format appears to be similar to ours described here. They assumed two binding domains. At one (A), equivalent to our 5-HT binding site, 5-HT, methysergide and ICI 169,369 compete. At the second (allosteric) site, methysergide and ICI 169,369 compete and binding of methysergide causes a change in the state of domain A equivalent to the $R \rightleftharpoons R'$ conversion proposed by Kaumann and Frenken [1]. A good fit of this model to their data for rat tail was obtained with pK values of 9 and 9.4 for methysergide at the 5-HT and allosteric sites respectively and pK values of 8.4 for ICI 169,369 at both sites.

Table 3 (above) shows that we obtained with our model rather similar values for the affinities of methysergide at the 5-HT and allosteric sites on rat tail artery (pKs about 9.4, 8.4). We have not used the model to estimate the effects of ICI 169,369 on rat tail artery. However, on calf coronary artery, we obtained values of 9.4 and 9.2 for methysergide and 9.0 and 9.3 for ICI 169,369 at the 5-HT and allosteric sites respectively. The discrepancy between our findings and those of Lemoine and Teng probably reflects, in part, differences between tissues (see eg Table 3) and the presence of prazosin in their experiments. However, it also probably reflects important differences between the two models in the way the influence of the allosteric site on the 5-HT site is defined (simple Michaelis-Menten dependence on methysergide concentrations in Lemoine and Teng's model; equation 5 in our model) and in the transfer functions associated with R and R' [not stated by Lemoine and Teng; g and g' (equation 7) in our scheme]. The more complicated formulations we adopted were required in order to simulate, with a single model, experiments with agents of varying relative potency as deactivators and also the properties of calf coronary artery where methysergide produced a marked rightward broadening of the 5-HT concentration-effect curve (see eg Figure 2) which appears not prazosin-sensitive [6].

It is also worth noting that our present model fits the experimental data better than a simpler model based on classical, but time-dependent, competitive interactions between 5-HT, and "activators" and "deactivators". In such a model, the insurmountability of a deactivator like methysergide is only apparent, reflecting very slow dissociation together with relatively rapid equilibration of 5-HT with the same binding sites during a cumulative dose-response curve.

We have analysed such an "incomplete equilibrium" model [27] and found that it can indeed simulate some of the effects of deactivators and activators on 5-HT-induced tension. Thus, preincubation of the 5-HT binding sites with a slowly associating/dissociating deactivator results in some binding of that ligand to the 5-HT sites. If a concentration-effect curve to 5-HT is then performed relatively fast (i.e. so that deactivator binding cannot completely re-equilibrate at each 5-HT concentration), there is a depression of the maximum response to 5-HT ($Resp_{max}$) which depends on deactivator concentration (as in Figure 3 above, left panel). This effect is prevented by the simultaneous presence of a rapidly-equilibrating activator during the preincubation (as in Figure 3, right panel). However, in three respects this model is quantitatively inconsistent with experimental observations. High deactivator concentrations completely, rather than partly, abolish the response to 5-HT. The dependence of $Resp_{max}$ on log[Deactivator] is much too steep. The rightward shift in the 5-HT dose-response curve produced by the deactivator is at least 10-fold less than that observed with the same depression of $Resp_{max}$.

5. Conclusion

We have analysed the role and properties of some arterial $5\text{-}HT_2$ receptors. Human coronary artery has both $5\text{-}HT_2$ receptors and non-$5\text{-}HT_2$ receptors. 5-HT-induced contractions are mediated predominantly by $5\text{-}HT_2$ receptors in non-atheromatous artery. In atheromatous coronary artery, on the other hand, 5-HT-induced contractions appear to be mediated mainly by non-$5\text{-}HT_2$ receptors.

In calf coronary artery and rat tail artery, 5-HT-induced contractions are mediated mainly by $5\text{-}HT_2$ receptors. Some antagonists cause surmountable and simple competitive blockade. Other antagonists, designated deactivators, cause blockade that can be only partially surmounted by 5-HT. Several competitive surmountable antagonists, designated activators, can reverse or prevent the depression of maximum 5-HT induced contractions caused by deactivators. A two-state $R \rightleftharpoons R'$ system, that is allosterically modulated, has been proposed for the interactions of 5-HT, activators and deactivators with the $5\text{-}HT_2$ receptor by Kaumann and Frenken [1]. Fast and slow 5-HT responses are assumed to be mediated by R and R' respectively.

We have now formalised this system by assuming that the conversion of R into R' is facilitated by the association of deactivators with the allosteric site. Activators are assumed to act simply by preventing the association of deactivators with the allosteric site. Some ligands are assumed to act both at the allosteric site, as partial deactivators, and also to compete with 5-HT for the R state of the receptor. With appropriate choice of parameters, concentration-effect curves for 5-HT and their modifications by activators and deactivators were satisfactorily simulated with the above assumptions.

This model predicts that the overall affinities of 5-HT for R and R' are the same, suggesting that the R' state is less efficiently coupled to a biochemical cascade than is the R state. Alternatively, cascades activated by occupied R and R' may be different. The parameters obtained by fitting the model to experimental data yield similar affinities of a partial deactivator for the allosteric site and for the R-state, suggesting that the allosteric site resembles the receptor or is part of it. The 5-HT_2 receptors of rat tail artery appear more resistant to conversion from R into R' than the 5-HT_2 receptors of calf coronary artery. Recently Connor et al. [29] have confirmed the co-participation of 5-HT_2 and non-5-HT_2 receptors in 5-HT-induced contraction in human coronary artery.

Acknowledgement

We are grateful to colleagues of the Surgical Unit at Papworth Hospital, Everard, for providing human heart tissue.

References

1. Kaumann AJ, Frenken M (1985): A paradox: the 5-HT_2 receptor antagonist ketanserin restores the 5-HT-induced contraction depressed by methysergide in large coronary arteries of calf. Allosteric regulation of 5-HT_2 receptors. *Naunyn-Schmiedeberg's Arch Pharmacol* 328: 295—300.
2. Peroutka SJ, Snyder SH (1979): Multiple serotonin receptors: Differential binding of [³H]-5-hydroxytryptamine [³H]lysergic acid diethylamide and [³H]-spiroperidol. *Mol Pharmacol* 16: 687—699.
3. Clancy M, Maayani S (1985): 5-Hydroxytryptamine receptor in isolated rabbit aorta. Characterisation with tryptamine analogs. *J Pharmacol Exp Ther* 233: 761—769.
4. Frenken M, Kaumann AJ (1987): Interconversion into a low active state protects vascular 5-HT_2 receptors against irreversible antagonism by phenoxybenzamine. *Naunyn-Schmiedeberg's Arch Pharmacol* 335: 481—490.
5. Van Nueten JM, Janssen PAJ, van Beck J, Xhonneux R, Verbeuren TJ, Vanhoutte PM (1981): Vascular effects of ketanserin (R 41468), a novel antagonist of 5-HT_2 serotonergic receptors. *J Pharmacol Exp Ther* 218: 217—230.
6. Kaumann AJ (1983): Yohimbine and rauwolscine inhibit 5-HT_2 receptors. *Naunyn-Schmiedeberg's Arch Pharmacol* 333: 149—154.
7. Freedman SB, Chierchia S, Rodriguez-Plaza L, Burgiardini R, Smith G, Maseri A (1984): Ergonovine-induced myocardial ischaemia: no role for serotonergic receptors? *Circulation* 70, 178—183.
8. Frenken M, Kaumann AJ (1985): Ketanserin causes surmountable antagonism of 5-hydroxytryptamine-induced contractions in large coronary arteries of dog. *Naunyn-Schmiedeberg's Arch Pharmacol* 328: 301—303.
9. Frenken M, Kaumann AJ (1986): Surmountable antagonism by ketanserin of 5-hydroxy-tryptamine-induced contractions in dog basilar artery. *Br J Pharmac* 89: 550P.
10. Gaddum JH, Hameed KA (1954): Drugs which antagonize 5-hydroxytryptamine. *Br J Pharmac* 9: 240—248.
11. Kaumann AJ (1989): The allosteric 5-HT_2 receptor system, in: Fozard J (ed) *The peripheral actions of 5-hydroxytryptamine.* Oxford University Press pp. 45—71.
12. Kaumann AJ, Frenken M (1988): ICI 169,369 is both a competitive antagonist and an allosteric activator of the arterial 5-hydroxytryptamine₂ receptor system. *J Pharmacol Exp Ther* 245: 1010—1015.
13. Lemoine H, Kaumann AJ (1986): Allosteric properties of 5-HT_2 receptors in tracheal smooth muscle. *Naunyn-Schmiedeberg's Arch Pharmacol* 333: 91—97.
14. Sampford KA, Kaumann AJ (1988): ICI 169,369 is both a competitive antagonist and activator of the 5-HT_2 receptor system of guinea-pig trachea. *Br J Pharmacol* 95: 775P.

15. Frenken M, Kaumann AJ (1987): Allosteric properties of the 5-HT$_2$ receptor system of the rat tail artery — Ritanserin and methysergide are not competitive 5-HT$_2$ receptor antagonists but allosteric modulators. *Naunyn-Schmiedeberg's Arch Pharmacol* 335: 359—366.

16. Blackburn TP, Thornber CW, Pearce RJ, Cox B (1988): In vitro pharmacology of ICI 170,809 — a new 5-HT$_2$ antagonist. Abstract. *FASEB Journal* 5(2): A 1404.

17. Frenken M, Kaumann AJ (1989): Dimethylation of the activator ICI 169,369 results in a high-affinity partial deactivator, ICI 170,809, of the arterial 5-HT$_2$ receptor system. *J Pharmacol Exp Ther* 250: 707—713.

18. Kaumann AJ (1987): A two-state model for the 5-HT$_2$ receptor. *Biol Chem Hoppe-Seyler* 368: 1131—1132.

19. Cohen ML, Fuller RW, Kurz KD (1983): LY 53857, a selective and potent serotonergic (5-HT$_2$) receptor antagonist does not lower blood pressure in spontaneously hypertensive rat. *J Pharmacol Exp Ther* 227: 327—332.

20. Barrett VJ, Leff P, Martin GR, Richardson PJ (1986): Pharmacological analysis of the interaction between Bay K8644 and 5-HT in rabbit aorta. *Br J Pharmac* 87: 487—494.

21. Frenken M, Kaumann AJ (1988): Effects of tryptamine mediated through 2 states of the 5-HT$_2$ receptor in calf coronary artery. *Naunyn-Schmiedeberg's Arch Pharmacol* 337: 484—492.

22. Kaumann AJ (1988): A two-state model for the 5-HT$_2$ receptor: Effects of α-adrenoceptor ligands. *J Cardiovasc Pharmacol* 11 (suppl 1): S88—S92.

23. Doyle VM, Creba JA, Ruegg UT, Hoyer D (1986): Serotonin increases production of inositol phosphates and mobilises calcium via the 5-HT$_2$ receptor in A$_7$r$_5$ smooth muscle cells. *Naunyn-Schmiedeberg's Arch Pharmacol* 333: 98—103.

24. Lemoine H, Pohl V, Teng KJ (1988): Serotonin (5-HT) stimulates phosphatidyl inositol (P$_i$) hydrolysis only through the R-state of allosterically regulated 5-HT$_2$ receptors in calf tracheal smooth muscle. *Naunyn-Schmiedeberg's Arch Pharmacol* 337: R103.

25. Nakaki T, Roth BL, Chuang DM, Costa E (1985): Phasic and tonic components in 5-HT$_2$ receptor-mediated rat aorta contraction. Participation of Ca^{++} channels and phospholipase C. *J Pharmacol Exp Ther* 234: 442—446.

26. Lemoine H, Teng KJ (1989): A mathematical model describing the allosteric regulation of peripheral 5-HT$_2$-receptors. *Naunyn-Schmiedeberg's Arch Pharmacol* 339: R97.

27. Kaumann AJ, Brown AM (1989): Differences between allosterism and incomplete equilibrium in the 5-HT$_2$ system. *Naunyn-Schmiedeberg's Arch Pharmacol* 339: R97.

28. Frenken M, Kaumann AJ (1984): Interaction of ketanserin and its metabolite ketanserinol with 5-HT$_2$-receptors in pulmonary and coronary arteries of calf. *Naunyn-Schmiedeberg's Arch Pharmacol* 326: 334—339.

29. Connor HE, Feniuk W, Humphrey PPA (1989): 5-Hydroxytryptamine contracts human coronary arteries predominantly via 5-HT$_2$ receptor activation. *Eur J Pharmacol* 161: 91—94.

XI. An analysis of unsurmountable antagonism to 5-hydroxytryptamine in the isolated perfused rat kidney: evidence for pseudoirreversible inhibition

D. A. CRAIG, A. G. ORNSTEIN and D. E. CLARKE

1. Introduction

Many 5-hydroxytryptamine (5-HT) antagonists give rise to unsurmountable antagonism. Unlike competitive antagonism, unsurmountable antagonism is not limited to a single mechanism, and therefore its utility for receptor identification, characterization, and classification is at best limited. In general, however, the mechanistic bases of unsurmountable antagonism have not received rigorous attention. The objectives of this chapter are to document instances of unsurmountable antagonism, to discuss possible mechanisms involved, and to present data suggesting that pseudoirreversible antagonism best explains unsurmountable antagonism of 5-HT-induced vasoconstriction in the isolated perfused rat kidney. Finally, the utility of antagonist probes for receptor classification will be discussed.

Unsurmountable antagonism describes antagonism in which the inhibitory effects of the antagonist cannot be overcome by increasing the agonist concentration [1]. The concentration-effect curves to the agonist are rotated dextrally, and the maximum response is reduced.

2. Occurrence of unsurmountable antagonism

Table 1 lists selected examples of 5-HT receptor antagonists which have been reported to exhibit unsurmountable antagonism. For comparison, examples of competitive interactions for these drugs are also given. From the drugs and tissues presented, it can be seen that all three 5-HT receptor subtypes (5-HT$_1$-like, 5-HT$_2$ and 5-HT$_3$), as defined by Bradley et al. [2], express unsurmountable antagonism. The occurrence of unsurmountable antagonism is seen to be high with some drugs (e.g. cyproheptadine), whereas competitive kinetics is displayed most frequently by others (e.g. trazodone). In general, high affinity at 5-HT receptors is associated with the expression of unsurmountable antagonism. Likewise, unsurmountable antagonism seems to

P.R. Saxena, D.I. Wallis, W. Wouters and P. Bevan (eds), Cardiovascular Pharmacology of 5-Hydroxytryptamine, pp. 143—155.
© 1990 *Kluwer Academic Publishers. Dordrecht* —

Table 1. Drug antagonism toward 5-HT in several tissues.

Drug	Antagonism	Tissue[a–n]	Reference
Lysergide (LSD)	Unsurmountable	a, b	1, 4
	Competitive	—	
Methysergide	Unsurmountable	a, c, e—i, k—m	3, 5, 9, 13—16, 18, 19, 21
	Competitve	b, d, h, i	4, 7, 8, 10, 11, 17
Trazodone	Unsurmountable	d	8
	Competitive	a—c, g, h	3, 4, 5, 10
			19, 21
Cyproheptadine	Unsurmountable	d, i—m	5, 7, 8, 14, 16, 18,
	Competitive	b	11, 20
Ketanserin	Unsurmountable	a, d, h, j	5, 8, 10, 16
	Competitive	b, e—h	5, 9, 10, 12, 17
Metergoline	Unsurmountable	i, m	13, 21
	Competitive	c	6
ICS 205—930	Unsurmountable	n	22, 23
	Competitive	n	24

[a–n] a, rat uterus; b, rabbit aorta; c, rat stomach fundus; d, canine coronary artery; e, calf coronary artery; f, calf pulmonary artery; g, rabbit jugular vein; h, rat caudal arteries; i, canine basilar artery; j, rat kidney (vasoconsriction); k, canine saphenous vein; l, rabbit jugular vein (endothelial cells); m, human basilar artery; n, vagus nerve or ganglia (nodose, superior cervical).

be associated more frequently with some tissues (e.g. coronary and basilar arteries), whereas competitive antagonism appears most often in others (e.g. rabbit aorta). Thus, the expression of unsurmountable antagonism appears to involve both ligand and tissue determinants.

3. Mechanisms of unsurmountable antagonism

Figure 1 illustrates three mechanisms of unsurmountable antagonism which are of current interest and which may operate in functional pharmacological studies.

Multiple receptor sites for 5-HT in tissues may lead to unsurmountable antagonism when the antagonist binds selectively or preferentially to one particular receptor subtype. For example, contraction of isolated blood vessels by 5-HT may occur as the resultant of contraction and relaxation (e.g. endothelium-dependent relaxation). Antagonism toward the contractile response will give depressed concentration-effect curves to 5-HT and the expression of unsurmountable antagonism. The concept of multiple receptor sites as a possible reason for unsurmountable antagonism has been raised by Feniuk [5] and Bradley et al. [2].

Pseudoirreversible antagonism describes the situation in which the disso-

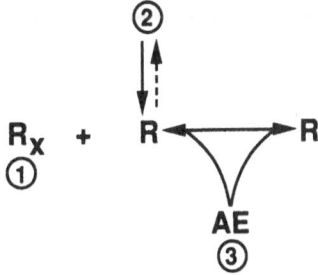

Figure 1. Some mechanisms of unsurmountable antagonism: 1. Multiple receptors for 5-HT. One or more receptors (R_x) for 5-HT may exist which oppose the response elicited by the 5-HT receptor of interest (R). A selective or preferential affinity of an antagonist for R may lead to the expression of unsurmountable antagonism. 2. Pseudoirreversible antagonism. The antagonist binds to the 5-HT receptor (R), but under the experimental conditions its slow dissociation rate constant ($\rightarrow$) prevents the expression of competitive kinetics. 3. Allosteric modulation. The antagonist may act at the allosteric effector (AE) site to promote a low affinity state of the 5-HT receptor (R′) and the expression of unsurmountable antagonism. (Other ligands at AE may promote the formation of R from R′, and act as competitive antagonists at R). See text for further details.

ciation rate constant of the antagonist from the receptor is slow, and as a consequence, the agonist and antagonist fail to reach equilibrium under the time constraints imposed experimentally. The available receptor pool for the agonist is diminished, and unsurmountable antagonism is expressed. In tissues exhibiting a receptor reserve for the agonist, parallel dextral shifts in the concentration-effect curve to the agonist will precede the expression of unsurmountable antagonism. Thus, behaviourally, pseudoirreversible anta-gonism may appear identical to irreversible antagonism. However, given enough time, pseudoirreversible antagonists will dissociate from the receptor, and equilibrium with the agonist will be reached. Even so, in functional systems, it is often impossible to measure protracted responses to the agonist due to the intervention of fade. The tissue component of fade (uncoupling of receptors, loss of agonist due to uptake) represents an important tissue factor predisposing preparations to the expression of unsurmountable antagonism, whereas the magnitude of the dissociation rate constant of the antagonist from the receptor is a drug determinant. Taylor et al. [13] have evoked pseudoirreversible antagonism to explain unsurmountable antagonism by metergoline toward 5-HT-induced contraction of canine basilar artery, and Doggrell [25] has used the same argument for unsurmountable antagonism toward 5-HT by ketanserin and mianserin in rat aorta.

Allosteric modulation of 5-HT receptors has been proposed recently by Kaumann and Frenken [26–29] and is discussed by Kaumann in this book [Chapter X]. As illustrated in Figure 1, the concept involves a change in the state of the 5-HT receptor via an allosteric effector site (receptor ?). In essence three interlinked sites are proposed: 1. A high affinity state of the 5-HT receptor (R), 2. A low affinity state of the 5-HT receptor (R′), 3. An allosteric effector site (AE). Theoretically, compounds may act at one or more of the three sites. Some 5-HT receptor antagonists are considered to act at AE to promote the R' form of the 5-HT receptor, thereby inducing unsurmountable antagonism when receptor reserve for the agonist is limited or absent. In contrast, other 5-HT receptor antagonists, which act as competitive antagonists at the R form, may also act at AE to promote the conversion of R' to the R form, thereby evoking the opposite effect of unsurmountable antagonists. Competitive antagonists may function, therefore, to reverse the effects of unsurmountable antagonists. De Chaffoy de Courcells et al. [30] have also proposed an allosteric model to explain unsurmountable antagonism at platelet 5-HT$_2$ receptors. Two binding sites are postulated (agonist and antagonist), and as with the Kaumann model, competitive inhibitors can displace unsurmountable antagonists and vice versa.

Intrinsically, allosteric models are more complex mechanistically than multiple receptors or pseudoirreversible inhibition as they depend upon changes in state of the 5-HT receptor and agonism by 5-HT antagonists at putative allosteric effector sites.

4. Unsurmountable antagonism in the isolated perfused rat kidney

The isolated perfused rat kidney gives dose-dependent vasoconstrictor responses to bolus injections of 5-HT, and this preparation has been utilized to analyze the mechanism or mechanisms of unsurmountable antagonism by 5-HT receptor antagonists [31].

4.1 Experimental

Briefly, kidneys were perfused at a constant rate (6 ml.min^{-1}) with Krebs solution (37°, pH 7.4), and perfusion pressure recorded. Cocaine (30 μM) was present in the Krebs solution to inhibit neuronal and extraneuronal uptake of 5-HT [26]. Exposure of kidneys to pargyline (100 μM for 30 min), followed by wash-out (30 min), did not affect the dose-effect curves to 5-HT. Therefore, this treatment was not used routinely. However, pargyline was utilized in experiments in which the relative potency of 5-HT and 5-HT analogues was measured, because the biophase concentration of non-polar analogues of 5-HT (e.g. tryptamine) has been shown to be limited by oxidative deamination [20]. Prazosin (0.1 μM) was also included in the Krebs solution in view of the direct and indirect actions of 5-HT at alpha-adrenoceptors [5, 6, 32]. In this regard it should be noted that vasoconstriction to norepinephrine in the isolated perfused rat kidney is mediated by alpha$_1$-adrenoceptors [16, 31]. Under control conditions, prazosin (0.1 μM) did not affect the dose-response curve to 5-HT. However, prazosin was retained in the Krebs solution to guard against alpha$_1$-adrenoceptor agonism with higher doses of 5-HT, such as would be required to overcome dextral shifts with antagonists. Also, some analogues of 5-HT exhibit agonism at alpha-adrenoceptors [20].

4.2   *Unsurmountable versus competitive antagonism*

Experiments with seven 5-HT receptor antagonists gave results consistent with unsurmountable antagonism in that the dose-effect curves to 5-HT were rotated dextrally and the maximum responses were reduced. No parallel shift in the dose-response curves to 5-HT preceeded these changes. The following compounds, listed with their respective IC$_{50}$ values (concentration producing 50% reduction in the maximum response to 5-HT), behaved as unsurmountable antagonists: metergoline (0.07 nM); methiothepin (0.08 nM); cyproheptadine (0.5 nM); methysergide (2.0 nM); ketanserin (3.2 nM); mesulergine (3.2 nM); and spiroperidol (4.9 nM). Dose-effect curves to 5-HT in the absence and presence of metergoline (0.03 − 1 nM) are shown in Figure 2. In contrast, (−)-propranolol acted as a competitive antagonist in

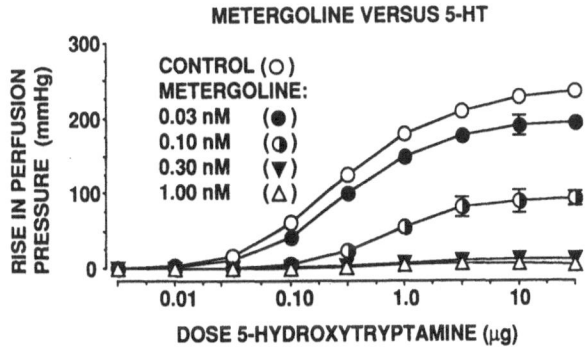

Figure 2. The effect of metergoline on the dose-effect curve to 5-HT in the isolated perfused rat kidney. A control dose-effect curve to 5-HT was constructed in each kidney before perfusion with metergoline. A second dose-effect curve to 5-HT was commenced 1 hr after the start of perfusion with metergoline. The number of kidneys studied is as follows: control (n = 17); metergoline, 0.03 nM (n = 4); 0.1 nM (n = 4); 0.3 nM (n = 6); 1.0 nM (n = 3). Each point is the mean value ± SE and is only illustrated where larger than the symbol. (Figure from reference 31.)

that it evoked parallel, dextral shifts in the dose-effect curves to 5-HT without affecting the maximum response. A Schild regression of the data is shown in Figure 3. A pA$_2$ value for (−)-propranolol of 6.5 with a slope of 0.98 (95% confidence limits: 0.8−1.2) was computed.

148 D. A. Craig, A. G. Ornstein and D. E. Clarke

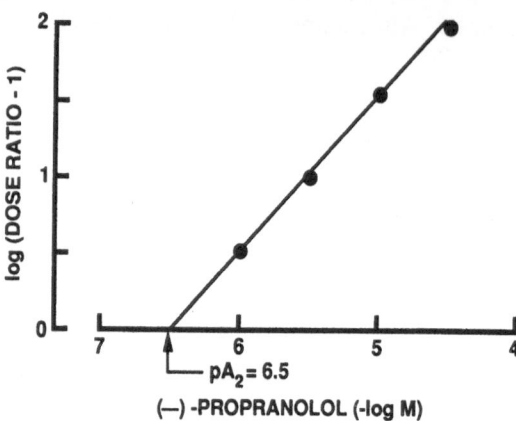

Figure 3. Arunlakshana and Schild [35] plot for (−)-propranolol versus 5-HT. (Figure from reference 31.)

4.3 *Multiple receptors*

Multiple receptor sites for 5-HT might explain unsurmountable antagonism with metergoline and the other antagonists. Although the interaction between (−)-propranolol and 5-HT obeyed competitive kinetics, suggesting the involvement of a single receptor population, it does not prove it. (−)-Propranolol might possess the same ratio of affinities as 5-HT for multiple sites. To explore further the possibility of multiple receptors, experiments were performed with analogues of 5-HT which discriminate between receptor subtypes. The following order and relativity of agonist potency was obtained: 5-HT (1.0) > 5-methoxytryptamine (5-MT) (0.5) > alpha-methyl-5-hydroxytryptamine (alpha-M-5-HT) (0.3) > tryptamine (T) (0.05) > 5-carboxamidotryptamine (5-CT) (0.01). In addition, (−)-propranolol gave the following pA_2 values versus the same agonists: 5-HT (6.45), 5-MT (6.52), alpha-M-5-HT (6.37), T (6.69), and 5-CT (6.2). Other experiments, using phenoxybenzamine, gave an estimated equilibrium dissociation constant for 5-HT of 185 nM, and a similar equilibrium dissociation constant (211 nM) was estimated using the 5-HT dose-effect curve depressed by metergoline (0.1 nM; Figure 2). Taken together, the results suggest the presence of a single receptor population for 5-HT-induced vasoconstriction in the isolated perfused kidney which fits criteria defining the 5-HT_2 subtype [2, 32].

4.4 *Pseudoirreversible antagonism versus allosteric receptor modulation*

Comparative time-course experiments with metergoline (0.1 nM) and (−)-propranolol (10 μM) revealed that metergoline behaved as a slow on-set, slow off-set antagonist toward 5-HT, whereas (−)-propranolol behaved as a fast on-set, fast off-set antagonist. With metergoline, 1 hr was required for inhibition of 5-HT responses to approach maximum, whereas inhibition of 5-HT responses with (−)-propranolol was maximal within 5 min. Similarly, inhibition by metergoline was not reversed fully by perfusion with drug-free Krebs solution for 1 hr (Figure 4), whereas less than 5 min was required to reverse completely the inhibitory effect of (−)-propranolol.

The fast on-set, fast off-set rate of (−)-propranolol is consistent with the expression of competitive antagonism in a perfused system, where the time for equilibration of 5-HT with its receptor is brief following bolus injection. With metergoline, however, its slow kinetics, coupled with the brief response time for 5-HT, suggests pseudoirreversible antagonism as the operative mechanism. Allosteric modulation for metergoline cannot be ruled out, but if operative, the onset is uncharacteristically slow for this type of modulatory mechanism. In addition, experiments with phenoxybenzamine demonstrated little or no receptor reserve for 5-HT. These data, and the apparent 'tight-binding' of metergoline, favour the expression of pseudoirreversible antagonism and militate against a role for allosteric modulation.

Other experiments demonstrated that (−)-propranolol (30 μM) can protect 5-HT responses from inhibition by metergoline (0.3 μM). However, these data may be interpreted either as evidence of 5-HT$_2$ receptor protection by (−)-propranolol or as evidence for protection at an allosteric effector site (Figure 1). Behaviourally, pseudoirreversible antagonism and allosteric modulation share much in common, and experimentally they are difficult to discriminate.

The experiment illustrated in Figure 4 was devised in a further attempt to distinguish between these two mechanisms. The results show that (−)-propranolol (3 μM), perfused in the presence of metergoline (0.1 nM), restored responses to 5-HT to the same extent as wash-out of metergoline with metergoline-free Krebs solution (compare Figure 4C with 4D). Furthermore, the dose-effect curve to 5-HT in the presence of both (−)-propranolol and metergoline is displaced dextrally and parallel to the wash-out curve. A pA$_2$ value of 6.57 for (−)-propranolol was calculated. A similar result was obtained when the experiment was repeated using a higher concentration of metergoline (0.3 μM), except that the magnitude of the 5-HT restorations by wash-out and (−)-propranolol (3 μM) were less. In this experiment, a pA$_2$ value of 6.65 for (−)-propranolol was calculated between the wash-out and (−)-propranolol/metergoline curves.

Figure 4 also shows that mechanisms other than, or additional to, simple agonism at 5-HT$_2$ receptors are operative with high doses of 5-HT (30 to 3000 μg). 5-HT analogues evoked the same pattern of responses and the

150   *D. A. Craig, A. G. Ornstein and D. E. Clarke*

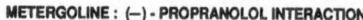

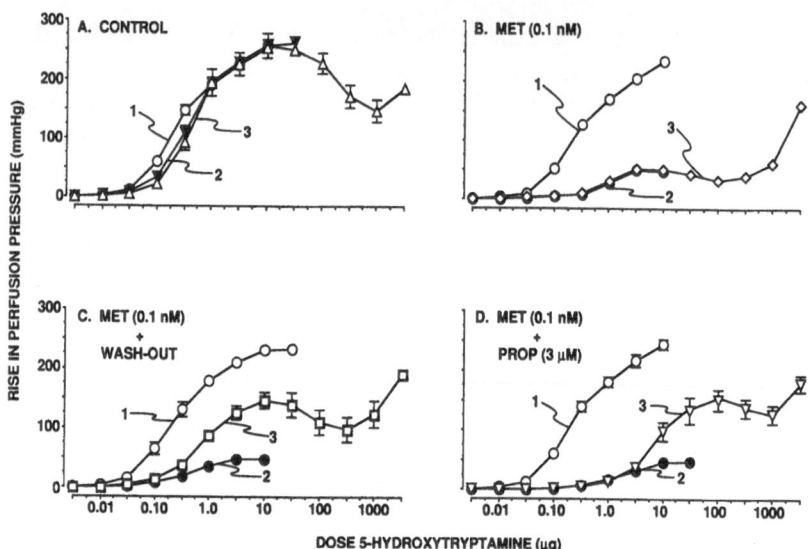

Figure 4. Interaction between metergoline (MET) and (—)-propranolol (PROP) on the dose-effect curve to 5-HT. A. Three control curves to 5-HT, with 1 hr intervals between curves. B. As in A, but MET (0.1 nM) was added to the perfusion fluid after completion of the first dose-effect curve to 5-HT. C. As in B, but MET (0.1 nM) was removed from the perfusion fluid after completion of the second dose-effect curve to 5-HT (wash-out). D. As in B, but PROP (3 μM) was added to the perfusion fluid after completion of the second dose-effect curve to 5-HT. The number of kidneys studied is as follows: A (n = 5), B (n = 6), C (n = 8) and D (n = 5). Each point is the mean value ± SE and is only illustrated where larger than the symbol. (Figure from reference 31.)

second phase of vasoconstriction occurred at the same doses as for 5-HT (1000 and 3000 μg). The mechanism or mechanisms of the second vasoconstrictor phase and the preceding diminished responsiveness to 5-HT, remain for determination. It is clear, however, that they are not induced by metergoline as a result of allosteric modulation [compare 26, 28, 29] because they are present in control preparations. The responses to 5-HT (1000—3000 μg) proved to be insensitive to metergoline (0.3 nM), (—)-propranolol (30 μM), prazosin (0.1 μM), phentolamine (10 μM) and phenoxybenzamine (1 μM for 15 min).

Figure 5 illustrates a third set of experiments in which wash-out of metergoline (0.1 nM) and its interaction with (—)-propranolol (3 μM) were studied. The key difference between this experiment and the previous experiment is that the dose-effect curves to 5-HT were commenced 5 min after the start of washing out the metergoline and 5 min after the start of the metergoline/(—)-propranolol interaction (instead of 60 min as illustrated in Figure 4). Neither wash-out of metergoline nor (—)-propranolol reversed the depressed responses to 5-HT. A pA$_2$ value for (—)-propranolol of 6.46 was calculated from the dose-ratio between the third curves in Figure 5A and 5B.

The simplest explanation for the results described is that metergoline acts

METERGOLINE : (−) - PROPRANOLOL INTERACTION

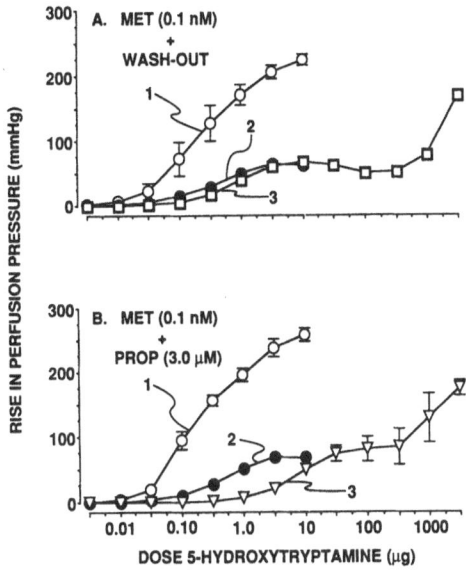

Figure 5. Interaction between metergoline (MET) and (−)-propranolol (PROP) on the dose-effect curve to 5-HT. A and B correspond to panels C and D, respectively, in figure 4, except that the third dose-effect curve to 5-HT was commenced 5 min (instead of 1 hr) after wash-out (panel A) and 5 min (instead of 1 hr) after the start of perfusion with (−)-propranolol (panel B). A (n = 3) and B (n = 3). Each point is the mean value ± SE and is only illustrated where larger than the symbol. (Figure from reference 31.)

as a pseudoirreversible antagonist. It may be assumed that partial recovery of 5-HT responses after wash-out for 1 hr reflects the slow dissociation rate constant of metergoline from the 5-HT$_2$ receptor resulting in a partial recovery of receptors for agonism by 5-HT. Reassociation of metergoline with the 5-HT$_2$ receptor would approach zero, due to dilution and continued wash-out. (−)-Propranolol mimics wash-out by virtue of its faster kinetics, on and off the receptor. As metergoline dissociates and frees some of the receptors, (−)-propranolol occupies the freed receptors and effectively protects them from renewed block by metergoline. 5-HT$_2$ receptors so occupied by (−)-propranolol interact competitively with 5-HT, and the resultant dose-effect curve to 5-HT is displaced dextrally to the wash-out curve by an appropriate shift determined by the pA$_2$ value for (−)-propranolol at the 5-HT$_2$ receptor.

Restorations of the vasoconstrictor responses to 5-HT which are of equal magnitude, whether effected by wash-out or (−)-propranolol, are difficult to explain via an allosteric model, except on a coincidental basis. Furthermore, the time-dependency for reversal of 5-HT responses favours pseudoirreversible antagonism rather than allosteric receptor modulation. Control experiments demonstrated that neither wash-out nor (−)-propranolol can reverse dose-effect curves to 5-HT depressed by phenoxybenzamine (instead of metergoline). Indeed, the remaining dose-effect curve to 5-HT, generated after prior exposure to phenoxybenzamine (either 1 μM for 15 min or 0.3 μM for 15 min), was antagonized competitively by (−)-propranolol, giving pA$_2$ values of 6.2 and 6.42, respectively. These results differ from those obtained by Kaumann and Frenken [27] in calf pulmonary artery, where ketanserin was found to restore 5-HT responses depressed by phenoxybenzamine. The authors suggested the pre-existence of a low affinity state of the 5-HT$_2$ receptor in calf pulmonary arteries, which can be transformed allosterically by ketanserin to the high affinity state.

The attractiveness of pseudoirreversible inhibition as the operative mechanism for unsurmountable antagonism in the isolated perfused rat kidney may be summarized as follows:

a) Pseudoirreversible inhibition is a simple explanation that does not require the postulation of an allosteric effector site or a change in the state of the 5-HT receptor.

b) Pseudoirreversible inhibition is consistent with the slow kinetics of metergoline and may be expected with other potent antagonists of 5-HT in systems where spare receptors for 5-HT are limited or absent, and where the time-response relationship to 5-HT is brief (due to fade, removal by perfusion, or other means).

c) Pseudoirreversible antagonism is consistent with the reversal of metergoline-induced inhibition of 5-HT by both wash-out and (−)-propranolol (a fast on-set, fast off-set competitive antagonist at the 5-HT$_2$ receptor). Wash-out and (−)-propranolol exhibited the same time-dependency and magnitude of reversal versus metergoline, and the dose-ratios measured between 5-HT dose-effect curves restored by wash-out and those restored by (−)-propranolol (3 μM) are consistent with the pA$_2$ value for (−)-propranolol at the 5-HT$_2$ receptor. Furthermore, the concordance of pA$_2$ values for (−)-propranolol, whether estimated in the presence or absence of metergoline, suggest that metergoline failed to change the state of remaining 5-HT$_2$ receptors.

d) Pseudoirreversible inhibition with metergoline, methiothepin, cyproheptadine, methysergide, ketanserin, mesulergine, and spiperone is consistent with the high affinity of these antagonists for 5-HT$_2$ receptors, as measured in both functional and ligand binding studies [31, 33, 34], especially when coupled with a limited receptor reserve for 5-HT.

e) Pseudoirreversible inhibition by metergoline is supported by the finding that metergoline and phenoxybenzamine yielded similar estimates of the equilibrium dissociation constant for 5-HT. This suggests a direct interaction of metergoline with the 5-HT$_2$ receptor independent of secondary or additional influences.

Some of the above points may also explain the data of others. For example, de Chaffoy de Courcelles [30] measured responses to 5-HT only 40 s after application of 5-HT to platelets versus antagonists with half-lives of dissociation ranging from 4.8 to 160 min. Thus, it is unlikely that equilibrium between agonist and antagonist was obtained. On the other hand, it should be recalled that unsurmountable antagonism is not constrained to a single mechanism, and can be expected to exhibit a drug, tissue and species dependency.

4.5 *Accessory binding sites*

Accessory binding sites for antagonists may be one of the more important factors determining tissue differences. Accessory binding sites are postulated to be located outside the restricted domain of the actual 5-HT binding site on its receptor protein. When present, antagonist molecules, which are usually of large molecular size, may bind tightly to accessory sites, and may act as pseudoirreversible antagonists. Differences in affinity of antagonists for a given receptor may vary between tissues depending upon the presence or absence of accessory binding sites in the local environment.

Because of the many factors which can intervene to prevent antagonists from behaving in a simple competitive fashion, we concur with Leff and Martin [32] that agonist 'fingerprints' may have a more general utility for receptor definition. In the present study, the $5\text{-}HT_2$ receptor was defined primarily upon the order and relative potency of 5-HT and related analogues, coupled with an estimate of the K_A value for 5-HT. Even so, it is difficult to define a receptor in the absence of a competitive antagonist. In this regard, (−)-propranolol suggested that 5-HT and its analogues acted at a single site.

5. Conclusions

Unsurmountable antagonism is a common occurrence in the 5-HT field. The present studies, conducted in the isolated perfused rat kidney, favour pseudoirreversible antagonism as the operative mechanism over multiple receptor-mediated responses or allosteric receptor modulation. Behaviourally, pseudoirreversible antagonism and allosteric receptor modulation are similar and are difficult to discriminate experimentally. However, pseudoirreversible antagonism is intrinsically less complicated than allosteric receptor modulation, which involves the postulation of an allosteric binding site, in addition to the 5-HT receptor, which in turn, undergoes changes in state. However, it must be stressed that unsurmountable antagonism is not constrained to a single mechanism and, in this regard, is not only drug dependent but also dependent upon the tissue, species and experimental conditions.

Acknowledgements

This work was supported by NIH Grant NS24871.

References

1. Gaddum JH, Hameed KA, Hathaway DE, Stephens FF (1955): Quantitative studies of antagonists for 5-hydroxytryptamine. *Quart J Exp Physiol* 40: 49—74.
2. Bradley PB, Engel G, Feniuk W, Fozard JR, Humphrey PPA, Middlemiss DN, Mylecharane EJ, Richardson BP, Saxena PR (1986): Proposals for the classification and nomenclature of functional receptors for 5-hydroxytryptamine. *Neuropharmacol* 25: 563—576.
3. Wrigglesworth SJ (1983): Heterogeneity of 5-hydroxytryptamine receptors in the rat uterus and stomach strip. *Br J Pharmacol* 80: 691—697.
4. Black JW, Brazenor RM, Gerskowitch VP, Leff P(1983): The problem of insurmountable antagonism in 5-hydroxytryptamine receptor classification. *Br J Pharmacol* 80: 607P.
5. Feniuk W (1984): An analysis of 5-hydroxytryptamine receptors mediating contraction of isolated smooth muscle. *Neuropharmacol* 23: 1467—1472.
6. Cohen M, Schenck KW, Colbert W, Wittenauer L (1985): Role of $5-HT_2$ receptors in serotonin-induced contractions of nonvascular smooth muscle. *J Pharmacol Exp Ther* 232: 770—774.
7. Brazenor RM, Angus JA (1981): Ergotamine contracts isolated canine coronary arteries by a serotonergic mechanism: No role for alpha adrenoceptors. *J. Pharmacol. Exp. Ther* 218: 530—536.
8. Brazenor RM, Angus JA (1982): Actions of serotonin antagonists on dog coronary artery. *Eur J Pharmacol* 81: 569—576.
9. Kaumann AJ, This Book.
10. Leff P, Martin GR (1986): Peripheral $5-HT_2$-like receptors. Can they be classified with available antagonists? *Br J Pharmacol* 88: 585—593.
11. Apperley E, Humphrey PPA, Levy GP (1976): Receptors for 5-hydroxytryptamine and noradrenaline in rabbit isolated ear artery and aorta. *Br J Pharmacol* 58: 211—221.
12. Chang J-Y, Owman C (1987): Involvement of specific receptors and calcium mechanisms in serotonergic contractile response of isolated cerebral and peripheral arteries from rats. *J Pharmacol Exp Ther* 242: 629—636.
13. Taylor EW, Duckles SP, Nelson DL (1986): Dissociation constants of serotonin agonists in the canine basilar artery correlate to K_i values at the $5-HT_{1A}$ binding site. *J Pharmacol Exp Ther* 236: 118—125.
14. Peroutka SJ (1984): Vascular serotonin receptors. Correlation with $5-HT_1$ and $5-HT_2$ binding sites. *Biochem Pharmacol* 33: 2349—2353.
15. Muller-Schweinitzer E, Engel G (1983): Evidence for mediation by $5-HT_2$ receptors of 5-hydroxytryptamine-induced contraction of canine basilar artery. *Naunyn-Schmiedeberg's Arch Pharmacol* 324: 287—292.
16. Charlton KG, Johnson TD, Clarke DE (1984): Vasoconstrictor and norepinephrine potentiating action of 5-hydroxykynuramine in the isolated perfused rat kidney: involvement of serotonin receptors and $alpha_1$-adrenoceptors. *Naunyn-Schmiedeberg's Arch Pharmacol* 328: 154—159.
17. Bradley PB, Humphrey PPA, Williams RH (1983): Are vascular 'D' and '$5-HT_2$' receptors for 5-hydroxytryptamine the same? *Br J Pharmacol* 79: 295P.
18. Apperley E, Feniuk W, Humphrey PPA, Levy GP (1980): Evidence for two types of excitatory receptor for 5-hydroxytryptamine on dog isolated vasculature. *Br J Pharmacol* 68: 215—224.
19. Leff P, Martin CR, Morse JM (1987): Differential classification of vascular smooth muscle and endothelial cell 5-HT receptors by use of tryptamine analogues. *Br J Pharmacol* 91: 321—331.
20. Stollak JS, Furchgott RF (1983): Use of selective antagonists for determining the types of receptors mediating the actions of 5-hydroxytryptamine and tryptamine in the isolated rabbit aorta. *J Pharmacol Exp Ther* 224: 215—221.

21. Foster C, Whalley ET (1982): Analysis of the human basilar arterial strip compared with rat aortic strip in vitro. *Naunyn-Schmiedeberg's Arch Pharmacol* 319: 12—17.

22. Ireland SJ, Tyers MB (1987): Pharmacological characterization of 5-hydroxytryptamine-induced depolarization of the isolated vagus nerve. *Br J Pharmacol* 90: 229—238.

23. Round A, Wallis DF (1986): The depolarizing action of 5-hydroxytryptamine on rabbit vagal afferent and sympathetic neurones in vitro and its selective blockade by ICS 205-930. *Br J Pharmacol* 88: 485—494.

24. Richardson BP, Engel G, Donatsch P, Stadler PA (1985): Identification of serotonin M-receptor subtypes and their specific blockade by a new class of drugs. *Nature* 316: 126—131.

25. Doggrell SA (1987): Differential antagonism of initial fast and secondary slow contractile responses of the rat isolated aorta to 5-hydroxytryptamime by mianserin and ketanserin. *J Auton Pharmacol* 7: 157—164.

26. Kaumann AJ, Frenken M (1985): A paradox: the $5-HT_2$-receptor antagonist ketanserin restores the 5-HT-induced contraction depressed by methysergide in large coronary arteries of calf. Allosteric regulation of $5-HT_2$ receptors. *Naunyn-Schmiedeberg's Arch Pharmacol* 328, 295—300.

27. Frenken M, Kaumann AJ (1987): Interconversion into a low active state protects vascular $5-HT_2$ receptors against irreversible antagonism by phenoxybenzamine. *Naunyn-Schmiedeberg's Arch Pharmacol* 335: 481—490.

28. Frenken M, Kaumann AJ (1988): Effects of tryptamine mediated through 2 states of the $5-HT_2$ receptor in calf coronary artery. *Naunyn-Schmiedeberg's Arch Pharmacol* 337: 484—492.

29. Kaumann AJ, Frenken M (1988): ICI 169,369 is both a competitive antagonist and an allosteric activator of the arterial 5-hydroxytryptamine$_2$ receptor system. *J Pharmacol Exp Ther* 245: 1010—1015.

30. de Chaffoy de Courcelles D, Leysen J, Roevens P, Van Belle H (1986): The serotonin-S$_2$ receptor: A receptor transducer coupling model to explain insurmountable antagonist effects. *Drug Dev Res* 8: 173—178.

31. Bond RA, Ornstein AG, Clarke DE (1988): Unsurmountable antagonism to 5-HT results from pseudoirreversible inhibition rather than multiple receptors or allosteric receptor modulation. *J Pharmacol Exp Ther* In press.

32. Leff P, Martin GR (1988): The classification of 5-hydroxytryptamine receptors. *Med Res Rev* 8: 187—202.

33. Hoyer D, Engel G, Kalkman HO (1985): Molecular pharmacology of 5-HT$_1$ and 5-HT$_2$ recognition sites in rat and pig membrances: Radioligand binding studies with [^{3}H] 5-HT, [^{3}H] 8-OH-DPAT, (—)-[^{125}I] iodocyanopindolol, [^{3}H] mesulergine and [^{3}H] ketanserin. *Eur J Pharmacol* 118: 13—23.

34. Leysen JE (1985): Serotonergic binding sites, pp. 43—62 in: Vanhoutte PM (ed) *serotonin and the cardiovascular system*. New York: Raven Press.

35. Arunlakshana O, Schild HO (1959): Some quantitative uses of drug antagonism. *Br. J. Pharmacol* 14: 48—58.

XII. Tryptamine fingerprints in the classification of 5-hydroxytryptamine receptors

G. R. MARTIN, P. LEFF and S. J. MACLENNAN

1. Introduction

In a series of recent studies [1—4] we have investigated the utility of tryptamines in the classification of 5-hydroxytryptamine (5-HT) receptors. These studies have shown that in situations where conventional antagonists are unable to provide reliable quantitative information, 'fingerprints' comprising tryptamine affinity and relative efficacy estimates can improve the rigour with which 5-HT receptors are classified. A particular advantage of this approach is that it enables receptors to be identified positively. This is in contrast to the scheme proposed by Bradley et al. [5] in which, for example 5-HT$_1$-like receptors are defined by a high agonist potency ($\geqslant$5-HT) of 5-carboxamidotryptamine (5-CT), susceptibility to blockade by the nonselective antagonist methiothepin and a resistance to blockade by ketanserin and MDL 72222. In our view, application of such exclusion criteria establishes what the receptor is not rather than what it is.

Here we consider the case of a 5-HT receptor mediating contraction of the rabbit saphenous vein and show how the use of antagonists for exclusion purposes leaves its classification equivocal. We then illustrate how, using the tryptamine fingerprinting approach, the receptor is positively defined and, at the same time, differentiated from other 5-HT receptor types.

2. Methods

Lateral saphenous veins were obtained from male New Zealand White rabbits (2.5—3.0 kg) killed by injecting pentobarbitone sodium (60 mg/kg, i.v.). Changes in tissue isometric force were recorded from vascular ring preparations (3—5 mm) suspended between tungsten wire hooks in 20 ml organ baths containing Krebs solution [6] at 37 °C and gassed with 95%O_2:5%CO_2. A force of 2g was applied to each preparation and re-established after a period of 30 min. During this interval, tissues were

P.R. Saxena, D.I. Wallis, W. Wouters and P. Bevan (eds), Cardiovascular Pharmacology of 5-Hydroxytryptamine, pp. 157—162.
© 1990 Kluwer Academic Publishers, Dordrecht —

exposed to pargyline (500 μM), an irreversible inhibitor of MAO, and phenoxybenzamine (0.3 μM) which irreversibly occluded α-adrenoceptors and prevented the sympathetic neuronal uptake of 5-HT. After washout of excess inhibitors agonist concentration-effect curves were constructed cumulatively. Antagonist effects were studied after a 60 min contact time. Estimates of agonist affinity and efficacy and of antagonist affinity were obtained using direct model-fitting procedures [3].

3. Results

3.1. Analysis of the 5-HT receptor in rabbit saphenous vein

In rings of rabbit saphenous vein 5-HT (0.001—1.0 μM) produced concentration-dependent contractions which were resistant to blockade by mepyramine (0.3 μM), atropine (0.3 μM), prazosin (0.3 μM) and idazoxan (1.0 μM) excluding the involvement of histamine H_1 receptors and muscarinic receptors and confirming no role for either α_1- or α_2-adrenoceptors. The response curve to 5-HT was also unaffected by MDL 72222 (1.0 μM), but was shifted to the right in parallel by methiothepin (0.01 μM; Δp[A_{50}] = 1.44 $\pm$ 0.17) and also by ketanserin (0.3 μM; Δp[A_{50}] = 0.44 $\pm$ 0.07). Further analysis of the latter interaction showed that the antagonism by ketanserin (0.3 — 30.0 μM) was non-competitive in nature yielding a non-linear Schild plot: the mean concentration-ratios obtained were 4.9 [0.3 μM], 44.7 [3 μM] and 53.7 [30 μM]. Moreover the antagonism was independent of the agonist used, similar concentration-ratios being obtained with the selective 5-HT$_1$-like receptor agonist GR43175. These results were not exclusive to ketanserin since the non-selective 5-HT receptor antagonist spiperone (0.3 — 30 μM) also produced surmountable blockade of 5-HT effects with concentration-ratios of 1.7 [0.3 μM], 4.3 [3 μM] and 12.6 [30 μM]. Once again antagonism was agonist-independent as evidenced by the comparable blockade of GR43175-induced contractions.

Like 5-HT and GR43175, 5-CT and methysergide were agonists at the receptor in the rabbit saphenous vein. Their potencies, expressed as p[A_{50}] values, decreased in the order: 5-CT(8.3) > 5-HT(7.8) > GR43175(6.6) > methysergide (6.4) and their maximum effects (relative to 5-HT) were: 5-HT (1.00) = 5-CT (1.06) = GR43175 (0.95) > methysergide (0.58). Evidently methysergide behaves as a partial agonist with respect to 5-HT at this receptor type.

3.2. Tryptamine "fingerprinting"

The affinities and relative efficacies of 5-HT, 5-CT, 5-methyltryptamine (5-MeT), ($\pm$)α-Me-5-HT and N,N-dimethyltryptamine (N,N-DMT) at the

5-HT receptor in rabbit saphenous vein were obtained using the method of partial irreversible receptor occlusion [7]. Direct operational model-fitting of agonist concentration-effect curves before and after receptor inactivation with benextramine tetrahydrochloride (1 μM for 30 min) provided the estimates summarised in Table 1. The Table also shows for comparison the affinity and relative efficacy values obtained for the same set of tryptamines at three other types of 5-HT receptor.

4. Discussion

The unifying scheme proposed by Bradley et al. [5] for classifying and naming 5-HT receptors is now widely accepted and has served to focus and consolidate 5-HT receptor research. In this study we attempted to classify the 5-HT receptor mediating contraction of the rabbit saphenous vein in accordance with these recommendations. Resistance to antagonism by MDL 72222 and susceptibility to blockade by ketanserin, spiperone and methiothepin infers a 5-HT$_2$ classification, but this is contradicted by the results with the agonists. These imply that the receptor is 5-HT$_1$-like. Indeed, the high agonist potency of 5-CT relative to 5-HT, the activity of GR43175 and the partial agonism demonstrated by methysergide suggests identity of the receptor in rabbit saphenous vein with the 5-HT$_1$-like receptor described in dog saphenous vein [8, 9]. However, the latter receptor is not blocked by micromolar concentrations of either ketanserin or spiperone. This raises two possibilities; either the receptors in the two tissues are different and are effectively differentiated by these antagonists or they are in fact the same, in which case the antagonists must be regarded as unreliable probes for classifying them. We have shown previously [6] that antagonists like ketanserin display variable affinities at the same 5-HT receptor type and have argued that such ligands, which bear little or no chemical relation to the endogenous agonist 5-HT, might bind to sites not recognised by 5-HT and consequently provide misleading information for classification. The ability of such drugs to distinguish the receptors in dog and rabbit saphenous vein, when agonists fail to do so, might be explained in these terms.

For these reasons we have turned our attention to the use of ligands which retain a close chemical identity to 5-HT. This approach uses information on agonists as well as antagonists and therefore provides information about the cognitive and transducer roles that receptors have. Furthermore, the use of hormone analogues emphasises a physiological definition for the term receptor [10] and consequently minimises the risk of simply classifying drug binding sites. The practical utility and economy of this method is illustrated in Table 1. Here, the affinities and relative efficacies of just five tryptamines provide unique fingerprints which not only enable the positive identification of the receptor in rabbit saphenous vein, but at the same time differentiate it from three other 5-HT receptor types regardless of their current appellation.

Table 1. Tryptamine affinity (pK_A) and relative efficacy (τ) 'fingerprints' for the 5-HT receptors in rabbit aorta (RbA), saphenous vein (RbSV) and jugular vein with (RbJV + E) and without (RbJV − E) endothelium.

Receptor			Affinity order								
Assay	Type										
RbA	5-HT$_2$	pK_A	5-HT	>	α-me-5-HT	>	5-MeT	>	N,N-DMT	>	5-CT
			6.92		6.59		6.28		6.09		5.90
		τ	1.00		0.79		0.59		0.18		0.35
RbSV	5-HT$_1$-like?	pK_A	5-CT	>	5-HT	>	5-MeT	>	N,N-DMT	>	α-me-5-HT
			7.53		7.12		6.43		5.82		5.68
		τ	0.98		1.00		1.00		0.65		0.93
RbJV + E*	5-HT$_1$-like?	pK_A	5-HT	>	α-me-5-HT	>	5-CT	>	5-MeT	>	N,N-DMT
			8.36		8.14		7.51		7.17		6.57
		τ	1.00		1.04		0.95		1.14		0.50
RbJV − E*	5-HT$_1$-like	pK_A	5-CT	>	5-HT	>	N,N-DMT	>	5-MeT	>	α-me-5-HT
			6.66		6.20		5.94†		5.67		<4.50
		τ	4.70		1.00		<0.10		0.53		—

† pK_B by Schild analysis

* from [4, 5]

Key; 5-CT = carboxamidotryptamine; 5-MeT = 5-methyltryptamine; N,N-DMT = N,N-dimethyltryptamine; α-me-5-HT = (±) α-methyl-5-HT.

By extending these studies further to provide a fingerprint for the 5-HT$_1$-like receptor in dog saphenous vein, it should be possible to ascertain with confidence the identity or otherwise of this receptor with other types of 5-HT receptor including that which mediates contraction of the rabbit saphenous vein.

5. Conclusions

An increasing number of reports describe 5-HT receptors which cannot be allocated to the 5-HT$_1$-like, 5-HT$_2$ or 5-HT$_3$ classes; this also appears to be the case for the 5-HT receptor mediating contraction of the rabbit saphenous vein. We suggest that this problem is due largely to the emphasis that the current nomenclature scheme places upon negative criteria for classification. As illustrated here, "fingerprints" comprising tryptamine affinity and efficacy estimates provide a quantitative and secure basis for classification, allowing different receptors types to be defined positively. As such this approach complements and extends the present scheme for classifying 5-HT receptors.

References

1. Leff P, Martin GR, Morse JM (1986): The classification of peripheral 5-HT$_2$-like receptors using tryptamine agonist and antagonist analogues. *Br J Pharmacol* 89: 493–499.
2. Leff P, Martin GR, Morse JM (1987): Differential classification of vascular smooth muscle and endothelial cell 5-HT receptors by use of tryptamine analogues. *Br J Pharmacol* 91: 321–331.
3. Martin GR, Leff P, Cambridge D, Barrett VJ (1987): Comparative analysis of two types of 5-hydroxytryptamine receptor mediating vasorelaxation: differential classification using tryptamines. *Naunyn-Schmiedeberg's Arch Pharmacol* 336: 365–375.
4. Martin GR, Leff P, MacLennan SJ, Dougall I (1988): Three types of 5-HT$_1$-like receptor recognised by tryptamine affinity and efficacy "fingerprints". *Br J Pharmacol* 95: 626P.
5. Bradley PB, Engel G, Feniuk W, Fozard JR, Humphrey PPA, Middlemiss DN, Mylecharane EJ, Richardson BP, Saxena PR (1986): Proposals for the classification and nomenclature of functional receptors of 5-hydroxytryptamine. *Neuropharmacol* 25: 563–576.
6. Leff P, Martin GR (1986): Peripheral 5-HT$_2$-like receptors. Can they be classified with the available antagonists? *Br J Pharmacol* 88: 585–593.
7. Furchgott RF (1966): The use of β-haloalkylamines in the differentiation of receptors and determination of dissociation constants of receptor-agonist complexes. *Adv Drug Res* 3: 21–55.
8. Feniuk W, Humphrey PPA, Perren MJ, Watts AD (1985): A comparison of 5-hydroxytryptamine receptors mediating contraction in rabbit aorta and dog saphenous vein: evidence for different receptor types obtained by use of selective agonists and antagonists. *Br J Pharmacol* 86: 697–704.
9. Humphrey PPA, Feniuk W, Perren MJ, Connor HE, Oxford AW, Coates IH, Butina D (1988): GR43175, a selective agonist for the 5-HT$_1$-like receptor in dog isolated saphenous vein. *Br J Pharmacol* 94: 1123–1132.

10. Stephenson RP (1975): Interactions of agonists and antagonists with their receptors, pp. 15—28 in: Warcel M, Vassort G (eds), *Les colloques de l'institute de la santé et de la recherche medicale. Smooth Muscle Pharmacology and Physiology.* Vol. 50.

Neurophysiology and
Neuropharmacology

XIII. Central neuronal responses and 5-hydroxytryptamine receptors

M. H. T. ROBERTS and M. DAVIES

1. Introduction

Most evidence for a role of 5-hydroxytryptamine (5-HT) in hypertension points to an action on the blood vessel wall [1] but many compounds acting on 5-HT receptors also penetrate the blood-brain barrier and central neuronal receptors to 5-HT significantly affect sympathetic outflows [2, 3]. Undoubtedly, the central actions at 5-HT receptors of some antihypertensive agents are of relevance to their therapeutic actions. Until recently the actions of 5-HT on central neurones have been ill defined and controversial due to the lack of a proper framework of receptor definition and a lack of drugs which discriminate between receptor types. Selective agonists and antagonists have been developed in the last decade and the proposed classification of 5-HT receptor types by Bradley et al. [4] has enabled studies of central functional receptors to 5-HT. However, lack of selective antagonists at the 5-HT_1-like receptor continues to inhibit proper definition of 5-HT actions in the CNS.

2. Historical perspective

Early studies of 5-HT actions on central neurones were conducted on cortical neurones in the cat anaesthetised with barbiturate [5]. Potent depressant effects were reported which were resistant to antagonism by lysergide (LSD). Further studies by Roberts and Straughan [6] revealed dual effects of 5-HT on cortical neurones in the brain of unanaesthetised cats (encephale isole) or cats anaesthetised with fluothane. They reported that apart from the potent depression of neuronal activity by 5-HT, many cells responded with a slower, longer latency excitation. Only the excitatory response was antagonised reversibly and surmountably by LSD, methysergide or cinanserin. Intravenous barbiturate (sodium thiopentone) very signifi-

P.R. Saxena, D.I. Wallis, W. Wouters and P. Bevan (eds), Cardiovascular Pharmacology of 5-Hydroxytryptamine, pp. 165—176.
© 1990 *Kluwer Academic Publishers, Dordrecht* —

cantly reduced the occurrence of excitatory responses to 5-HT [7]. The two populations of responses and the effectiveness of antagonists on only one of them suggested two receptor types. The excitatory receptor had characteristics resembling the 'D' receptor of Gaddum and Picarelli [8]. Subsequent studies have extensively confirmed the existence of both excitatory and depressant responses to 5-HT in neocortex of cat and rat [9—13] and also in brainstem neurones [14—19]. Both types of response have also been observed on thalamic neurones [20], striatal neurones [21] and in the dorsal horn of the spinal cord [22, 23]. In other areas of the brain however, only depressant effects of 5-HT have been observed. This is the case on hippocampal, amygdaloid, lateral geniculate and dorsal raphe neurones [24—29]. Spinal and facial motoneurones conversely reveal only facilitatory effects of 5-HT [30—34].

In 1974 Bennett and Aghajanian [35] used the radioligand binding technique to study central 5-HT binding sites. They observed that [^{3}H] LSD demonstrated a stereoselective, saturable and reversible binding which was most dense in areas known to receive a large 5-HT innervation. Subsequently LSD was found to bind to two distinct sites. [^{3}H] 5-HT at nanomolar concentrations bound to one site [36] and [^{3}H] spiperone was more selective for a second site. Peroutka and Snyder [37] named these sites 5-HT$_1$ and 5-HT$_2$ respectively. Significant advances were rapidly made with the pharmacology of these binding sites and the knowledge has facilitated the study of functional receptors. It is important to remember however, that binding studies do not identify the efficacy of a drug nor discriminate between full or partial agonists or antagonists. It is a mistake to equate a binding site with a pharmacological receptor until full pharmacological characterisation of the functional response is complete.

5-HT$_1$ binding sites may be identified by their high (nanomolar) affinity for 5-HT. 5-HT$_2$ sites have micromolar affinity for 5-HT but nanomolar affinity for spiperone [38]. Antagonists of 5-HT (compounds which bind selectively to 5-HT$_3$ sites are discussed later) all have a higher affinity for the 5-HT$_2$ site than for the 5-HT$_1$ sites. Agonists tend to have greater affinity for the 5-HT$_1$ site. Incomplete awareness of this has led to some errors of interpretation concerning the functional effects of both agonists and antagonists. 5-Methoxytryptamine (5-MeOT) is an agonist with a K_i (affinity) for the 5-HT$_1$ site of 11 nM and for the 5-HT$_2$ site of 2,700 nM. It is highly selective for the 5-HT$_1$ site. Its affinity compares with a K_i of 5-HT for the 5-HT$_1$ site of 3.8 nM and for the 5-HT$_2$ site of 2,700 nM [39]. Thus, although the difference in affinity of 5-MeOT for the 5-HT$_1$ and 5-HT$_2$ sites is very large, this is also true for 5-HT itself and the probability of 5-MeOT acting selectively in the CNS is about the same as the probability of 5-HT acting selectively in the CNS. It cannot be assumed that functional responses to 5-MeOT are necessarily at the 5-HT$_1$ site anymore than it can be assumed that 5-HT acts at only the 5-HT$_1$ site. In fact, behavioural studies by Green et al. [40] have demonstrated quite clearly that some effects of 5-HT$_1$

selective agonists are due to actions at 5-HT$_2$ sites. The problem with antagonists is not so great. Ketanserin, for example, has a K$_i$ at the 5-HT$_1$ site of more than 1,000 nM and at the 5-HT$_2$ site a K$_i$ of 2.1 nM [38]. Thus the selectivity of this antagonist is of the same order of magnitude as the selectivity of the agonists. However, ketanserin will bind readily to the 5-HT$_2$ site and easily displace 5-HT which binds with low affinity. It is very unlikely that ketanserin will competitively displace the high affinity binding of 5-HT from the 5-HT$_1$ site. Ketanserin is very likely to block functional responses to 5-HT$_2$ binding and will not be an antagonist at 5-HT$_1$ sites. Other antagonists also show greatest affinity for 5-HT$_2$ sites but are less selective, having moderate affinities for the 5-HT$_1$ sites. Nevertheless, compounds like me-thysergide, methiothepin and metergoline which have K$_i$ values at 5-HT$_1$ sites of 99, 62 and 20 nM respectively [38], will displace the high affinity binding of 5-HT from this site (K$_i$ 3.8 nM) only at high concentrations. Selective antagonism of responses due to 5-HT$_1$ binding cannot be expected with any of the known antagonists therefore.

The 5-HT$_1$ binding sites have been subdivided into at least A, B, C and D subgroups on the basis of the relative affinities of agonists and antagonists [41—43]. To some extent, these subdivisions represent species differences in binding. The 5-HT$_{1B}$ binding site seems to be a rodent site and the 5-HT$_{1D}$ receptor is found in humans, cow and pig [44, 45]. 5-HT$_{1C}$ sites are found most densely in the choroid plexus [39]. 5-HT$_{1A}$ and 5-HT$_{1B}$ sites may be discriminated by 8-OH-DPAT which binds with high affinity to the 5-HT$_{1A}$ site (pK$_D$ 8.7, [39]) and with lower affinity to the 5-HT$_{1B}$ and 5-HT$_{1C}$ sites. 5-carboxamidotryptamine (5-CT) is a high affinity binding ligand at both 5-HT$_{1A}$ and 5-HT$_{1B}$ sites but has at least 100 fold less affinity for the 5-HT$_{1C}$ site [39].

This brief summary of 5-HT binding in the CNS has made no reference to 5-HT$_3$ binding sites because such binding was not thought to be present until December 1987, [46] when it was reported to be found concentrated in cortical and limbic areas. Before this report only functional responses to 5-HT$_3$ receptor activation were known. However, as these responses included anxiolytic [47] and a centrally mediated antiemetic activity, [48] as well as actions on the heart and peripheral neurones, the existence of central binding sites had been confidently predicted.

At the same time as the binding studies in CNS tissue were being conducted, the pharmacology of the actions of 5-HT on a wide range of behavioural responses and peripheral tissues was being studied. These studies are the subject of other reviews in this volume and will not be reiterated here. Importantly, however, Bradley et al. [4] defined the functional receptors to 5-HT by surveying these data. They used terminology very similar to that used in binding studies which, as stated above, can be misleading. 5-HT$_2$ receptors were defined as receptors with a pharmacology very similar indeed to that for 5-HT$_2$ binding sites i.e. no preferentially selective agonist was known and responses were easily blocked by ketanserin, cyproheptadine or methysergide. 5-HT$_1$-like receptors were acknowledged to be a heterogenous group, but were not subdivided due to a lack of antagonists selective for the subgroups. Antagonism of these receptors on various tissues was reported with high doses of methysergide and methiothepin, but they were resistant to ketanserin and cyproheptadine. The last functional receptor type defined [4] was the 5-HT$_3$ receptor, which was potently and selectively antagonised by MDL 72222 and ICS 205-930, both essentially inactive at 5-HT$_1$-like and 5-HT$_2$ receptors. 2-methyl 5-HT was a relatively selective agonist.

All these functional receptor types have been shown to mediate different behavioural responses and presumably therefore have actions upon central neurones. 5-HT$_1$-like receptors mediate the "5-HT behavioural syndrome", e.g. reciprocal forepaw treading; 5-HT$_2$ receptors mediate 5-HTP-induced head twitch and wet dog shake; 5-HT$_3$ receptors have recently been reported to be involved in the anxiolytic effects of GR 38032F [47] and the antiemetic effects of BRL 24924 [49] and GR 38032F [50]. Both compounds are very selective and potent 5-HT$_3$ antagonists. However, a clearly defined role for any of these receptor types in controlling the activity or excitability of central neurones has not been established until very recently.

The pharmacological study of functional 5-HT receptors on central neurones was taking place during the same period when the binding studies and the behavioural and peripheral tissue studies outlined above were occurring. Aghajanian led the field. As a result of an intensive series of experiments with microelectrodes recording in several areas of the brain, he proposed a classification of central 5-HT receptor types: S1, S2 and S3 [51]. The S1 receptor mediates the facilitatory effects of 5-HT on facial motoneurones; methysergide, cinanserin, metergoline and cyproheptadine were all found to be antagonists at this receptor. The S2 receptor mediates the depressant effects of 5-HT in areas postsynaptic to 5-HT neurones and particularly neurones in the limbic system and secondary visual areas; several 5-HT antagonists were found to be weak or ineffective and LSD acted as a weak or partial agonist. The S3 receptor mediates the depressant effects of 5-HT on serotoninergic cell bodies in the dorsal raphe nucleus; 5-HT antagonists are ineffective and LSD acted as a potent agonist.

It is difficult to relate the receptor classification of Aghajanian [51] to that of Bradley et al. [4], because the latter was based on new selective compounds which were not available when the bulk of the work was done which gave rise to Aghajanian's classification. It has been suggested that the actions of 5-HT on spinal and facial motoneurones [30—34] which are blocked by several antagonists, are likely to be due to 5-HT$_2$ receptors. However, the antagonists available before 1982 were much less selective for the 5-HT$_2$ receptor and more recent studies (see below) question this conclusion. S2 and S3 are presumably variants of 5-HT$_1$-like receptors although definitive data were lacking both for inclusion in the 5-HT$_1$-like group (agonist effects of 5-CT; antagonism by methiothepin or methysergide) and for exclusion of 5-HT$_3$ receptors (effects of the selective 5-HT$_3$ receptor antagonists).

It will be noted that Aghajanian included no receptor type responsible for excitation of neurones in forebrain and brainstem by 5-HT. This is because such responses were rarely seen in his experiments [26] and yet they have been extensively reported by other laboratories [6, 9—23]. The technical differences between the experiments or the nature of an intervening artifact have been studied without satisfactory resolution; the pH of drug solutions [52] or the anaesthetic state of the animals are unlikely causes of the different observations. The excitatory effects of 5-HT, which have been seen in many parts of the neuraxis, can be selectively and reversibly antagonised suggesting they are due to a drug-receptor interaction. It has been suggested that the depressant effects of 5-HT represent "a true synaptic action" of 5-HT [26], but for similar reasons the excitatory effects of 5-HT also seem to represent a true synaptic action. Thus, Briggs [53] found that a high proportion of cells excited by 5-HT in the rat brainstem were also excited by electrical stimulation of the hindbrain raphe nuclei in the region of the cell bodies which contain 5-HT. Both synaptic and 5-HT-induced excitation of cells was blocked by LSD. Jones [54—56] demonstrated the inhibition and excitation of cells in rat cortex following stimulation of raphe medianus. The excitatory synaptic response was strongly reduced by inhibition of 5-HT synthesis with para-chlorophenylalanine and enhanced by the 5-HT precursors 1-tryptophan and 5-hydroxytryptophan, or the selective 5-HT uptake blockers fluoxetine or zimelidine. Methysergide was an effective antagonist. Intracellular studies have also revealed that stimulation of dorsal raphe evokes excitatory postsynaptic potentials in the neostriatum which are reduced or abolished by para-chlorophenylalanine [57]. It seems essential that any system of classification of central 5-HT receptor types must account for the excitatory responses to 5-HT which may be readily and selectively antagonised.

3. Recent work

The paucity of studies of central neuronal responses to the new selective agonists and antagonists of 5-HT led us to apply these compounds by microiontophoresis to brainstem and spinal neurones in the rat anaesthetised with fluothane [58—60]. Brainstem cells were found to be either excited or depressed by iontophoretic application of 5-HT. Pontamine sky blue was ejected from the electrodes after the studies and a tendency was found for those cells in the midline of the brainstem to be excited and for those 0.5 mm or more lateral to the midline to be depressed by 5-HT. As studies were conducted at the level of nucleus raphe magnus and obscurus, this suggests that cells in the hindbrain raphe were excited by 5-HT. This observation confirms that of Llewelyn et al. [19], but at first sight seems at variance with the data reported by some investigators [24, 29, 61, 62]. However, that is not so because in all these investigations, cells in the dorsal raphe nucleus referred to simply as "raphe neurons" were studied. Studies of dorsal raphe cells in our laboratory confirm the reports by others that 5-HT is exclusively depressant on these cells [63]. It seems unlikely to us, however, that 5-HT depresses the activity of all serotonin-containing neurones (S3 receptor, [51]), because cells in the region of hindbrain raphe are excited by 5-HT. However, these data should be interpreted with great caution because it has not been demonstrated conclusively that all of the particular cells studied in the raphe nuclei contain 5-HT. At least 70% do not.

The brainstem cells excited by 5-HT were occasionally, but weakly, excited by the 5-HT_1-like agonists 5-CT and 8-OH-DPAT [58]. Potency comparisons between the effects of drugs applied by microiontophoresis are notoriously difficult, but radiolabelled drugs were used to determine the transport numbers and therefore the rates at which the agonists were released from the microelectrodes. There were no significant differences between the release of any of these drugs. It seems, therefore, that both 5-CT and 8-OH-DPAT are less potent than 5-HT at the excitatory receptor on brainstem neurones. The absolute potency of the compounds cannot be determined from these experiments.

Antagonists were studied by iontophoretic application and were given intravenously as well. Although intravenous administration is not without problems due to uncertain penetration of the blood-brain barrier, many of these compounds are known to have behavioural or other central effects following systemic administration. It is necessary to know at least the order of magnitude of antagonist potency in absolute terms to determine if 5-HT_1-like or 5-HT_2 receptors are blocked. This is because few of the antagonists are totally selective for one of the receptor types and at higher doses may compete for binding at several sites. Ketanserin readily blocked the excitatory responses of brainstem neurones to 5-HT. Glutamate and noradrenaline excitations were not prevented and responses to 5-HT returned some time after ketanserin applications were stopped. Ketanserin (200 μg kg^{-1} i.v.) selectively reduced excitatory responses to iontophoretically applied 5-HT by more than 50%. The $alpha_1$ adrenoceptor blocking actions of ketanserin were not responsible for this [58]. The potency of ketanserin suggests that excitatory responses are mediated by a 5-HT_2 receptor. Methysergide is also potent at the 5-HT_2 receptor and antagonised excitatory responses selectively with intravenous doses of about 1 mg kg^{-1}. These antagonists are not very active at 5-HT_3 receptors and, further, MDL 72222 had no selective action upon responses to 5-HT even when applied with doses of 1 mg kg^{-1}. This dose is 25 times larger than the dose required to block the von Bezold-Jarisch reflex bradycardia [64] and strongly suggests that 5-HT_3 receptors are not involved in these particular responses to 5-HT.

It may be concluded from these data that the excitatory effects of 5-HT on brainstem neurones are mediated by 5-HT_2 receptors. The weak agonist actions of 5-CT and 8-OH-DPAT may seem to reduce confidence in this conclusion, but 5-CT has some, albeit low, affinity for 5-HT_2 binding sites and in the rabbit aorta, 5-CT acts on 5-HT_2 receptors, being only 26 times less potent than 5-HT [65]. Thus, the weak effects of 5-CT on the excitatory receptor may simply be due to an expected weak action upon 5-HT_2 receptors.

On those brainstem neurones depressed by 5-HT, 5-CT and 8-OH-DPAT were very potent agonists [59]. As explained above, these differences cannot be due to some physical artifact of drug release from the electrode and must reflect a genuine high comparative potency of the 5-HT_1-like receptor agonists at the depressant 5-HT receptor. It should be noted that a high correlation existed between the effects of 5-CT, 8-OH-DPAT and 5-HT. Cells excited by 5-HT responded very weakly and mostly not at all, to these agonists and all cells depressed by 5-HT were depressed by the agonists. Ketanserin was ineffective as an antagonist of the depressant effects of 5-HT even when applied iontophoretically for periods of 2 hours or intravenously with doses up to 2 mg kg^{-1}. It is unlikely therefore that depression is mediated by 5-HT_2 receptors. This conclusion is similar to that reached by others who studied the effects of ketanserin on cells depressed by 5-HT in cortex, hippocampus and dorsal raphe [66, 67]. MDL 72222 was also ineffective when given with i.v. doses up to 1 mg kg^{-1}, which indicates that 5-HT_3 receptors do not mediate the depressant response. There is no preferentially effective 5-HT_1-like antagonist and full proof that the depressant response is due to the action of 5-HT at 5-HT_1-like receptors cannot be offered. However, the potent actions of 5-CT, 8-OH-DPAT and the lack of effect of ketanserin and MDL 72222 makes the involvement of 5-HT_1-like receptors very probable. Methysergide and methiothepin are antagonists which have high affinity at 5-HT_2 receptors, but have only about 10–30 fold less affinity for some of the 5-HT_1-like receptors [38]. This has led Bradley et al. [4] to suggest that they may be useful antagonists to discriminate 5-HT_1-like receptors. Given iontophoretically to neurones, high currents of methysergide have membrane stabilising actions which depress the amplitude of the action potential. Very high intravenous doses of methysergide (30 mg kg^{-1}) do not do this and abolish the depressant effects of 5-HT. Cells continued to respond to control agonists (GABA or glutamate), but recovery of the responses to 5-HT was not seen following these high doses [59]. Methiothepin has a greater discimination ratio between 5-HT_1-like and 5-HT_2 receptors than methysergide [38], but it has not proved possible to obtain a selective antagonism of depressant responses to 5-HT with this compound (Moody et al., unpublished). It is difficult to interpret the effects of such very high doses of methysergide but the results are compatible with depressant responses being due to 5-HT acting at a 5-HT_1-like receptor.

There are two reports that metergoline is an effective antagonist of the depressant effects of 5-HT on cortical neurones [68, 69]. Metergoline failed to block the depressant effects of 5-HT on brainstem neurones [59], however, and this may indicate that the depressant receptors on these two cell types are different. This would be extremely interesting as Aghajanian [51] has come to a similar conclusion using quite different drugs. Involvement of the 5-HT_{1C} binding site in these responses seems unlikely as mesulergine was not an effective antagonist (Moody et al., unpublished).

4. Conclusions

It would be a serious oversimplification of the data outlined above to conclude that excitation of central neurones is mediated by 5-HT_2 receptors and that depression is mediated by 5-HT_1-like receptors. This is illustrated by the study of spinal motoneurones [60]. The studies were conducted upon a physiologically identified, homogenous population of alpha motoneurones in vivo. Iontophoretically applied 5-HT always raised the excitability of these cells as did electrical stimulation of nucleus raphe obscurus. 5-CT was a very potent agonist at this excitatory 5-HT receptor although 8-OH-DPAT was without effect. Ketanserin failed to block the effects of 5-HT selectively, as did the 5-HT_1 ligand cyanopindolol. Methysergide, however, was a very effective agonist when given iontophoretically or intravenously at 2—3 mg kg^{-1}. MDL 72222 was not effective. Very similar data have been obtained in vitro using the hemisected neonate spinal cord [70], which show, in addition, that spiperone, mesulergine and cyproheptadine are effective antagonists [71]. It may be concluded that the facilitatory effects of 5-HT on motoneurones are due to a 5-HT_1-like receptor which is different from the 5-HT_1-like receptor in the brainstem. Although these differences are very marked: the responses they mediate are different; the potency of methysergide is different; and the effects of 8-OH-DPAT are different, there is no basis for subdivision of the receptor types into the A or B subdivisions of the binding site classification. It is true that 5-HT_1 binding sites with high affinity for 8-OH-DPAT are 5-HT_{1A} and those with low affinity are 5-HT_{1B}, but agonist potency differences are insufficient to define functional receptors. In addition the receptor on motoneurones does not resemble the 5HT_{1B} binding site as the 5HT_{1B} ligand, RU 24969 is inactive [71]. The considerable potency difference of methysergide as an antagonist at the two receptors may be a good basis for defining the difference between them. Further studies of other antagonists may reveal more definitive characteristics of the two 5-HT_1-like functional receptors, which depress brainstem neurones and excite motoneurones, respectively.

References

1. Vanhoutte PM, Luescher TF (1986): Serotonin and the blood vessel wall. *J Hypertension* 4 (suppl 1): S29—S35.
2. Chalmers JP, Pilowski PM, Minson JB, Kapoor V, Mills E, West MJ (1988): Central serotonergic mechanisms in hypertension. *Am J Hypertension* 1: 79—83.
3. Ramage AG, Fozard JR (1987): Evidence that the putative 5HT 1A receptor agonists,

8-OH-DPAT and ipsapirone, have a central hypotensive action that differs from that of clonidine in anaesthetised cats. *Eur J Pharmacol* 138: 179—191.

4. Bradley PB, Engel G, Feniuk W, Fozard J, Humphrey PPA, Middlemiss DN, Mylecharane EJ, Richardson BP, Saxena PR (1986): Proposals for the classification and nomenclature of functional receptors for 5-hydroxytryptamine. *Neuropharmacology* 25: 563—576.

5. Krnjevic K, Phillis JW (1963): Actions of certain amines on cerebral cortical neurones. *Br J Pharmacol Chemother* 20: 471—490.

6. Roberts MHT, Straughan DW (1967): Excitation and depression of cortical neurones by 5 Hydroxytryptamine. *J Physiol (Lond)*. 193: 269—294.

7. Johnson ES, Roberts MHT, Straughan DW (1969): The responses of cortical neurones to monoamines under differing anaesthetic conditions. *J Physiol (Lond.)* 203: 261—280.

8. Gaddum JH, Picarelli ZP (1957): Two kinds of tryptamine receptor. *Br J Pharmac Chemother* 12: 323—328.

9. Bradshaw CM, Roberts MHT, Szabadi E (1974): Effects of imipramine and desipramine on the responses of single cortical neurones to noradrenaline and 5 Hydroxytryptamine. *Br J Pharmacol* 52: 349—358.

10. Szabadi E, Bradshaw CM, Bevan P (1977): Excitatory and depressant neuronal responses to noradrenaline, 5-hydroxytryptamine and mescaline: the role of the baseline firing rate. *Brain Res* 126: 580—583.

11. Jones, RSG, Roberts MHT (1979): Potentiation of responses to monoamines by antidepressants after destruction of monoamine afferents. *Br J Pharmacol* 65: 501—510.

12. Jones RSG, Boulton AA (1980): Tryptamine and 5-hydroxytryptamine: actions and interactions on cortical neurons in the rat. *Life Sci* 27: 1849—1856.

13. Bradshaw CM, Stoker MJ, Szabadi E (1983): Comparison of neuronal responses to 5-Hydroxytryptamine, noradrenaline and phenylephrine in the cerebral cortex: effects of haloperidol and methysergide. *Neuropharmacology* 22: 677—683.

14. Boakes RJ, Bradley PB, Briggs I, Dray A (1970): Antagonism of 5-hydroxytryptamine by LSD-25 in the central nervous system: a possible basis for the actions of LSD-25. *Br J Pharmacol* 40: 202—218.

15. Couch JR (1970): Responses of neurons in the raphe nuclei to serotonin, norepinephrine and acetylcholine and their correlation with an excitatory synaptic input. *Brain Res* 19: 137—150.

16. Couch JR (1976): Further evidence for a possible excitatory serotonergic synapse on raphe neurons of pons and lower midbrain. *Life Sci* 19: 761—768.

17. Hosli L, Tebecis AK, Schonwetter HP (1970): Monoamines, LSD and brain stem reticular neurones. *Experientia* 26: 7.

18. Bradley PB, Briggs, I (1974): Further studies on the mode of action of psychotomimetic drugs: antagonism of the excitatory actions of 5-hydroxytryptamine by methylated derivatives of tryptamine. *Br J Pharmacol* 50: 345—354.

19. Llewelyn MB, Azami J, Roberts MHT (1983): Effects of 5-Hydroxytryptamine applied into nucleus raphe magnus on nociceptive thresholds and neuronal firing rate. *Brain Res* 258: 59—68.

20. Tebecis AK (1970): Effects of monoamines and amino acids on medial geniculate neurones of the cat. *Neuropharmacology* 9: 381—391.

21. York DH (1970): Possible dopaminergic pathway from substantia nigra to putamen. *Brain Res* 20: 233—247.

22. Belcher G, Ryall RW, Schaffner R (1978): The differential effects of 5-Hydroxytryptamine, noradrenaline, and raphe stimulation on nociceptive and non-nociceptive dorsal horn interneurones in the cat. *Brain Res* 151: 307—321.

23. McCall RB (1983): Serotonergic excitation of sympathetic preganglionic neurones: a microiontophoretic study. *Brain Res* 289: 121—127.

24. Haigler HJ, Aghajanian GK (1974): Lysergic acid diethylamide and serotonin: a com-

parison of effects on serotonergic neurons and neurons receiving a serotonergic input. *J Pharm Exp Ther* 18: 688—699.

25. Haigler HJ, Aghajanian GK (1974): Peripheral serotonin antagonists: failure to antagonise serotonin in brain areas receiving a prominent serotonergic input *J Neural Trans* 35: 257—273.

26. Haigler HJ, Aghajanian GK (1977): Serotonin receptors in brain. *Fed Proc* 36: 2159—2164.

27. Segal M (1976): 5-HT antagonists in rat hippocampus. *Brain Res* 103: 161—166.

28. Wang RY, Aghajanian GK (1977): Inhibition of neurones in the amygdala by dorsal raphe stimulation: mediation through a direct serotonergic pathway. *Brain Res* 120: 85—102.

29. Blier P, de Montigny C (1983): Effects of quipazine on pre- and postsynaptic serotonin receptors: single cell studies in the rat CNS. *Neuropharm* 22: 495—499.

30. Barasi S, Roberts MHT (1974): The modification of lumbar motoneurone excitability by stimulation of a putative 5-Hydroxytryptamine pathway. *Br J Pharmacol* 52: 339—348.

31. McCall RB, Aghajanian GK (1979): Serotonergic facilitation of facial motoneuron excitation. *Brain Res* 169: 11—27.

32. McCall RB, Aghajanian GK (1980): Pharmacological characterization of serotonin receptors in the facial motor nucleus: a microiontophoretic study. *Eur J Pharmacol* 65: 175—183.

33. Parry O, Roberts MHT (1980): Responses of motoneurones to 5-Hydroxytryptamine. *Neuropharmacology* 19: 515—518.

34. White SR, Neuman RS (1980): Facilitation of spinal motoneurone excitability by 5-hydroxytryptamine and noradrenaline. *Brain Res* 188: 119—127.

35. Bennett JL, Aghajanian GK (1974): d-LSD binding to rat brain homogenates: a possible relationship to serotonin receptors. *Life Sci* 15: 1935—1944.

36. Bennett JP, Snyder SH (1976): Serotonin and lysergic acid diethylamide binding in rat brain membranes. Relationship to post synaptic serotonin receptors. *Molec Pharmacol* 12: 373—389.

37. Peroutka SJ, Snyder SH (1979): Multiple serotonin receptors: Differential binding of [3H] 5-hydroxytryptamine, [3H] lysergic acid diethylamide and [3H] spiroperidol. *Molec Pharmacol* 16: 687—699.

38. Leysen JE, Awouters F, Kennis L, Laduron PM, Vandenberg J, Janssen PAJ (1981): Receptor binding profile of R 41 468, a novel antagonist at 5-HT receptors. *Life Sci* 28: 1015—1022.

39. Engel G, Gothert M, Hoyer D, Schlicker E, Hillenbrand K (1986): Identity of inhibitory presynaptic 5-hydroxytryptamine (5HT) autoreceptors in the rat brain cortex with 5HT1B binding sites. *Nauynyn-Schmiedeberg's Arch Pharmacol* 322: 1—7.

40. Green AR, Hall JE, Rees AR (1981): A behavioural study in rats of 5-hydroxytryptamine receptor agonists and antagonists, with observations on structure-activity requirements for the agonists. *Br J Pharmacol* 73: 703—719.

41. Pedigo NW, Yamamura HI, Nelson DL (1981): Discrimination of multiple 3H 5-hydroxytryptamine binding sites in rat brain by neuroleptics. *J Neurochem* 36: 220—226.

42. Deshmukh PP, Nelson DL, Yamamura HI (1982): Localisation of 5HT1 receptor subtypes in rat brain by autoradiography. *Fed Proc* 41: 6238.

43. Pazos A, Hoyer D, Palacios JM (1984): The binding of serotonergic ligands to the porcine choroid plexus: characterisation of a new type of serotonin recognition site. *Eur J Pharmacol* 106: 539—546.

44. Hoyer D, Engel G, Kalkman HO (1985): Molecular pharmacology of 5HT 1 and 5HT 2 recognition sites in rat and pig brain membranes: Radioligand binding studies with [3H]5HT, [3H]8-OH-DPAT, (−)[125 I]iodocyanopindolol, [3H]mesulergine and [3H]ketanserin. *European J Pharmacol* 118: 13—23.

45. Hoyer D, Pazos A, Probst A, Palacios JM (1986): Serotonin receptors in the human

brain. 1 Characterisation and autoradiographic localisation of 5HT 1A sites. Apparant absence of 5HT 1B sites. *Brain Res* 376: 85—96.

46. Kilpatrick GJ, Jones BJ, Tyers MB (1987): Identification and distribution of 5HT 3 receptors in rat brain using radioligand binding. *Nature* 330: 746—748.

47. Jones BJ, Oakey NR, Tyers MB (1987): The anxiolytic activity of GR 38032F, a 5HT 3 receptor antagonist in the rat and cynomolgus monkey. *Br J Pharmacol* 90: 90P.

48. Carmichael J, Cantwell BMJ, Edwards CM, Rapeport WG, Harris AL (1988): The serotonin type 3 receptor antagonist BRL 43694 and nausea and vomiting induced by cisplatin. *Br Med J* 297: 110—111.

49. Andrews PLR, Hawthorn J (1987): Evidence for an extra-abdominal site of action for the 5HT 3 receptor antagonist BRL 24924 in the inhibition of radiation-evoked emesis in the ferret. *Neuropharmacology* 26: 1367—1370.

50. Costall B, Domeny AM, Gunning SJ, Nayor RJ, Tatersall FD, Tyers MB (1987). GR 38032F: a potent and novel inhibitor of cisplatin-induced emesis in the ferret. *Br J Pharmacol* 90: 90P.

51. Aghajanian GK (1981): The modulatory role of serotonin at multiple receptors in brain. pp. 156—185 in: Jacobs BL, Gelperin A (eds), *Serotonin neurotransmission and behaviour.* Cambridge: MIT Press.

52. Bevan P, Bradshaw CM, Roberts MHT, Szabadi E (1973): Effects of pH on the release of noradrenaline from micropipettes. *J pharm Pharmac* 25: 1007—1008.

53. Briggs I (1977): Excitatory responses of neurones in rat bulbar reticular formation to bulbar raphe stimulation and to iontophoretically applied 5-hydroxytryptamine and their blockade by LSD-25. *J Physiol* 265: 327—340.

54. Jones RSG (1982): Responses of cortical neurones to stimulation of nucleus raphe medianus: a pharmacological analysis of the role of indoleamines. *Neuropharmacology* 21: 511—520.

55. Jones RSG, Broadbent J (1982): Differential effects of fluoxetine and zimelidine on the uptake of 5-hydroxytryptamine and tryptamine by cortical slices and on responses of cortical neurones to stimulation of the nucleus raphe medianus. *Eur J Pharmacol* 81: 681—685.

56. Jones RSG, Broadbent J (1982): Further studies on the role of indoleamines in the responses of cortical neurones to stimulation of nucleus raphe medianus: effects of indoleamine precursor loading. *Neuropharmacology* 21: 1273—1277.

57. Park MR, Gonzales-Vegas JA, Kitai ST (1982): Serotonergic excitation from dorsal raphe stimulation recorded intracellularly from rat caudate-putamen. *Brain Res* 243: 49—58.

58. Davies M, Wilkinson LS, Roberts MHT (1988) Evidence for excitatory 5-HT 2 receptors on rat brainstem neurones. *Br J Pharmacol* 94: 483—491.

59. Davies M, Wilkinson LS, Roberts MHT (1988): Evidence for depressant 5HT 1-like receptors on rat brainstem neurones. *Br J Pharmacol*: 94: 492—499.

60. Roberts M, Davies M, Girdlestone D, Foster GA (1988): Spinal motoneurone responses to stimulation of raphe obscurus, application of 5-hydroxytryptamine (5HT) and 5HT receptor agonists and antagonists. *Brit J Pharmacol* 95: 437—448.

61. Montigny, C de, Aghajanian GK (1977): Preferential action of 5-methoxytryptamine and 5-methoxydimethyltryptamine on presynaptic serotonin receptors: a comparative ionto-phoretic study with LSD and serotonin. *Neuropharmacology* 16: 811—815.

62. Yarborough GG, Singh DK, Pettibone DJ (1984): A comparative electrophysiological and biochemical assessment of serotonin (5-HT) and a novel 5-HT agonist (MK-212) on central serotonergic receptors. *Neuropharmacology* 23: 1271—1277.

63. Paterson I (1985): The actions of Beta carbolines on single neurones in the central nervous system. PhD thesis. University of Wales.

64. Fozard JR (1984): MDL 72222: a potent and highly selective antagonist at neuronal 5-hydroxytryptamine receptors. *Naunyn-Schmiedeberg's Arch Pharmacol* 326: 36—44.

65. Feniuk, W, Humphrey PPA, Perren MJ, Watts AD (1985): A comparison of 5-hydroxy-tryptamine receptors mediating contraction in rabbit aorta and dog saphenous vein: evidence for different receptor types obtained by use of selective agonists and antagonists. *Br J Pharmacol* 86: 697—704.

66. Lakoski JM, Aghajanian GK (1985): Effects of ketanserin on neuronal responses to serotonin in the prefrontal cortex, lateral geniculate and dorsal raphe nucleus. *Neuropharmacology* 24: 265—273.

67. Mason R (1985): Characterisation of 5HT sensitive neurones in the rat CNS using iontophoresed 8-OH-DPAT and ketanserin. *Br J Pharmacol* 86: 433P.

68. Sastry BSR, Phillis JW (1977): Metergoline as a selective 5-hydroxytryptamine antagonist in the cerebral cortex. *Can J Pharmac* 55: 130—135.

69. Jones RSG (1982): A comparison of the responses of cortical neurons to iontophoretically applied tryptamine and 5-hydroxytryptamine in the rat. *Neuropharmacology* 21, 209—214.

70. Connell LA, Wallis DI (1988): Responses to 5-hydroxytryptamine evoked in the hemisected spinal cord of the neonate rat. *Br J Pharmacol* 94: 1101—1114.

71. Connell LA, Wallis DI (1989): 5-hydroxytryptamine depolarises neonatal rat motoneurones via a receptor unrelated to an identified binding site. *Neuropharmacology* 28: 625—634.

XIV. 5-Hydroxytryptamine and related drugs and autonomic ganglia

D. I. WALLIS and P. ELLIOTT

A cardiovascular response to 5-HT will be evoked if, amongst other actions, the amine increases impulse traffic in sympathetic neurones causing vasoconstriction or in autonomic neurones which alter cardiac output. In addition, cardiovascular responses will be modified if 5-HT modulates the output of transmitter at the neuroeffector junction. Cardiovascular actions may also result from 5-HT affecting the afferent limb of reflex pathways.

Many autonomic ganglia are readily excited by 5-HT or transmission through them is modified. The evidence for this has been reviewed extensively [1, 2, 3, 4, 5]. In this chapter, I believe it is more appropriate to consider briefly the multiplicity of 5-HT actions, to highlight certain of them and consider their possible physiological significance, and indicate the directions in which future experimental work may move. Although these reviews describe a considerable variety of effects of 5-HT on autonomic neurones, it is apparent that there still remains much to be understood. Thus, although 5-HT can excite both pre- and postganglionic autonomic neurones and is capable of modulating transmitter release both at ganglionic synapses and at the neuroeffector junction, the observations derive from a narrow range of species and from a limited number of end organs, mainly certain blood vessels. Investigation mostly depends upon electrophysiological techniques, which can range from examination of population responses from many neurones through intracellular studies on single cells to measures of single channel currents in channels associated with $5-HT_3$ receptors. Despite the responsiveness of the rabbit superior cervical ganglion (scg) to 5-HT, it is known that a substantial proportion of the cells are insensitive to the amine [6, 7]. Recent developments in the categorization of sympathetic neurones, in which 3 major neurochemical groups have been described [8] and correlated with differences in firing characteristics, membrane currents and control of end-organs, [9, 10] have not been paralleled by studies showing whether neurones of different functional types have any differential sensitivity to 5-HT.

P.R. Saxena, D.I. Wallis, W. Wouters and P. Bevan (eds), Cardiovascular Pharmacology of 5-Hydroxytryptamine, pp. 177—190.
© 1990 *Kluwer Academic Publishers, Dordrecht —*

1. Sites of action on autonomic neurones

It appears that 5-HT receptors and associated ion channels may be present on most, or perhaps all, of the surface membrane of certain sympathetic neurones with non-myelinated axons. Parasympathetic neurones, excepting the neurones of the enteric plexuses, have received less attention and only occasional reference will be made to parasympathetic pathways. The sites of action on sympathetic neurones may be (a) postsynaptic, where a soma-dendritic post-synaptic potential may be set up, (b) axonal, where depolarizing effects have been observed on both preganglionic and postganglionic sympathetic axons, and (c) presynaptic, on nerve terminals within the ganglion and at nerve terminals at the neuroeffector junction, where the functional effect is an alteration in transmitter release. Each action is associated with a particular type of 5-HT receptor, and different types of receptor may be found on different areas of the same neurone or class of neurones. The development of selective agonists and antagonists and the proposed classification of 5-HT receptor types [11] has allowed a dissection of these actions; both 5-HT_3 and 5-HT_1-like receptors are present on these neurones, but 5-HT_2 receptors have not been identified.

2. Investigating presynaptic actions of 5-HT on autonomic neurones

A presynaptic action of 5-HT within a ganglion will manifest itself as an alteration of transmission through the ganglion. The effects of 5-HT on transmitter release at the neuroeffector junction, which are known at different sites to be both facilitatory and inhibitory, are beyond the scope of this chapter to discuss and are dealt with elsewhere in this volume. The extensive literature describes effects of 5-HT on transmission in autonomic ganglia which are variable and inconsistent [4, 5]. This is likely to be due to a number of factors. Firstly, altered transmission will be the resultant of both presynaptic and postsynaptic action on the ganglion; secondly, transmitter release to a particular cell may be depressed, unaltered or, possibly, facilitated [4]; and, thirdly, the postganglionic actions may include one or both of depolarization (excitation) or hyperpolarization (inhibition). Thus, it is less surprising that both depression and facilitation of ganglionic transmission in response to 5-HT have been reported from both in vivo and in vitro experiments [12, 13, 14, 15, 16]. Of interest in a cardiovascular context is the substantial facilitation of transmission observed in the rat stellate ganglion which is induced by 5-HT [17], although whether this action results in an increase in cardiac output was not examined. These electrophysiological studies employed extracellular recording techniques, but, as discussed by Wallis and Dun [4], these are not incisive enough to distinguish a presynaptic from a postsynaptic site of modulation of transmission. Rather, individual routes of transmission through ganglia need to be examined in circumstances, if possible, where the function of the ganglion cell can be established. Very little, if any, work of this kind has been done. However, intracellular recording to examine epsps evoked by preganglionic stimulation and assessment of the number of acetylcholine quanta released (quantal analysis) can identify presynaptic actions. Such methods have revealed an inhibition of nicotinic transmission in the rabbit scg [4, 18], while in bullfrog lumbar sympathetic ganglia low concentractions (1–30 μm) of 5-HT enhance acetylcholine release and higher concentrations (100–1000 μm) depress it. The receptors responsible for these actions can only be characterized with selective agonists and antagonists. Our preliminary results suggest that a 5-HT$_1$-like receptor underlies the presynaptic depression of transmission (Figure 1). Transmission of an orthodromic action potential to certain cells is sensitive to blockade by 5-HT, RU 24969 and 5-carboxamidotryptamine (each applied at a concentration of 10 μm). With the stimulation level set to generate an epsp in the cell of just great enough amplitude consistently to trigger an action potential (controls), failure of transmission (to leave an epsp only or a spike initiated after a longer latency) occurs in the presence of the agonists. As yet we have not tested other concentrations of agonist. Since the agonists produced no discernible change in the membrane potential or membrane properties of the ganglion cells, we interpret these effects as a reduction in the amount of acetylcholine released by the preganglionic neurone as a result of some presynaptic action of the amines. Dun and Karczmar [19] have demonstrated that the presynaptic action of 5-HT on this ganglion is to reduce the number of quanta of acetylcholine released by the preganglionic action potential.

Assessment of transmitter release depends upon statistical methods to determine the size of the effect produced by a single quantum of transmitter. Quantal analysis of epsp amplitude is complicated or (invalidated) when the synaptic input to many sympathetic neurones is examined because of the high degree of convergence onto these cells. Further, a substantial number of synaptic inputs appear to be insensitive to 5-HT [4, 18, our unpublished data]. Another approach which we have adopted is to see whether these 5-HT$_1$-like receptors, which are on the presynaptic nerve terminal and, therefore, may also be distributed over the axonal membrane, may be studied in terms of an axonal action. A method devised by Elliott [20] assumes that the presynaptic action is one which, directly or indirectly, decreases calcium entry and thus reduces transmitter release. The axonal compound action potential of the cervical sympathetic nerve may be converted to a Ca spike by superfusion with a medium containing tetrodotoxin to block Na currents, 4-aminopyridine to block voltage-gated K currents and an increased extracellular concentration of Ca (Figure 2). After total block of the axonal compound action potential with tetrodotoxin, a regenerative spike re-appears in the presence of 4-aminopyridine. This has a higher threshold, longer latency and duration, and the characteristics of a Ca spike [20]. The spike persisted when external Ca was replaced with Sr or Ba, but was

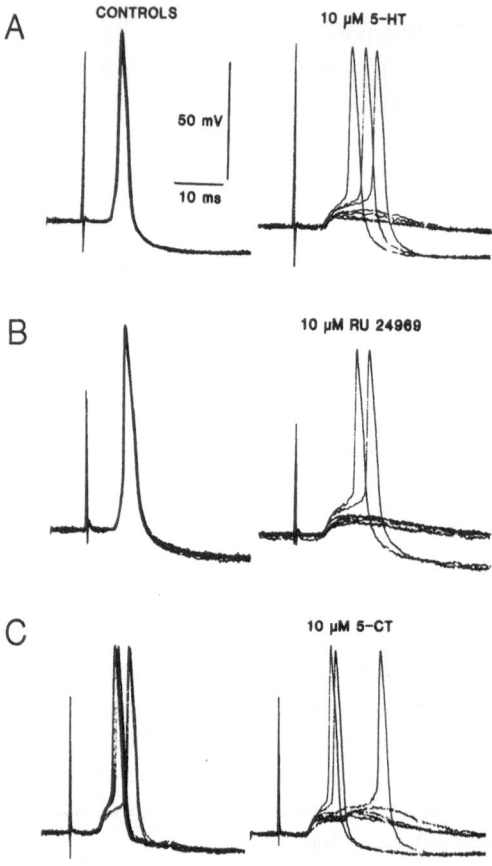

Figure 1. Transmission failure produced by 5-HT and selective agonists for 5-HT$_1$-like receptors in rabbit superior cervical ganglion. Note that in these cells the amines caused no discernible change in membrane potential so that it was assumed that the altered transmission was due to some presynaptic action. I—V curves were constructed to confirm absence of a post-synaptic effect (not shown).

Transmission was tested by applying a repeated stimulus to the pre-ganglionic trunk just supra-threshold for the initiation of an action potential at a frequency of 0.5 Hz. Actions of 10 μM 5-HT, RU 24969 and 5-CT. The traces show seven consecutive superimposed sweeps A, resting membrane potential −56 mV, presynaptic stimulation 0.1 ms, 15 V, 0.5 Hz; B, the same cell following 20 minutes wash-out; C, resting membrane potential −60 mV, presynaptic stimulation 0.1 ms, 6 V, 0.5 Hz and the effect of 5-CT on a different cell.

blocked by the addition of the following inorganic Ca channel blockers (in descending order of potency): Cd > Pa > Ni > Co > Mn > Mg [20]. In the experiment illustrated, the amplitude of the Ca spike was reduced by 5-HT in a concentration- related manner. A concentration as low as 0.01 μM could induce such an effect. This action was seen during blockade of any 5-HT$_3$ receptors with ICS 205—930. Whether a 5-HT$_1$-like receptor mediates this effect we cannot yet say, nor do we know whether 5-HT acts directly to reduce Ca influx or indirectly reduces spike amplitude by, say, activating a K

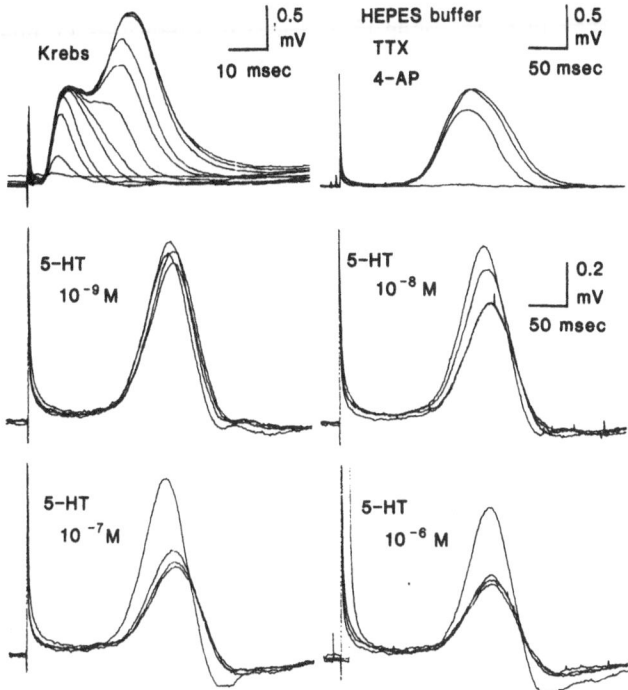

Figure 2. Conversion of compound action potential of rabbit cervical sympathetic axons to Ca spike and reduction in Ca spike amplitude by 5-HT. Chart records from oscilloscope digital store.

Upper row (left): Na spike in Krebs solution evoked by a stimulus of 7.5 V, pulse durations 0.01 to 0.3 msec, 0.2 Hz; (right): after superfusion in modified saline (HEPES buffer, 0.5 μM TTX, 1 mM 4-amino-pyridine, 4-AP), the Na spike disappeared and, on increasing the stimulus voltage (20, 30, 40 or 50 V, 0.01 Hz), was replaced by a spike of longer latency and duration (Ca spike). Note slower time base. Elliott has confirmed that a similar procedure in rat axons leads to development of a spike dependent upon calcium.

Middle and lower rows: the amplitude of the Ca spike was reduced on superfusion with 5-HT (10^{-9} to 10^{-6} M) in a concentration-dependent manner. Experiments were done following blockade of 5-HT$_3$ receptors with ICS 205-930 (10^{-7} M). The largest response in each panel is the control, the other traces show the gradual reduction of the Ca spike during the 5-HT superfusion period of 300 s. The Ca spike recovered on washing — largest response in succeeding panels.

current. Nevertheless, 5-HT action on Ca-spike amplitude may serve as a useful model of presynaptic 5-HT actions on which quantitative pharmacology may be attempted.

3. Responses of ganglion cells to 5-HT

It may be noted, in passing, that the cell bodies of preganglionic sympathetic neurones are depolarized [21] and/or excited by 5-HT [22, 23] and that this excitatory effect is blocked by methysergide [21, 24], cyproheptadine [21], cinanserin [24] and metergoline [25]. There is a dense 5-HT innervation of the lateral horn [26, 27], but no 5-HT-mediated epsps seem to have been identified in these cells. However, a full pharmacological characterization of the 5-HT response remains to be made. In contrast, the responses to 5-HT of sympathetic ganglion cells have been well documented. Since these are discussed extensively in a forthcoming review [5], their features will only be summarised here. The major action of 5-HT on sympathetic ganglion cells is to elicit a substantial, phasic depolarization, which is generated by the opening of channels permeable to Na and K ions [5, 28, 29]. The 5-HT_3 receptor involved has been characterized by a range of antagonists, including novel 5-HT_3 receptor antagonists, e.g. MDL 72222, ICS 205-930, GR 38032F, quipazine, metoclopramide [2, 3, 4, 5, 30, 31]. Intracellular recording has served to confirm results from studies in which the recording of population responses has allowed a quantitative pharmacological approach [see 5].

Receptors which are probably identical [2, 3, 5] are found on parasympathetic ganglion cells [32], visceral (vagal) primary afferent neurones and on various murine clonal cell lines (N1E-115 neuroblastoma, NG 108—15 neuroblastoma x glioma clone and NCB-20 neuroblastoma x Chinese hamster brain clone cells). These cultured cells have been studied with patch clamp techniques [33] and the inward current evoked by 5-HT has been shown to be carried by monovalent cations [34]. 5-HT-induced currents are antagonised by the 5-HT_3 receptor antagonists, quipazine [35], MDL 72222, ICS 205—930 [36] and GR 38032F [37]. A binding site corresponding to the 5-HT_3 receptor has been identified in NIE-115 cells [38]. The significance of these studies is that neuronal clonal cell lines may provide a model for the study of 5-HT_3 receptors and the associated ion channel. Single channel currents have now been measured in at least two laboratories and the channel opened by the 5-HT_3 receptor proposed to be one of low conductance [e.g. about 1 pS] [37] or of high conductance [about 140 pS] [39].

Surface extracellular recordings made in vivo from cat scg revealed a triphasic response to 5-HT [14, 40]. This consisted of a rapid depolarization, a hyperpolarization and, finally, a late depolarization. Recently, intracellular records have clarified the nature of these potential changes indicating that rapid and slow depolarizing responses occur in different, and sometimes the same, individual ganglion cells and correspond to the surface potential changes. Some sympathetic neurones display a slow depolarization to 5-HT and some a slow depolarization following a fast depolarization; the slow depolarization is mediated by an, as yet, uncharacterized receptor [41, 42], whereas the fast depolarization is 5-HT_3 receptor-mediated [41, 42]. Slow depolarizing responses evoked by 5-HT have been identified in guinea-pig coeliac, inferior mesenteric and superior cervical ganglion cells [5, 41, 42]. In a sample of 120 guinea-pig coeliac ganglion cells, 43% responded with a fast depolarization alone, 30% responded with a fast and slow depolarization and 25% responded with a slow depolarization alone. Slow responses to 5-HT last seconds or minutes and are accompanied by a decrease in membrane conductance in many cells, i.e. their ionic mechanism is one where channels close in response to 5-HT [43, 44]. They are blocked by methysergide, but are insensitive to MDL 72222, quipazine and metoclopramide [42]. Dun and his colleagues [44] have suggested that there is a physiological event related to the slow depolarization. The slow depolarizations shared several characteristics with synaptic responses evoked by repetitive orthodromic stimulation in about 60% of coeliac ganglion cells which exhibited a non-cholinergic epsp. Further, immunohistofluorescence techniques revealed that many coeliac ganglion cells are surrounded by a network of 5-HT-immunoreactive fibres [43, 44], although in another study the presence of 5-HT-containing nerve fibres could not be confirmed [9]. The possibility remains that 5-HT may act as a neurotransmitter for the slow non-cholinergic epsp in the coeliac ganglion. Indeed, there is a rather striking parallel between the modes of action of acetylcholine (ACh) and 5-HT at sympathetic ganglion cells. The nicotinic response to ACh and the fast response to 5-HT are remarkably similar in their ionic features, while the slow response to 5-HT parallels in some ways the muscarinic response to ACh. If fast synaptic responses to 5-HT were eventually discovered, then 5-HT might mediate fast and slow modes of ganglionic transmission as does ACh [42].

The hyperpolarization is not easily investigated in single cells [5], but study of population responses from rat scg has identified it as mediated by a $5-HT_1$-like receptor [45]. Hyperpolarizations induced by 5-HT can arise secondarily to a preceding depolarization as a result of electrogenic extrusion of Na ions or the activation by Ca of Ca-gated K potassium currents [5]. The direct hyperpolarizing action has been characterized by Ireland and Jordan [45, 46]. It was also elicited by 5-carboxamidotryptamine and was blocked reversibly by spiperone and in a manner incompatible with competitive antagonism by ($\pm$)-cyanopindolol [46].

More subtle effects of 5-HT on sympathetic ganglion cells have yet to be placed in a pharmacological context or clearly related to physiological function. Thus, in guinea-pig coeliac ganglion cells associated with control of gastro-intestinal motility, 5-HT has been shown to suppress a slow Ca-activated K current [9]. This current causes a prolonged after-hyperpolarization following the spike and may determine the characteristic firing pattern of the cell [9]. A second example has been described in bull-frog sympathetic ganglion cells, where 5-HT appears to decrease the affinity of the ACh molecule for its recognition site at the receptor-ion channel complex [47, 48], thus acting as an endogenous antagonist.

4. 5-HT$_3$ receptors on sympathetic preganglionic and post-ganglionic axons

The presence of 5-HT$_3$ receptors mediating a depolarization of the axons of ganglion neurones [49] is, perhaps, not unexpected in view of their soma-dendritic location and their location on the terminal nerve membrane at certain neuroeffector junctions (e.g. rabbit heart [2], nictitating membrane [50]). On preganglionic neurones, as discussed above, receptors within the spinal cord and those modulating transmitter release within the ganglion appear likely to be 5-HT$_1$-like in so far as they can be classified at this stage. It was, therefore, a surprise for us to identify a fast depolarizing response to 5-HT in the preganglionic axons of the rabbit cervical sympathetic nerve which was clearly mediated by 5-HT$_3$ receptors [51]. Using an extracellular recording technique, 5-HT depolarizations were demonstrated which showed marked tachyphylaxis and were blocked reversibly by MDL 72222, ICS 205-930 and SDZ 206-830 in nanomolar concentrations or lower; 2-methyl-5-HT mimicked the action of 5-HT [51, 52]. The receptor profile appeared similar to that for the 5-HT$_3$ receptor on the terminals of sympathetic nerves innervating the heart [2, 3, 53].

5. Parasympathetic ganglia

Excitatory effects of 5-HT have been identified on the parasympathetic innervation of the bladder in dog, rat and cat [54, 55, 56, 57], although at low concentrations 5-HT may depress transmission in cat ganglia [56] and in rabbit ciliary ganglia [58]. 5-HT can evoke release of a non-cholinergic, non-adrenergic neurotransmitter (probably a purine) from parasympathetic neurones in the guinea-pig bladder [59], while a depolarization of parasym-pathetic ganglion cells mediated by 5-HT$_3$ receptors has been recorded intracellularly [32]. 5-HT$_3$ receptors have been identified on the terminals of the parasympathetic innervation of rat bronchi [60] and rabbit heart [61]. However, the receptors on parasympathetic neurones in the mouse bladder, which facilitate transmission, are not 5-HT$_3$ receptors but appear to be 5-HT$_1$-like [62].

6. General considerations

This brief survey of the effects of 5-HT on autonomic ganglia raises some general questions about possible sources of 5-HT, about its function in relation to the cardiovascular system and about the association between particular responses and particular receptors.

6.1 *Are there sources of 5-HT which can activate autonomic neurones?*

There is an increasing body of evidence that 5-HT may be available to influence autonomic neurones from a number of sources, including plasma 5-HT derived from platelets, 5-HT released from paracrine cells (mast and SIF cells) and 5-HT stored in nerve fibres. Although plasma levels of unbound 5-HT are normally low [63, 64], 5-HT may be released from platelets on damage of blood vessel walls and, for instance, during a migraine attack. The platelets of migraineurs lose some 30—40% of their 5-HT content at the onset of a migraine attack [see 65]. 5-HT may be released from mast cells [66] or from small intensely fluorescent (SIF) cells within ganglia [see 4]. Using immunohistochemical techniques, SIF cells in the rat scg [67], in guinea-pig prevertebral sympathetic ganglia [67], in parasympathetic [68] and in trigeminal ganglia [69] have been identified as 5-HT-containing. The innervation by 5-HT-containing nerve fibres of the lateral horn of the spinal cord has already been mentioned; it is unclear, however, whether these make direct synaptic contract with preganglionic sympathetic neurones [see 4]. Innervation of sympathetic ganglia by 5-HT-containing nerves is more debatable (see above). However, since there are known to be 5-HT-containing neurones in intramural ganglia of the intestine (see chapter by Gershon, Mawe & Branchek), and since, in addition, various intramural ganglionic neurones give off collaterals to prevertebral ganglia [70] this is a distinct possibility.

6.2 *What could be the functions of so many diverse actions of 5-HT?*

Clearly, there is a multiplicity of sites of action for 5-HT within autonomic pathways which indicates that 5-HT has the potential for modulating cardiovascular reflexes in a number of ways. The mechanisms described above include those which would facilitate discharge, either phasically or tonically, along cardiovascular reflex pathways, but also those which would reduce such discharge. There is the capability for fine-tuning of the system. However, is it the case that cardiovascular effects, in the inact animal or man, have been ascribed in particular to an interaction of intrinsic 5-HT with autonomic ganglia? To my knowledge cardiovascular effects have not been so ascribed, in part because the conditions under which a physiological or a pathophysiological release of 5-HT occurs are poorly understood. In vivo experiments, in which physiological or pathophysiological alterations in cardiovascular function can be shown to be caused by an action of intrinsic 5-HT on autonomic pathways are required to answer the point. The multiplicity of potential sites of interaction does not mean, necessarily, that most of these regulatory mechanisms will be redundant. In the first place, multiple safeguard of action is a common principle in biology. It may be that some of these sites of interaction are brought into play when other regulatory mechanisms start to fail. An associated idea is that the recruitment of some of these modulatory mechanisms occurs in certain pathologies. As discussed above, there may be a selectivity in the distribution of 5-HT receptors on certain functional pathways, e.g. to the heart or to arterio-venous anastomoses in skeletal muscle, which has yet to be fully elucidated.

6.3   Is equation of functional effect and 5-HT receptor type of any value?

When dealing with the complexities of the nervous system, there is a temptation to link a functional action with a particular type of 5-HT receptor in any tissue where this kind of response occurs. If the ionophore or effector mechanism and the receptor are independent entities this clearly does not follow. Strictly, differentiation of the receptors should be based, if possible, on equilibrium dissociation constants of competitive antagonists, although the rank order of agonist potencies may be a further discriminating feature. Electrophysiologists in particular are prone to the view that a different mode of action suggests involvement of a different receptor. As discussed more fully elsewhere [5], it may be the case that $5\text{-}HT_3$ receptors on sympathetic, parasympathetic and enteric ganglion cells and on primary afferent neurones are homologous and all linked to the same ionophore. One might speculate that the membrane components responsive to 5-HT may normally involve association of particular sorts of recognition site with particular sorts of operant sub-unit. However, although 5-HT receptors reducing transmitter release may all be considered $5\text{-}HT_1$-like, there are differences reported between 5-HT receptors inhibiting noradrenaline release in different tissues [71, 72] and between these and 5-HT receptors inhibiting ACh release in the guinea-pig ileum [73]. The receptor reducing ACh release in sympathetic ganglia is also $5\text{-}HT_1$-like (see above), but whether it is homologous with any of these presynaptic receptors has yet to be established. It may be premature to discuss this in respect of presynaptic receptors, since it is not known whether the mechanism by which transmitter release is reduced may not also differ at these different sites.

Acknowledgements

The recent experimental work by the authors described in this chapter was supported by Wellcome Trust Grants to D. I. Wallis.

References

1. Wallis DI (1981): Neuronal 5-hydroxytryptamine receptors outside the central nervous system. *Life Sci* 29: 2345—2355.

2. Fozard JR (1984): Neuronal 5-HT receptors in the periphery. *Neuropharmacology* 23: 1473—1486.
3. Richardson BP, Engel G (1986): The pharmacology and function of 5-HT$_3$, receptors. *Trends Neurosci* 9: 424—428.
4. Wallis DI, Dun NJ (1989): Presynaptic action of 5-hydroxytryptamine on autonomic ganglia, (in press) in: Feigenbaum JJ, Hanani M (eds), *Presynaptic regulation of neurotransmitter release*. London and Tel Aviv: Freund Publishing Co.
5. Wallis, DI (1989): Interaction of 5-HT with autonomic and sensory neurones, pp. 220—246 in Fozard JR, (ed), *The peripheral actions of 5-hydroxytryptamine*. Oxford: Oxford University Press.
6. Wallis DI, North RA (1978): Intracellular recording of responses of rabbit superior cervical ganglion cells to 5-hydroxytryptamine applied by iontophoresis. *Neuropharmacology* 17: 1023—1028.
7. Skok V, Selyanko AA (1979): Acetylcholine and serotonin receptors in mammalian sympathetic ganglion neurones, pp. 248—253 in: Brooks CMcC, Koizumi K, Sato A (eds), *Integrative functions of the autonomic nervous system*. Tokyo: University of Tokyo Press.
8. Macrae IM, Furness JB, Costa M (1986): Distribution of subgroups of noradrenaline neurones in the coeliac ganglion of the guinea-pig. *Cell and Tissue Res* 244: 173—180.
9. Cassell JF, McLachlan EM (1987): Two calcium-activated potassium conductances in a subpopulation of coeliac neurones of guinea-pig and rabbit. *J Physiol* 394: 331—349.
10. McLachlan EM (1987): Functional specialization of membrane properties of sympathetic post-ganglionic neurones, pp. 1—10 in: Polosa C, Calaresu F (eds), *Organization of the Autonomic Nervous System: Central and peripheral mechanisms*. New York: Alan Liss.
11. Bradley PB, Engel G, Fenuik W, Fozard J, Humphrey PPA Middlemiss DN, Mylecharane EJ, Richardson BP, Saxena PR (1986): Proposals for the classification and nomenclature of functional receptors for 5-hydroxytryptamine. *Neuropharmacology* 25: 563—576.
12. Trendelenburg U (1956): The action of 5-hydroxytryptamine on the nictitating membrane and on the superior cervical ganglion of the cat. *Br J Pharmacol Chemother* 11: 74—80.
13. DeGroat WC, Volle RL (1966): The actions of the catecholamines on transmission in the superior cervical ganglion of the cat. *J Pharmacol exp Ther* 154: 1—13.
14. Haefely W (1974): The effects of 5-hydroxytryptamine and some related compounds on the cat superior cervical ganglion in situ. *Naunyn-Schmiedeberg's Arch Pharmacol* 281: 145—165.
15. DeGroat WC, Lalley PM (1973): Interaction between picrotoxin and 5-hydroxytryptamine in the superior cervical ganglion of the cat. *Br J Pharmacol* 48: 233—244.
16. Wallis DI, Woodward B (1974): The facilitatory actions of 5-hydroxytryptamine and bradykinin in the superior cervical ganglion of the rabbit. *Br J Pharmacol* 51: 521—531.
17. Hertzler EC (1961): 5-hydroxytryptamine and transmission in sympathetic ganglia. *Br J Pharmacol Chemother* 17: 406—413.
18. Dun NJ, Karczmar AG (1981): Evidence for a presynaptic inhibitory action of 5-hydroxytryptamine in a mammalian sympathetic ganglion. *J Pharmacol exp Ther* 217: 714—718.
19. Hirai K, Koketsu K (1980): Presynaptic regulation of the release of acetylcholine by 5-hydroxytryptamine. *Br J Pharmacol* 70: 499—500.
20. Elliott P, Marsh SJ, Brown DA (1989): Inhibition of Ca-spikes in rat preganglionic cervical sympathetic nerves by sympathomimetic amines. *Br J Pharmacol* 96: 65—76.
21. Ma RC, Dun NJ (1986): Excitation of lateral horn neurons of the neonatal rat spinal cord by 5-hydroxytryptamine. *Developmental Brain Research* 24: 89—98.
22. De Groat WC, Ryall RW (1967): An excitatory action of 5-hydroxytryptamine on sympathetic preganglionic neurones. *Exp Brain Res* 3: 299—305.
23. Coote JH, MacLeod VH, Fleetwood-Walker S, Gilbey MP (1981): The response of individual sympathetic preganglionic neurones to microelectrophoretically applied endogenous monoamines. *Brain Res* 215: 135—145.

24. Kadzielawa K (1983): Antagonism of the excitatory effects of 5-hydroxytryptamine on sympathetic preganglionic neurones and neurones activated by visceral afferents. *Neuropharmacology* 22: 19—27.

25. McCall RB (1983): Serotonergic excitation of sympathetic preganglionic neurones: a microiontophoretic study. *Brain Res* 289: 121—127.

26. Dahlstrom A, Fuxe K (1964): Evidence for the existence of monoamine-containing neurons in the central nervous system. I. Demonstration of monoamines in the cell bodies of brainstem neurons. *Acta physiol Scand* 62, Suppl. 232: 1—55.

27. Dahlstrom A, Fuxe K (1965): Evidence for the existence of monoamine-containing neurons in the central nervous system. II. Experimentally-induced changes in the intraneuronal amine levels of bulbospinal neuron systems. *Acta physiol Scand* 64, Suppl. 247: 1—36.

28. Wallis DI, Woodward B (1975): Membrane potential changes induced by 5-hydroxytryptamine in the rabbit superior cervical ganglion. *Br J Pharmacol* 55, 199—212.

29. Wallis DI, North RA (1978): Intracellular recording of responses of rabbit superior cervical ganglion cells to 5-hydroxytryptamine applied by iontophoresis. *Neuropharmacology* 17, 1023—1028.

30. Ireland SJ, Straughan DW, Tyers MB (1982): Antagonism by metoclopramide and quipazine of 5-hydroxytryptamine-induced depolarizations of the rat isolated vagus nerve. *Br J Pharmacol* 75: 16P.

31. Brittain RT, Butler A, Coates H, Fortune DH, Hagan R, Hill JM, Humber DC, Humphrey PPA, Hunter DC, Ireland SJ, Jack D, Jordan CC, Oxford A, Tyers MB (1987): GR 38032F, a novel selective 5-HT$_3$ receptor antagonist. *Br J Pharmacol* 90: 87P.

32. Akasu T, Hasuo H, Tokimasa T (1987): Activation of 5-HT$_3$ receptor subtypes causes rapid excitation of rabbit parasympathetic neurones. *Br J Pharmacol* 91: 453—455.

33. Guharay F, Usherwood PNR (1981): Characterisation of the effects of 5-hydroxytryptamine on NIE-115 neuroblastoma cells. *Br J Pharmacol* 74: 294—295P.

34. Neijt HC, Vijverberg HPM, van den Bercken J (1986): The dopamine response in mouse neuroblastoma cells is mediated by serotonin 5-HT$_3$ receptors. *Eur J Pharmacol* 127: 271—274.

35. Peters J, Usherwood PNR (1983): 5-hydroxytryptamine responses of murine neuroblastoma cells. Ions and putative antagonists. *Br J Pharmacol* 80: 532P.

36. Neijt HC, Te Duits IJ, Vijverberg HPM (1988): Pharmacological characterisation of serotonin 5-HT$_3$ receptor-mediated electrical response in cultured mouse neuroblastoma cells. *Neuropharmacology* 27: 301—307.

37. Lambert JJ, Peters JA, Hales TG, Dempster J (1989): The properties of 5-HT$_3$ receptors in clonal cell lines studied by patch-clamp techniques. *Br J Pharmacol* 97: 27—40.

38. Hoyer D, Neijt HC (1988): Identification of serotonin 5-HT$_3$ recognition sites in membranes of NIE-115 neuroblastoma cells by radioligand binding. *Mol. Pharmacol* 33: 303—309.

39. Guharay F, Ramsay RL, Usherwood PNR (1985): 5-hydroxytryptamine-activated single-channel currents recorded from murine neuroblastoma cells. *Brain Res* 340: 325—332.

40. Machova J, Boska D (1969): The effects of 5-hydroxytryptamine, dimethylphenylpiperazinium and acetylcholine on transmission and surface potential in the cat sympathetic ganglion. *Eur J Pharmacol* 7, 152—158.

41. Wallis DI, Dun JN (1988): A comparison of fast and slow depolarizations evoked by 5-HT in guinea-pig coeliac ganglion cells in vitro. *Br J Pharmacol* 93: 110—120.

42. Wallis DI, Dun NJ (1987): Fast and slow depolarizing responses of guinea-pig coeliac ganglion cells to 5-hydroxytryptamine. *J Auton Nerv System* 21: 185—194.

43. Kiraly M, Ma RC, Dun NJ (1983): Serotonin mediates a slow excitatory potential in mammalian coeliac ganglion. *Brain Res* 275: 378—383.

44. Dun NJ, Kiraly M, Ma RC (1984): Evidence for a serotonin-mediated slow excitatory potential in the guinea-pig coeliac ganglia. *J Physiol* 351: 61—76.

45. Ireland SJ (1987): Origin of 5-hydroxytryptamine-induced hyperpolarization of the rat superior cervical ganglion and vagus nerve. *Br J Pharmacol* 92: 407—416.

46. Ireland SJ, Jordan CC (1987): Pharmacological characterization of 5-hydroxytryptamine-induced hyperpolarization of the rat superior cervical ganglion. *Br J Pharmacol* 92: 417—427.

47. Akasu T, Kirai K, Koketsu K (1981): 5-hydroxytryptamine controls ACh-receptor sensitivity of bullfrog sympathetic ganglion cells. *Brain Res* 211: 217—220.

48. Koketsu K, Akasu T, Miyagawa M, Hirai K (1982): Modulation of nicotinic transmission by biogenic amines in bullfrog sympathetic ganglia. *J. Auton Nerv System* 6: 47—53.

49. Nash HL, Wallis DI (1981): Effects of divalent cations on responses of a sympathetic ganglion to 5-hydroxytryptamine and 1,1-dimethyl-4-phenyl piperazinium. *Br J Pharmacol* 73: 759—772.

50. Adler-Graschinsky E (1983): Dual presynaptic effects of 5-hydroxytryptamine on peripheral noradrenergic synapses. *J Auton Pharmacol* 3: 303—315.

51. Elliott P, Wallis DI (1988): 5-HT depolarizations of rabbit cervical sympathetic axons: mediation by 5-HT$_{3B}$ receptors? *Br J Pharmacol* 93: 93P.

52. Elliott P, Wallis DI (1988): The depolarizing action of 5-hydroxytryptamine on rabbit isolated preganglionic cerivcal sympathetic nerves. *Naunyn-Schmiedeberg's Arch Pharmacol* 338: 608—615.

53. Fozard JR, Mobarok Ali ATM (1978): Receptors for 5-hydroxytryptamine on the sympathetic nerves of the rabbit heart. *Naunyn-Schmiedeberg's Arch Pharmacol* 301: 223—235.

54. Gyermek L (1962): Action of 5-hydroxytryptamine on the urinary bladder of the dog. *Arch Int Pharmacod Ther* 87: 137—144.

55. Vanov S (1965): Responses of the rat urinary bladder in situ to drugs and to nerve stimulation. *Br J Pharmacol* 24: 591—600.

56. Saum WR, De Groat WC (1973): The actions of 5-hydroxytryptamine on the urinary bladder and on vesical autonomic ganglia in the cat. *J Pharmacol Exp Ther* 185: 70—83.

57. Saxena PR, Heiligers J, Mylecharane EJ, Tio R (1985): Excitatory 5-hydroxytryptamine receptors in the cat urinary bladder are of the M- and 5-HT$_2$ type. *J Auton Pharmacol* 5: 101—107.

58. Tatsumi H, Katayama Y (1987): The actions of 5-hydroxytryptamine in the rabbit ciliary ganglion. *J Auton Nerv System* 20: 137—145.

59. Burnstock G, Cocks T, Crowe R, Kasakov K (1978): Purinergic innervation of the guinea-pig urinary bladder. *Br J Pharmacol* 63: 125—138.

60. Aas P (1983): Serotonin-induced release of acetylcholine from neurons in the bronchial smooth muscle of the rat. *Acta physiol Scand* 117: 477—480.

61. Fozard JR (1984): MDL 72222: A potent and highly selective antagonist at neuronal 5-hydroxytryptamine receptors. *Naunyn-Schmiedeberg's Arch Pharmacol* 326: 36—44.

62. Holt SE, Cooper M, Wyllie JH (1986): On the nature of the receptor mediating the action of 5-hydroxytryptamine in potentiating responses of the mouse urinary bladder strip to electrical stimulation. *Naunyn-Schmiedeberg's Arch Pharmacol* 334: 333—340.

63. Garattini S, Valzelli L (1965): Serotonin. Elsevier, Amsterdam.

64. Franzen F, Eysell K (1969): Biologically active amines found in man. Pergamon, Oxford.

65. Fozard JR (1985): "Vascular neuroeffector mechanisms", pp. 321. Elsevier, Amsterdam.

66. Johnson AR, Erdos EG (1973): Release of histamine from mast cells by vasoactive peptides. *Proc Soc Exp Biol and Med* 142: 1252—1256.

67. Verhofstad AAJ, Steinbusch HWM, Penke B, Varga J, Joosten HWJ (1981): Serotonin-immunoreactive cells in the superior cervical ganglion of the rat. Evidence for the existence of separate serotonin- and catecholamine-containing small ganglionic cells. *Brain Res* 212: 39—49.

68. Neel DS, Parsons RL (1986): Catecholamine, serotonin and substance P-like peptide containing intrinsic neurones in the mud puppy parasympathetic cardiac ganglion. *J Neurosci* 6: 1970—1975.

69. Moskowitz MA, Reinhard JF, Romero J, Melamed E, Pettibone DJ (1979): Neurotransmitters and the fifth cranial nerve. Is there a relation to the headache phase of migraine? Lancet ii, 883—885.
70. Jule Y, Krier J, Szurszewski JH (1983): Patterns of innervation of neurones in the inferior mesenteric ganglion of the cat. *J Physiol* 344: 293—304.
71. Engel G, Gothert M, Müller-Schweinitzer E, Schlicker E, Sistonen L, Stadler PA (1983): Evidence for common pharmacological properties of [^{3}H] 5-hydroxytryptamine binding sites, presynaptic 5-hydroxytryptamine autoreceptors in CNS and inhibitory presynaptic 5-hydroxytryptamine receptors on sympathetic nerves. *Naunyn Schmiedeberg's Arch Pharmacol* 324: 116—124.
72. Charlton KG, Bond RA, Clarke DE (1986): An inhibitory prejunctional 5-hydroxytryptamine-1-like receptor in the isolated perfused rat kidney; apparent distinction from the 5-hydroxytryptamine-1A, 5-hydroxytryptamine-1B and 5-hydroxytryptamine-1C subtypes. *Naunyn-Schmiedeberg's Arch Pharmacol* 332: 8—15.
73. Fozard JR, Kilbinger H (1985): 8-OH-DPAT inhibits transmitter release from guinea-pig enteric cholinergic neurones by activating 5-HT$_{1A}$ receptors. *Br J Pharmacol* 86: 601P.

XV. 5-Hydroxytryptaminergic neurotransmission in the gut

MICHAEL D. GERSHON, GARY M. MAWE and
THERESA A. BRANCHEK

1. Intrinsic enteric neurons are part of a complex and autonomous nervous system

The enteric nervous system (ENS) is quite different in structure, complexity, organization, and function from other divisions of the autonomic nervous system (for reviews see [1—3]). Unlike the sympathetic and parasympathetic divisions, most enteric neurons receive no direct innervation from the central nervous system (CNS). Despite this relative lack of input from the CNS, the ENS can mediate reflex activity. To have this capability, the ENS must contain intrinsic primary afferent neurons, a variety of interneurons, and motor neurons. Thus, enteric ganglia cannot be considered to be simple relays. In addition, like the CNS, the ENS has many different types of neuron, defined either by established or putative neurotransmitter content or by shape. This complexity must be borne in mind when interpreting the effects of neuroactive compounds on the gastrointestinal tract.

2. 5-Hydroxytryptamine (5-HT) is a transmitter in the enteric nervous system

The largest store of 5-HT in the body is contained in the gut and, within the bowel, most of the 5-HT is contained within enteroendocrine cells (EC) of the gastrointestinal mucosa [4]. Nevertheless, indirect evidence was obtained as early as 1965 suggesting that there are neurons in the myenteric plexus that utilize 5-HT as a transmitter and that these putative serotoninergic neurons might function in the mediation of the peristaltic reflex [5]. Observations made in the period following this initial suggestion have satisfied all of the criteria needed to establish 5-HT as an enteric neurotransmitter. For example, even after removal of the mucosa, significant amounts of 5-HT remain in the gut wall [6]. These amounts, 57—110 ng/g in the small intestine [7—10] and ~ 500 ng/g, in the cecum [11, 12], are large if it is considered that the neural tissue in which the 5-HT is concentrated makes up only a

P.R. Saxena, D.I. Wallis, W. Wouters and P. Bevan (eds), Cardiovascular Pharmacology of
5-Hydroxytryptamine, pp. 191—210.

small proportion of the mucosa-free preparations of bowel wall. The actual concentration of 5-HT in the myenteric plexus is probably similar to or greater than that of 5-HT in the brain.

The identity of the cells in which 5-HT is stored was first demonstrated cytochemically by aldehyde-induced fluorescence [7, 13—15]. Moreover, 5-HT is present in the ENS of a large number of vertebrates, indicating that enteric serotoninergic neurons arose early in vertebrate ontogeny [16—20]. More recently, 5-HT-containing neurons in the myenteric plexus have been demonstrated immunocytochemically in many different mammals using a variety of anti-5-HT sera and monoclonal antibodies [21—29]. These 5-HT-containing neurons must be intrinsic to the gut, because they persist in long-term organotypic tissue cultures of bowel, even after the mucosa and extrinsic nerves have degenerated [15, 30]. The morphology of enteric 5-HT-containing neurons grown in culture is very similar to their morphology *in situ* [24]. In addition to their storage of 5-HT itself, enteric serotoninergic neurons contain a binding protein, SBP [31, 32], that is also found in the serotoninergic neurons of the brain [33, 34]. Another site where SBP is found is the 5-HT-containing parafollicular cells of the thyroid gland, which are derived from the same region of the neural crest as are the neurons of the ENS [35, 36]. SBP appears to be a component of the synaptic vesicles of serotoninergic neurons, since it is released by a Ca^{2+}-dependent mechanism, along with 5-HT, from stimulated enteric neurons [32, 37, 38]. The vesicular localization of SBP is supported by the observations that the protein moves proximo-distally in axons by fast transport and that SBP is concentrated in vesicular fractions derived from the CNS [39] and the thyroid [36]. The concentration of 5-HT in enteric neurons has been estimated to be about 7mM (~ 60 fmol/cell) [40]. Since the amine is probably stored entirely in synaptic vesicles where it is protected from degradation, its intravesicular concentration must be still higher. Conceivably the binding of intravesicular 5-HT by SBP may serve to reduce osmotic pressure within serotoninergic synaptic vesicles.

Enteric neurons take up ^3H-5-HT [7, 41]. This uptake is saturable, has a K_M of about 0.7 μM, a Q_{10} (27—37°C) of 3.6, and is energy dependent. ^3H-5-HT uptake is also Na^+-dependent, inhibited as an exponential function of the $[K^+]_0$, and sensitive to $[Ca^{2+}]_0$. Affinity of compounds for the ^3H-5-HT uptake site is much reduced when the alkyl amino group of 5-HT is substituted and when the 5-hydroxyl group on the indole ring is missing or masked [42]. Ring-hydroxylated analogues of 5-HT compete with ^3H-5-HT for entry into enteric neurons and are taken up by them. The uptake of some of these analogues can be demonstrated by histofluorescence [43], immunocytochemistry [21, 22], and electron microscopy [44, 45]. Although cell bodies of enteric 5-HT-containing neurons also take up ^3H-5-HT, the uptake is mainly into axon terminals [27, 44]. Like that of central serotoninergic neurons, the uptake of 5-HT by enteric neurons is inhibited specifically by fluoxetine [46] and zimelidine [10].

Evidence that enteric serotoninergic neurons contain tryptophan hydroxylase has been provided by the observations that ^{3}H-5-HT and ^{3}H-5-hydroxyindole acetic acid are synthesized from ^{3}H-L-tryptophan by mucosa-free strips of intestinal wall [12, 15]. ^{3}H-L-tryptophan is also metabolized to ^{3}H-5-HT and ^{3}H-5-hydroxyindole acetic acid by enteric 5-HT-containing neurons in tissue cultures [15]. As in the CNS, this biosynthesis of ^{3}H-5-HT from ^{3}H-L-tryptophan is inhibited by p-chlorophenylalanine. An antiserum raised against tryptophan hydroxylase purified from raphe neurons has also been found to demonstrate neurons in the gut [47], although the specificity of this antiserum has been questioned [3]. Although the production of ^{3}H-5-hydroxyindole acetic acid suggests that 5-HT is catabolized by monoamine oxidase (MAO) in enteric neurons, an alternate route of 5-HT metabolism, conversion of 5-HT to 5-HT-O-glucuronide, also exists [48]. The biosynthesis of 5-HT from L-tryptophan by enteric neurons is facilitated by the presence of a saturable uptake mechanism ($K_M \sim 50 \ \mu$M) for L-tryptophan [49].

5-HT is released from stimulated gastric neurons by activation of the vagus nerves [50, 51]. Both exogenous ^{3}H-5-HT [32, 52] and endogenous 5-HT [9, 37] are also released by electrical stimulation of neurons of the myenteric plexus of the small intestine. This release is Ca^{2+}-dependent and is inhibited by tetrodotoxin. 5-HT release from the bowel has been detected during peristalsis [53], suggesting, as does other evidence, that enteric serotoninergic neurons function in the mediation of the peristatic reflex [54]. The release of 5-HT from enteric neurons can also be provoked by application of tryptamine [10]. In contrast to the release of the amine by electrical stimulation, the release of 5-HT by tryptamine is Ca^{2+}-independent.

3. 5-HT has many actions on the gut

Enteroendocrine cells release 5-HT tonically and in response to vagal stimulation [25, 55] or increases in intraluminal pressure [56, 57]. In order for 5-HT to act as a neurotransmitter, therefore, it is necessary that myenteric neurons be insulated from mucosal 5-HT. In fact, when 5-HT is applied to the serosal surface of the bowel the peristaltic reflex is blocked, probably because of desensitization of ganglionic 5-HT receptors [58]. In contrast, application of 5-HT to the intestinal mucosa activates the peristaltic reflex, apparently by stimulating the mucosal processes of intrinsic enteric sensory neurons. An intraenteric barrier that prevents the 5-HT released from the mucosal epithelium from affecting myenteric neurons has been demonstrated by introducing ^{3}H-5-HT into the intestinal lumen [37]. The barrier appears to be located between the submucosa and the muscularis externa, but has not been linked to a specific structure. The effect of 5-HT on the bowel thus depends on how the amine is applied.

Application of 5-HT may affect the enteric epithelium, muscle, or neurons. For example, crypt cells are stimulated to secrete Cl⁻ by 5-HT [59—62]. A portion of this response is indirect and is mediated by sub-mucosal neurons, which are stimulated by 5-HT [62—64]. Smooth muscle is also directly excited by 5-HT [65—67]; however, the responsiveness of smooth muscle shows a wide regional and species variation [51, 67, 68]. Enteric neuronal actions of 5-HT include excitation both of extrinsic afferent nerve fibers [69—72] and intrinsic primary afferent neurons [56—58]. 5-HT also stimulates cholinergic ganglion cells leading to contraction of the muscularis externa [51, 66—68, 73—76] and muscularis mucosa [77], activates intrinsic inhibitory non-adrenergic, non-cholinergic ganglion cells [51, 67, 68, 76, 78], and presynaptically inhibits the release of acetylcholine [79, 80]. Physiological responses in which an action of 5-HT has been implicated include vagal relaxation of the stomach [51], vagal relaxation of the lower esophageal sphincter [81], post-train synaptic excitation of myenteric ganglion cells [82], ascending excitation in the colon [78, 83], descending inhibition of vagal excitation of the colon [54], cholera toxin-induced enteric secretion [63], and modulation of the migrating myoelectric complex [84, 85].

Actions of 5-HT on single enteric neurons have been extensively analyzed. Myenteric neurons have been classified physiologically into 4 groups [86—89]. Type I/S neurons have a high input resistance, spike repeatedly during the injection of depolarizing current pulses, show anodal break excitation, display tetrodotoxin-sensitive somal spikes, and lack prolonged hyperpolarizing afterpotentials. Type II/AH cells have a low input resistance, do not spike repeatedly during the injection of depolarizing current, do not display anodal break excitation, but manifest tetrodotoxin-resistant action potentials and prolonged hyperpolarizing afterpotentials (the AH). Type III/NS neurons have a low input resistance, do not spike at all in response to injection of depolarizing current pulses, but show prominent cholinergic, nicotinic excitatory postsynaptic potentials (EPSPs) that do not trigger action potentials. A fourth type of cell is inexcitable when first impaled with a recording micropipette, but during prolonged impalement behaves like a type II/AH neuron. 5-HT induces a long lasting depolarization in type II/AH neurons that is associated with an increased input resistance (the "slow response") and also blocks the AH [90—94]. These effects of 5-HT are due to inhibition of the Ca^{2+}-activated K^+ conductance that is responsibel for the AH. 5-HT has a similar effect on neurons of the submucosal plexus [95]. As a consequence of this slow response, the cells become hyperexcitable. 5-HT also may induce a rapid depolarization of myenteric or submucosal neurons that is associated with a fall in input resistance [94—96]. This response is short in duration and appears to be mediated by an increased Na^+ conductance. Both the short-lived and the slow responses to 5-HT are blocked by receptor desensitization using prolonged exposures to high concentrations of 5-HT itself. More rarely, a hyperpolarization, associated with a decrease in input resistance, may be evoked by application of 5-HT. No responses of type III/NS neurons to 5-HT have been reported.

4. There are specific receptors for 5-HT on enteric neurons

4.1. *Neural receptors for 5-HT are different from those on muscle*

One of the earliest attempts to analyze the effects of 5-HT was made by Gaddum and Picarelli [66] on the basis of mechanical responses of the guinea pig ileum to 5-HT. Responses that were antagonized by morphine were considered to be mediated by "M" receptors, while those that were blocked by dibenzyline were attributed to "D" receptors. "M" receptors are located on neurons and their activation causes the contraction of the gut indirectly through the release of acetylcholine [67, 75, 76]. In pharmacological studies, therefore, "M" receptor-mediated responses to 5-HT have been defined as those that are blocked by anti-muscarinic agents or tetrodotoxin [67, 76, 97, 98]. "D" receptors are located on smooth muscle [67]; therefore, "D" receptor-mediated responses to 5-HT are blocked neither by anti-muscarinic agents nor tetrodotoxin. It is probable that "D" receptors are similar to $5-HT_2$ receptors; however, "M" receptors correspond neither to $5-HT_1$ nor $5-HT_2$ receptors [99—101].

4.2 *"M" receptors are not a homogeneous class*

The observation that 5-HT has multiple actions on single enteric neurons mediated by different ion channels suggests that there must be more than a single type of enteric neuronal 5-HT receptor. Moreover, enteric serotoninergic neurons are all interneurons acting in an extremely complex nervous system [1—3]. Addition of 5-HT to a segment of bowel in vitro, therefore, is likely to activate many different types of neuron. As a result, it is impossible to evaluate the complete nature of the neural response to 5-HT, or drugs that effect 5-HT receptors, from measurements of the final output of the ENS in the form of muscle contraction. Contractile responses reflect the net result of what may be a complex pattern of changes in the activity of enteric microcircuits. To characterize enteric neural receptors for 5-HT, therefore, it is preferable to evaluate the actions of compounds on individual enteric neurons that have been impaled with a microelectrode, especially if this is done in combination with radioligand binding assays.

Two dipeptides, N-hexanoyl- and N-acetyl-5-hydroxytryptophyl-5-hydroxytryptophan amide (5-HTP-DP), specifically antagonize slow responses of myenteric type II/AH neurons to 5-HT [94]. 5-HTP-DP antagonizes neither the muscarinic, nor the substance P-mediated, long-lived responses of myenteric type II/AH neurons, which, in their ionic mechansim, resemble the slow response to 5-HT. 5-HTP-DP also fails to affect fast EPSPs, nicotinic responses to acetylcholine, or short-lived responses to 5-HT [94, 96]. Slow responses to 5-HT in neither myenteric nor submucosal neurons are affected by the $5-HT_3$ receptor antagonist, ICS 205—930. In contrast, short-lived responses to 5-HT of both myenteric [96] and submucosal neurons [95] are blocked by ICS 205—930. These observations suggest that at least two different classes of enteric neural 5-HT receptor can be defined through the use of 5-HTP-DP and ICS 205—930. The receptor responsible for the slow response to 5-HT, at which 5-HTP-DP is a specific antagonist, has been called a 5-HT$_{1P}$ receptor, while that responsible for the short-lived, ICS 205-930-sensitive response, is a member of the 5-HT$_3$ receptor category [95, 96, 102, 103]. The slow response to 5-HT can be mimicked by hydroxylated indalpines and resposes to these compounds are antagonized by 5-HTP-DP, but not by ICS 205—930; therefore, hydroxylated indalpines are agonists at 5-HT$_{1P}$ receptors. On the other hand, 2-methyl-5-HT is able to mimic the short-lived response to 5-HT and this effect of 2-methyl-5-HT can be blocked by ICS 205—930; therefore, 2-methyl-5-HT is an agonist at 5-HT$_3$ receptors. At higher concentrations, however, 2-methyl-5-HT loses specificity and also has an action at 5-HT$_{1P}$ sites. Recently, a substituted benzamide, BRL 24924, has been observed to inhibit slow responses to 5-HT; therefore it is an antagonist of 5-HT$_{1P}$ receptor-mediated responses. BRL 24924 appears to be more potent, but less specific than 5-HTP-DP, since, unlike 5-HTP-DP, it is able to depress short-lived (5-HT$_3$ receptor-mediated) responses to 5-HT at a 10-fold higher concentration than that required to block the slow response.

Other classes of compounds have been reported to be antagonists of 5-HT at "M" receptors. These include the benzoyltropine analogues [104], the indoletropanyl esters [98] and the substituted benzamides [105]. All of these substances have in common the ability to antagonize atropine-and tetrodotoxin-sensitive contractions of the bowel in response to 5-HT. It is thus clear that the site of action of these antagonists lies within the ENS; however, the fact that these drugs block neural actions of 5-HT does not establish which of the types of neuronal 5-HT receptor is acted upon. The "M" receptor, as noted earlier, is not a single class. 5-HT$_{1P}$ and 5-HT$_3$ effects must be separately analyzed and distinguished. In doing so, it must be remembered that measurements of the final common output of the ENS depend on the activities of motor neurons and can mask the effect the compounds may have on interneurons. Effects on interneurons, however, are of considerable importance, because however difficult they may be to evaluate in isolated preparations of strips of guinea-pig intestine, they may determine the in vivo action of the drugs on the bowel.

4.3 Enteric neuronal 5-HT$_{1P}$ receptors can be characterized by using either ^{3}H-5-HT or ^{3}H-5-hydroxyindalpine

Radioligand binding techniques have recently been applied to the study of enteric neuronal 5-HT receptors using either ^{3}H-5-HT or ^{3}H-5-hydroxyindalpine (5-OHIP) as ligands [106—108]. The binding of ^{3}H-5-HT to a membrane fraction derived from neurons of the myenteric plexus is saturable and dissociable, with a K_D that ranges in different species between 1.4 and 3.7 nM. The dissociation rate constant of the ^{3}H-5-HT-receptor complex (K_{-1}) is about 0.11/min and the association rate constant (K_{+1}) is about 7.5 × 10^7 mol/min. The kinetic estimate of the K_D, K_{-1}/K_{+1}, 1.5 nM, is close to that obtained from analysis of saturation isotherms. Moreover, the Hill coefficient is 0.96; therefore, there is probably a single high affinity ^{3}H-5-HT binding site with no positive or negative cooperativity. A similar high affinity binding site ($K_D = 7.6$ nM) has been detected in enteric neuronal membranes using the 5-HT$_{1P}$ receptor agonist, ^{3}H-5-OHIP. The binding of ^{3}H-5-HT or ^{3}H-5-OHIP is not inhibited by compounds known to combine with receptors for other neurotransmitters, with 5-HT$_1$, 5-HT$_2$, or 5-HT$_3$ receptors, or with ^{3}H-5-HT uptake sites (see Table 1); therefore, the binding of ^{3}H-5-HT or ^{3}H-5-OHIP to enteric membranes is specific. In contrast, the binding of ^{3}H-5-HT to enteric neuronal membranes is antagonized by dipeptides of 5-HTP and by hydroxylated indalpines, which are antagonists or agonists, respectively, at 5-HT$_{1P}$ receptors [94, 96, 102, 108]. The high affinity receptor for ^{3}H-5-HT in isolated enteric neuronal membranes, therefore, is different from the 5-HT receptors that have previously been described in the brain and is not the receptor which is responsible for those enteric actions of 5-HT that can be antagonized by benzoyltropine analogues [104] or indoletropanyl esters [98]. It is likely to be the 5-HT$_{1P}$ receptor which is responsible for those actions of 5-HT that are antagonized by 5-HTP-DP.

The structure-activity requirements for antagonism of ^{3}H-5-HT binding to enteric neuronal membranes (5-HT$_{1P}$ receptors) have many similarities to those previously reported for activity at enteric neural 5-HT receptors [68, 76, 97, 109]. For example, hydroxylated tryptamines can evoke neuronally mediated enteric contractions, while tryptamine itself neither mimics nor antagonizes neuronally mediated responses to 5-HT [68, 76, 97, 109]. Similarly, the binding of ^{3}H-5-HT to enteric neuronal membranes from rabbit, guinea pig, or mouse bowel is antagonized only by those tryptamines that are ring-hydroxylated. Analogues that bear other ring substituents, or tryptamine itself, are inactive against the binding of ^{3}H-5-HT [96, 106—108]. Similarly, substitutions on the aliphatic amino group of 5-HT yield compounds that retain both the ability to act on neuronal 5-HT receptors and their ability to interfere with the binding of ^{3}H-5-HT. The failure of "classical" 5-HT antagonists, such as D-lysergic acid diethylamide, methysergide, cyproheptadine, metergoline, and cinanserin to compete with ^{3}H-5-HT for binding to enteric neuronal membranes also parallels the inability of these same compounds to antagonize neuronally mediated responses of the bowel (or other peripheral organs) to 5-HT [68, 76, 97, 109—111]. One exception is 5-methoxytryptamine, which has been reported to be a 5-HT "M" receptor agonist [97, 112], but fails to block the binding of ^{3}H-5-HT to enteric neuronal membranes [106]. 5-Methoxytryptamine, however, produces a long-lasting depolarization of enteric neurons with a conductance change (increase) opposite to that seen in the slow response to 5-HT, and which is

Table 1. Compounds that have been assayed and that have failed to inhibit the binding of ^{3}H-5-HT or ^{3}H-5-OHIP to enteric neuronal membranes.

Compound	Selectivity
atropine	muscarinic
BRL 43969	5-HT$_3$
butaclamol	dopamine
5-carboxyimidotryptamine	5-HT$_1$
cimetidine	histamine (H$_2$)
cinanserin	5-HT$_1$
cocaine	5-HT$_3$
codeine	opiate
cyproheptadine	5-HT$_2$; histamine (H$_1$)
D-lysergic acid diethylamide	5-HT$_1$; 5-HT$_2$: dopamine
diphenhydramine	histamine (H$_1$)
domperidone	dopamine
fluoxetine	uptake of 5-HT
gaboxadol (THIP)	GABA
8-hydroxy-di-n-propylaminotetralin (8-OH-DPAT)	5-HT$_{1A}$
hexamethonium	nicotinic
ICS 205—930	5-HT$_3$
indalpine	uptake of 5-HT
ketanserin	5-HT$_2$
MDL 72222	5.HT$_3$
metergoline	5-HT$_1$; 5-HT$_2$
5-methoxytryptamine	5-HT$_1$
methysergide	5-HT$_1$; 5-HT$_2$
metoclopramide	5-HT$_3$; dopamine
mianserin	5-HT$_1$; 5-HT$_2$; histamine (H$_1$)
morphine	opiate
muscimol	GABA
nalorphine	opiate
naloxone	opiate
naltrexone	opiate
nicotine	nicotinic
6-nitroquipazine	5-HT$_1$
phentolamine	α-adrenoceptor
pirenipirone	5-HT$_2$
propranolol	5-HT$_{1B}$; β-adrenoceptor
quipazine	5-HT$_1$; 5-HT$_2$; 5-HT$_3$
RU 24929	5-HT$_{1B}$
spiroperidol	5-HT$_{1A}$; 5-HT$_2$; dopamine
thebaine	opiate
trazodone	5-HT$_1$; uptake of 5-HT
zimelidine	uptake of 5-HT

longer-lasting than that seen in the short-lived response to 5-HT. The receptor acted upon by 5-methoxytryptamine, therefore, is probably neither a 5-HT$_{1P}$ nor a 5-HT$_3$ receptor. The observation that tryptamine, which is an agonist at muscle receptors for 5-HT, and methysergide, which is an antagonist [76], fail to block binding of ^{3}H-5-HT [106], further argues that the binding sites are neuronal and not smooth muscle receptors for 5-HT. Tryptamine has been shown to act on enteric 5-HT-containing neurons in an unusual manner. Application of tryptamine leads first to activation and then desensitization of enteric neuronal 5-HT receptors by releasing endogenous 5-HT in a Ca^{2+}-independent manner [10]. While the 5-HT-releasing properties of tryptamine provide a useful tool for the study of enteric serotoninergic mechanisms, its mode of action also should lead to caution in interpreting the effects of compounds on intact strips of gut. Direct effects of compounds on 5-HT receptors have to be distinguished from indirect effects mediated through the release of endogenous 5-HT from serotoninergic neurons in enteric ganglia.

The location of binding sites for ^{3}H-5-HT and ^{3}H-5-OHIP in peripheral tissues has been visualized by radioautography [102—106]. The properties of the binding of these radioligands in radioautographs are identical to those found by rapid filtration for their binding to enteric neuronal membranes [96, 102, 106—108]; therefore, radioautographs demonstrate the 5-HT$_{1P}$ receptor. The development of enteric neuronal 5-HT receptors has been studied by radioautography [102]. 5-HT$_{1P}$ receptors first appear in the fetal murine bowel on day E14, when they extend from the stomach to the mid-jejunum. The receptors then spread to more anal segments of the gut, but do not reach the distal colon until two days after birth. The terminal bowel does not contain 5-HT$_{1P}$ receptors until the animals are weaned (about the end of the third postnatal week). In contrast, enteric serotoninergic neurons develop at day E12 in the foregut and are present in the terminal bowel by day E15 [26, 113]. Enteric serotoninergic neurons thus predate 5-HT$_{1P}$ receptors in the timing of their appearance. 5-HT$_{1P}$ receptors are therefore not required for the development of serotoninergic neurons; however, it is possible that enteric serotoninergic neurons are necessary in order for 5-HT$_{1P}$ receptors to appear or to be maintained. Knowledge of what capabilities are acquired by the colon in the period around weaning. when 5-HT$_{1P}$ receptors are acquired, may provide considerable insight into their function.

The distribution of ^{3}H-5-HT and ^{3}H-5-OHIP binding sites, determined by radioautography, is consistent with a neuronal location of 5-HT$_{1P}$ receptors. Binding sites are found, not only in the myenteric and submucosal plexuses, but also in the lamina propria of the enteric mucosa, just underneath the epithelium [102, 108]. These mucosal binding sites coincide in location with the subepithelial plexus of nerve fibers. Although the resolution of radioautographs is not sufficient to allow 5-HT$_{1P}$ receptors to be localized to these nerve fibers, the mucosal ^{3}H-5-HT binding sites have been found to be virtually absent from segments of mutant bowel that are congenitally aganglionic [114]. Intrinsic neurons are totally missing in the terminal colon of the lethal spotted (*ls/ls*) mouse [113], but the aganglionic zone is heavily innervated by the enteric projections of neurons whose cell bodies lie external to the bowel [115]. While some axons of intrinsic myenteric neurons, the cell bodies of which are located in the more proximal ganglionated region of the gut, do enter the aganglionic region, the mucosa of the aganglionic segments contains few processes of intrinsic neurons and probably no processes of intrinsic submucosal neurons. The relative paucity of 5-HT$_{1P}$ receptors in the mucosa of the aganglionic colon of the *ls/ls* mouse, therefore, strongly suggests that these receptors are normally found on mucosal intrinsic nerve fibers, as well as on enteric ganglion cells. A functional role for 5-HT receptors on mucosal axons in the initiation of the peristaltic reflex has been postulated [56—58]. Application of pressure to the mucosal surface of the gut releases 5-HT from enteroendocrine cells, where it reaches the lamina propria and stimulates intrinsic mucosal afferent nerve processes. The location of mucosal 5-HT$_{1P}$ receptors is consistent with the possibility that they are the receptors upon which 5-HT released from enteroendocrine cells acts. ^{3}H-5-HT does not bind to isolated mucosal epithelial cells [116], and the epithelium itself is not radioautographically labeled by ^{3}H-5-HT or ^{3}H-5-OHIP. 5-HT$_{1P}$ receptors, consequently, are probably not located on the intestinal epithelium.

There is a very good correlation between the structure of compounds that antagonize the binding of ^{3}H-5-HT or ^{3}H-5-OHIP and the structure of compounds that are able physiologically to interact with 5-HT$_{1P}$ receptors [94, 96, 102]; thus, substances that inhibit the specific binding of these radioligands either mimic or block the slow response of myenteric II/AH neurons to 5-HT. For example, the selective 5-HT$_{1P}$ antagonist, 5-HTP-DP, effectively blocks the binding of ^{3}H-5-HT and ^{3}H-5-OHIP as do hydroxylated indalpines, which mimic the slow response to 5-HT [96]. In contrast, ICS 205—930, which blocks the fast, but not the slow response to 5-HT, fails to interfere with the binding of ^{3}H-5-HT or ^{3}H-5-OHIP. 2-Methyl-5-HT is a more potent agonist at 5-HT$_3$ than at 5-HT$_{1P}$ receptors, but as predicted from its 5-HT$_{1P}$ effect, 2-methyl-5-HT is a weak antagonist of the binding of ^{3}H-5-HT. Neurons of the submucosal plexus have recently been reported to display two depolarizing responses to 5-HT, one short lived and the other long lasting, essentially identical to those found in neurons of the myenteric plexus [95]. As is the case in the myenteric plexus, these responses can also be differentiated on the basis of their differing ionic mechanisms and sensitivity to blockade by ICS 205—930. Only the fast response can be antagonized by this 5-HT$_3$ receptor antagonist.

4.4   *Functions of 5-HT receptors in the bowel*

For many years research on the role played by 5-HT in the physiology of the ENS was complicated by the paucity and non-specificity of antagonists of neuronal actions of 5-HT and by the assumption that all neurally mediated 5-HT responses involved a single 5-HT receptor. Slow EPSPs in myenteric type II/AH neurons, resembling the slow response to 5-HT, and sensitive to methysergide were reported by Wood and Mayer [90], who suggested that 5-HT might be *the* mediator of these responses. However, methysergide is not a specific antagonist at enteric neuronal 5-HT receptors. It also decreases the height of cholinergic fast EPSPs in both type I/S and type II/AH neurons. Methysergide does not block nicotinic responses to acetylcholine itself; thus, its effect on fast EPSPs is due to antagonism of the release of ACh. If the drug can inhibit the release of one transmitter the possibility exists that it can also antagonize the release of another; therefore, the ability of methysergide to inhibit slow EPSPs does not constitute definitive evidence that slow EPSPs are mediated by 5-HT. Its action could be presynaptic as easily as postsynaptic. Moreover, 5-HT is only one of several neuroactive substances found in the ENS that can mimic slow EPSPs. The response is also mimicked by ACh acting at muscarinic cholinoceptors receptors [117], by substance P [118—120], bombesin, cholecystokinin, gastrin releasing peptide, vasoactive intestinal polypeptide and somatostatin, as well as by histamine [89]. More specific antagonists than methysergide are needed to establish a substance as a neurotransmitter.

Recent evidence has confirmed that the original suggestion of Wood and Mayer [90] that 5-HT mediates slow EPSPs is correct; however, it now appears that 5-HT is likely to be only one of several substances that can mediate these responses. Which transmitter is involved probably depends on which presynaptic neurites are stimulated and from which follower cells records are made. Every type II/AH neuron in which a slow EPSP can be elicited by stimulating interganglionic fiber tracts in the myenteric plexus has been demonstrated to be covered by many serotoninergic synapses [121]. No similar study has been made of neurons showing slow EPSPs to determine if they receive synapses from peptidergic or cholinergic neurons. Nevertheless, it should be noted in this regard that enteric serotoninergic axons are extremely numerous in interganglionic fiber tracts, but their terminals are relatively sparse within ganglia [27]. In contrast, substance P-immunoreactive fibers are short and more numerous in ganglia than in connectives [3]. As a result, stimulation of interganglionic fiber tracts would be expected to activate serotoninergic axons selectively, while focal intraganglionic stimulation would be predicted to stimulate substance P-containing neurons. This difference in distribution probably accounts for the ability of intraganglionic stimuli to elicit slow EPSPs in surgically prepared islands of ganglia that have been depleted of 5-HT [93]. It is more difficult to evoke slow EPSPs in such preparations, but the response does not disappear. On the other hand, when endogenous 5-HT is depleted by tryptamine there is a complete loss of slow, but not fast, EPSPs in myenteric type II/AH cells in response to stimulation of interganglionic fiber tracts [10]. Strong evidence that slow EPSPs are mediated by 5-HT has also been provided by analyses of the effects of 5-HTP-DP on these responses [94]. 5-HTP-DP, a specific 5-HT$_{1P}$ antagonist, blocks both slow EPSPs and slow responses to 5-HT; nevertheless, the neurons still respond to ACh or substance P in the presence of the drug.

Unlike methysergide, 5-HTP-DP does not reduce the size of fast EPSPs; consequently, there is no reason to believe that its antagonism of slow EPSPs is due to a decrement in the release of transmitter or to a non-specific action on a transmitter other than 5-HT. It can be concluded that 5-HT is one of many neurotransmitters in the ENS and that one of its functions is to mediate slow EPSPs in myenteric type II/AH neurons. The fact that neurons of the myenteric plexus have additional 5-HT receptors makes it likely that 5-HT will be discovered to play other roles in the ENS besides just the one that is now known. Wood [89] has proposed that 5-HT-containing neurons, which are relatively few in number and which all project proximo-distally for long distances [21, 27], are responsible for a "feed-forward" activation of synaptic circuits that mediate the descending wave of orad contraction that is part of the peristaltic reflex. In this view, there are two distinct types of slow synaptic excitation in the bowel: one, a 5-HT-mediated slow EPSP, which serves to facilitate the movement of activity down the bowel, and the other, a peptide-mediated slow EPSP that propagates activity circumferentially in locally contracted regions. The portion of this postulate that concerns 5-HT requires that 5-HT-containing neurons make synapses on one another, so that descending chains of serotoninergic neurons can spread activation distally. The existence of such 5-HT-5-HT synapses has been demonstrated [27, 121]. The portion of the hypothesis that concerns peptides requires that the peptide-containing neurons that might be responsible for evoking slow EPSPs in the circumferential direction be both more numerous and shorter than 5-HT-containing neurons; substance P-containing neurons fulfill these requirements. [2, 3].

A paradigm that may prove useful in distinguishing functional roles of 5-HT acting through different receptors is gastric emptying. $5-HT_3$ antagonists such as ICS 205—930 have been shown to enhance the rate of gastric emptying of glycerin-coated beads [122]. We have recently found that BRL 24924 antagonizes $5-HT_{1P}$ receptor-mediated effects on myenteric neurons, but is a poor antagonist of those responses that are mediated by $5-HT_3$ receptors [123]. The murine stomach has a large number of $5-HT_{1P}$ receptors [102]. We thus studied the interactions of BRL 24924 with enteric neuronal 5-HT receptors. The investigation utilized intracellular recordings from single neurons of the guinea pig myenteric plexus, analyses of the binding of ^3H-5-HT to enteric neuronal membranes, and the determination of the effects of the compound on the rate of emptying of a ^{51}Cr-labeled liquid meal from the murine stomach. Effects of BRL 24924 were compared to those of the known $5-HT_3$ receptor antagonist, ICS 205—930 [123, 124]. BRL 24924 was found to have no direct effect on single enteric neurons and not to be an agonist at either $5-HT_{1P}$ or $5-HT_3$ receptors. BRL 24924 blocked slow responses to exogenous 5-HT and slow EPSPs evoked by the release of endogenous 5-HT, both of which are mediated by $5-HT_{1P}$ receptors. In contrast, BRL 24924 had no effect on slow responses of myenteric neurons to SP; therefore, it does not prevent slow responses, but antagonizes only those mediated by 5-HT. BRL 24924 (1.0 μM) did not block the 5-HT$_3$ receptor-mediated fast responses. BRL 24924, as well as ICS 205–930, failed to compete with ^{3}H-5-HT for binding to enteric neurons (assessed by filtration or radioautography). Since BRL 24924 does not interact with the 5-HT recognition site of the 5-HT$_{1P}$ receptor, its ability to antagonize specifically responses mediated by this receptor is likely to be due to an action on the coupling of the receptor to the responses it mediates. BRL 24924, but not ICS 205–930, enhanced the rate of emptying of a liquid meal from the murine stomach. As a working hypothesis, we have proposed that intrinsic inhibitory neurons of the murine stomach may be tonically activated (slow EPSPs induced) by serotonergic neurons acting through 5-HT$_{1P}$ receptors. The difference in the activity of ICS 205–930 in the murine vs guinea pig stomach may be attributable to a species difference. Alternatively, the action of ICS 205–930 may be centrally mediated and dependent on the type of meal investigated. For example, centrally administered ICS 205–930 has been shown to enhance gastric emptying in the guinea pig [125] and naloxone enhances gastric emptying of a fat-containing, but not a fat-free, liquid meal [126].

5. Conclusions

Since it was first suggested in 1965 that 5-hydroxytryptamine (5-HT) might be an enteric neurotransmitter [5], that role has been confirmed by many studies (see [103]). 5-HT has now been accepted as an enteric neurotransmitter. A great deal has been learned about the cellular biology of enteric serotoninergic neurons and the role played by 5-HT in the physiology of the gut. The cell bodies of enteric serotoninergic neurons are located in ganglia in the myenteric plexus; all of them are interneurons and they send extremely long axonal projections both down the gut in a predominantly oral-anal direction and to the ganglia of the submucosal plexus. 5-HT is synthesized within the bowel from L-tryptophan, is released along with a specific 45 kDa binding protein SBP, and is inactivated by the high affinity, Na$^+$-dependent neural re-uptake of the amine. 5-HT re-uptake is specifically inhibited by drugs, such as fluoxetine or zimelidine. Because 5-HT has many sites of action in the bowel, it has proved difficult to ascertain which of the many putative functional activities that have been proposed for 5-HT in the gut are of physiological significance. Electrophysiological examination of the effects of 5-HT on single enteric neurons has facilitated analysis of its role as a transmitter in the enteric nervous system (ENS). Two of these effects, a prolonged depolarization associated with a decreased K$^+$ conductance (the slow response) and a short-lived depolarization associated with a rise in Na$^+$ conductance (the fast response) have been linked to specific 5-HT receptors [96]. The slow response is mediated by 5-HT$_{1P}$ receptors; these receptors are characterized by a high affinity for ^{3}H-5-HT (K$_D$ $\cong$ 3 nM) and no or little affinity for compounds that specifically act at other subtypes of 5-HT_1, 5-HT_2, or 5-HT_3 receptor. The 5-HT_{1P} receptor has been demonstrated by radioautography to be present in the ganglia of both enteric plexuses and in the lamina propria of the mucosa. Since very few 5-HT_{1P} receptors are present in the mucosa in segments of gut derived from *ls/ls* mice, which are congenitally aganglionic, the receptor appears to be located on the mucosal projections of intrinsic enteric nerves. Hydroxylated indalpines are agonists and dipeptides of 5-hydroxytryptophan (5-HTP-DP) are antagonists at 5-HT_{1P} receptors. More recently, BRL 24924 has also been found to be a relatively specific antagonist at 5-HT_{1P} receptors. 5-HT is a transmitter responsible for slow EPSPs evoked in type II/AH neurons of the myenteric plexus by stimulation of interganglionic fiber tracts and these responses to the endogenous release of 5-HT are mediated by 5-HT_{1P} receptors. Slow EPSPs can thus be blocked by 5-HT_{1P} antagonists, such as 5-HTP-DP or BRL 24924. Because of the gastrokinetic action of BRL 24924, it has been proposed that 5-HT may provide a tonic activation of intrinsic inhibitory neurons. The fast response to 5-HT is mediated by 5-HT_3 receptors; therefore, the fast response is mimicked by 2-methyl-5-HT and antagonized by ICS 205—930. No physiological activity has yet been found that can be assigned to the activation of enteric neural 5-HT_3 receptors. Although impressive progress has been made toward understanding the function of enteric 5-HT, a number of unresolved questions remain. These provide reason to believe that the future of research on the enteric and other peripheral actions of 5-HT will supply both excitement and controversy, as this research has done in the past.

Acknowledgements

Work presented in this review was supported in part by grants NS 12969, NS 15547, NS 22637, and NS 07062 from the National Institutes of Health. Additional support was provided by the Council for Tobacco Research and the Pharmaceutical Manufacturer's Association Foundation.

References

1. Gershon MD (1981): The enteric nervous system. *Ann Rev Neurosci* 4: 227—272.
2. Costa M, Furness JB, Llewellyn-Smith I (1987): Histochemistry of the enteric nervous system, pp. 1—41 in: Johnson LR (ed), *Physiology of the Gastrointestinal Tract* Vol 1, 2nd edition. New York: Raven Press.
3. Furness JB, Costa M (1987): *The Enteric Nervous System* pp. 65—69. New York: Churchill Livingston.
4. Erspamer V (1966): Occurrence of indolealkylamines in nature, pp. 132—181 in: Erspamer V (ed), *Handbook of Experimental Pharmacology* Vol 19, 5-Hydroxytryptamine and Related Indolealkylamines. New York: Springer-Verlag.

5. Gershon MD, Drakontides AB, Ross LL (1965): Serotonin: synthesis and release from the myenteric plexus of the mouse intestine. *Science* 149: 197—199.
6. Feldberg W, Toh CC (1953): Distribution of 5-hydroxytryptamine (serotonin, enteramine) in the wall of the digestive tract. *J Physiol London* 119: 352—362.
7. Robinson R, Gershon MD (1971): Synthesis and uptake of 5-hydroxytryptamine by the myenteric plexus of the small intestine of the guinea pig. *J Pharmacol Exp Ther* 179: 29—41.
8. Juorio AV, Gabella G (1974): Noradrenaline in the guinea-pig alimentary canal: regional distribution and sensitivity to denervation and reserpine. *J Neurochem* 221: 851—858.
9. Holzer P, Skofitsch G (1984): Release of endogenous 5-hydroxytryptamine from the myenteric plexus of the guinea-pig isolated small intestine. *Br J Pharmacol* 81: 381—386.
10. Takaki M, Mawe GM, Barasch J, Gershon MD (1985b): Physiological responses of guinea-pig myenteric neurons secondary to the release of endogenous serotonin by tryptamine. *Neurosci* 16: 223—240.
11. Legay C, Faudon M, Héry F, Ternaux JP (1983a): 5-HT metabolism in the intestinal wall of the rat. I The Mucosa. *Neurochem Intl* 5: 721—727.
12. Legay C, Faudon M, Héry F, Ternaux JP (1983b): 5-HT metabolism in the intestinal wall of the rat. II. The nerves plexuses-interactions between 5-HT containing cells. *Neurochem Intl* 5: 571—577.
13. Feher E (1974): Effect of monoamine oxidase inhibitory on the nerve elements of the isolated cat ileum. *Acta Morphologica Acad Sci Hung* 22: 249—263.
14. Feher E (1975): Effects of monoamine oxidase inhibition on the nerve elements of the isolated cat's ileum. *Verh Anat Ges* 69: 477—482.
15. Dreyfus CF, Bornstein MB, Gershon MD (1977a): Synthesis of serotonin by neurons of the myenteric plexus *in situ* and in organotypic tissue culture. *Brain Res* 128: 109—123.
16. Baumgarten HG, Björklünd A, Lachenmayer L, Nobin A, Rosengren E (1973): Evidence for existence of serotonin-, dopamine- and noradrenaline-containing neurons in the gut of Lampetra fluviatilis. *Z Zellforsch* 141: 33—54.
17. Goodrich JT, Bernd P, Sherman DL, Gershon MD (1980): Phylogeny of enteric serotonergic neurons. *J Comp Neurol* 190: 15—28.
18. Watson AHD (1979): Fluorescent histochemistry of the teleost gut: evidence for the presence of serotonergic neurons. *Cell Tissue Res* 197: 155—164.
19. Anderson C (1983): Evidence for 5-HT containing intrinsic neurons in the teleost intestine. *Cell Tis Res* 230: 377—386.
20. Salimova N (1978): Localization of biogenic monoamines in Amphioxus *Brachiostoma lanceolatum. Dokl Aca Sci* USSR 242: 939—941.
21. Costa M, Furness JB, Cuello AC, Verhofstad AAJ. Steinbusch HWJ, Elde RP (1982): Neurons with 5-hydroxytryptamine-like immunoreactivity in the enteric nervous system: Their visualization and reactions to drug treatment. *Neuroscience* 7: 351—363.
22. Furness JB, Costa M (1982): Neurons with 5-hydroxytryptamine-like immunoreactivity in the enteric nervous system: Their projections in the guinea pig small intestine. *Neurosci* 7: 341—350.
23. Legay C, Saffrey MJ, Burnstock G (1984): Coexistence of immunoreactive substance P and serotonin in neurons of the gut. *Brain Res* 302: 379—382.
24. Saffrey MJ. Legay C, Burnstock G (1984): Development of 5-hydroxytryptamine-like immunoreactive neurons in cultures of the myenteric plexus from the guinea-pig caecum. *Brain Res* 304: 105—116.
25. Grønstad KO, DeMagistris L, Dahlström A, Nilsson O, Price B, Zinner MJ, Jaffe BM, Ahlman H (1985): The effects of vagal nerve stimulation on endoluminal release of serotonin and substance P into the feline small intestine. *Scand J Gastroenterol* 20: 163—169.

26. Rothman TP, Gershon MD (1982): Phenotypic expression in the developing murine enteric nervous system. *J Neurosci* 2: 381—393.
27. Gershon MD, Sherman DL (1987): Noradrenergic innervation of serotoninergic neurons in the myenteric plexus. *J Comp Neurol* 259: 193—210.
28. Nada O, Toyohara T (1987): An immunohistochemical study of serotonin-containing nerves in the colon of rats. *Histochem* 86: 229—232.
29. Kurian SS, Feri GL, Demeg J, Polak JM (1983): Immunocytochemistry of serotonin-containing nerves in the human gut. *Histochem* 78: 523—529.
30. Dreyfus CF, Sherman D, Gershon MD (1977b): Uptake of serotonin by intrinsic neurons of the myenteric plexus grown in organotypic tissue culture. *Brain Res* 128: 109—123.
31. Jonakait GM, Tamir H, Rapport MM, Gershon MD (1977): Detection of a soluble serotonin binding protein in the mammalian myenteric plexus and other peripheral sites of serotonin storage. *J Neurochem* 28: 277—284.
32. Jonakait GM, Tamir H, Gintzler AR, Gershon MD (1979): Release of [³H] serotonin and its binding protein from enteric neurons. *Brain Res* 174: 55—69.
33. Tamir H, Huang IL (1974): Binding of serotonin to soluble protein from synaptosomes. *Life Sci* 14: 83—93.
34. Tamir H, Kuhar MJ (1975): Association of serotonin-binding protein with projections of the midbrain raphe nuclei. *Brain Res* 83: 164—172.
35. Barasch JM, Mackey H, Tamir H, Nunez EA, Gershon MD (1987a): Induction of a neural phenotype in a serotonergic endocrine cell derived from the neural crest. *J Neurosci* 7: 2874—2883.
36. Barasch JM, Tamir H, Nunez EA, Gershon MD (1987b): Serotonin-storing secretory granules from thyroid parafollicular cells. *J Neurosci* 7: 4017—44033.
37. Gershon MD, Tamir H (1981a): Release of endogenous 5-hydroxytryptamine from resting and stimulated enteric neurons. *Neuroscience* 6: 2277—2286.
38. Gershon MD, Tamir H (1981b): Serotonin binding protein: role in transmitter storage in central and peripheral serotonergic neurons, pp. 37—50 in: Haber B, Gabay S, Issidorides M, Alivisatos S (eds), *Serotonin*. New York: Plenum Publishing Co.
39. Tamir H, Gershon MD (1979): Storage of serotonin and serotonin binding protein in synaptic vesicles. *J Neurochem* 33: 35—44.
40. Gershon MD (1982): Enteric serotonergic neurons, pp. 363—399 in: Osborne N (ed), *Biology of serotonergic neurotransmission*. New York: John Wiley and Sons.
41. Gershon MD, Altman RF (1971): An analysis of the uptake of 5-hydroxytryptamine by the myenteric plexus of the small intestine of the guinea-pig. *J Pharmacol Exp Ther* 179: 29—41.
42. Gershon MD, Robinson R, Ross LL (1976): Serotonin accumulation in the guinea pig's myenteric plexus: ion dependence, structure activity relationship, and the effect of drugs. *J Pharmacol Exp Ther* 198: 548—561.
43. Jönsson G Fuxe K, Hamberger B, Hökfelt T (1969): 6-Hydroxytryptamine-a new tool in monoamine fluorescence histochemistry. *Brain Res* 13: 190—195.
44. Gershon MD, Sherman DL (1982a): Selective demonstration of serotonergic neurons and terminals in electron micrographs: Loading with 5,7-dihydroxytryptamine and fixation with NaMnO₄. *J Histochem and Cytochem* 30: 769—773.
45. Gershon MD, Sherman DL (1982b): Identification of and interactions between noradrenergic and serotonergic neurites in the myenteric plexus. *J Comp Neurol* 204: 407—421.
46. Gershon MD. Jonakait GM (1979): Uptake and release of 5-hydroxytryptamine by enteric serotonergic neurons: effects of fluoxetine (Lilly 110140) and chlorimipramine. *British J Pharmacol* 66: 7—9.
47. Gershon MD, Dreyfus CF, Pickel VM, Joh TH, Reis DJ (1977): Serotonergic neurons in the peripheral nervous system: Identification in gut by immunohistochemical localization of tryptophan hydroxylase. *Proc Natl Acad Sci (USA)* 74: 3086—3089.
48. Gershon MD, Ross LL (1966): Radioisotopic studies of the binding, exchange and

distribution of 5-hydroxytryptamine synthesized from its radioactive precursor. *J Physiol (London)* 186: 451—476.

49. Gershon MD, Dreyfus CF (1980): Stimulation of tryptophan uptake into enteric neurons by 5-hydroxytryptamine: a novel form of neuromodulation. *Brain Res* 184: 229—233.

50. Paton WDM, Vane JR (1963): An analysis of the response of the isolated stomach to electrical stimulation and to drugs. *J Physiol (London)* 165: 10—46.

51. Bülbring E, Gershon MD (1967): 5-Hydroxytryptamine participation in the vagal inhibitory innervation of the stomach. *J Physiol (Lond)* 192: 823—846.

52. Schulz R, Cartwright C (1974): Effect of morphine on serotonin release from the myenteric plexus of the guinea pig. *J Pharmacol Exp Ther* 190: 420—430.

53. Gwee MCE, Yeoh TS (1968): The release of 5-hydroxytryptamine from rabbit small intestine *in vitro. J Physiol (London)* 194: 817—825.

54. Julé Y (1980): Nerve-mediated descending inhibition in the proximal colon of the rabbit. *J Physiol (London)* 159: 361—368.

55. Ahlman H, Lundberg J, Dahlström A, Kewenter J (1976): A possible vagal adrenergic release of serotonin from enterochromaffin cells in the cat. *Acta Physiol Scand* 98: 366—375.

56. Bülbring E, Crema A (1958): Observations concerning the action of 5-hydroxytryptamine on the peristaltic reflex. *Br J Pharmacol* 13: 444—457.

57. Bülbring E, Lin RCY (1958): The effect of intraluminal application of 5-hydroxytryptamine and 5-hydroxytryptophan on peristalsis, the local production of 5-hydroxytryptamine and its release in relation to intraluminal pressure and propulsive activity. *J Physiol (Lond)* 140: 381—407.

58. Bülbring E, Crema A (1959): the release of 5-hydroxytryptamine in relation to pressure exerted on the intestinal mucosa. *J Physiol (Lond)* 146: 381—407.

59. Sheerin HE (1979): Serotonin action on short circuit current and ion transport across isolated rabbit ileal mucosa. *Life Sci* 24: 1609—1616.

60. Donowitz M, Tai Y-H, Asarkof N (1980): Effect of serotonin on active electrolyte transport in rabbit ileum, gall bladder, annd colon. *Amer J Physiol* 239: G463—G472.

61. Hardcastle J, Hardcastle PET, Redfern JS (1981): Action of 5-hydroxytryptamine on intestinal transport in the rat. *J Physiol (Lond)* 320: 41—55.

62. Cooke HJ, Carey HV (1985): Pharmacological analysis of 5-hydroxytryptamine actions on guinea pig ileal mucosa. *Eur J Pharmacol* 111: 329—337.

63. Cassuto J, Jodal M, Tuttle R, Lundgren O (1982): 5-Hydroxytryptamine and cholera secretion. *Scand J Gastroenterol* 17: 695—703.

64. Cooke HJ (1987): Neural and humoral regulation of small intestinal electrolyte transport, pp. 1307—1350 in: Johnson LR (ed), *Physiology of the Gastrointestinal Tract* Vol. 2. New York: Raven Press.

65. Vane JR (1957): A sensitive method for the assay of 5-hydroxytryptamine. *Br J Pharmacol Chemother* 12: 344—349.

66. Gaddum JH, Picarelli ZP (1957): Two kinds of tryptamine receptor. *Br J Pharmacol Chemother* 12: 323—328.

67. Gershon MD (1967): Effects of tetrodotoxin on innervated smooth muscle preparations. *Br J Pharmacol* 29: 259—279.

68. Costa M, Furness JB (1979b): The sites of action of 5-HT in nerve muscle preparations from guinea-pig small intestine and colon. *Br J Pharmacol* 65: 237—248.

69. Paintal AS (1964): Effects of drugs on vertebrate mechanoreceptors. *Pharmacol Rev* 16: 341—380.

70. Lew WYW, Longhurst JC (1986): Substance P, 5-hydroxytryptamine and bradykinin stimulate abdominal visceral afferents. *Am J Physiol* 250: R465—R473.

71. Ireland SJ, Tyers MB (1987): Pharmacological characterization of 5-hydroxytryptamine-induced depolarization of the rat isolated vagus nerve. *Br J Pharmacol* 90: 229—238.

72. Wallis DI, Stansfeld CE, Nash HL (1982): Depolarizing responses recorded from

nodose ganglion cells in the rabbit evoked by 5-hydroxytryptamine and other substances. *Neuropharmacol* 21: 31—40.

73. Brownlee G, Johnson ES (1963): The site of the 5-hydroxytryptamine receptor in the peristaltic reflex. *Br J Pharmacol* 13: 444—457.

74. Harry J (1963): The action of drugs on the circular muscle strip from the guinea pig isolated ileum. *Br J Pharmacol Chemother* 20: 399—417.

75. Vizi VA, Vizi ES (1978): Direct evidence for acetylcholine releasing effect of serotonin in the Auerbach's plexus. *J Neural Transm* 42: 127—138.

76. Drakontides AB, Gershon MD (1968): 5-HT receptors in the mouse duodenum. *Br J Pharmacol* 33: 480—492.

77. Kamikawa Y, Shimo Y (1983): Indirect action of 5-hydroxytryptamine on the isolated muscularis mucosa of the guinea pig oesophagus. *Br J Pharmacol* 78: 103—110.

78. Furness JB, Costa M (1973): The nervous release and the action of substances which affect intestinal muscle through neither adrenoreceptors nor cholinoreceptors. *Phil Trans Roy Soc Series B* 265: 123—133.

79. North RA, Henderson C, Katayama Y, Johnson SM (1980): Electrophysiological evidence of presynaptic inhibition of acetylcholine release by 5-hydroxytryptamine in the enteric nervous system. *Neuroscience* 5: 581—586.

80. Sanger GJ (1985): Three different ways in which 5-hydroxytryptamine can affect cholinergic activity in guinea-pig isolated ileum. *J Pharm Pharmacol* 37: 584—586.

81. Rattan S, Goyal RK (1978): Evidence of 5-HT participation in vagal inhibitory pathway to opossum LES. *Am J Physiol.*

82. Dingeldine R, Goldstein A (1976): Effect of synaptic transmission blockade on morphine action in the guinea pig myenteric plexus. *J Pharmacol Exp Ther* 196: 97—106.

83. Costa M, Furness JB (1976): The peristaltic reflex: an analysis of the nerve pathways and their pharmacology. *Naunyn-Schmiedeberg's Arch Pharmacol* 294: 47—60.

84. Ormsbee HS, Silver DA, Hardy FE (1984): Effects of 5-hydroxytryptamine on the migrating myoelectric complex in the canine intestine. *J Pharmacol Exp Ther* 231: 436—440.

85. Davidson HI, Pilot MA (1986): Does endogenous neuronal 5-hydroxytryptamine influence canine intestinal motility. *J Physiol (Lond)* 376: 49P.

86. Holman ME, Hirst GDS, Spence I (1972): Preliminary studies of the neurons of Auerbach's plexus using intracellular microelectrodes. *Aust J Exp biol Med* 50: 795—801.

87. Nishi S, North RA (1973): Intracellular recording from the myenteric plexus of the guinea pig ileum. *J Physiol (London)* 231: 471—491.

88. Hirst GDS, Holman ME, Spence I (1974): Two types of neurons in the myenteric plexus of duodenum in the guinea-pig. *J Physiol (London)* 236: 303—326.

89. Wood JD (1987): Physiology of enteric neurons, pp. 1—41 in: Johnson LR (ed), *Physiology of the Gastrointestinal Tract* Vol. 1, 2nd edition. New York: Raven Press.

90. Wood JD, Mayer CJ (1979): Serotonergic activation of tonic-type enteric neurons in guinea pig small bowel. *J Neurophysiol* 422: 582—593.

91. Johnson SM, Kayatama Y, North RA (1980a): Slow synaptic potentials in neurons of the myenteric plexus. *J Physiol (London)* 301: 505—516.

92. Johnson SM, Katayama Y, North RA (1980b): Multiple actions of 5-hydroxytryptamine on myenteric neurons of the guinea-pig ileum. *J Physiol (London)* 304: 459—479.

93. Bornstein J, North RA, Costa M, Furness JB (1984): Excitatory synaptic potentials due to activation of neurons with short projection in the myenteric plexus. *Neurosci* 11: 723—731.

94. Takaki M, Branchek T, Tamir H, Gershon MD (1985a): Specific antagonism of enteric neural serotonin receptors by dipeptides of 5-hydroxytryptophan: Evidence that serotonin is a mediator of slow synaptic excitation in the myenteric plexus. *J Neuroscience* 5: 1769—1780.

95. Surprenant A, Crist J (1988): Electrophysiological characterization of functionally distinct 5-HT receptors on guinea-pig submucous plexus. *Neuroscience* 24: 283—295.

96. Mawe GM, Branchek T, Gershon MD (1986): Peripheral neural serotonin receptors: Indentification and characterization with specific agonists and antagonists. *Proc Nat Acad Sci (USA)* 83: 9799—9803.

97. Fozard JR, Mobarok Ali ATM (1978): Receptors for 5-hydroxytryptamine on sympathetic nerves of the rabbit heart. *Naunyn-Schmeideberg's Arch Pharmacol* 301: 224—235.

98. Richardson BP, Engel G, Donatsch P, Stadler PA (1985): Identification of serotonin M-receptor subtypes and their specific blockade by a new class of drugs. *Nature* 316: 216—131.

99. Engel G, Hoyer D, Kalkman HO, Wick MB (1984): Identification of $5-HT_2$-receptors on longitudinal muscle of the guinea-pig ileum. *J Recept Res* 4: 113—126.

100. Richardson BP, Engel G (1986): The pharmacology and functions of $5-HT_3$ receptors. *Trends in Neurosci* 9: 424—428.

101. Bradley PB, Engel G, Feniuk W, Fozard JR, Humphrey PPA, Middemiss DN, Mylecharane EJ, Richardson BP, Saxena PR (1986): Proposals for the classification and nomenclature of functional receptors for 5-hydroxytryptamine. *Neuropharmacology* 25: 563—576.

102. Branchek T, Mawe G, Gershon MD, (1988): Characterization and localization of a peripheral neural 5-hydroxytryptamine receptor subtype with a selective agonist, ^{3}H-5-hydroxyindalpine. *J Neuroscience* 8: 2582—2595.

103. Gershon MD, Mawe G, Branchek T (1988): 5-Hydroxytryptamine and enteric neurons, pp. 247—264 in: Fozard JR (ed), *The Peripheral Actions of 5-HT*. UK: Oxford Press.

104. Fozard JR (1984): Neuronal 5-HT receptors in the periphery. *Neuropharmacology* 23: 1473—1486.

105. Sanger GJ (1987): Increased gut cholinergic activity and antagonism of 5-hydroxytrypt-amine M-receptors by BRL 24924: potential clinical importance of BRL 24924. *Br J Pharmac* 91: 77—87.

106. Branchek TA, Kates M, Gershon MD (1984a): Enteric receptors for 5-hydroxytrypt-amine. *Brain Res* 324: 107—118.

107. Gershon MD, Takaki M, Tamir H, Branchek T (1985): The enteric neural receptor for 5-hydroxytryptamine. *Experientia* 41: 863—868.

108. Branchek TA, Gershon MD (1987): Development of neural receptors for serotonin in the murine bowel. *J Comp Neurol* 258: 597—610.

109. Gyermek L (1966): Drugs which antagonize 5-hydroxytryptamine and release indolealkylamines, pp. 471—528 in: Erspamer (ed), *Handbüch der experimentellen Pharmakologie XIX*. New York: Springer-Verlag.

110. Humphrey PPA (1983): Pharmacological characterization of cardiovascular 5-hydroxy-tryptamine receptors, pp. 237—242 in: Bevan JA, Maxwell RA, Shibata S, Fujiwara M, Muhri K, Toda N (eds), *Proceedings of IV International Sumposium on Vascular Neuroeffector Mechanisms*. New York: Raven Press.

111. Humphrey PPA, Feniuk W, Watts AD (1983): Prejuctional effects of 5-hydroxytrypta-mine on noradrenergic nerves in the cardiovascular system. *Fed Proc* 42: 218—222.

112. Fozard JR (1985): 5-Methoxytryptamine (5-MeOT) discriminates between excitatory neuronal 5-hydroxytryptamine (5-HT) receptors in the guinea-pig ileum. *J Pharmacol* 16: 498.

113. Rothman TP, Gershon MD (1984): Regionally defective colonization of the terminal bowel by the precursors of enteric neurons in lethal spotted mutant mice. *Neuroscience* 12: 1293—1311.

114. Branchek T, Rothman T, Gershon MD (1984b): Serotonin receptors on the processes of intrinsic enteric neurons: Reduction in the aganglionic bowel of the *ls/ls* mouse. *Soc Neurosci Abstr* 10:1097.

115. Payette RF, Tennyson VM, Pham TD, Mawe GM, Pomeranz H, Rothman TP, Gershon

MD (1978): Origin and morphology of nerve fibers in the aganglionic colon of the lethal spotted (*ls/ls*) mutant mouse. *J Comp Neurol* 257: 237—252.

116. Gaginella TS, Rimele TJ, Wietecha M (1983): Studies on rat intestinal epithelial cell receptors for serotonin and opiates. *J Physiol* 335: 101—111.

117. North RA, Tokimasa T (1982): Muscarinic potentials in guinea-pig myenteric plexus neurons. *J Physiol (London)* 333: 151—156.

118. Katayama Y, North RA (1978): Does substance P mediate slow synaptic excitation within the myenteric plexus? *Nature(London)* 274: 387—388.

119. Katayama Y, North RA, Williams JT (1979): The action of substance P on neurons of the myenteric plexus of the guinea-pig small intestine. *Proc R Soc Lond* 206: 191—208.

120. Johnson SM, Katayama Y, Morita K, North RA (1981): Mediators of slow synaptic potentials in the myenteric plexus of the guinea pig ileum. *J Physiol (London)* 320: 175—186.

121. Erde S, Sherman D, Gershon MD (1985): Morphology of the serotonergic innervation of physiologically identified cells of the guinea pig myenteric plexus. *J Neuroscience* 5: 617—633.

122. Bucheit KH, Costall B, Engel G, Gunning SJ, Naylor RJ, Richardson BP (1985): 5-Hydroxytryptamine receptor antagonism by metaclopramide and ICS 205—930 in the guinea-pig leads to enhancement of contractions of stomach muscle strips induced by electrical field stimulation and facilitation of gastric emptying in vivo. *J Pharm Pharmac* 37: 664—667.

123. Mawe GM, Branchek T, Gershon MD (1989): Blockade of 5-HT mediated enteric slow EPSP$_s$ by BRL24924: Gastrokinetic effects. *Am J Physiol* 257: G386–G396.

124. Branchek T, Mawe G, Gershon MD (1988): Actions of BRL 24924 on enteric neurons: Role of 5-HT$_{1P}$ receptors. *Abstract Symp* "Cardiovasular Pharmacology of Serotonin", The Netherlands, Amsterdam.

125. Costall B, Kelly ME, Naylor RJ, Tan CCW, Tattersall FD (1986): 5-hydroxytryptamine M-receptor antagonism in the hypothalamus facilitates gastric emptying in the guinea pig. *Neuropharmacol* 125: 1293—1296.

126. Fioramonti J, Fargas MJ, Bueno L (1988): Involvement of endogenous opiates in regulation of gastric emptying of fat test meals in mice. *Am J Physiol* 18: G158—G161.

XVI. Presence of 5-hydroxytryptamine in adrenergic nerves of the brain circulation: its role in sympathetic neurotransmission and regulation of the cerebral vessel wall

CHRISTER OWMAN, JING-YU CHANG and JAN ERIK HARDEBO

1. Introduction

It has for long been believed that 5-hydroxytryptamine (5-HT) plays an aetiological role in some important cerebral vascular disorders, such as migraine and vasospasm following subarachnoid hemorrhage [1—6]. This is related to the strong vasoconstrictor action of 5-HT on brain vessels in vitro [7, 8]. When infused into the carotid artery, it reduces cerebral blood flow in many brain regions, provided the blood-brain barrier is opened or monoamine oxidase is inhibited. The response seems to be partly associated with a decrease in cerebral metabolism [9—11].

Since 5-HT-containing nerve fibers have been found in the wall of cerebral vessels, the possibility that 5-HT may act as a neurotransmitter to regulate cerebral circulation has received considerable attention in recent years. Our own studies have mainly focused on various aspects of the distribution and origin of the 5-HT nerve fibers, the receptor mechanisms mediating vasoconstriction, its neuronal uptake and release, and the interaction of the indole with other vasoconstrictor substances.

2. Origin and distribution of 5-HT-containing nerve fibers in cerebral arteries

The first report of a possible serotoninergic innervation of cerebral vessels appeared more than a decade ago on the basis of autoradiographic methods [12]. With the development of antisera against 5-HT, specific and highly sensitive immunohistochemical techniques have been developed [13] making it possible to visualize directly 5-HT immunoreactive nerve fibers in association with cerebral arteries from various species, including man [14—22]. Biochemical measurements of the 5-HT content of cerebral vessels by high performance liquid chromatography (HPLC) also support the existence of

P.R. Saxena, D.I. Wallis, W. Wouters and P. Bevan (eds), Cardiovascular Pharmacology of 5-Hydroxytryptamine, pp. 211—230.
© 1990 *Kluwer Academic Publishers, Dordrecht* —

the indolamine in the cerebrovascular bed, including pial vessels of different size and cerebral microvessels [23—26].

Attempts to trace the origin of the 5-HT nerve fibers have led to conflicting results. Thus, Edvinsson et al. [16] and Scatton et al. [25], measuring 5-HT content with HPLC in the fine vessels from the brain surface, have reported that raphe nuclei lesions markedly reduce 5-HT content, whereas superior cervical ganglionectomy does not alter it. The result was supported by the finding [27] that [³H]-5-HT uptake was attenuated in rat cerebral artery preparations following raphe lesion, while no change occurred with superior cervical ganglionectomy. Tsai et al. [28] have described a possible pathway connecting the middle cerebral artery and the raphe nuclei in cat by retrograde tracing.

Evidence against central 5-HT innervation has also accumulated recently. Thus, Alafaci et al. [18] demonstrated that 5-HT immunoreactive nerve fibers disappear after superior cervical ganglionectomy in the gerbil, confirmed also for cerebral arteries of rat and rabbit [20, 21, 29]. This would suggest that the superior cervical gangion (SCG), besides being the major source of sympathetic innervation in cerebral vessels, may also be the origin of the cerebrovascular 5-HT fibers. Observations supporting this hypothesis are the recent discovery of 5-HT immunoreactivity in small intensely fluorescent (SIF) cells of SCG from adult rat [21, 30], as well as in some main neurons of the SCG in newborn rats and in the adult ganglion following loading with 5-HT precursor [31, 32]. Sah and Matsumoto [33] have even demonstrated that cultured principal neurons of newborn rat SCG can synthesize, take up and release 5-HT. Although 5-HT immunoreactive neurons can no longer be demonstrated in the SCG of adult rat, Cowen et al. [20] suggested that the 5-HT terminals around arteries still maintain their ability to synthesize and store the indolamine even in adult life. The groups of Levitt and Duckles [26] and Saito and Lee [29] have examinined rabbit basilar arteries and confirmed that 5-HT present in the cerebrovascular system is largely accumulated into sympathetic nerve fibers, suggesting the indole is not an authentic, but an alternative, transmitter stored in the sympathetic nerve terminals [21]. Between these two positions Marco et al. [24] propose a dual innervation, based on measurement of the 5-HT concentration in cat cerebral arteries, showing that both raphe lesion and superior cervical ganglionectomy significantly reduce the indole content.

3. Uptake and accumulation of 5-HT in cerebrovascular nerves

In addition to its presence in serotoninergic nerves, the indole is frequently taken up into sympathetic fibers. In 1964 Owman [34] described the accumulation of endogenous 5-HT by sympathetic nerves of rat pineal gland, an uptake which changes according to the circadian rhythm. Subsequently, Thoa et al. [35] demonstrated the ability of sympathetic nerve terminals in the guinea-pig vas deferens to take up and store exogenous 5-HT. Numerous subsequent reports confirm the efficient uptake of 5-HT into sympathetic nerve terminals of the vascular system, not only at high concentrations where uptake may be unspecific [36—38], but also at relatively low concentrations [26, 29, 39]. The 5-HT can be released upon either electrical stimulation or pharmacological challenges and subsequently induces vasoconstriction.

Since 5-HT immunoreactive nerve fibers have been visualized in cerebral arteries, it would be natural to assume that 5-HT is accumulated in serotoninergic nerve fibers. However, most recent studies do not favour this assumption. Thus, Verbeuren et al. [39], using 30 nM [^{3}H]-5-HT which is below the threshold for nonspecific uptake [40], found considerable 5-HT accumulation in sympathetic nerve fibers of dog cerebral and peripheral arteries. The accumulation was abolished by chemical sympathectomy and 5-HT could be displaced by tyramine, a drug believed to displace noradrenaline from sympathetic storage sites. Similar findings in rabbit basilar artery strongly indicate that most of the 5-HT is taken up by sympathetic, rather than by truly serotoninergic, nerve fibers [26].

Recently Saito and Lee [29], combining immunohistochemical and in vitro pharmacological methods, showed that 5-HT can be visualized immunohistochemically in rabbit basilar artery only following immersion fixation, when the indole may be taken up by sympathetic fibers during the dissection procedure. An uptake of 5-HT by sympathetic nerve fibers can be seen by immunohistochemistry even at a concentration of 10 nM. Following incubation with a higher concentration (1 μM), nerve stimulation evokes a neurogenic vasoconstriction as a result of the release of the indole from sympathetic nerve terminals. It should be mentioned that a vasoconstriction induced by putative, endogenous 5-HT has been reported in canine forelimb vasculature as well as in rabbit vertebral artery [14, 41], suggesting that 5-HT could act as an authentic neurotransmitter in these tissues. However, this has not been confirmed in studies on rabbit basilar artery [17, 26].

In contrast to the hypothesis of sympathetic uptake of 5-HT, other studies favour the presence of a specific serotoninergic system in cerebral arteries. The results by Amenta et al. [27] have already been mentioned. Edvinsson et al. [17] incubated rat pial vessels with 10^{-7} M [^{3}H]-5-HT and suggested that it was taken up, at least partly, into serotoninergic nerves. Considering the concentration of [^{3}H]-5-HT used in the study — 100 nM compared to 10 and 30 nM as used by Verbeuren et al. [39] and by Levitt and Duckles [26] — it may be difficult to exclude involvement of sympathetic nerves. Kinetic studies of 5-HT uptake into pial arteries of rat and rabbit by Scatton et al. [25] gave K_m values of 0.27 and 2.2 μM, respectively; they concluded that the uptake was serotoninergic in nature. Unfortunately, sympathectomized controls were not included in these experiments.

4. Sympathetic origin of 5-HT-containing nerves supplying pial vessels

Nerve fibers showing 5-HT immunoreactivity have been demonstrated in cerebral arteries from mouse, rat, gerbil, guinea-pig, cat, rabbit, monkey [14, 17, 19, 20, 22], as well as in humans [15]. In our own recent studies, 5-HT immunoreactive fibers were visualized in all branches of the circle of Willis in guinea-pig [42], and in the basilar artery of rat [43]. The pattern of 5-HT fiber distribution in guinea-pig (Figure 1) resembled that of noradrenergic fibers: the most dense network was found in the anterior cerebral arteries, followed by middle cerebral and posterior cerebral arteries, and the basilar artery was among the most sparsely supplied vessels.

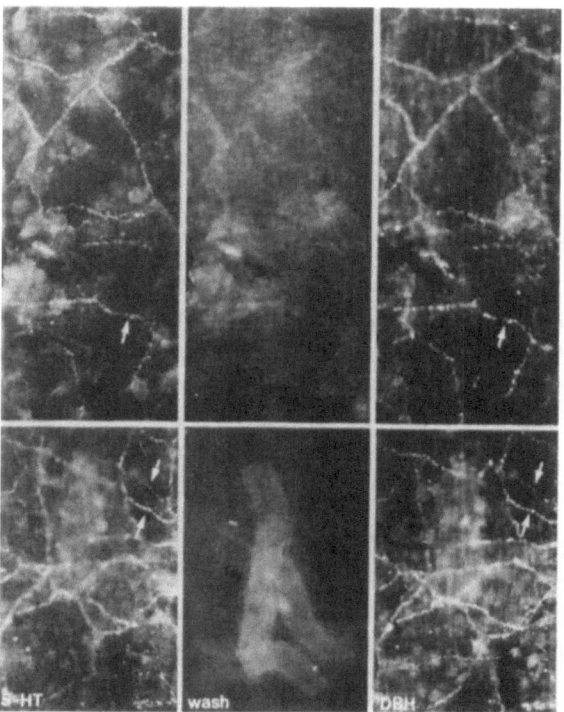

Figure 1. Elution-restaining experiment on pial arteries from guinea-pig showing 5-HT immunofluorescence, the result of elution in the presence of sulphuric acid and potassium permanganate, followed by immunoreaction for the specific enzyme in noradrenaline synthesis, DBH. The results demonstrate that 5-HT and DBH are co-localized in the same nerve fibers, as evidenced by the identity of single varicosties (see arrows). In these sequential staining and photographic procedures it is difficult to identify in the microscope the same focal planes within the fairly thick, vascular whole-mounts; for this reason two complementary vascular regions were chosen as examples. Magnification, X250.

Immunohistochemical demonstration of 5-HT was more difficult in rat cerebral arteries than in guinea-pig vessels. In untreated rats, a weak 5-HT-like immunoreactivity was inconsistently observed in nerve fibers of the basilar artery and its adjoining area. When 5-HT concentration was increased by loading the animal with tryptophan together with the monoamine oxidase inhibitor, nialamide, a clearly visible plexus of 5-HT immunoreactive fibers could be demonstrated in the basilar and vertebral arteries with a high degree of reproducibility, whereas the other parts of the circle of Willis still reacted negatively. A positive immunoreactivity in all parts of the circle of Willis could only be achieved after incubating the vessels with 1 nM 5-HT plus 30 μM nialamide for 60 min in vitro.

The SCG is the major source of sympathetic innervation to cerebral arteries. Since previous studies had suggested the presence of 5-HT neurons in the SCG, superior cervical ganglionectomy was undertaken to see if it affected the 5-HT nerve fibers in the pial vascular system. In guinea-pig [42], 5-HT nerve fibers disappeared totally from all parts of the pial vessels studied one week after operation. Unilateral sympathectomy resulted in elimination of immunoreactive nerve fibers from the ipsilateral part of the vasculature. To exclude possible innervation from other sympathetic ganglia, such as the stellate, decentralization of SCG was performed. No change in the distribution of 5-HT nerve fibers could be detected after this operation, indicating that the SCG is the major source for the 5-HT fibers distributed in the large pial arteries. However, no main neurons in the SCG reacted with 5-HT antiserum, even after preloading the animal with tryptophan following monoamine oxidase inhibition.

In rat [43], ganglionectomy abolished 5-HT fibers in the basilar, superior cerebellar and vertebral arteries in most cases. After incubation with 5-HT in vitro, 5-HT immunoreactive fibers were observed to form dense networks in the pial arteries in all parts at the base of the brain. Unilateral sympathectomy led to the disappearance of these immunoreactive fibers from the ipsilateral side. One week after bilateral ganglionectomy, no or only very few fibers were visible in the lower part of the basilar and vertebral arteries in the majority of animals following incubation with 5-HT. That a few nerve fibers remained is not surprising, considering the variation among individual animals [44, 45]. Nerve fibers in the vertebro-basilar system may be derived not only from the SCG but also from the stellate ganglia [46]. Cowen et al. [19, 20], using sympathetic ganglionectomy to investigate 5-HT as well as noradrenergic fibers in gerbil and rat, report varying results in basilar and vertebral arteries. Because of this variability, it does not necessarily follow that immunoreactive nerve fibers remaining after removal of the SCG constitute serotoninergic nerves orginating from the central raphe nuclei. Napoleone et al. [46] found a few, yellow-fluorescent nerve fibers with the formaldehyde method in the basilar artery and other parts of the circle of Willis after superior cervical ganglionectomy, and claimed that they were serotoninergic. Considering they administered the precursor, 5-hydroxytryptophan, which can be transformed to 5-HT even in noradrenergic fibers, it is most likely that the nerve fibers were residual sympathetic fibers deriving from ganglia other than the SCG.

Although the possibility of a specific serotoninergic innervation from sources other than the sympathetic system cannot be excluded, these sources could only represent a small proportion of 5-HT fibers in the pial vessels, and their physiological significance may therefore be questionable. This idea is reinforced by the uptake and release experiments discussed later. Our data are consistent with the results of Alafaci et al. [18] and Saito and Lee [29], indicating peripheral sources for the 5-HT innervation in pial arteries of gerbil and rabbit.

As most experiments in favour of a central innervation have been performed in the rat, species diferences have to be taken into consideration. Uptake studies were performed in order to investigate further the origin of 5-HT fibers in pial vessels in the rat [47]. Blood-free arteries from rat were incubated with [^{3}H]-5-HT (10 to 300 nM) for periods from 5 to 60 min. 5-HT uptake was significantly reduced after superior cervical ganglionectomy (Figure 2), which agrees well with other observations [26] using chemical denervation of rabbit basilar artery. On the other hand, lesion of the raphe nuclei verified by HPLC measuremet of 5-HT and 5-hydroxyindoleacetic acid contents in various brain regions, was virtually without effect on 5-HT uptake in pial vessels (Figure 2). This finding is opposite to that of Amenta et al. [27] whose raphe lesion experiments caused significat decrease in 5-HT uptake, whereas excision of the SCG had no effect at all. The contradictory results are hard to explain. Although we worked with identical tritium

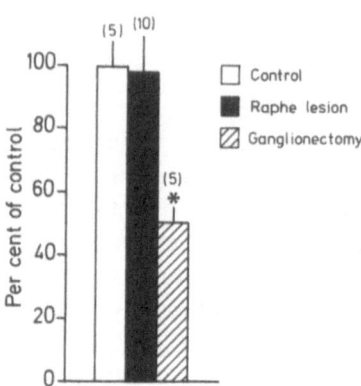

Figure 2. The effects on rats of stereotaxic lesions of the raphe complex, or bilateral removal of the superior cervical sympathetic ganglia, on pial arterial uptake of 100 nM tritated 5-HT compared to controls. Values are means ± SEM, number of animals in parenthesis. There is no effect of the raphe lesion, whereas uptake in vitro is approximately halved (analysis of variance: *p < 0.05) following sympathectomy. Remaining accumulation in the sympathectomized vessels corresponds well with the non-neuronal uptake of tracer into the vasculature.

concentrations and the same species, the type of vessel preparation used for analysis was not identical.

The varying results regarding the possibility of a central or a peripheral 5-HT innervation of cerebral vessels could be attributed to different vascular regions studied. Inasmuch as the data supporting a central innervation are obtained from cerebral microvessels or small pial vessels [23, 25], the possibility should not be excluded that the sympathetic innervation might primarily be associated with large pial vessels.

5. Are sympathetic nerves to brain vessels truly serotoninergic or 5-HT-containing adrenergic fibers?

Since our data strongly indicate that the 5-HT fibers originate largely from the SCG in both guinea-pig and rat, failure to visualize 5-HT neurons in the SCG focuses attention on the nature of these 5-HT immunoreactive fibers. Are they truly serotoninergic nerve fibers or does the immunoreactivity represent 5-HT uptake by adrenergic nerve fibers? Two approaches were followed to clarify this issue. One utilized the elution-restaining method to observe the relationship between 5-HT and adrenergic nerve fibers [42, 48]; the other attempted to distinguish the nerve fibers through the use of neurotoxic agents [21, 43]. Noradrenergic fibers were visualized immunohistochemically through the presence of the specific enzyme, dopamine-β-hydroxylase (DBH).

In guinea-pig, coexistence of 5-HT- and DBH-like immunoreactivity was established in pial arteries (Figure 1). Coexistence was substantiated by examining the identical, detailed location of the nerve varicosities. The neurotoxic agents, 5,6-dihydroxytryptamine (5,6-DHT) and 6-hydroxydopamine (6-OHDA), were used to distinguish serotoninergic and sympathetic nerve terminals on the basis of their selective toxicity towards 5-HT and noradrenergic systems, respectively [49—51]. In the rat, administration of 5,6-DHT (200 μg i.c.v.) one week beforehand left the 5-HT fibers in the basilar artery intact, whereas 6-OHDA (250 μg i.c.v.) completely abolished 5-HT immunoreactive fibers within one week. The results imply that the 5-HT immunoreactive fibers running in pial vessels may not represent an authentic serotoninergic innervation, but reflect that 5-HT is taken up by sympathetic nerve terminals and thus is co-localized with noradrenaline, as had been demonstrated in guinea-pig pial arteries.

Since uptake may contribute to the presence of 5-HT in the pial vessels, as discussed above, two experiments were designed to explore this mechanism. An attempt was made to investigate if a low concentration of 5-HT could be taken up into sympathetic nerve terminals and subsequently released by electrical or pharmacological stimulation [43]. Experiments were also undertaken to study the kinetic properties of the 5-HT uptake into sympathetic nerve terminals [47].

6. Characterization of the 5-HT uptake into cerebrovascular sympathetic nerves

The 5-HT concentrations generally used in uptake studies in the CNS may be divided into high (>100 nM), at which involvement of catecholamine uptake systems cannot be avoided, and low (<100 nM), when uptake is thought to be specifically by serotoninergic systems [40, 52, 53]. Although in many studies higher concentrations of 5-HT have been applied to prove its uptake into sympathetic nerves, especially in the case of release studies [36—38], many have used relatively low concentrations, down to 10 nM [26, 29]. In our immunohistochemical studies, substantial accumulation of 5-HT was found in sympathetic nerve fibers even during incubation with a concentration of 1 nM.

Numerous experiments have confirmed the accumulation of 5-HT by sympathetic nerves, but little attention has been paid to the kinetic properties of this uptake in peripheral organs, partly due to the difficulties in distinguishing between neuronal and extraneuronal uptake. Denervation seems the only reliable way to eliminate neuronal uptake in cerebral arteries, based on our previously mentioned immunohistochemical experiments. Therefore, superior cervical sympathectomy served as a blank and the difference between the intact and sympathectomy groups was regarded as the neural uptake.

Saturable uptake processes operating against concentration gradients were found for both noradrenaline and 5-HT [47], with almost identical K_m values, whereas the V_{max} value was ten times higher for NE than for 5-HT (Figure 3). This, and the observation that reserpine treatment markedly inhibited uptake of noradrenaline (by about 50%) but had little effect on 5-HT (whose uptake was reduced by some 15%), indicate that the two amines are stored by different mechanisms intra-axonally. By analogy, neuropeptide Y, another mediator stored in cerebrovascular sympathetic nerves [48] is also resistant to reserpine, whereas 6-OHDA, which abolishes the 5-HT immunoreactivity from pial sympathetic fibers [21, 43], markedly depletes neuropeptide Y from the nerves [54—56]. The K_m values obtained were consistent with those for 5-HT and noradrenaline uptakes in both central and peripheral nervous systems [57—62]. The K_m value for 5-HT was also identical with that reported by Scatton et al. [25] in their 5-HT uptake study on rat cerebral arteries (although they attributed it to uptake into specific serotoninergic nerves). Non-radioactive 5-HT and noradrenaline inhibited uptake of [^{14}C]-noradrenaline and [^{3}H]-5-HT in a concentration-dependent manner, with IC_{50} values quite similar to the K_m values for 5-HT and noradrenaline uptakes. On the other hand, noradrenaline and 5-HT showed no interaction with each other in the accumulation at extraneuronal sites, suggesting that the uptake$_2$ process was independent for these two amines. Further, the uptake$_2$ blocker, corticosterone, was more potent in inhibiting 5-HT than noradrenaline uptake into the extraneuronal sites.

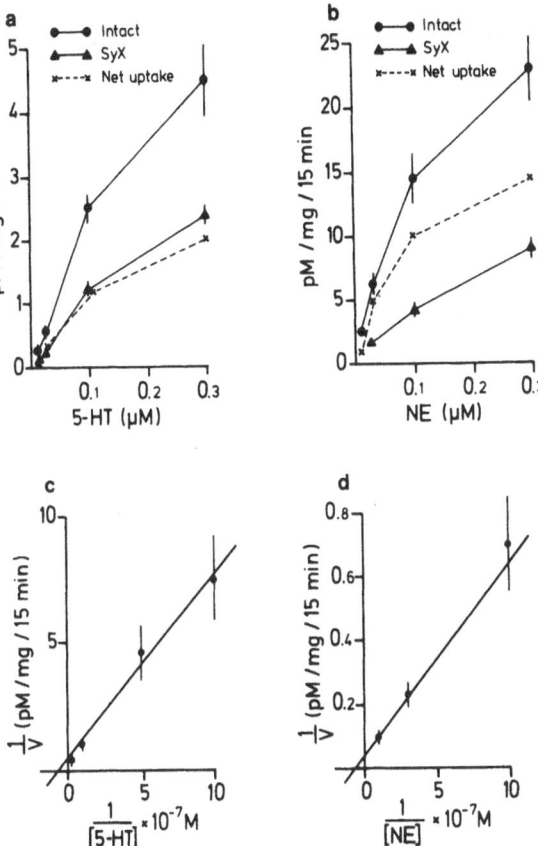

Figure 3. Accumulation of (a) [³H]-5-HT and (b) [¹⁴C]-noradrenaline in rat pial arteries incubated for 15 min in the presence of increasing amine concentrations. The net uptake was obtained by subtracting the uptake in sympathectomized (SyX) arteries from the total uptake in intact vessels of non-operated animals. The Lineweaver-Burke plots from the experiments with (c) 5-HT and (d) noradrenaline were used to calculate K_m and V_{max}. Values are means ± SEM, preparations from 3—6 animals were used at each concentration.

There is a general consensus that 5-HT and catecholamines are taken up separately in the brain [40, 52, 53, 63, 64], but no evidence for the coexistence of these two biogenic amines in the CNS. However, it may not be possible to extrapolate from brain to peripheral sympathetic nervous system, where the nerves differ substantially in structure and function.

Paroxetine and desipramine are selective in their inhibition of amine uptake [47]. Paroxetine has a higher potency in blockade of 5-HT than noradrenaline uptake; the reverse order was found for desipramine. Levitt and Duckles [26], however, showed that another selective 5-HT uptake blocker, fluoxetine, had similar potency in inhibiting 5-HT and noradrenaline uptake in rabbit basilar artery. Fluoxetine inhibits 5-HT uptake (IC_{50} 0.7 μM) in rat pial artery preparations [25] and rabbit basilar artery with similar potency [26]. Paroxetine is much more potent than fluoxetine in inhibiting

5-HT uptake in the CNS (IC_{50} 0.4 and 15 nM, respectively). On the other hand, Magnussen et al. [65] have shown that paroxetine is a weak inhibitor of noradrenaline uptake, (IC_{50} 1 μM), in contrast to our study where IC_{50} values for 5-HT and noradrenaline uptake were 0.03 and 52.4 nM, respectively. The different results could be due, among other things, to the different preparations used. Thus, it is possible that a high affinity transport site for 5-HT susceptible to paroxetine is located in sympathetic nerve terminals; alternatively, a specific serotoninergic uptake system may be present in the cerebral vessels [25, 27].

7. Electrically-induced release of 5-HT from cerebrovascular sympathetic fibers

The 5-HT accumulating in the cerebrovascular sympathetic nerve fibers may have originated from several local sources. Within the brain, the central raphe nuclei project to widespread areas where serotoninergic terminals come close to cerebral vessels, especially in the case of the raphe pallidus nucleus in the brain stem located immediately adjacent to the basilar artery. In the blood stream, 5-HT released from the enterochromaffin cell system of the intestine can reach a concentration of about 10—100 nM [65a, 66, 67], which is much higher than we used in the previously mentioned incubation study. The plasma concentration of 5-HT is enough for uptake into sympathetic nerve terminals, but the existence of a blood-brain barrier would make this uptake into cerebrovascular nerves less prominent [68]. On the other hand, 5-HT is synthesized in the endothelial cells of cerebral vessels [68, 69], allowing possible transport of 5-HT into the vascular smooth musculature or adventitial layer in which sympathetic nerve fibers terminate. 5-HT might also originate from mast cells, which contain large amounts of 5-HT in some species. These cells are located close to the cerebral vessels [70, 71] and may synthesize and release 5-HT which can be taken up by the sympathetic nerve terminals [72].

The reported reduction of perivascular 5-HT following raphe lesions [16, 25] is consistent with this nucleus representing the source for 5-HT which, following diffusion into the extracellular space and cerebrospinal fluid, is taken up into the perivascular sympathetic fibers. If this is the case, it emphasizes that caution has to be exercised when interpreting results from lesions of a brain nucleus in terms of the origin of a particular fiber system.

An important question is whether 5-HT, taken up by perivascular sympathetic fibers, can be liberated from the nerves. In a series of experiments [43], 3 nM tritiated 5-HT was used to preincubate rat pial arteries to investigate whether the indolamine could be released from perivascular fibers upon electrical or pharmacological activation after exposure to a near physiological concentration [65a]. It was found that release of tritium increased by more than 100% upon stimulation (Figure 4). The liberation

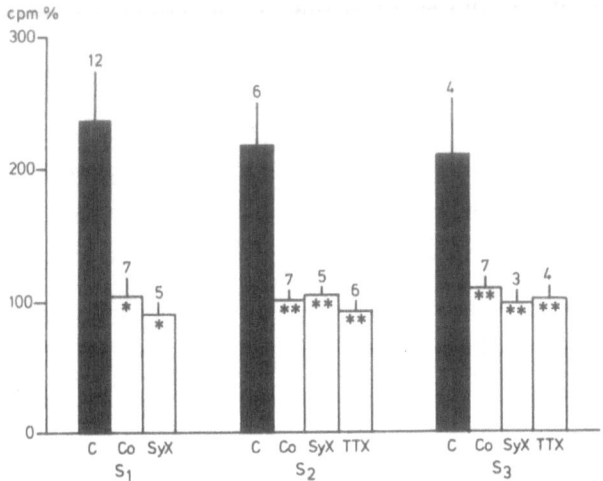

Figure 4. Fractional release of tritium from rat pial arteries during three 2-min periods of electrical field stimulation (S_1-S_3), following preincubation with 3 nM of [^{3}H]-5-HT, 30 μM nialamide, 100 μM ascorbic acid and 30 μM Na$_2$Ca EDTA. The efflux was expressed as percent change compared with the mean cpm value from three 2-min periods before each period of stimulation or drug exposure. Electrical activation markedly increases the tritium efflux in control preparations (C). No increase is seen when stimulation is carried out with preparations preincubated in the presence 10 μM cocaine (Co) or following surgical sympathectomy (SyX), or if stimulation is performed in the presence of 0.3 μM tetrodotoxin (TTX). Values are means ± SEM, number of preparations is indicated. Analysis of variance: *p < 0.05, **0.001 < p <0.01.

was associated with sympathetic nerve terminals, because (1) the effect was totally abolished by tetrodotoxin, (2) potassium and tyramine also induced marked release of tritium from the preparation, the latter by entering sympathetic nerve terminals and displacing 5-HT from its storage sites, and (3) all effects were abolished or greatly inhibited by superior cervical ganglionectomy or by preincubation with radioactive 5-HT in the presence of cocaine.

8. Characterization of the cerebrovascular 5-HT receptors

The results show that 5-HT may be efficiently taken up into pial sympathetic fibers at concentrations close to those prevailing in the environment of the fibers, from where it may be released upon activation. Following release, 5-HT may act directly on the vessel wall, or it may interact with the liberation of noradrenaline and/or its effect on the vessel.

Experiments on isolated pial arteries from rat and guinea-pig with various 5-HT receptor agonists and antagonists were performed to characterize the 5-HT receptors [73]. In the rat, 5-HT induced pronounced vasoconstriction of the basilar artery with an EC_{50} value of about 300 nM (Figure 5a). The contraction was competitively antagonized by the selective 5-HT$_2$ receptor antagonist, ketanserin (Figure 5a), with a pA$_2$ value of 9.31, which was identical to the $-\log K_d$ value for ketanserin binding to 5-HT$_2$ receptors in brain tissue [74]. Moreover, the selective 5-HT$_1$ receptor agonist, 5-carboxamidotryptamine (5-CT), contracted the vessels less effectively, the EC_{50} value being about 16 times higher than that of 5-HT. This is consistent with results in rabbit aorta [75], where a 20 times lower potency of 5-CT was considered an indicator for involvement of 5-HT$_2$ rather than 5-HT$_1$-like receptors in the vasoconstriction. Methiothepin, propranolol and mesulergine, albeit used to characterize subtypes of 5-HT$_1$-like receptor, all have affinity for 5-HT$_2$ receptors [76—78]. Accordingly, they all inhibited the

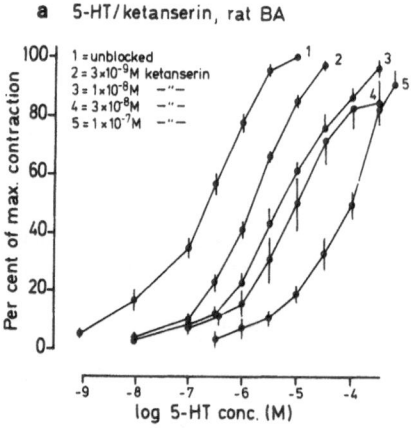

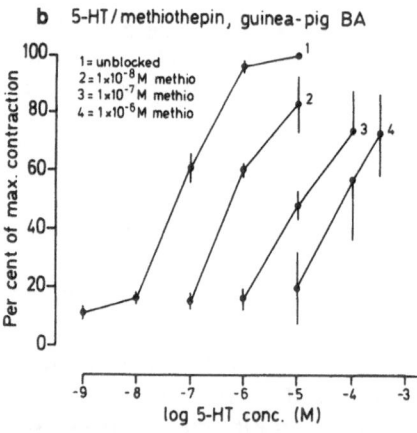

Figure 5. Concentration-response curves (means ± SEM; n = 4 — 8) for 5-HT tested on basilar artery (BA) from (a) rat and (b) guinea-pig. The results suggest (see text) that the 5-HT receptor in the former artery is of the 5-HT$_2$ type whereas contraction in the latter is mediated by 5-HT$_1$-like receptors.

5-HT-induced vasoconstriction in rat basilar artery with potencies corresponding to their binding affinities to 5-HT$_2$ receptors. The data taken together suggest that 5-HT$_2$ receptors are involved in the 5-HT-induced vasoconstriction in this artery.

In contrast, 5-HT receptors in guinea-pig basilar artery (Figure 5b) are different because the EC$_{50}$ value for vasoconstriction was lower compared with rat (48 and 300 nM, respectively), in line with the high affinity of the indole for 5-HT$_1$-like receptors in brain tissue [79]. 5-CT contracted the vessel with a potency even higher than that of 5-HT (16 nM), different from the situation in the rat. The selective 5-HT$_{1A}$ receptor agonist, 8-hydroxy-2-(di-n-propy-lamino) tetralin (8-OH-DPAT), which strongly contracts canine basilar artery [80, 81] exhibited a negligible vasoconstrictor effect in guinea-pig and rat vessels. The 5-HT receptor antagonists ketanserin, propranolol (which acts as a 5-HT$_{1B}$ blocker [82, 83]), and mesulergine (which antagonizes 5-HT$_{1C}$ receptors [84]) displayed poor ability to block 5-HT-induced vasoconstriction in guinea-pig basilar artery. The only compound tested that could substantially block the vasoconstriction was methiothepin (Figure 5b): at concentrations from 0.01 to 1 μM this antagonist shifted the concentration-response curves to 5-HT to the right, with a pA$_2$ value of 8.74. Similar results have been reported for dog saphenous vein and coronary artery [85, 86]. The results from guinea-pig basilar artery fit very well the criteria proposed by Bradley et al. [87] for classifying 5-HT$_1$-like receptors.

9. Interaction of 5-HT and noradrenaline in pial vasoconstriction

The potentiating effect of 5-HT on the vasoconstriction evoked by vasoactive substances appears to be a non-specific phenomenon. Apart from noradrenaline, it can also amplify vasoconstriction induced by histamine, prostaglandin F$_{2a}$, thromboxane A$_2$ as well as angiotension II. In view of the coexistence and probable corelease of 5-HT and noradrenaline in pial arteries, the interaction of the two amines in cerebral vessels may represent an important physiological mechanism. Because the basilar artery of rats did not constrict in response to noradrenaline, we chose guinea-pig for the experiments investigating the postjunctional vasomotor interaction between 5-HT and noradrenaline [88].

The results show (Figure 6) that 5-HT at low concentration (3 nM) greatly enhances the noradrenaline-induced vasoconstriction to about 200—300% of control level. The potentiating effect could not be blocked by ketanserin, but was substantially inhibited by methiothepin, indicating that 5-HT$_1$-like receptors which also mediate 5-HT-induced vasoconstriction play a major role in the potentiating action of 5-HT. The amplification could not be blocked by methysergide, another 5-HT$_1$-like receptor antagonist. On the contrary, methysergide itself augmented the noradrenaline-induced vasoconstriction to a similar extent as 5-HT, consistent with the partial agonist effect of methysergide at 5-HT$_1$ receptors [8, 89, 90]. A potentiating effect of

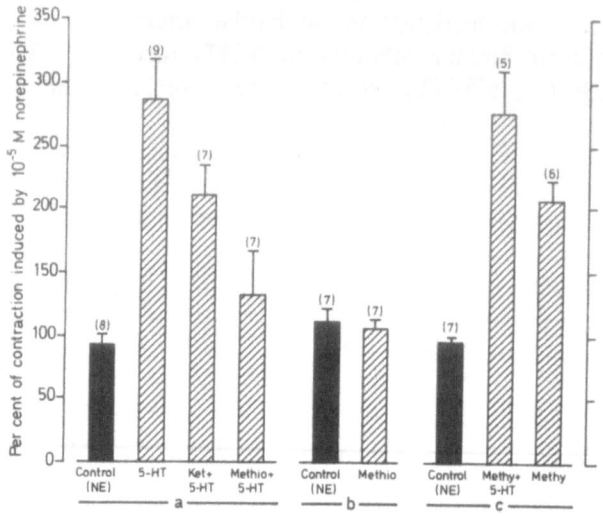

Figure 6. Potentiating effect of 3 nM 5-HT on the contractile response induced by 10 μM noradrenaline. The potentiation is not significantly affected by 3 nM ketanserin (Ket), but is antagonized by the same concentraton of methiothepin (Methio). (b) Methiothepin itself has no antagonistic effect on the noradrenaline response. (c) Methysergide (Methy; 1 μM) does not inhibit the 5-HT-induced potentiation of the noradrenergic contraction, but when given alone it mimicks the amplifying effect of 5-HT. In the calculations the mean amplitude of the contractile response to noradrenaline — before and after the test with 5-HT plus noradrenaline — was taken as 100%. The noradrenaline response before adding 5-HT, as well as the net contractile response to noradrenaline immediately after 5-HT had been added, were compared with this mean value. In this way it was possible to determine the control values (filled bars). Values shown are means ± SEM, number of vessels tested in parenthesis.

methysergide has also been found in various peripheral arteries [41, 91—93], suggesting that methysergide may act on 5-HT receptors to enhance the vasoconstriction induced by noradrenaline.

It can be assumed that the 5-HT taken up by a high affinity, low capacity transport system located in cerebrovascular sympathetic nerve terminals can be released together with noradrenaline. Although 5-HT is probably liberated in lower concentration than the "host transmitter" noradrenaline, it may still be efficacious in enhancing the otherwise weak vasoconstrictor effect of noradrenaline.

10. Conclusions

5-HT can be demonstrated by immunohistochemistry in plexuses of nerve fibers surrounding arteries at the base of the brain. Subsequent immunohistochemical visualization of adrenergic nerves through the specific enzyme, dopamine-β-hydroxylase, has revealed that 5-HT is, in fact, stored in sympathetic nerves. Accordingly, the 5-HT-containing nerves disappear following superior cervical ganglionectomy or treatment with the neurotoxic agent, 6-hydroxydopamine. The 5-HT present seems to be taken up locally, probably from the cerebrospinal fluid, by an efficient axonal transport process and is then accumulated in a reserpine-resistant pool. Once taken up into the cerebrovascular sympathetic fibers, 5-HT appears to function as a "false transmitter" releasable by electrical field stimulation of the perivascular nerves or through potassium depolarization, as well as by treatment with the indirectly-acting sympathomimetic agent, tyramine. 5-HT activates specific receptors in the vascular smooth musculature to cause strong vasoconstriction and, in subliminal concentrations, it markedly amplifies the α-adrenoceptor mediated contraction of noradrenaline. Both responses to 5-HT appear to be mediated by the same subtype of 5-HT receptor.

It is suggested that 5-HT, besides its direct vasoconstrictor effect, acts to "economize" sympathetic neurotransmission in cerebrovascular sympathetic nerves (like similarly co-stored neuropeptide Y). This may be of both physiological and pathophysiological importance in the neurogenic control of cerebral blood flow.

Acknowledgements

Supported by grant No. 14X-732/5680 from the Swedish Medical Cell Research Council. Excellent word processing by Ms Maud Mårtensson is highly appreciated.

References

1. Deshmukh VD, Harper AM (1973): The effect of serotonin on cerebral and extracerebral blood flow with possible implications in migraine. *Acta Neurol Scand* 49: 649—658.
2. Allen GS, Henderson LM, Chou SN, French LA (1974): Cerebral arterial spasm. Part 2: *In vitro* contractile activity of serotonin in human serum and CSF on the canine basilar artery, and its blockage by methysergide and phenoxybenzamine. *J Neurosurg* 40: 442—450.
3. Sjaastad O (1975): The significance of blood serotonin levels in migraine. *Acta Neurol Scand* 51: 200—210.
4. Owman Ch, Edvinsson L, Olin T, Sahlin Ch, Svendgaard N-Aa (1979): Pathophysiology of cerebral vasospasm: Transmitter changes in perivascular sympathetic nerves, and increased pial artery sensitivity to norepinephrine and serotonin, pp. 295—305 in: Price T R, Nelson E (eds), *Cerebrovascular Disease*. New York: Raven Press.
5. Pickard JD, Perry S (1984): Spectrum of altered reactivity of isolated cerebral arteries following subarachnoid haemorrhage — response to potassium, pH, noradrenaline, 5-hydroxytryptamine, and sodium loading. *J Cereb Blood Flow Metab* 4: 599—609.
6. Fozard JR (1985): 5-Hydroxytryptamine in the pathophysiology of migraine, pp. 321—328 in: Bevan JA, Godfraind T, Maxwell RA, Stoclet JC, Worcel, W (eds), *Vascular Neuroeffector Mechanisms*. Amsterdam: Elsevier.
7. Edvinsson L, Hardebo JE, Owman Ch (1978): Pharmacological analysis of 5-hydroxy-

tryptamine receptors in isolated intracranial and extracranial vessels of cat and man. *Circ Res* 42: 143—151.

8. Hardebo JE, Edvinsson L, Owman Ch, Svendgaard N-Aa (1978): Potentiation and antagonism of serotonin effects on intracranial and extracranial vessels. *Neurology* 28: 64—70.

9. Harper AM, MacKenzie ET (1977): Cerebral circulatory and metabolic effects of 5-hydroxytryptamine in anaesthetised baboons. *J Physiol* 271: 721—733.

10. Eidelman BN, Mendelow AD, McCalden TA, Bloom DS (1978): Potentiation of cerebrovascular response to intra-arterial 5-hydroxytryptamine. *Am J Physiol* 234: H300—H304.

11. Grom JJ, Harper AM (1983): The effects of serotonin on local cerebral blood flow. *J Cereb Blood Flow Metab* 3: 71—77.

12. Chan-Palay V (1976): Serotonin axons in the supra- and subependymal plexuses and in the leptomeninges: their roles in local alterations of cerebrospinal fluid and vasomotor activity. *Brain Res* 102: 103—130.

13. Steinbusch HWM, Verhofstad AAJ, Joosten HWJ (1978): Localization of serotonin in the central nervous system by immunohistochemistry: Description of a specific and sensitive technique and some applications. *Neuroscience* 3: 811—819.

14. Griffith SG, Lincoln J, Burnstock G (1982): Serotonin as a neurotransmitter in cerebral arteries. *Brain Res* 247: 388—392.

15. Griffith SG, Burnstock G (1983): Immunohistochemical demonstration of serotonin in nerves supplying human cerebral and mesenteric blood vessels. *Lancet* 1: 561—562.

16. Edvinsson L, Degueurce A, Duverger D, MacKenzie ET, Scatton B (1983): Central serotonergic nerves project to the pial vessels of the brain. *Nature* 306: 55—57.

17. Edvinsson L, Birath E, Uddman R, Lee TJF, Duverger D,Mackenzie ET, Scatton B (1984): Indoleaminergic mechanisms in brain vessels: Localization, concentration, uptake and in vitro responses of 5-hydroxytryptamine. *Acta Physiol Scand* 121: 291—299.

18. Alafaci C, Cowen T, Crockard HA, Burnstock G (1986): Cerebral perivascular serotonergic fibres have a peripheral origin in the gerbil. *Brain Res Bull* 16: 303—304.

19. Cowen T, Alafaci C, Crockard HA, Burnstock G (1986): 5-HT-containing nerves to major cerebral arteries of gerbil originate in the superior cervical ganglia. *Brain Res* 384: 51—59.

20. Cowen T, Alafaci C, Crockard HA, Burnstock G (1987): Origin and postnatal development of nerves showing 5-hydroxytryptamine-like immunoreactivity supplying major cerebral arteries of the rat. *Neurosci Lett* 78: 121—126.

21. Chang J-Y, Owman Ch (1986): Immunohistochemical and pharmacological studies on serotonergic nerves and receptors in brain vessels. *Acta Physiol Scand* 127 suppl. 552: 49—53.

22. Chang J-Y, Hardebo JE, Owman Ch, Sahlin Ch, Svendgaard N-Aa (1987): Nerves containing serotonin, its interaction with noradrenaline and characterization of serotonergic receptors in cerebral arteries of monkey. *J Auton Pharmacol* 7: 317—329.

23. Reinhard JF, Liebmann JE, Schlosberg AJ, Moskowitz MA (1979): Serotonin neurons project to small blood vessels in the brain. *Science* 206: 85—87.

24. Marco EJ, Belfagon G, Salaices M, Sanchez-Ferrer C, Marin J (1985): Serotonergic innervation of cat cerebral arteries. *Brain Res* 338: 137—139.

25. Scatton B, Duverger D, L'Hereux R, Serrano A, Fage D, Nowicki JP, MacKenzie ET (1985): Neurochemical studies on the existence, origin and characteristics of the serotonergic innervation of small pial vessels. *Brain Res* 345: 219—229.

26 Levitt B, Duckles SP (1986): Evidence against serotonin as a vasoconstrictor neurotransmitter in the rabbit basilar artery. *J Pharmacol Exp Ther* 238: 880—885.

27 Amenta F, De Rossi M, Mione MC, Geppetti P (1985): Characterization of ^{3}H-5-hydroxytryptamine uptake within rat cerebrovascular tree. *Eur J Pharmacol* 112: 181—186.

28. Tsai SH, Lin SZ, Wang SD, Liu JC, Shih CJ (1985): Retrograde localization of the innervation of the middle cerebral artery with horseradish peroxidase in cats. *Neurosurgery* 16: 463—467.

29. Saito A, Lee TJ-F (1987): Serotonin as an alternative transmitter in sympathetic nerves of large cerebral arteries of the rabbit. *Circ Res* 60: 220—228.

30. Verhofstad AAJ, Steinbusch HWM, Penke B, Varga J, Joosten HWJ (1981): Serotonin-immunoreactive cells in superior cervical ganglion of the rat: Evidence for the existence of separate serotonin and catecholamine containing small ganglionic cells. *Brain Res* 212: 39—49.

31. Häppölä O, Päivärinta H, Soinila S, Steinbusch HWM (1986):Pre- and postnatal development of 5-hydroxytryptamine-immunoreactive cells in the superior cervical ganglion of the rat. *J Auton Nerv Syst* 15: 21—31.

32. Häppölä O, Soinila S, Lahtinen T, Joh TH, Steinbusch HWM (1987): Immunohistochemical localization of 5-hydroxytryptamine in principal neurons and nerve fibers of the rat superior cervical ganglion. *Neuroscience* 22 (suppl.): S813.

33. Sah DWY, Matsumoto SG (1987): Evidence for serotonin synthesis, uptake and release in dissociated rat sympathetic neurons in culture. *J Neurosci* 7: 391—399.

34. Owman Ch (1964): Sympathetic nerves probably storing two types of monoamines in the rat pineal gland. *Int J Neuropharmacol* 2: 105—112.

35. Thoa NB, Eccleston D, Axelrod J (1969): The accumulation of C^{14} serotonin in the guinea-pig vas deferens. *J Pharmacol Exp Ther* 169: 68—73.

36. Kawasaki H, Takasaki K (1984): Vasoconstrictor response induced by 5-hydroxytryptamine released from vascular adrenergic nerves by periarterial nerve stimulation. *J Pharmacol Exp Ther* 229: 816—822.

37. Cohen RA (1984): Platelet-induced neurogenic coronary contractions due to accumulation of the false neurotransmitter, 5-hydroxytryptamine. *J Clin Invest* 75: 286—292.

38. Paiva MQ, Caramona M, Osswald W (1984): Intra- and extraneuronal metabolism of 5-hydroxytryptamine in the isolated saphenous vein of the dog. *Naunyn-Schmiedeberg's Arch Pharmacol* 325: 62—68.

39. Verbeuren TJ, Jordaens EH, Herman AG (1983): Accumulation and release of ^{3}H-5-hydroxytryptamine in saphenous veins and cerebral arteries of dog. *J Pharmacol Exp Ther* 226: 579—588.

40. Ross SB (1982): The characteristics of serotonin uptake systems, pp. 159—195 in: Osborne NN (ed), *Biology of Serotonergic Transmission*. John Wiley & Sons Ltd: Chichester, New York, Brisbane, Toronto.

41. Jandhyala BS, Kivlighn SD (1987): Antagonism by methysergide of neurogenic vasoconstriction in the dog forelimb. *Fed Proc* 46: 276—280.

42. Chang J-Y, Owman Ch, Steinbusch HWM (1988): Evidence for coexistence of serotonin and noradrenaline in sympathetic nerves supplying brain vessels of guinea-pig. *Brain Res* 438: 237—246.

43. Chang J-Y, Ekblad E, Kannisto P, Owman Ch (1989): Serotonin uptake into cerebrovascular nerve fibers of rat, visualization by immunohistochemistry, disappearance following sympathectomy, and release during electrical stimulation. *Brain Res* 492: 79—88.

44. Kajikawa H (1968): Flourescence histochemical studies on the distribution of adrenergic nerve fibers to intracranial blood vessels. *Arch Jap Chir* 37: 473—484.

45. Kajikawa H (1969): Mode of the sympathetic innervation of the cerebral vessels demonstrated by the fluorescent histochemical technique in rat and cat. *Arch Jap Chir* 38: 227—235.

46. Arbab MAR, Delgado TJ, Wiklund L, Svendgaard N-Aa (1989): Stellate ganglion innervation of the vertebro-basilar arterial system demonstrated in the rat with anterograde and retrograde WGA-HRP tracing. *Brain Res* 445: 175—180.

47. Chang J-Y, Hardebo JE, Owman Ch (1989): Kinetic studies on uptake of serotonin and noradrenaline into pial arteries of rats. *J Cereb Blood Flow Metab* in press.

48. Owman Ch, Chang J-Y, Ekblad E, Steinbusch HWM (1987): Immunohistochemical investigation of the relationship between different neuropeptides and amine transmitters in monkey and guinea-pig cerebral arteries, pp. 355—370 in: Nobin A, Owman Ch, Arneklo-Nobin B (eds), *Neuronal Messengers in Vascular Function*. Elsevier: New York, Oxford, Amsterdam.

49. Breese GR, Traylor TD (1970): Effect of 6-hydroxydopamine on brain norepinephrine and dopamine: Evidence for selective degeneration of catecholamine neurons. *J Pharmacol Exp Ther* 174: 413—420.

50. Baumgarten HG, Evetts KD, Holman RB, Iversen LL, Vogt M, Wilson G (1972): Effect of 5,6-hydroxytryptamine on monoaminergic neurones in the central nervous system of the rat. *J Neurochem* 19: 1587—1597.

51. Björklund A, Horn AS, Baumgarten HG, Nobin A, Schlossberger HG (1975): Neurotoxicity of hydroxylated tryptamines: Structure-activity relationships. 2. In vitro studies on monoamine uptake inhibition and uptake impairments. *Acta Physiol Scand* (suppl.) 429: 31—60.

52. Shaskan EG, Snyder SH (1970): Kinetics of serotonin accumulation into slices from rat brain: Relationship to catecholamine uptake. *J Pharmacol Exp Ther* 175: 404—418.

53. Kuhar MJ, Roth RH, Aghajanian G (1972): Synaptosomes from forebrains of rats with midbrain raphe lesions: Selective reduction of serotonin uptake. *J Pharmacol Exp Ther* 181: 36—45.

54. Lundberg JM, Terenius L, Hökfelt T, Martling CR, Tatemoto K, Mutt V, Polak J, Bloom S, Goldstein M (1982): Neuropeptide Y (NPY)-like immunoreactivity in peripheral noradrenergic neurons and effects of NPY on sympathetic function. *Acta Physiol Scand* 116: 477—480.

55. Lundberg JM, Saria A, Hökfelt T, Franco-Cereceda A, Terenius L (1985): Tissue-specific depletion of NPY-like immunoreactivity by reserpine. *Acta Physiol Scand* 123: 363—365.

56. Stjernquist M, Owman Ch (1987): Interaction of noradrenaline, NPY and VIP with the neurogenic cholinergic response of the rat uterine cervix in vitro. *Acta Physiol Scand* 131: 553—562.

57. Lightman SL, Iversen LL (1969): The role of uptake$_2$ in the extraneuronal metabolism of catecholamines in the isolated rat heart. *Br J Pharmacol* 37: 638—649.

58. Ross SB, Renyi AL (1969): Inhibition of the uptake of tritiated 5-hydroxytryptamine in brain tissue. *Eur J Pharmacol* 7: 270—277.

59. Ross SB, Renyi AL (1975): Tricylic antidepressant agents. I. Comparison of the inhibition of the uptake of ^{3}H-noradrenaline and ^{14}C-5-hydroxytryptamine into crude synaptosome preparations of the midbrain-hypothalamus region of the rat brain. *Acta Pharmacol Toxicol* 36: 382—394.

60. Gershon MD, Altman KF, (1971): Analysis of the uptake of 5-hydroxytryptamine by the myenteric plexus of small intestine of the guinea-pig. *J Pharmacol Exp Ther* 179: 29—41.

61. Alm P, Owman Ch, Sjöberg N-O, Thorbert G (1979): Uptake and metabolism of ^{3}H-norepinephrine in uterine nerves of pregnant guinea-pig. *Am J Physiol* 236: C277—C285.

62. Koevary SB, Azmitia EC, McEvoy RC (1983): Rat pancreatic serotonergic nerves: Morphologic, pharmacological and physiological studies. *Brain Res* 265: 328—332.

63. Fuxe K, Ungerstedt U (1968): Histochemical studies on the distribution of catecholamines and 5-hydroxytryptamine after intraventricular injection. *Histochemie* 13: 16—28.

64. Iversen LL (1970): Neuronal uptake processes for amines and amino acids, pp. 109—132 in: Costa E, Giacobini E (eds), *Advances in Biochemical Psychopharmacology*. Vol. 2. New York: Raven Press.

65. Magnussen I, Tønner K, Engbaek F (1982): Paroxetine, a potent selective long-acting inhibitor of synaptosomal 5-HT uptake in mice. *J Neural Transm* 55: 217—226.

65a. Engbaek F and Voldby B (1982): Radioimmunoassay of serotonin (5-hydroxytryptamine) in cerebrospinal fluid, plasma and serum. *Clin Chem* 28: 624—628.

66. Crawford N (1965): Systemic venous platelet-bound and plasma free serotonin levels in non-carcinoid malingancy. *Clin Chem Acta* 12: 274—281.

67. Genefke IK, Garel A, Mandel P (1968): Factors influencing free serotonin in human plasma. *Clin Chem Acta* 20: 61—67.

68. Hardebo JE, Owman Ch (1980): Barrier mechanisms for neurotransmitter monoamines and their precursor at the blood-brain interface. *Ann Neurol* 8: 1—11.
69. Maruki C, Spatz M, Ueki Y, Nagatsu I, Bembry J (1984): Cerebrovascular endothelial cell culture: Metabolism and synthesis of 5-hydroxytryptamine. *J Neurochem* 43: 316—319.
70. Edvinsson L, Cervós-Navarro J, Larsson L-I, Owman Ch, Rönnberg A-L (1977): Regional distribution of mast cells containing histamine, dopamine, or 5-hydroxytryptamine in mammalian brain. *Neurology* 27: 878—883.
71. Dimitriadou V, Aubineau P, Taxi J, Seylaz J (1987): Ultrastructural evidence for a functional unit between nerve fibers and type II cerebral mast cells in the cerebral vascular wall. *Neuroscience* 22: 621—630.
72. Green JP, (1966): Synthesis, uptake and binding of histamine and 5-hydroxytrytamine in mast cells, pp. 125—145 in: Euler US von, Rosell S, Uvnäs B (eds), *Mechanisms of Release of Biogenic Amines*. Oxford: Pergamon Press.
73. Chang J-Y, Owman Ch (1989): Cerebrovascular serotonergic receptors mediating vasoconstriction: Further evidence for the existence of $5-HT_2$ receptors in rat and $5-HT_1$-like receptors in guinea-pig basilar arteries. *Acta Physiol Scand* 136: 59—67.
74. Leysen JE, Niemegeers CJE, Van Nueten JM, Laduron PM (1982): [3H] Ketanserin (R41 468) a selective [3H] ligand for serotonin$_2$ receptor binding sites. *Mol Pharmacol* 21: 301—314.
75. Feniuk W, Humphrey PPA, Perren MJ, Watts AD (1985): A comparison of 5-hydroxytryptamine receptors mediating contraction in rabbit aorta and dog saphenous veins: Evidence for different receptor types obtained by use of selective agonists and antagonists. *Br J Pharmacol* 86: 697—704.
76. Leysen JE, Awouters F, Kennis L, Laduron PM, Vandenberk J, Janssen PAJ (1981): Receptor binding profile of R41 468, a novel antagonist at $5-HT_2$ receptors. *Life Sci* 28: 1015—1022.
77. Hoyer D (1985): Characterization of multiple serotonin (5-HT) recognition sites in rat and pig brain membranes by radioligand binding. *Naunyn-Schmiedeberg's Arch Pharmacol* 329: R82.
78. Engel G, Göthert M, Hoyer D, Schlicker E, Hillenbrand K (1986): Identity of inhibitory presynaptic 5-hydroxytryptamine (5-HT) autoreceptors in the rat brain cortex with $5-HT_{1B}$ binding sites. *Naunyn-Schmiedeberg's Arch Pharmacol* 332: 1—7.
79. Peroutka SJ, Snyder SH, (1979): Multiple serotonin receptors: Differential binding of [3H]-5-hydroxytryptamine, [3H]-lysergic acid diethylamide and [3H]-spiroperidol. *Mol Pharmacol* 16: 687—699.
80. Taylor EW, Duckles SP, Nelson DL (1986): Dissociation constants of serotonin agonists in the canine basilar artery correlate to K_i values at the $5-HT_{1A}$ binding site. *J Pharmacol Exp Ther* 236: 118—125.
81. Peroutka SJ, Noguchi M, Tolner DJ, Allen GS (1983): Serotonin-induced contraction of canine basilar artery: Mediation by $5-HT_1$ receptors. *Brain Res* 259: 327—330.
82. Middlemiss DN, Blakeborough L, Leather SR (1977): Direct evidence for an interaction of β-adrenergic blockers with the 5-HT receptor. *Nature* 267: 289—290.
83. Middlemiss DN, (1984): Stereospecific blockade at [3H] 5-HT binding sites and at 5-HT autoreceptor by propranolol. *Eur J Pharmacol* 101: 289—293.
84. Pazos A, Hoyer D, Palacios JM (1985): The binding of serotonergic ligands to the porcine choroid plexus: Characterization of a new type of serotonin receptor site. *Eur J Pharmacol* 106: 539—546.
85. Apperley E, Humphrey PPA (1986): The interaction of 5-hydroxytryptamine and methysergide with methiothepin at "$5-HT_1$-like" receptors in dog saphenous vein. *Br J Pharmacol* 87: 131P.
86. Cohen RA (1986): Contractions of isolated canine coronary arteries resistant to S_2-serotonergic blockade. *J Pharmacol Exp Ther* 237: 548—552.

87. Bradley PB, Engel G, Feniuk W, Fozard JR, Humphrey PPA, Middlemiss DN, Mylecharane EJ, Richardson BP, Saxena PR (1986): Proposals for the classification and nomenclature of functional receptors for 5-hydroxytryptamine. *Neuropharmacology* 25: 563—576.

88. Chang J-Y, Owman Ch (1989): Serotonin potentiates noradrenaline-induced vasoconstriction through 5-HT$_1$ type receptors in guinea-pig basilar artery. *J Cereb. Blood Flow Metab* 9: 713—716.

89. Apperley E, Feniuk W, Humphrey PPA, Levy GP (1980): Evidence for two types of ^{3}H-5-hydroxytryptamine uptake within rat cerebrovascular tree. *Eur J Pharmacol* 112: 181—186.

90. Peroutka SJ (1984): 5-HT receptor sites and functional correlates. *Neuropharmacology* 23: 1489—1492.

91. Saxena PR (1972): The effects of antimigraine drugs on the vascular response by 5-hydroxytryptamine and related biogenic substances on the external carotid bed of dog: Possible pharmacological implications to their antimigraine action. *Headache* 12: 44—54.

92. Carroll PR, Ebeling PW, Glover WE (1974): The responses of the human temporal and rabbit ear artery to 5-hydroxytryptamine and some of its antagonists. *Aust J Exp Biol Med Sci* 52: 813—823.

93. Tsuji T, Chiba S (1984): Potentiating effect of methysergide on norepinephrine-induced constriction of isolated internal carotid artery of the dog. *Japan J Pharmacol* 34: 95—100.

Blood Pressure Regulation
and Hypertension

XVII. Cardiovascular reflexes and 5-hydroxytryptamine

DANIEL S. McQUEEN

1. Introduction

The effects of 5-hydroxytryptamine (5-HT) on the cardiovascular system are complex and very variable [1], which is not surprising given that the amine can act directly on specific 5-HT receptors in the heart and blood vessels, inhibit transmitter release from adrenergic nerves, amplify the activity of mediators on vascular smooth muscle, displace noradrenaline from adrenergic nerve terminals, release endothelium-dependent relaxant factor(s), facilitate platelet aggregation, and, in addition, can also activate sensory receptors in the cardiopulmonary system and carotid bifurcation, thereby reflexly affecting the cardiovascular system [2, 3, 4]. This chapter focuses on certain sensors that are activated by 5-HT to cause reflex cardiovascular changes, and reviews what is known about the type(s) of 5-HT receptor involved in evoking these reflexes.

2. Species variability

Inter-species differences in cardiovascular responses to exogenous 5-HT are commonly reported. For example, Page [5] found that 5-HT was depressor in anaesthetised cats, but primarily pressor, though occasionally with an initial transient depressor component, in dogs. In anaesthetized rats a triphasic effect on systemic arterial blood pressure (B.P.) was obtained [6], with an initial transient fall followed by a small pressor response which was succeeded by a more marked and prolonged hypotension (see Figure 1). After ganglion blockade or pithing, 5-HT elicited only large pressor responses. Page and McCubbin [1] commented that pressor responses could be obtained with 5-HT when basal arterial pressure is low, whereas vasodepression occurred when pressure was high, and they coined the term 'amphibaric' to describe the variable effects of 5-HT on B.P.

Species differences were also evoked to explain why 5-HT stimulated

P.R. Saxena, D.I. Wallis, W. Wouters and P. Bevan (eds), Cardiovascular Pharmacology of
5-Hydroxytryptamine, pp. 233–245.
© 1990 Kluwer Academic Publishers, Dordrecht —

carotid body chemoreceptors in dogs but not in cats [7]. However, 5-HT has subsequently been shown to excite chemoreceptors in cats, and it is worth considering briefly whether there are fundamental species differences in responsiveness to 5-HT. The overall effect of 5-HT on the cardiovascular system is the net result of actions (some facilatory, some inhibitory) at different sites. Tachyphylaxis can develop to pressor responses when intervals between doses are short (< 5–10 min), and vascular responsiveness can change during the course of an experiment. In addition, biological variability, differences in operator technique, dose, route, and speed of administering 5-HT (fast injection gives different responses in comparison with slow infusion of the same dose), variable influence of anaesthetic agents, and respiratory changes which reflexly affect the cardiovascular responses [8] can all contribute to variations in responses within and between species. Thus, although fundamental species differences may exist, in the intact animal interspecies variability to 5-HT may be more a consequence of physiological differences in systems under given experimental conditions (e.g. sympathetic tone higher in anaesthetized cats in comparison with dogs [1]), with the same fundamental actions of 5-HT on individual elements making a different contribution to the overall response.

3. Sensory receptors

Sensory receptors play an important role in cardiovascular regulation [8–14], and it is known that certain cardiopulmonary and carotid sensory receptors can be activated by exogenous 5-HT to cause cardiovascular reflexes [6, 12, 15, 16]; the sensory receptors shown schematically in Figure 1 will be considered individually in the following sections. The physiological significance of these reflexes is still a matter for debate [13, 14], but the introduction of selective antagonists [17, 18] has enabled advances to be made in characterising the type(s) of 5-HT receptor [19] involved in the reflexes, and should help to clarify the physiological or pathophysiological role of 5-HT and its receptors at these sensory sites.

3.1 Carotid body arterial chemoreceptors

Most attention will be given to reviewing the actions of 5-HT on carotid sensory receptors because more evidence is available for these sensors than there is for cardiopulmonary receptors, reflecting the fact that the former are more accessible and relatively easier to study. In addition, 5-HT is found in the carotid body glomus cells apposed to the sensory nerve terminals, which is suggestive of a physiological role for 5-HT at this site. Two types of sensory receptor are present in the carotid bifurcation, arterial chemoreceptors in the carotid body, and arterial baroreceptors in the carotid artery [9].

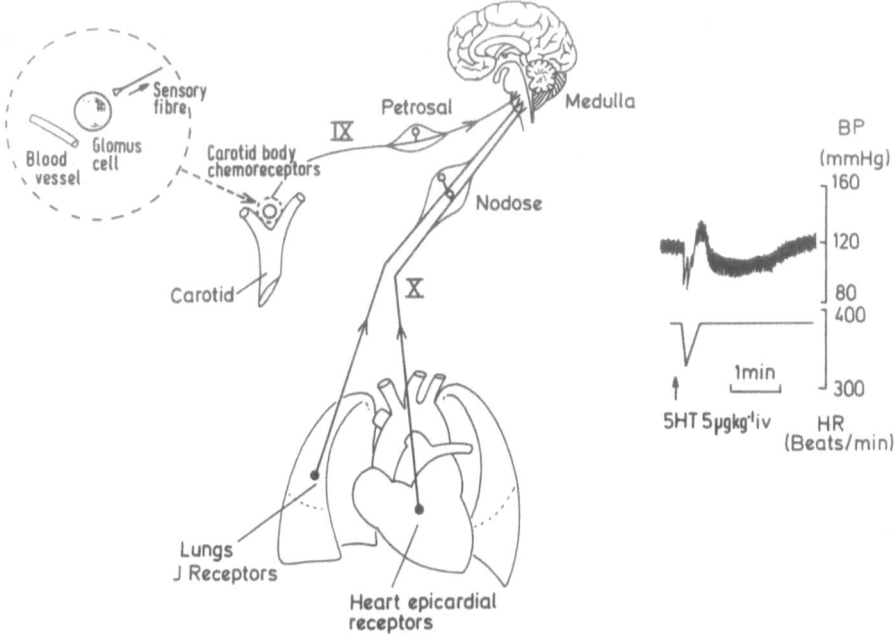

Figure 1. Schematic for the sensory receptors activated by 5-HT to evoke cardiovascular reflexes. *Carotid chemoreceptors*: A and C fibres run in IX cranial nerve, with cell bodies in the petrosal ganglion. 5-HT causes bradycardia (contribution to early depressor/bradycardia phase of the triphasic effect of injected 5-HT seen in many species — illustrated by the inset from an anaesthetized rat) by reflex increase in vagal activity; also sympathetic vasoconstriction which contributes to the secondary pressor phase — hyperventilation also occurs. *Epicardial and ventricular* cardiac receptors and pulmonary *J* receptors: mainly in C fibre afferents of the vagus (X) nerve with cell bodies in nodose ganglion. 5-HT causes reflex bradycardia and hypotension — also hypoventilation. Increased efferent vagal activity and decreased sympathetic tone are responsible for most of the initial depressor/bradycardia phase.

Although 5-HT has been shown to stimulate some barosensory afferents [20], this action has not been studied in detail and may be secondary to contraction of smooth muscle in the arterial walls rather than a direct action on the sensory receptors [9, 10]. In contrast, there have been a number of studies relating to the actions of 5-HT on chemoreceptors, particularly those in the carotid body. The chemoreceptors of the aortic bodies are qualitatively similar to those of the carotid body in responsiveness to 5-HT [12] but they evoke much weaker reflexes and appear to be non-functional in some species (e.g. rat [21, 22]). Since most of the literature is concerned with carotid chemoreceptors, these will be given detailed consideration.

3.1.1 *Presence of 5-HT in the carotid body*
Relatively large quantities of 5-HT have been found in the carotid bodies of various species, including man, using techniques such as fluorimetry [23],

H.P.L.C. [24] and immunohistochemistry [25, 26]; 5-HT is located in dense-cored vesicles of some glomus or type 1 cells which are "pre-synaptic" to the sensory terminals (see Figure 1). Recent work by Perrin et al. [26] shows that 5-HT is the main amine in the carotid bodies of infants, which may indicate a greater importance in neonatal than in adult life.

Preliminary results from low-resolution autoradiographic studies with [^{3}H]-5-HT indicate that binding is present in slices of carotid body incubated with the radioligand, and that it is denser if the carotid nerve is cut chronically (see Figure 2). If binding sites can be equated with pharmaco-logical receptors (a moot point), then the fact that the sensory fibres will have degenerated on the sectioned side means the receptors are associated with non-neural elements, probably glomus cells; they may, of course, also be on the afferent nerves too, by analogy with vagal afferents (see below). The denser binding may mean that denervation leads to up-regulation of receptors. Further studies involving high-resolution analysis and use of

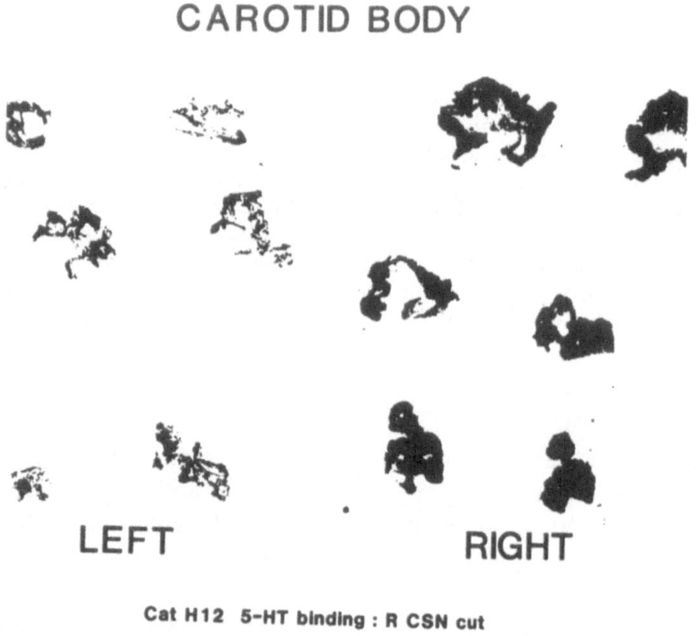

CAROTID BODY

LEFT   RIGHT

Cat H12 5-HT binding : R CSN cut

Figure 2. Autoradiograms from sections of cat carotid body incubated with [^{3}H] 5-HT demonstrating the presence of 5-HT binding sites (presumed receptors). The right carotid nerve was cut 8 days before fixation and sections from the chronically denervated right carotid body show denser binding of the ligand than obtained on the intact left side — which received the same exposure. Thus, 5-HT receptors are apparently up-regulated following chronic denervation, and must be located on non-sensory nerve structures within the carotid body (type I cells (glomus), type II cells; blood vessels) which survive the sectioning (Dashwood, McQueen & Molony, unpublished data).

radioligands selective for different types of 5-HT receptor should help to establish which elements in the carotid body are associated with specific 5-HT receptors.

3.1.2 *5-HT-induced chemoreceptor reflexes*
Cardiovascular and respiratory reflexes can be evoked by 5-HT acting on chemoreceptors in the carotid body in most species and generally consist of bradycardia, hypotension followed by hypertension, and hyperventilation [8, 9, 16, 28]; they are observed when the sympathetic ganglioglomerular nerves to the carotid body are cut, showing that chemoexcitation is not secondary to ganglion stimulation [16]. The changes in heart rate, cardiac output and peripheral vascular resistance are variable and difficult to predict because much depends on the strength of the concomitant hyperventilation, which can override the primary chemoreflex [8]. Data are, rather unusually, also available from studies in man [29]: a rapid intracarotid injection of 5-HT, but not a slower infusion, stimulated the chemoreceptors and caused reflex hyperventilation; surgical removal of the carotid body abolished the hyperventilation.

Black et al [7] found species differences in responsiveness of carotid chemoreceptors to 5-HT and concluded that dog but not cat chemoreceptors are stimulated by the amine. They commented on the apnoea that could be evoked by stimulation of the nodose ganglion, presumably affecting vagal afferents from the lungs (see also 29), which can mask chemoreceptor-induced reflex hyperpnoea. Because of difficulties in interpreting reflex effects, more direct evidence concerning actions of 5-HT at the sensory receptors was needed and is provided by neural recordings. Direct recording of chemoreceptor neural discharge from single or few-functional fibres in the carotid nerve makes it possible to show more clearly the effects of 5-HT on the chemosensors, and this has been the basis of most recent studies.

3.1.3 *Neural recordings of chemosensory discharge — effects of 5-HT*
5-HT usually has a bi- or tri-phasic effect on chemosensory discharge [20, 30, 31] with an initial transient excitation (seen in about half the experiments) followed by a period of depression which is succeeded by a more prolonged increase in frequency (see Figure 3; also [27] for a review). These effects can be obtained in most species, but the initial transient chemoexcitation is very prone to tachyphylaxis. The dose of 5-HT and the rate at which it is injected appears to determine the relative contribution of excitation/ depression, and low doses are usually depressant [30]. The same general pattern is observed with the in vitro carotid body preparation where there are no vascular actions to complicate interpretation [32].

3.1.4 *Characterisation of 5-HT receptors in the carotid body*
The neural response to 5-HT in anaesthetized cats in unaffected by atropine, methysergide or gramine [20] but the excitatory component can be blocked

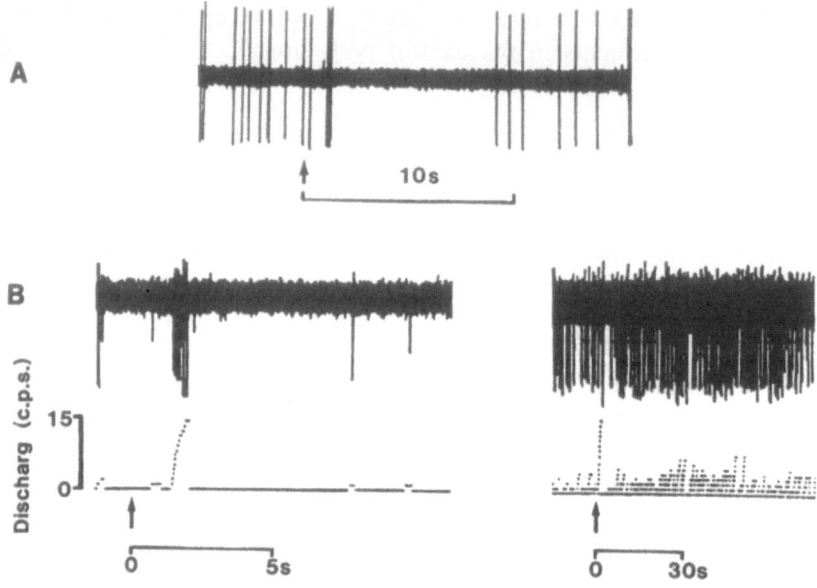

‘ure 3. Neural recordings illustrating responsiveness of cat carotid chemoreceptors to a close-arterial injection of 25 nmoles 5-HT at arrow.

A. Single chemoreceptor fibre showing a brief burst of activity followed by a period of relative depression. The ganglioglomerular (sympathetic) nerves were cut in this experiment, precluding any ganglion-stimulant action of 5-HT from altering blood flow and thereby indirectly increasing discharge. The excitation is also too fast (occurring within the 2s injection period) to allow a vascular explanation. *B.* Multiunit recording in a separate experiment with intact ganglioglomerular nerves. The ramp is the output from a window discriminator, reset every 1s. Left side shows transient excitation, followed by depression in response to 5-HT; right panel is the same test at slower sweep speed demonstrating the delayed chemoexcitation which is generally more prominent when the sympathetics are intact, and may be secondary to vasoconstriction. Anaesthetized animals artificially ventilated with air and paralysed by gallamine. *A* modified from [27], *B* modified from [31].

by α-flupenthixol — higher doses also blocked the chemodepression [27]. In dogs the excitatory effect of 5-HT is reduced by D-tubocurarine and the inhibitory response blockade by dihydroergotamine [30] — however D-tubocurarine also antagonised excitatory responses to noradrenaline and dopamine, which might reflect non-specific channel-block; dihydroergotamine is not a very specific agent. There are a few other reports relating to the effects of antagonists, but they do not merit detailed consideration because it is only recently that consistent data have been obtained following the advent of new and selective antagonists.

Initial experiments with the 5-HT_3 receptor antagonist MDL 72222 clearly demonstrated that the initial rapid but transient chemoexcitation obtained following intracarotid injection of 5-HT in 56% of cat chemoreceptor recordings (see Figure 3) was virtually abolished by the antagonist, suggesting that 5-HT_3 receptors were involved in the response [31]. The chemodepression observed in all recordings, even those in which there was no transient excitation, was also greatly reduced by MDL 72222, whereas the delayed somewhat variable chemoexcitation was unaffected. Ketanserin, a 5-HT_2 antagonist, had no significant effect on the excitation or depression, but reduced the delayed increase in discharge (Figure 3), which may be secondary to local vasoconstriction within the carotid body. These findings were confirmed using a different 5-HT_3 antagonist, namely ICS 205—930 (see Figure 4), which also blocked the initial chemoexcitation, as well as the depression evoked by 5-HT in cats, and similar results have been obtained with this antagonist in rats [33].

The use of agonists for characterising pharmacological receptors is less satisfactory, but 2-methyl 5-HT, an agonist which is 'selective' for 5-HT_3 receptors, caused chemodepression equal to or greater than that caused by 5-HT, although it was less active in causing chemoexcitation. These actions were antagonised by MDL 72222 [34], as were those of phenylbiguanide, which has been used as a probe for identifying cardiopulmonary sensory receptors [2, 12]; the fact that its actions on the chemoreceptors are antagonised by MDL 72222 [35] and ICS 205—930 (Figure 4) strongly suggests phenylbiguanide is a 5-HT_3 agonist (see evidence below from

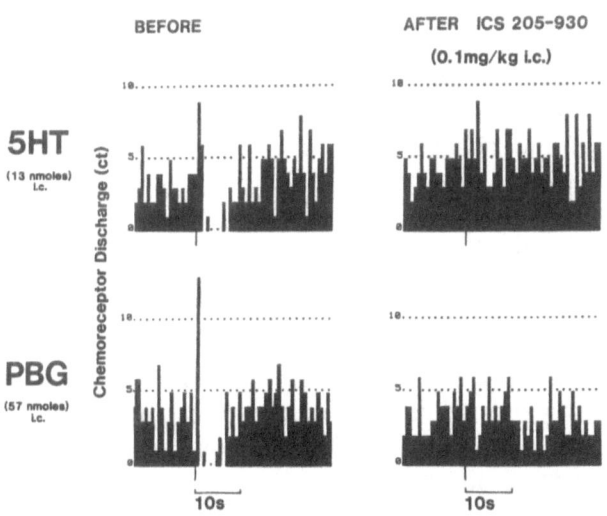

Figure 4. Counts of chemoreceptor discharge (2 units) illustrating the transient chemoexcitation and subsequent depression evoked by intra-carotid (i.c.) injection of 5-HT or phenylbiguanide (PBG) — at marks — in an anaesthetised cat with intact ganglioglomerular (sympathetic) nerves. After a single injection of ICS 205—930 (which had no significant effect on basal discharge) the excitation and the depression caused by both drugs were greatly reduced, and this provides evidence that their actions involved 5-HT_3 receptors within the carotid body. The anaesthetized animal was artificially ventilated with air and paralysed by gallamine (McQueen & Mir, unpublished data related to [24]).

cardiopulmonary receptors which supports this hypothesis). The finding that a combination of 5-HT$_2$ and 5-HT$_3$ receptor antagonists can substantially reduce the responsiveness of the cat carotid chemoreceptors to locally injected 5-HT [31] would appear to eliminate the possibility of actions at 5-HT$_1$ receptors. However, a few preliminary experiments involving 8-OH-DPAT and RU24969, agonists at 5-HT$_{1A}$ and 5-HT$_{1B}$-like receptors respectively, have provided surprising results by showing that 8-OH-DPAT causes chemodepression, which is unaffected by MDL 72222, whereas RU24969 causes delayed chemoexcitation [34]. More detailed studies are needed to confirm these preliminary observations and to determine whether there are 5-HT$_1$ receptors in the carotid body which can influence discharge.

3.1.5 Physiological significance of 5-HT receptors in the carotid body

Results with MDL 72222 [31] showed that this 5-HT$_3$ antagonist had no significant effect on responsiveness of the cat chemoreceptors under either normoxic condition or in response to physiological stimulation by hypoxia, although responses to exogenous 5-HT were greatly reduced. However, recent experiments with ICS 205–930 (10 μg kg^{-1}) injected during steady-state hypoxia reveal a dose-related depression ($\sim$ 30%) in discharge (unpublished) which could mean that endogenous 5-HT contributes to chemoexcitation. The fact that ICS 205–930 causes antagonism, whereas MDL 72222 does not, may be due to differences in antagonist potency or specificity, but might also be due to actions of ICS 205–930 at additional sub-types of 5-HT$_3$ receptor, e.g. 5-HT$_{3C}$ [18]. However, it could also be the consequence of a non-specific channel-blocking action with high doses of ICS 205–930 [36], although responses to the chemoexcitant acetylcholine [27] were unaffected by the dose of antagonist used (unpublished). Again, further studies are needed to clarify this aspect.

Considerable advances have recently been made in characterising the 5-HT receptors of the carotid body. Use of selective antagonists should facilitate studies on the role(s) of 5-HT in the carotid body under normal and pathophysiological conditions and show the extent to which 5-HT may be involved in evoking or modulating cardiovascular and other reflex activity from this sensory organ. Further information should come from biophysical and biochemical studies to determine what ion channels (e.g. Na$^+$, K$^+$) and messenger systems are involved.

3.2 Cardiopulmonary receptors

Stimulation of certain sensory receptors in the heart and lungs with small diameter vagal afferent fibres generally causes reflex bradycardia, hypotension, tachypnoea and nausea. These effects are brought about by increased efferent vagal activity and a concomitant reduction in sympathetic tone. Most of the receptors are technically difficult to isolate for pharmacological and physiological studies, and consequently interpretation of the effects of substances such as 5-HT is problematic because more than one sensory receptor is usually involved [14]. Probably the best known reflex (bradycardia, hypotension and apnoea) is the Bezold (or Bezold-Jarisch) reflex caused by veratridine or veratrum alkaloids acting mainly on the heart; this reflex actually involves actions of the alkaloids at a variety of cardiac receptors, including left and right ventricular pressure receptors, left atrial type A and type B receptors, right atrial type A, and epicardial receptors [3]; the overall effect is the algebraic summation of these actions. Injected 5-HT appears to act mainly on the epicardial/ventricular receptors of the heart which have C fibres afferents [14], as does phenylbiguanide [3]. Reflex bradycardia, hypotension and apnoea are evoked (but not the latter in dogs or man [3]), which is best described as a Bezold-like reflex, to distinguish it from the true (more potent) Bezold reflex elicited by the action of veratrum alkaloids on a wider range of cardiac sensors. In contrast to the carotid chemoreceptors, little is known about the structure of epicardial receptors which are present on the surface and in the walls of the left and right ventricles; they are stimulated, physiologically or pathophysiologically, by increased atrial or ventricular pressure. There is evidence that ventricular sensors are tonically active and may modulate vasomotor tone, particularly that to the kidney [14]. Glutamatergic synapses located within the brain stem appear to be involved in the vagal reflex pathway [3].

3.2.1 *Characterisation of 5-HT receptors associated with epicardial and ventricular sensory receptors*

5-HT and phenylbiguanide can cause depolarisation in rat isolated vagus nerve preparations which is antagonised by metoclopramide [38], and both agonists cause abrupt bradycardia and hypotension when injected i.v., i.e. a Bezold-like reflex. This effect is also blocked by metoclopramide [39], suggesting involvement of a common 5-HT receptor sub-type which may be expressed along the course of the nerve fibres as well as at the terminals and cell bodies, assuming the actions in vivo are on the same fibres as those recorded in vitro. Fozard [40] found that the 5-HT_3 antagonist MDL 72222 antagonised a Bezold-like reflex evoked by 5-HT in anaesthetized rats; doses of ICS 205—930 as low as 1 μg kg^{-1} had similar effects and also antagonised the 5-HT-induced reduction of the C fibre action potential in desheathed rat vagus nerve [41]. Recent results with MDL 72222 and ICS 205—930 on 5-HT-induced depolarisation of the rat vagus [42] support involvement of a 5-HT_3 type of receptor associated with vagally-innervated epicardial receptors, but direct electrical recording is needed to verify this in vivo and to established the role of these receptors, and of 5-HT, in cardiovascular regulation under normal and pathophysiological (e.g. heart failure) conditions.

3.3 Pulmonary J (deflation) receptors

Various pulmonary receptors exist which have profound reflex effects on respiration when activated, and some also cause cardiovascular changes [11—16]. 5-HT and phenylbiguanide have been shown, by direct electrical recording from vagal afferents, to activate type J (juxta-pulmonary capillary) receptors situated in the interstitium of alveolar walls close to pulmonary capillaries [2, 3, 12]. A certain amount of information is available concerning their morphology and it appears that increased pulmonary capillary pressure, such as occurs during exercise (particularly at high altitude), sudden left heart failure, anaphylaxis, or pulmonary embolism leads to oedema which activates the free nerve endings of these receptors by distension [3, 12]. Volatile anaesthetics also activate them [12]. In animals bradycardia and hypotension result, accompanied by rapid shallow breathing. Breathlessness and muscle weakness is reported in man — victims of the Bhopal gas tragedy died of pulmonary oedema and survivors complained of severe muscle weakness in addition to dry cough and breathlessness, symptoms which can be attributed to J receptor activation [43]. The extent, if any, to which endogenous 5-HT is involved in activating J receptor remains to be established.

3.3.1 Characterization of 5-HT receptors associated with J receptors
In anaesthetized rabbits 5-HT or phenylbiguanide injected into the right atrium cause bradycardia, hypotension and rapid shallow breathing which is the typical pattern evoked by stimulating J receptors; the responses are antagonised by MDL 72222, and it was concluded that MDL 72222-sensitive reflexes evoked by 5-HT and phenylbiguanide emanate from pulmonary vagal afferents [44]. The rapid shallow breathing caused by pulmonary embolism in anaesthetized rabbits was also antagonised by MDL 72222 [45]. These results with MDL 72222 and phenylbiguanide plus earlier evidence with 5-HT and PBG [2], strongly suggests that $5-HT_3$ receptors are associated with these sensory receptors, but further experiments are needed to provide direct neuropharmacological evidence that this is the case.

In rats [D Met^{2}DPro^5] enkephalinamide (an enkephalin analog) evokes the typical J receptor reflex and it was demonstrated by recording from vagal afferents that J receptors were activated; naloxone antagonised the opioid induced reflex without affecting responses to phenylbiguanide [46]. This raises the question of whether 5-HT and opioids share a common mechanism for activating J receptors, and whether opioids might act via 5-HT (methysergide had no effect, but would a selective $5-HT_3$ antagonist block the opioid's action?).

4. Conclusion

A start has been made in characterising 5-HT receptors involved in evoking cardiovascular reflexes via the sensors reviewed, and further studies with selective agonists and antagonists are required. Basic questions remain to be answered: does 5-HT act directly as a transmitter or modulator on its own, or are co-transmitters (? peptides) involved; is long-term 5-HT (over minutes or hours) action more important than transient effects studied in most experiments; are there subtypes of 5-HT$_3$ receptor at sensory sites; is the role of 5-HT greater in neonates than adults; do 5-HT and its associated receptors function mainly under pathophysiological conditions; what biophysical and biochemical changes occur at the sensors in response to 5-HT; how does local release/presence of 5-HT in tissues correlate with alterations in sensory nerve discharge; could tachyphylaxis to 5-HT (seen with transient chemoexcitation in particular) be the consequence of opioid release and of physiological significance [e.g. 47]? Use of selective drugs (e.g. agonists, antagonists, uptake blockers, depletors) should advance knowledge concerning the role of 5-HT at sensory receptors involved in cardiovascular regulation and could be important in helping to understand and treat various disorders.

References

1. Page IH, McCubbin JW (1953): The variable arterial pressure response to serotonin in laboratory animals and man. *Circ Res* 1: 354—362.
2. Paintal AS (1955): Impulses in vagal afferent fibres from specific pulmonary deflation receptors. The response of these receptors to phenyl diguanide, potato starch, 5-hydroxytryptamine and nicotine, and their role in respiratory and cardiovascular reflexes. *Q J Exp Physiol* 40: 89—111.
3. Paintal AS (1973): Sensory mechanisms involved in the Bezold-Jarisch reflex. *Australian J Exp Biol &Med Sci* 51: 3—15.
4. Hollenberg NK (1988): Serotonin and vascular responses. *Ann Rev Pharmacol Toxicol* 28: 41—59.
5. Page IH (1952): The vascular action of natural serotonin, 5- and 7-hydroxytryptamine and tryptamine. *J Pharmacol Exp Ther* 105: 58—73.
6. Salmoiraghi GC, Page IH, McCubbin JW (1956): Cardiovascular and respiratory response to intravenous serotonin in rats. *J Pharmacol Exp Ther* 118: 477—481.
7. Black AMS, Comroe JH Jr, Jacobs L (1972): Species difference in carotid body response of cat and dog to dopamine and serotonin. *Am J Physiol* 223: 1097—1102.
8. Daly M de B (1985): Chemoreceptor reflexes and cardiovascular control. *Acta Physiol Pol* 36: 4—20.
9. Heymans C, Neil E (1958): 'Reflexogenic areas of the cardiovascular system', pp. 271. London, Churchill.
10. Ginzel KH (1975): The importance of sensory nerve endings as sites of drug action. *NS Arch Pharmacol* 288: 29—56.
11. Mancia G, Lorenz RR, Shepherd JT (1976): Reflex control of circulation by heart and lungs. *Inter Rev Physiol Cardiovascular Physiol II* 9: 111—144.

244   *D. S. McQueen*

12. Paintal AS (1977): Effects of drugs on chemoreceptors, pulmonary and cardiovascular receptors. *Pharmac Ther Bull* 3: 41—63.
13. Donald DE, Shepherd JT (1978): Reflexes from the heart and lungs: physiological curiosities or important regulatory mechanisms. *Cardiovasc Res* 12: 446—469.
14. Thoren P (1979): Role of cardiac vagal C-fibres in cardiovascular control. *Rev Physiol Biochem Pharmacol* 86: 1—94.
15. Dawes GS, Mott JC, Widdicombe JG (1951): Respiratory and cardiovascular reflexes from the heart and lungs. *J Physiol* 115: 258—291.
16. Ginzel KH (1958): The effects of 5-hydroxytryptamine on peripheral receptors of cardiovascular and respiratory reflexes, pp. 131—135 in: Lewis GP (ed.), *5-Hydroxytryptamine*. London: Pergamon.
17. Richardson BP, Engel G, Donatsch P, Stadler PA (1985): Identification of serotonin M-receptor subtypes and their specific blockade by a new class of drugs. *Nature* 316: 126—131.
18. Richardson BP, Engel G (1986): The pharmacology and function of 5-HT$_3$ receptors. *Trends in Neurosci* 9: 424—428.
19. Bradley PB, Engel G, Feniuk W, Fozard JR, Humphrey PPA, Middlemiss DN, Mylencharane EJ, Richardson BP, Saxena PR (1986): Proposals for the classification and nomenclature of functional receptors for 5-hydroxytryptamine. *Neuropharmacol* 25: 563—576.
20. Nishi K (1975): The action of 5-hydroxytryptamine on chemoreceptor discharges of the cat's carotid body. *Br J Pharmacol* 55: 27—40.
21. Sapru HN, Krieger AJ (1977): Effect of 5-hydroxytryptamine on the peripheral chemoreceptors in the rat. *Res Comm Chem Path Pharmacol* 16: 245—250.
22. Sapru HN, Krieger AJ (1977): Carotid and aortic chemoreceptor function in the rat. *J Appl Physiol* 42: 344—348.
23. Chiocchio SR, Biscardi AM, Tramezzani JH (1967): 5-Hydroxytryptamine in the carotid body of the cat. *Science* 158: 790—791.
24. McQueen DS, Mir AK (1984): Changes in carotid body amine levels and effects of dopamine on rats treated neonatally with capsaicin. *Br J Pharmacol* 83: 909—918.
25. Gronblad M, Liesi P, Rechardt L (1983): Serotonin-like immunoreactivity in rat carotid body. *Brain Res* 276: 348—350.
26. Perrin DG, Chan W, Cutz E, Madapallimattam A, Sole MJ (1986): Serotonin in human infant carotid body. *Experientia* 42: 562—564.
27. McQueen DS (1983): Pharmacological aspects of putative transmitters in the carotid body, pp. 149—196 in: Acker H, O'Regan RG (ed.), *Physiology of the peripheral arterial chemoreceptors*. Amsterdam: Elsevier.
28. McQueen DS, Ungar A (1971): On the direct and crossed components of reflex responses to stimulation of the carotid body chemoreceptors in the dog. *J Physiol* 219: 1—16.
29. Skinner SL, Whelan RF (1962): Carotid body stimulation by 5-hydroxytryptamine in man. *J Physiol* 162: 35—43.
30. Bisgard GE, Mitchell RA, Herbert DA (1979): Effects of dopamine, norepinephrine and 5-hydroxytryptamine on the carotid body of the dog. *Resp Physiol* 37: 61—80.
31. Kirby GC, McQueen DS (1984): Effects of the antagonists MDL 72222 and ketanserin on responses of cat carotid body chemoreceptors to 5-hydroxytryptamine. *Br J Pharmacol* 83: 259—269.
32. Eyzaguirre C, Koyano H (1965): The effects of some pharmacological agents on chemoreceptor discharges. *J Physiol* 178: 410—437.
33. Yoshioka M, Matsumoto M, Togashi H, Abe M, Tochihara M, Saito H (1987): The 5-hydroxytryptamine-induced increase in chemoreceptor afferent nerve discharge and its blockade by ICS 205—930 in the rat. *Res Comm Psych Psych & Behaviour* 12: 215—220.

34. Kirby GC, McQueen DS (1985): Effects of selective 5-hydroxytryptamine agonists on carotid body chemoreceptor discharge in anaesthetized cats. *Br J Pharmac* 86: 733P.
35. McQueen DS, Mir AK (1988): Involvement of 5-HT$_3$ receptors in responses of cat carotid body chemoreceptors to phenylbiguanide. *J Physiol* 401: 86P.
36. Scholtysik G. (1987): Evidence for inhibition by ICS 205—930 and stimulation by BRL 34915 of K$^+$ conductance in cardiac muscle. *N-S. Arch. Pharmacol* 335: 692—696.
37. Verberne AJM, Costa M, Lewis SJ, Louis WJ, Beart PM (1987): The N-Methyl-D-aspartate (NMDA) receptor antagonist MK-801, attenuates the Bezold-Jarisch reflex in the anaesthetized rat. *Neuropharmacology* 26: 1243—6.
38. Fortune DH, Ireland SJ, Tyers MB (1983): Phenylbiguanide minics the effects of 5-hydroxytryptamine on the rat isolated vagus nerve and superior cervical ganglion. *Br J Pharmacol* 79: 298P.
39. Collins DP, Fortune DH (1983): Phenylbiguanide mimics the Bezold-Jarisch effect of 5-HT in the rat. *Br J Pharmac* 80: 570P.
40. Fozard JR (1984): MDL 72222: a potent and highly selective antagonist at neuronal 5-hydroxytryptamine receptors. *N-S Arch Pharmacol* 326: 36—44.
41. Richardson BP, Engel G, Dontasch P, Stadler PA (1985): Identification of serotonin M-receptor subtypes and their specific blockade by a new class of drugs. *Nature* 316: 126—131.
42. Ireland SJ, Tyers MB (1987): Pharmacological characterisation of 5-hydroxytryptamine-induced depolarization of the rat isolated vagus nerve. *Br J Pharmac* 90: 229—238.
43. Paintal AS (1986): The significance of dry cough, breathlessness and muscle weakness. *Ind J Tuberculosis* 33: 51—55.
44. Armstrong DJ, Kay IS, Russell NJW (1986): The pulmonary chemoreflexes evoked by phenylbiguanide, diguanide and guanide. *J Physiol* 371: 115P.
45. Armstrong DJ, Kay IS, Russell NJW (1986): MDL 72222 antagonizes the reflex tachypneoic response to miliary pulmonary embolism in anaesthetized rabbits. *J Physiol* 381: 13P.
46. Sapru HN, Willette RN, Krieger AJ (1981): Stimulation of pulmonary J receptors by an enkephalin analog. *J Pharm Exp Ther* 217: 228—234.
47. Sicuteri F (1983): Is acute tolerance to 5-hydroxytryptamine opioid dependent? Its absence in migraine sufferers. *Cephalagia* 3: 187—190.

XVIII. 5-Hydroxytryptamine in central cardiovascular regulation

A. K. MIR and J. R. FOZARD

1. Central 5-hydroxytryptamine (5-HT) and its effects on the cardiovascular system

The existence of discrete 5-HT-containing neurones in the brain stem with extensive ramifications to neuroanatomical regions involved in cardiovascular regulation has been known for more than two decades [1]. Our understanding, however, of the intricate interactions of the 5-HT networks and central autonomic pathways has been rather slow to evolve [2—4]. Thus, despite substantial evidence implicating an important role for central 5-HT neurotransmission in blood pressure regulation, the precise nature of this role remains unclear.

Centrally administered 5-HT and its precursors have notoriously complex effects on both efferent autonomic nerve activity and blood pressure and heart rate. Thus, increases, decreases or biphasic changes in the above parameters have been observed with the effects varying qualitatively and quantitatively with the doses used, sites of injection and species [5—10]. It is now clear that this complexity reflects in large part the presence of multiple 5-HT receptor subtypes in the CNS for which 5-HT, by definition, is non-selective. It seems logical to suppose that the inhibitory and excitatory effects of centrally administered 5-HT on the central sympathetic control of blood pressure will be mediated via activation of different subtypes of 5-HT receptor.

Since the original division of central 5-HT receptors into 5-HT_1 and 5-HT_2 types by Peroutka and Snyder [11], data have appeared suggesting that at least four subtypes of the 5-HT_1 recognition site exist; these have been designated 5-HT_{1A}, 5-HT_{1B}, 5-HT_{1C} and 5-HT_{1D} (see for example [12]). The 5-HT_2 receptor has survived largely as originally defined. However, several subtypes of a further, functionally defined category of 5-HT receptor (5-HT_3; [13]) are believed to exist [14]. The availability of selective agonists and antagonists for certain of these subtypes [12, 13] has greatly facilitated both

P.R. Saxena, D.I. Wallis, W. Wouters and P. Bevan (eds), Cardiovascular Pharmacology of 5-Hydroxytryptamine, pp. 247—258.
© 1990 *Kluwer Academic Publishers, Dordrecht* —

the investigation and understanding of the mechanisms by which central 5-HT may alter cardiovascular function.

For reasons that are obvious from the above this review will *not* be concerned with the central effects of 5-HT or its precursor molecules. Rather, we would like to consider the evidence obtained with selective agonists/antagonists for particular 5-HT receptor subtypes mediating the *inhibitory* and *excitatory* effects of central 5-HT on autonomic and particularly sympathetic nervous activity and cardiovascular function. With regard to $5-HT_3$ receptors, although there is now ample direct evidence for their existence in brain [15] and there are several highly potent and selective $5-HT_3$ receptor antagonists and agonists now available as tools [15], there is as yet no good evidence suggesting a role for this particular receptor site in central cardiovascular control. This review, therefore, will focus primarily on the role of '5-HT_1-like' (particularly $5-HT_{1A}$) and $5-HT_2$ receptor involvement in the inhibitory and excitatory effects of 5-HT in the brain.

2. Inhibitory effects of central 5-HT; role of $5-HT_{1A}$ receptors

With respect to the *inhibitory* effects of central 5-HT receptor activation there is growing evidence for a key role for $5-HT_{1A}$ receptors in cardiovascular control. A number of compounds is now recognised to have both high affinity and selectivity for the $5-HT_{1A}$ receptor including 8-hydroxy-2-(di-n-propylamino)tetralin (8-OH-DPAT), N,N-dipropyl-5-carboxamidotryptamine (DP-5-CT), flesinoxan (DU 29373), 8-[4-(1,4-benzodioxan-2-ylmethylamino)-butyl]-8-azaspiro[4,5]decane-7,9-dione (MDL 72832), 8-[2-[2,3-dihydro-1,4-benzodioxin-2-y1)methylamino]ethyl]-8-azaspiro[4,5]-decan-7,9-dione (MDL 73005), 8-methoxy-2-(N-2-chlorethyl-N-n-propyl)amino tetralin (8-MeO-CLEPAT) and ipsapirone (TVX Q 7821) [16—22]. The above compounds manifest their functional effects either as full or partial agonists and have been used to explore the role of $5-HT_{1A}$ receptors in cardiovascular control. In particular, 8-OH-DPAT and flesinoxan show prominent cardiovascular effects in a number of species (Table 1). Both compounds induce falls in blood pressure in conscious and anaesthetized animals which are generally accompanied by bradycardia, the degree of bradycardia being species-dependent. Moreover, flesinoxan in preliminary clinical trials has been shown to lower blood pressure and heart rate in patients with essential hypertension [23].

2.1 *Evidence for a central site of action for 8-OH-DPAT and flesinoxan*

A fall in both blood pressure and heart rate in conscious animals is suggestive of a central site of drug action and compelling evidence for such a locus of action for 8-OH-DPAT and flesinoxan has been obtained. Thus, for

Table 1. Hypotension and bradycardia elicited by 5-HT$_{1A}$ receptor agonists in different experimental models.

Compound	Experimental model	References
8-OH-DPAT	Normotensive and spontaneously hypertensive rats	[20, 22, 26, 28, 38]
	Normotensive cats	[24, 25, 29, 30]
	Normotensive rabbits	[34]
	Renal hypertensive dogs	[67]
Flesinoxan	Spontaneously hypertensive rat	[68]
	Normotensive cats	[25, 31]
	Normotensive dogs	[68]
	Renal hypertensive rabbits	[68]
	Normotensive baboons	[68]
	Essential hypertensives	[23]

example, in the anaesthetized cat, direct administration of 8-OH-DPAT or flesinoxan into the central nervous system via either the vertebral arteries or the intracisternal cavity increases their hypotensive potency as compared to the intravenous route of administration [24, 25]. A similar increase in potency for the prototype centrally acting antihypertensive drug, clonidine, has been consistently observed following injection via the vertebral arteries [25]. In the rat, falls in blood pressure and heart rate are seen following intracisternal injections of 8-OH-DPAT although they do not exceed in magnitude or duration the responses to similar doses given by the intravenous route [26, 27]. In comparison, responses to 8-OH-DPAT elicited via the intracerebroventricular route are less prominent than those obtained via the intracisternal route [27]. Thus, in the rat, the cardiovascular effects of 8-OH-DPAT are likely to be mediated by an action at sites located in the brain stem which are not readily accessible from the lateral cerebral ventricle.

Perhaps the most direct evidence for a primarily central site of action for 8-OH-DPAT in the rat is provided by the selective (vis à vis clonidine) blockade of the cardiovascular responses to 8-OH-DPAT following intracisternal administration of the selective 5-HT$_{1A}$ receptor partial agonist, 8-MeO-CLEPAT; the dose used had no effect on the responses to 8-OH-DPAT when given by the intravenous route [20]. Further evidence supporting a central site of action is provided by the inability of 8-OH-DPAT to lower blood pressure in the angiotensin II- or vasopressin-blood pressure supported pithed rat [20, 28]; nor does it interfere in the periphery with sympathetic nervous transmission to the cardiovascular system [20].

Further evidence that the hypotension and bradycardia produced by 5-HT$_{1A}$ receptor agonists primarily reflects a centrally mediated decrease in sympathetic tone associated with an increase in vagal nerve activity comes from observations that 8-OH-DPAT and flesinoxan inhibit sympathetic nerve activity at doses that lower blood pressure [29—31] and their bradycardic effects can be blocked by atropine or vagotomy [28, 30, 31]. The inhibitory effects of 8-OH-DPAT and flesinoxan on sympathetic nerve activity are particularly marked at the level of the renal nerve; therefore, it is not surprising that central administration of 5-HT in the cat results in hypotension and bradycardia associated with a decrease in renal sympathetic nerve activity and that an increase in vagal tone is observed in the rat [32, 33].

Recent studies in the open chest rabbit emphasise the similarity of the haemodynamic changes induced by 8-OH-DPAT and flesinoxan [34]. The principal blood pressure lowering mechanism was widespread vasodilatation, particularly in the splanchnic circulation. Despite falls in heart rate and in myocardial contractile force, cardiac output changed minimally. Such a haemodynamic profile is quite different from that of direct peripheral vasodilators; however, it is similar to that seen with clonidine in the same model [34] and consistent with a central mechanism of action to reduce peripheral sympathetic tone and/or augment vagal tone.

Of the other selective 5-HT_{1A} receptor ligands, ipsapirone has only weak cardiovascular activity although, in the cat, the effects are qualitatively similar to those of 8-OH-DPAT [29]. Both MDL 72832 and MDL 73005 are reported to block selectively the cardiovascular effects of 8-OH-DPAT in the rat [21, 22]. In comparison to the effects of 8-OH-DPAT, the cardiovascular effect of DP-5-CT, the most potent and selective 5-HT_{1A} receptor agonist yet described [18], are quite different. Thus, DP-5-CT causes hypotension associated with reflex tachycardia in the conscious SH rat, and dose-related falls in blood pressure with no significant effects on heart rate in the pithed rat [35]. It is likely that the difference between DP-5-CT and 8-OH-DPAT reflects poor penetration of the former into the brain and thus an inability to activate the central 5-HT_{1A} receptors. Therefore, DP-5-CT is of limited usefulness for studying the functional consequences of *central* 5-HT_{1A} receptor activation *in vivo*. The nature of the receptor mediating the direct vasodilator action of DP-5-CT remains to be established; however, it is unlikely to be the 5-HT_{1A} receptor since it is not activated by 8-OH-DPAT nor is it blocked by MDL 72832 [35, 36].

2.2 *The receptor mediating the cardiovascular effects of 8-OH-DPAT and flesinoxan*

Strong evidence now exists implicating postsynaptic 5-HT_{1A} receptors as the sites mediating the cardiovascular effects of 8-OH-DPAT and flesinoxan. The inability of ketanserin and $1\alpha H, 3\alpha, 5\alpha H$-tropan-3-yl-3,5-dichlorobenzoate (MDL 72222) to block the cardiovascular effects of 8-OH-DPAT in the rat excludes the involvement of 5-HT_2 and 5-HT_3

receptors; whereas blockade with metergoline and methiothepin in the rat [20] and with methiothepin and pindolol in the cat [24] point to the involvement of a '5-HT$_1$-like' receptor. Direct evidence implicating the 5-HT$_{1A}$receptor comes from experiments where clear antagonism of the cardiovascular affects of 8-OH-DPAT was obtained with low doses of the selective 5-HT$_{1A}$ receptor partial agonist, 8-MeO-CLEPAT [20] and stereoselective blockade with the enantiomers of MDL 72832 [22]; in both cases blockade was selective vis à vis clonidine. Antagonism of the cardiovascular effects of flesinoxan has also been observed with 8-MeO-CLEPAT in the rat [37]. More recently, spiroxatrine, a powerful, although non-selective 5-HT$_{1A}$ receptor antagonist, has also been shown to antagonize the cardiovascular effects of 8-OH-DPAT and flesinoxan [37, 38].

With respect to the pre- or postsynaptic location of the 5-HT$_{1A}$ receptors involved in cardiovascular control, since treatment with parachlorophenylalanine (PCPA) does not effect the cardiovascular responses to 8-OH-DPAT in the rat, a post-synaptic localization of these receptor sites seems likely [20]. In this context, it is also important to note that in the rat, but not in the cat, an indirect catecholaminergic component to the mechanism of action of 8-OH-DPAT is present; hence, the effects of 8-OH-DPAT are susceptible to blockade with α_2-adrenoceptor antagonists and combined depletion of 5-HT and catecholamines with DL-α-fluoromethyldopa [20].

2.3   *Clinical significance of this novel antihypertensive principle*

The validity of agonist activity at 5-HT$_{1A}$ receptors as an antihypertensive principle is supported by the efficacy of flesinoxan in lowering blood pressure in essential hypertensives in a preliminary clinical study [23]. It is further supported by the finding that urapidil, a marketed antihypertensive drug with α_1-adrenoceptor antagonist properties [39], has appreciable potency and mixed agonist/antagonist effects at 5-HT$_{1A}$ receptors [40, 41]. In animal studies, the hypotensive activity of urapidil is primarily due to a reduction in total peripheral resistance, associated with sympathoinhibition and increase in vagal tone [42—44]. Moreover, the effects can be antagonized by spiroxatrine following injection into the intravertebral artery [45]. In cats, blood pressure and heart rate decreases are observed even after pretreatment with prazosin and these can be blocked with spiperone [46]. The above observations suggest that the antihypertensive effects of urapidil arise in part from activation of central 5-HT$_{1A}$ receptors.

Thus, activation of 5-HT$_{1A}$ receptors can be considered a novel antihypertensive principle. However, further evaluation in man will be required before the important question as to the relevance of the behavioural effects of 5-HT$_{1A}$ receptor agonists observed in experimental animals [47] can be properly assessed.

3. Inhibitory effects of central 5-HT; role of 5-HT$_2$ receptors

Recent evidence suggests that in the rat intrathecal administration of 5-HT at high doses produce inhibition of renal sympathetic nerve activity. The effect is mimicked by the putative selective 5-HT$_2$ receptor agonist, α-methyl-5-HT, in a dose-dependent manner and antagonised by ketanserin [10]; 8-OH-DPAT was not effective. The data suggest a sympathoinhibitory role for 5-HT$_2$ receptors at the spinal level in the rat. Such a possibility receives further support from the fact that the hypotensive responses to intrathecally administered 5-HT can be blocked by ritanserin given intravenously and the hypotensive responses to 5-methoxy-N-N-dimethyltryptamine following intravenous administration were blocked by intrathecal administration of ketanserin [48].

4. Excitatory effects of central 5-HT; role of 5-HT$_2$ receptors

There are numerous studies showing that central bulbospinal (ponto-medullary) 5-HT pathways exert, in addition to inhibitory effects, a tonic *excitatory* effect on sympathetic preganglionic neurones in the interomediola-teral cell column of the spinal cord (see above). The sympathoexcitatory effects of microiontophoretic application of 5-HT or electrical stimulation of the descending 5-HT neurones can be blocked by the "classical" 5-HT receptor antagonists, methysergide and metergoline [49–51]. The putative selective 5-HT$_2$ receptor agonist, 1-(2,5-dimethoxy-4-iodophenyl)-2-aminopropane (DOI) produces an increase in sympathetic nerve discharge and the effects can be inhibited by the 5-HT$_2$ receptor antagonists, ketanserin and 6-methyl-1-(1-metylethyl)ergoline-8-carboxylic acid (LY 53857) [52]. Many 5-HT$_2$ receptor antagonists such as cinanserin, methysergide, metergoline and notably ketanserin produce sympathoinhibition and in certain circumstances blood pressure lowering effects [9, 28, 53–55].

The above observations have led to speculation that central 5-HT$_2$ receptors may be involved in blood pressure regulation. However, there have been several recent observations which suggest that although 5-HT$_2$ receptor activation can result in sympatho-excitation, these receptor sites are not normally under tonic activation and a role in blood pressure maintenance is therefore questionable. Firstly, it is now considered that both the sympathoinhibitory [44, 55–57] and blood pressure lowering [58–60] effects of ketanserin are best explained by blockade of α_1-adrenoceptors rather than 5-HT$_2$ receptor blockade. Moreover, in the case of ritanserin, sympathoinhibition is seen only at high doses which also antagonise the pressor responses to phenylephrine, an α_1-adrenoceptor agonist [61]. Also in this context, certain other 5-HT receptor antagonists lower blood pressure in normotensive [59] or SH rats [60] at doses that best correlate with their α_1-adrenoceptor blocking potency. Moreover, the more selective 5-HT$_2$

receptor antagonists, such as 2-2(2-dimethylaminoethylthio)-3-phenylquinoline hydrochloride (ICI 169369) and LY 53857 do not produce either sympathoinhibition or falls in blood pressure [55, 61, 62]. Finally, antagonism of the sympathoexcitatory effects of 5-HT by non-selective 5-HT$_2$ receptor antagonists such as methysergide or metergoline cannot be taken as strong evidence for an effect mediated via 5-HT$_2$ receptors since it could also result from antagonist effects at '5-HT$_1$-like' sites (see below).

The mechanism by which ketanserin lowers blood pressure in man also remains controversial [63]. However, as more selective 5-HT$_2$ receptor antagonists are being investigated it is becoming increasingly evident that central 5-HT$_2$ receptor blockade is not an effective blood pressure lowering principle in man. For example, in recent studies, neither ritanserin [64] nor ICI 169369 [65] lowered blood pressure in hypertensive patients.

Recent evidence that activation of spinal 5-HT$_2$ receptors results in sympathoinhibition (see above) further underscores the difficulty in assigning a role for 5-HT$_2$ receptors in the maintenance of blood pressure. Furthermore, recent data suggest that sympathoexcitation can result from '5-HT$_1$-like' receptor activation as discussed below.

5. Excitatory effects of central 5-HT; role of '5-HT$_1$-like' receptors

Intrathecal administration of the selective '5-HT$_1$-like' receptor agonist, 5-carboxamidotryptamine (5-CT) mimics the sympathoexcitatory effects of low doses of 5-HT [10]. The 5-CT-induced increase in renal sympathetic nerve activity was dose-related over the range 25—200 μg and produced a maximum 600% increase in discharge. The effects of 5-HT were not antagonised by ketanserin, MDL 72222 or 3α-tropanyl-1H-indole-3-carboxylic acid ester (ICS 205—930), thus excluding a role for 5-HT$_2$ or 5-HT$_3$ receptors. It remains to be determined which subtype(s) of '5-HT$_1$-like' receptor mediate(s) the excitatory effects of 5-CT; however, it is unlikely to involve either the 5-HT$_{1A}$ site, since 8-OH-DPAT was inactive over a wide dose-range, or the 5-HT$_{1C}$ receptor, for which 5-CT has very low affinity [66].

6. Conclusions

It is probably fair to conclude that considerable progress has been made towards clarifying the utterly confusing situation that existed about eight years ago, when the last major review of the role of central 5-HT in cardiovascular control appeared [8]. There is little doubt that the recognition and definition of multiple receptor subtypes for 5-HT in the CNS and the availability of selective agonists/antagonists for certain of these receptors has been instrumental in being able to assign the mechanism of the *inhibitory* and *excitatory* effects of central 5-HT to pharmacologically distinct receptor subtypes.

It is now clear that central 5-HT$_{1A}$ receptors play a key role in mediating the *inhibitory* effects of 5-HT. Central 5-HT$_{1A}$ receptor activation results in a unique and interesting haemodynamic profile; hypotension and bradycardia associated with sympathoinhibition and an increase in vagal tone. That such a mechanism may be of therapeutic importance is suggested by the preliminary clinical results with flesinoxan in essential hypertension and by the findings that urapidil, a marketed drug with α_1-adrenoceptor antagonist activity, owes a significant component of its hypotensive activity in experimental animals to central 5-HT$_{1A}$ receptor activation.

Despite certain evidence for the involvement of 5-HT$_2$ receptors in mediating the *sympathoexcitatory* effects of 5-HT, there is no good evidence that these receptor sites are tonically activated. Moreover, both location of the site and species differences may complicate definition of a role for 5-HT$_2$ receptors in this respect, since in the rat activation of *spinal* 5-HT$_2$ receptors results in *sympathoinhibition*. Notwithstanding the ketanserin experience, it is becoming increasingly evident that selective 5-HT$_2$ receptor antagonism is *not* an effective means of lowering blood pressure in experimental animals or man. Thus, a role for central 5-HT$_2$ receptors in the maintenance or control of blood pressure appears unlikely.

Very recent data in the rat suggest that activation of '5-HT$_1$-like' receptor(s) results in *sympathoexcitation*. The nature of the subtype involved remains to be elucidated but it is unlikely to be either 5-HT$_{1A}$ or 5-HT$_{1C}$. Moreover, it remains to be shown if this receptor site is tonically activated and if selective blockade might form the basis of a novel antihypertensive mechanism.

References

1. Dahlstrom A, Fuxe K (1965): Evidence for the existence of monoamine neurones in the central nervous system II. Experimentally induced changes in the intraneuronal amine levels of bulbospinal neurone systems. *Acta Physiol Scand* 64 (suppl.) 247: 5—36.
2. Chalmers JR, Wing LMH (1975): Central serotonin and cardiovascular control. *Clin Exp Pharmac Physiol* 2 (suppl.): 195—200.
3. Korner PI (1971): Integrative neural cardiovascular control. *Physiological Reviews* 51: 312—367.
4. Chalmers JP, Pilowsky PM, Minson JB, Kapoor V, Mills E, West MJ (1988): Central serotonergic mechanisms in hypertension. *Am J Hypertens* 1, 79—83.
5. Bhargava KP, Tangri KK (1959): The central vasomotor effects of 5-hydroxytryptamine. *Br J Pharmacol* 14: 411—414.
6. Baum T, Shropshire AT (1975): Inhibition of efferent nerve activity by 5-hydroxytryptophan and centrally administered 5-hydroxytryptamine. *Neuropharmacology* 14: 227—233.
7. Krstic MK, Djurkovic D (1980): Analysis of cardiovascular responses to central administration of 5-hydroxytryptamine in rats. *Neuropharmacology* 19: 455—463.

8. Kuhn DM, Wolf WA, Lovenberg W (1980): Review of the role of the central serotonergic neuronal system in blood pressure regulation. *Hypertension* 2: 243—255.
   agonist, causes a biphasic blood pressure response and a bradycardia in the normotensive

9. McCall RB, Humphrey ST (1982): Involvement of serotonin in the central regulation of blood pressure: Evidence for a facilitating effect on sympathetic nerve activity. *J Pharmacol Exp Ther* 222: 94—102.

10. Yusof APM, Coote JH (1988): Excitatory and inhibitory actions of intrathecally administered 5-hydroxytryptamine on sympathetic nerve activity in the rat. *J Autonom Nerv Syst* 22: 229—236.

11. Peroutka SJ, Snyder SH (1979): Multiple serotonin receptors: Differential binding of [^{3}H]5-hydroxytryptamine, [^{3}H]lysergic acid diethylamide and [^{3}H]spiroperidol. *Mol Pharmacol* 16: 687—699.

12. Fozard JR (1987): 5-HT: The enigma variations. *Trends Pharmacol Sci* 8: 501—506.

13. Bradley PB, Engel G, Feniuk W, Fozard JR, Humphrey PPA, Middlemiss DN, Mylecharane EJ, Richardson B, Saxena PR (1986): Proposals for the classification and nomenclature of functional receptors for 5-hydroxytryptamine. *Neuropharmacology* 25: 563—575.

14. Richardson BP, Engel G (1986): The pharmacology and function of 5-HT$_3$ receptors. *Trends Neurol Sci* 5: 424—428.

15. Fozard JR (1989): Agonists and antagonists for 5-HT$_3$ receptors. Chapter VIII, this volume.

16. Middlemiss DN, Fozard JR (1983): 8-Hydroxy-2-(di-n-propylamino) tetralin discriminates between subtypes of the 5-HT recognition site. *Eur J Pharmacol* 90: 150—153.

17. Dompert WU, Glaser T, Traber J (1985): ^{3}H-TVX Q 7821: Identification of 5-HT$_1$ binding sites as targets for a novel putative anxiolytic. *Naunyn-Schmiedeberg's Arch Pharmacol* 328: 467—470.

18. Hagenbach A, Hoyer D, Kalkman HO, Seiler MP (1986): N-N-propyl-5-carboxamido-tryptamine (DP-5-CT) an extremely potent and selective 5-HT$_{1A}$ agonist. *Brit J Pharmacol* 87: 136P.

19. Bevan P, Ramage AG, Wouters W (1986): Investigation of the effects of DU 29373 on the cardiovascular system of the anaesthetised cat. *Br J Pharmac* 89: 506P.

20. Fozard JR, Mir AK, Middlemiss DN (1987): The cardiovascular response to 8-hydroxy-2-(di-n-propylamino) tetralin (8-OH-DPAT) in the rat: site of action and pharmacological analysis. *J Cardiovasc Pharmacol* 9: 328—347.

21. Hibert M, Mir AK, Maghioros G, Moser P, Middlemiss DN, Tricklebank MD, Fozard JR (1988): The pharmacological properties of MDL 73005 EF: a potent and selective ligand at 5-HT$_{1A}$ receptors. *Brit J Pharmacol* 93: 2P.

22. Mir AK, Hibert M, Tricklebank MD, Middlemiss DN, Kidd EJ, Fozard JR (1988): MDL 72832: a potent and stereoselective ligand at central and peripheral 5-HT$_{1A}$ receptors. *Eur J Pharmacol* 149: 107—120.

23. De Voogd JM (1988): Early clinical experience with flesinoxan, a new selective 5-HT$_{1A}$ agonist. *Cardiovascular Pharmacology of 5-HT*. Amsterdam: October 1988, Abst. P42.

24. Doods HN, Boddeke HWGM, Kalkman HO, Hoyer D, Mathy M-J, Van Zwieten PA (1988): Central 5-HT$_{1A}$ receptors and the mechanism of the central hypotensive effect of (+)8-OH-DPAT, DP-5-CT, R28935, and urapidil. *J Cardiovasc Pharmacol* 11: 432—437.

25. Wouters W, Tulp MTLP, Bevan P (1988): Flesinoxan lowers blood pressure and heart rate in cats via 5-HT$_{1A}$ receptors. *Eur J Pharmacol* 149: 213—223.

26. Martin GE, Lis EV (1985): Hypotensive action of 8-hydroxy-2-(di-n-propylamino) tetralin (8-OH-DPAT) in spontaneously hypertensive rats. *Arch Int Pharmacodyn* 273: 251—261.

27. Mir AK, Fozard JR (1987): Cardiovascular effects of 8-hydroxy-2-(di-n-propylamino)

tetralin (8-OH-DPAT), pp. 120—134 in: Dourish CT, Ahlenius S, Hutson PH (eds), *Brain 5-HT$_{1A}$ Receptors*. Chichester: Ellis Horwood.

28. Gradin K, Pettersson A, Hedner T, Persson B (1985): Acute administration of 8-hydroxy-2-(di-n-propylamino) tetralin (8-OH-DPAT), a selective 5-HT receptor Sprague-Dawley rat and the spontaneously hypertensive rat. *J Neural Transm* 62: 305—319.

29. McCall RB, Patel BN, Harris LT (1987): Effects of serotonin$_1$ and serotonin$_2$ receptor agonists and antagonists on blood pressure, heart rate and sympathetic nerve activity. *J Pharmacol Exp Ther* 242: 1152—1159.

30. Ramage AG, Fozard JR (1987): Evidence that the putative 5-HT$_{1A}$ receptor agonists, 8-OH-DPAT and ipsapirone, have a central hypertensive action that differs from that of clonidine in anaesthetized cats. *Eur J Pharmacol* 38: 179—191.

31. Ramage AG, Wouters W, Bevan P (1988): Evidence that the novel antihypertensive agent flesinoxan causes differential sympathoinhibition and also increases vagal tone by a central action. *Eur J Pharmacol* 151: 373—379.

32. Dalton DW, Feniuk W, Humphrey PPA (1986): An investigation into the mechanisms of the cardiovascular effects of 5-hydroxytryptamine in conscious normotensive and Doca-salt hypertensive rats. *J Auton Pharmac* 6: 219—229.

33. Coote JH, Dalton DW, Feniuk W, Humphrey PPA (1987): The central site of the sympatho-inhibitory action of 5-hydroxytryptamine in the cat. *Neuropharmacology* 26: 147—154.

34. Hof R, Fozard JR (1989): 8-OH-DPAT, flesinoxan and guanfacine: systemic and regional haemodynamic effects of centrally acting antihypertensive agents in anaesthetized rabbits. *Brit J Pharmacol* 96: 864—871.

35. Mir AK, Hibert M, Fozard JR (1987): Cardiovascular effects of N,N-dipropyl-5-carboxamidotryptamine, a potent and selective 5-HT$_{1A}$ receptor ligand, pp. 21—29 in: Nobin A, Owman C, Arneklo-Nobin B (eds.), *Neuronal Messengers in Vascular Function*. Amsterdam: Elsevier.

36. Fozard JR, Mir AK, Ramage AG (1989): 5-HT$_{1A}$ receptors and cardiovascular control, pp. 146—151, in Mylecharane EJ, Angus JA, De La Lande IS, Humphrey PPA (eds), Serotonin: Actions, Receptors, Pathophysiology. Proceedings of the 1987 IUPHAR Congress Satellite Meeting, Heron Island, Australia: London, MacMillan.

37. Dreteler GH, Wouters W, Saxena PR (1988): The effect of putative 5-HT$_{1A}$ antagonists on the cardiovascular response to flesinoxan in the rat. Cardiovascular Pharmacology of 5-HT, Amsterdam, October 1988, Abst. p. 34.

38. Dabire H, Cherqui C, Fournier B, Schmitt H (1987): Comparison of effects of some 5-HT$_1$ agonists on blood pressure and heart rate of normotensive anaesthetized rats. *Europ J Pharmacol* 140: 259—266.

39. Van Zwieten PA, De Jonge A, Wilffert B, Timmermans PBM WM, Beckeringh JJ, Thoolen MJMC (1985): Cardiovascular effects and interaction with adrenoceptors of urapidil. *Arch Int Pharmacodyn Ther* 276: 180—201.

40. Fozard JR, Mir AK (1987): Are 5-HT$_{1A}$ receptors involved in the antihypertensive effects of urapidil? *Br J Pharmac* 90: 24P.

41. Gross G, Hanft G, Kolassa N (1987): Urapidil and some analogues with hypotensive properties show high affinity for 5-hydroxytryptamine (5-HT) binding sites of the 5-HT$_{1A}$ subtype and for α_1-adrenoceptor binding sites. *Naunyn-Schmiedeberg's Arch Pharmacol* 336: 597—601.

42. Sanders KH, Jurna I (1985): Effects of urapidil, clonidine, prazosin and propranolol on autonomic nerve activity, blood pressure and heart rate in anaesthetized rats and cats. *Eur J Pharmacol* 110: 181—190.

43. Ramage AG (1986): A comparison of the effects of doxazosin and alfuzosin with those of urapidil on preganglionic sympathetic nerve activity in anaesthetised cats. *Eur J Pharmac* 129: 307—314.

44. Ramage AG (1988): Are drugs that act both on serotonin receptors and α_1-adrenoceptors more potent hypotensive agents than those that act only on α_1-adrenoceptors? *J Cardiovasc Pharmac* 11 (suppl. 1): S30—S34.

45. Kolassa N, Beller K-D, Bischler P, Kowallik P, Sanders KH (1988): Central serotonin-1A-receptor mediated hypotensive response to urapidil after peripheral administration. *Cardiovascular pharmacology of 5-HT.* Amsterdam October 1988, Abst. P27.

46. Ramage AG (1989): Evidence that spiperone reverses the additional sympathoinhibitory action of urapidil in anaesthetised prazosin pretreated cats. Chapter XXIX, this volume.

47. Tricklebank MD (1985): The behavioural response to 5-HT receptor agonists and subtypes of the central 5-HT receptor. *Trends Pharmacol Sci* 6: 403—407.

48. Berger A, Ramirez AJ (1988): Hypotensive spinal serotonergic effects are S_1 and S_2 receptors involved? *Hypertension* 11 (suppl. 1): 182—185.

49. Kadzielawa K (1983): Antagonism of the excitatory effects of 5-hydroxytryptamine on sympathetic preganglionic neurones and neurones activated by visceral afferents. *Neuropharmacology* 22: 19—27.

50. McCall RB (1984): Evidence for a serotonergic mediated sympathoexcitatory responses to stimulation of medullary raphe nuclei. *Brain Res* 311: 131—139.

51. McCall, RB (1983): Serotonergic excitation of sympathetic preganglionic neurons: microiontophoretic study. *Brain Res* 289: 121—127.

52. McCall RB, Harris LT (1988): $5-HT_2$ receptor agonists increase spontaneous sympathetic nerve activity. *Eur J Pharmacol* 151: 113—116.

53. Antonaccio MJ, Taylor DG (1977): Reduction in blood pressure, sympathetic nerve discharge and central evoked pressor response by methysergide in anaesthetised cats. *Eur J Pharmacol* 42: 331—338.

54. Tadepalli AS, Ho KW, Buckley JP (1979): Enhancement of reflex bradycardia following intracerebroventricular administration of methysergide in cats. *Eur J Pharmacol* 69: 85—93.

55. Ramage AG (1985): The effects of ketanserin, methysergide and LY 53857 on sympathetic nerve activity. *Eur J Pharmacol* 113: 295—303.

56. McCall RB and Schuette MR (1984): Evidence for an alpha$_1$ receptor mediated central sympathoinhibitory action of ketanserin. *J Pharmacol Exp Ther* 228: 704—710.

57. McCall RB, Harris DT (1987): Characterization of the central sympathoinhibitory action of ketanserin. *J Pharmacol Exp Ther* 241: 736—740.

58. Fozard JR (1982): Mechanism of the hypotensive effect of ketanserin. *J Cardiovasc Pharmacol* 4: 829—838.

59. Kalkman HO, Harms YM, Gelderen VM, van Batink HD, Timmermans PBMWM, Van Zwieten RA (1983): Hypotensive activity of serotonin antagonists; correlation with α_1-adrenoceptor and serotonin receptor blockade. *Life Sci* 32: 1499—1505.

60. Cohen MD, Fuller RW, Kurz KD (1983): Evidence that blood pressure reduction by serotonin antagonists is related to alpha receptor blockade in spontaneously hypertensive rats. *Hypertension* 5: 676—681.

61. Ramage AG (1988): Examination of the effects of some $5-HT_2$ receptor antagonists on central sympathetic outflow and blood pressure in anaesthetised cats. *Naunyn-Schmiedeberg's Arch Pharmacol* 338: 601—607.

62. Cohen ML, Fuller RW, Kurz KD (1983): LY 53857, a selective and potent serotonergic ($5-HT_2$) receptor antagonist, does not lower blood pressure in the spontaneously hypertensive rats. *J Pharmacol Exp Ther* 227: 327—332.

63. Vanhoutte PM, Ball SG, Berdeaux A, Cohen MD, Hedner T, McCall R, Ramage AG, Reimann IH, Richer C, Saxena PR, Schalekamp MADH, Struyker-Boudier HAJ, Symoens J, Van Neuten JM, Van Zwieten RA (1986): Mechanism of action of ketanserin in hypertension. *Trends Pharmacol Sci* 7: 58—59.

64. Hedner T, Persson B (1988): Experience with ketanserin and ritanserin in hypertensive patients. *J Cardiovasc Pharmacol* 11 (suppl. 1): S44—S48.

65. Scott AK, Chaudhury PR, Webster J, Petrie JC (1988): Selective 5-HT antagonist (ICI 169,369): lack of effect on blood pressure in hypertensive patients. *Brit J Clin Pharmacol* 25: P651.
66. Hoyer D (1989): Biochemical mechanisms of 5-HT receptor-effector coupling in peripheral tissues, pp. 72—99 in: Fozard JR (ed.), *The Peripheral Actions of 5-hydroxy-tryptamine.* Oxford University Press.
67. Di Francesco GF, Petty MA, Fozard JR (1988): Antihypertensive effects of 8-hydroxy-2-(di-n-propylamino) tetralin (8-OH-DPAT) in conscious dogs. *Eur J Pharmacol* 147: 287—290.
68. Wouters W, Bevan P (1988): 5-HT related drugs and hypertension. *Cardiovascular pharmacology of 5-HT,* Amsterdam October 1988, Abst. S23.

XIX. The central antihypertensive action of 5-hydroxytryptamine: The location of site of action

J. H. COOTE

1. Introduction

A great number of studies indicate that 5-hydroxytryptamine (5-HT) acts as a neurotransmitter or neuromodulator at sites in the CNS. Fluorescence histochemical and immunohistochemical studies have shown that 5-HT containing neurones originating in the brainstem project to a number of forebrain structures as well as to specific regions of mid brain, hind brain and spinal cord [1—8]. Furthermore, electrophysiological investigations have demonstrated both inhibitory and excitatory effects of 5-HT on spinal and brainstem neurones (see reviews [9—11]). From the many studies cited in these reviews it is clear that 5-HT neurones project to regions of the CNS intimately involved in cardiovascular regulation and that 5-HT could have excitatory or inhibitory actions at these sites. Sites which are of particular interest are the preoptic/anterior hypothalamus, the ventrolateral medulla and the dorsal medulla.

2. Cardiovascular effects of 5-HT injected into discrete brain areas

2.1 Pre-optic anterior hypothalamus

Injections of small amounts of 5-HT at a number of sites located in the preoptic nucleus and anterior hypothalamus leads to an increase in blood pressure with variable effects on heart rate [12]. It is very likely these effects are produced by 5-HT mimicking the actions of the numerous 5-HT containing terminals in these nuclei [4, 6, 13]. The two main sources of the 5-HT innervation of the forebrain are the dorsal and mid brain raphe nuclei [1, 2] but it is the dorsal raphe nucleus that provides the main excitatory influence on the neurones of the preoptic-anterior hypothalamic region. Thus, although electrical stimulation of either dorsal or median raphe nucleus produces a pressor response with no consistant change in heart rate in the anaesthetised

P.R. Saxena, D.I. Wallis, W. Wouters and P. Bevan (eds), Cardiovascular Pharmacology of 5-Hydroxytryptamine, pp. 259—270.
© 1990 *Kluwer Academic Publishers, Dordrecht* —

and unanaesthetised rat [14—17] and in anaesthetised cat [18] only the pressor response to dorsal raphe stimulation is abolished by lesioning the 5-HT neurones with the specific neurotoxin 5,7-dihydroxytryptamine (5,7-DHT [19]. This procedure does not produce a change in resting blood pressure but results in an enhanced pressor response to injection of 5-HT into the preoptic — anterior hypothalamus. In addition, treatment with fluoxetine (10 mg/kg i.v.), a 5-HT uptake inhibitor, enhances and prolongs the pressor response to dorsal raphe stimulation. Administrationn of the 5-HT antagonist 2-bromolysergic diethylamide into the region of the preoptic — anterior hypothalamus attenuates the dorsal raphe elicited pressor response. Furthermore, the pressor response can be abolished by transection rostral to the dorsal raphe and is reduced after treatment of the rats with bretylium or mecamylamine [15, 19, 20]. The evidence therefore strongly favours the idea that 5-HT neurones of the dorsal raphe nuclei project to neurones in the preoptic — anterior hypothalamus where they influence the activity of neurones leading to an increase in sympathetic nerve mediated vasoconstrictor tone.

Because of the closeness of the preoptic — anterior hypothalamus to the third ventricle, neurones are readily accessible to drugs given by the intracerebroventricular route (ICV). This may be of some importance since the ICV injection of 5-HT initially causes a dose related pressor response in anaesthetised or unanaesthetised rats and cats although this is followed by a fall in blood pressure [12, 17, 19, 21—29].

The pressor effect of ICV 5-HT is dependent on a central action mediated through spinal sympathetic vasoconstrictor outflows since it is accompanied by increases in sympathetic vasoconstrictor nerve activity [28, 29] abolished by transection of the spinal cord at C_1 and by the intravenous administration of phenoxybenzamine, bretylium or nicotine and reduced after bilateral adrenalectomy [23]. Other evidence supports the idea that the pressor effect of ICV 5-HT is dependent on forebrain structures at least in the cat since similar changes following ICV 5-HT are seen in this animal when access by 5-HT is confined to the lateral and third ventricles and it is absent when 5-HT is precluded from forebrain structures by injecting it directly into the IVth ventricle [28, 29]. Therefore, the most likely explanation at present for the pressor effect of ICV 5-HT is that it mimicks an excitatory action of endogenous transmitter on vasomotor neurones in the preoptic/anterior hypothalamus. This conclusion is supported by the observation that the pressor action of 5-HT injected into this forebrain region is prevented by interfering with cholinergic transmission by suppressing brain cholinesterase activity with physostigmine or by central administration of atropine or hemicholinium. These are procedures which, on their own are without effect on blood pressure suggesting that a cholinergic mechanism is activated by 5-HT [16, 30].

There also appears to be an important interaction between the 5-HT innervation and the catecholamine innervation of these preoptic-anterior hypothalamic neurones. Destruction of the ventral noradrenergic pathway by administration of 6-hydroxytryptamine (5 μg each side of ventral pons) reduced the content of noradrenaline in the anterior hypothalamus by 80% and induced an increase in arterial blood pressure and heart rate. The blood pressure of these hypertensive rats could be lowered by administration of the 5-HT antagonists methysergide (1—2 μg) and, to a lesser extent, ketanserin (1—2 μg), into the preoptic-anterior hypothalamus suggesting the maintenance of high blood pressure was due to release of a tonically active 5-HT innervation in this region. This idea was reinforced by the observation that the hypertension occurring after treatment with 6-OHDA in the ventral pons can be prevented by prior administration of 5,7-DHT (8 μg) into the medial forebrain bundle to decrease the 5-HT content of the anterior hypothalamus by 85% — a procedure which on its own had no effect on blood pressure [31].

In cat and DOCA salt hypertensive rat the pressor response and bradycardia and increases in renal sympathetic nerve activity followig ICV injection of 5-HT are mimicked by a number of 5-HT like agonists [27, 28]. In addition, the actions of 5-HT in both normotensive and hypertensive animals are reduced by ICV injection of the antagonist methysergide (5-HT$_1$/5-HT$_2$), but not by cyproheptadine (5-HT$_2$) or 3-dimethylamino-1-[IH-indole-3-yL]-1-propanone (CCI 19303; 5-HT$_3$) also given ICV [17, 27, 28]. These pharmacological experiments therefore suggest that the receptor involved inthe pressor action of ICV 5-HT is 5-HT$_1$-like in nature.

2.2 *Ventrolateral medulla*

There is now considerable evidence that structures in the ventrolateral medulla play an important role in cardiovascular control [32]. Lesions made close to the surface of the rostral ventrolateral medulla produce a profound fall in blood pressure [33] whilst electrical stimulation at similar sites evoked a rise in blood pressure and other cardiovascular changes [34—37]. Inactivation of neurones in this region by microinjection of inhibitory amino acids evokes a fall in blood pressure and decreases in sympathetic nerve activity [38—40]. On the contrary, microinjection of the amino acids, glutamate and D,L-homocysteic acid (DLH) to selectively excite neuronal perikarya, but not fibres of passage, produce rises in blood pressure when injected into a region which lies immediately caudal to the facial nucleus and adjacent to the inferior olive [34, 35, 37, 41]. This area has been identified as the nucleus paragigantocellularis lateralis (P.G.L.) [42, 43]. Further studies have shown that in the PGL there are separate populations of neurones which exert control over the heart and individual vascular beds. Thus, injection of DLH at one site causes changes in one vascular bed without effecting others [32, 44]. Similar differential effects have been documented for sympathetic nerve activity to different vascular beds [45, 46, 40].

This highly important region of the brainstem is particularly relevant to the present discussion because the neurones are close to the surface of the brain and therefore may be more readily affected by substances in the cerebrospinal fluid.

Neurones in PGL have a quite dense 5-HT innervation [6]; they are therefore a potential site for the central actions of 5-HT or of its agonists and antagonists. In recent work Lovick [47] has shown that microinjection of 5-HT (10−100 nmol) bilaterally into PGL of anaesthetised rats produces hypotension (5−57 mm Hg) and a bradycardia (6−126 bpm). The different pools of vasomotor neurones seem to be similarly affected by 5-HT since it reduced blood flow to hind limb muscle vascular bed and to kidney. These experiments so far suggest that 5-HT may have an inhibitory action on cardiovascular neurones of the ventrolateral medulla, although this needs to be substantiated by single unit recording from these cells.

2.3 Nucleus ambiguus

Changes in cardiac output are an important contributor to blood pressure control. The vagal cardioinhibitory neurones may therefore be a potential locus for the antihypertensive action of 5-HT or its agonists and antagonists.

Vagal preganglionic neurones innervating the heart are located in both the dorsal motor nucleus of the vagus and in the nucleus ambiguus of rabbit and rat [49, 48] but only in the nucleus ambiguus of cat [50]. 5-HT terminals surround the perikarya of neurones in both nuclei [6] and 5-HT immunoreactive boutons have been observed in close apposition to cardiac vagal motoneurones identified with HRP by retrograde labelling from cut cardiac vagal branches [51].

The action of 5-HT on cardiac vagal neurones is likely to be excitatory. In a recent preliminary study [51] it was shown that microinjection of 5-HT (25 ng − 2 μg) into the nucleus ambiguus of cats caused marked falls in heart rate an effect which was mimicked by similar microinjection of the 5-HT$_{1A}$ agonist 8-hydroxy-2-(di-n-propylamino) tetralin (8-OH-DPAT). Such experiments although at an early stage provide support for the contention that the decreases in cardiac output produced by the peripheral administration of a number of 5-HT agonists could be partly via a central action on cardiac vagal neurones [52−54]. Thus 8-OH-DPAT, isaspirone, and flexinoxan, given intravenously to anaesthetised cats, evoked, in addition to a sympathoinhibition, an increase in cardiac vagal tone by a likely CNS action. This conclusion is supported by data on the effects of 8-OH-DPAT in the rat [53]. 8-OH-DPAT (8-128 g/kg i.v.) caused dose related falls in blood pressure and heart rate which was blocked selectively by intracisternal or i.v. injection of putative 5-HT$_{1A}$ antagonists (8-methoxy-2-(N-2-chloroethyl-N-n-propyl) amino tetralin 8-MeO-CLEPAT), metergoline and by methiothepin). It was non selectively inhibited by substances which have in common some action at 5-HT$_1$ recognition sites, such as pindolol, cyanopindolol, spiperone and buspirone, yohimbine idazoxin and WY26392 and was unaffected by prazosin and cis-flupenthixol. In pithed rats 8 OH DPAT neither lowered blood pressure or heart rate nor affected the cardiovascular response to spinal sympathetic stimulation or to phenylephrine i.v. This clearly establishes that the cardiovascular response to i.v. 8-OH-DPAT in the rat is centrally mediated [53, 55]. Whether it is due to directly mimicking the actions of an endogenous 5-HT innervation of the cardiac vagal neurones remains to be established but encouraging signs are that in both rat and human nucleus ambiguus there is a preponderance of 5-HT$_{1A}$ binding sites [56, 57].

2.4 *Nucleus tractus solitarius (NTS)*

The NTS is the site of termination of afferent fibres from arterial baroreceptors and chemoreceptors [58]. As such it integrates several cardiovascular reflexes and modifications of synaptic transmission within the nucleus may lead to profound changes in arterial blood pressure and heart rate [59, 60].

Fibre terminals containing 5-HT, probably originating from cell bodies in nucleus raphe magnus are present in the nucleus [6, 7, 61] and 5-HT recognition sites of the 5-HT$_{1A}$ type predominate [56].

Microinjection of 5-HT (< 400 pmol, 0.1 μl) into the NTS around obex region of anaesthetised rats produced marked falls in arterial blood pressure (< 48 mm Hg) and heart rate (< 90 bpm). These effects are blocked by prior injection of the 5-HT antagonist metergoline (100 pmol), which according to the authors [61] produced no changes in arterial blood pressure or heart rate. However, two of the figures in their paper clearly indicate that after metergoline the heart rate was lower, though the baroreceptor reflex-mediated bradycardia following intravenous phenylephrine was not affected. These experiments suggest that in the anaesthetised rat the efficacy of the baroreceptor reflex is not dependent on a 5-HT innervation but that 5-HT can facilitate the normal reflex inhibitory influence mediated through the NTS.

Such an action may explain the findings in a recent study by Dalton (1987) which examined the changes in baroreceptor reflex effects on blood pressure, heart rate and renal nerve activity during the ICV application of 5-HT in anaesthetised cats. Electrical stimulation of both sinus nerves at a number of frequencies allowed the construction of stimulus response curves. Following ICV application of 5—HT (10 μg or 30 μg) there were larger falls in blood pressure and renal nerve activity at all stimulus frequencies compared to control although a large variability between animals prevented this reaching significance.

2.5 Area postrema

The area postrema is the most caudal of the circumventricular organs and lies on the dorsal surface of the medulla at the level of the obex. It is a region lying outside the blood brain barrier and it is probable that substances in the cerebrospinal fluid and blood plasma have ready access to neurones within this area [62, 63]. The area postrema also has numerous afferent nerve terminals which are immunoreactive to 5-HT antibody and these show a selective distribution to parts of the region [64, 65].

Electrical stimulation within the area postrema of the dog causes increases in arterial blood pressure and heart rate [66]. Angiotensin II infused via the vertebral artery in a number of animals acts specifically at the level of the area postrema to produce similar cardiovascular changes [67—70]. Ablation of the area postrema in the rat causes a substantial decrease in heart rate but surprisingly arterial blood pressure is unaltered [79].

Application of 5-HT to neurones in the area postrema of the dog causes them to increase their firing [71]. There have been no reports of cardiovascular effects of 5-HT microinjected into area postrema but in view of the above data increases in blood pressure and heart rate might be expected.

3. Cardiovascular effects of 5-HT after intracerebroventricular administration: the site of action

As referred to earlier, numerous studies have shown that in the conscious or anaesthetised rat or anaesthetised cat ICV administration of 5-HT produces an immediate pressor response [21, 22, 25] followed by prolonged decreases in blood pressure and heart rate [24—29] also accompanied by decreases in sympathetic nerve activity [29, 72].

When 5-HT is prevented having access to the hind brain by blocking the aqueduct of sylvius the depressor effect and bradycardia is absent leaving only the pressor effect and increase in renal sympathetic nerve activity. On the contrary when 5-HT is administered into the fourth ventricle the pressor response is absent [28, 29]. In view of the extensive data (see earlier) on the 5-HT mediated vasomotor influence of the preoptic — anterior hypothalamus it seems highly likely that neurones in this region of the forebrain are responsible for the pressor response to ICV 5-HT. The cardiovascular inhibitory effects of ICV 5-HT are dependent on hind brain structures since they do not occur when 5-HT is prevented from reaching the fourth ventricle and 5-HT injected into the fourth ventricle produces only decreases in blood pressure, heart rate and renal and splanchnic sympathetic nerve activity [28—29]. Application of 5-HT in similar doses to those given ICV either at various levels of the spinal cord using an intrathecal catheter passed down the subarachnoid space from the cisterna magna or directly onto the surface of the exposed ventral medulla did not produce changes in cardiovascular or sympathetic nerve activity. It therefore seemed reasonable for Coote et al. [29] to conclude that the important site for the effects of 5-HT lies some where accessible from the dorsal surface of the medulla. This indeed appeared to be the case because application of 5-HT directly onto the dorsal surface in the region of the NTS and obex produced marked decreases in blood pressure, heart rate and sympathetic nerve activity [28, 29]. Several factors now lead me to be cautious about the interpretation of this result.

Firstly, the decrease in arterial blood pressure produced by ICV 5-HT resulted from a substantial decrease in cardiac output (12%) with only a small decrease in total peripheral resistance (< 2%) despite large decreases in sympathetic activity to splanchnic and renal vascular beds. This suggests that vascular resistance via sympathetic vasoconstrictor activity was increasing in some other major tissue. Such a pattern of response is unlike that produced by baroreceptor activation or NTS stimulation [58, 73] indicating that 5-HT was not producing the cardiovascular changes by direct action only at this site.

The area postrema is also an improbable site for the depressor action of 5-HT because, as discussed earlier, activation of neurones in this region of the brain elicits increases in blood pressure and heart rate and 5-HT has excitatory actions on neurones there.

Structures in the ventral part of the medulla were arguably excluded because of the lack of effect of 5-HT applied on to the exposed surface. However, it is possible that penetration of 5-HT was impeded by accumulation of a surface layer of fibrin which in recent experiments we have noted occurs rapidly after exposing this region to air. An action of 5-HT via the ventral medulla could more easily explain the differential nature of the cardiovascular response to ICV 5-HT because of the separation of populations of target organ specified neurones. Hence the pattern of cardiovascular response to ICV 5-HT might be a consequence of how easily 5-HT reaches the vicinity of the different groups of neurones. How then can we explain the dramatic depressor response and bradycardia and inhibition of renal sympathetic nerve activity following direct application of 5-HT to the dorsal caudal medulla? Whilst some of the effects could be due to facilitation of the baroreceptor reflex (see section on NTS) it is also possible that some of the very large concentration of 5-HT leaked away and was carried to the unexposed ventral medullary surface where it could diffuse without being impeded by a fibrin membrane. There are many uncertainties in this explanation but, I feel it offers scope for further more rigorous experimental approaches which will give us a clearer understanding of the antihypertensive role of 5-HT.

266   J. H. Coote

4. Conclusions

The potential sites for the CNS mediated cardiovascular effects of 5-HT or its agonists and antagonists are illustrated in Figure 1. The picture that emerges is as follows.

1. *Pressor effects.* Endogenous 5-HT is likely to be excitatory to PO/AH neurones which in turn produce a purely vasomotor induced pressor response. Increases in both cardiac and vasomotor activity would be expected following release of 5-HT in the area postrema although this needs to be investigated.
2. *Depressor effects.* The actions of 5-HT at synapses in the NTS is likely to be facilitatory so augmenting the baroreceptor reflex and leading to falls in blood pressure and heart rate. It is also likely that 5-HT excites vagal cardiac neurones leading to bradycardia and a reduction in cardiac output and a fall in blood pressure. In contrast, preliminary studies suggest that the action of 5-HT on different populations of vasomotor neurones in the PGL is inhibitory leading to falls in blood pressure.
3. *5-HT receptors.* The predominant 5-HT receptor in each of these cardiovascular regions seems to be 5-HT_1-like in nature. Administration of 5-HT agonists or antagonists into the systemic circulation could allow them access to several or all of these sites provided they cross the blood brain barrier and this clearly is the case for 8-OH-DPAT. The resultant cardiovascular response would then be dependent on the concentration reaching each of the above sites and an algebraic summation of the pressor and depressor influences.

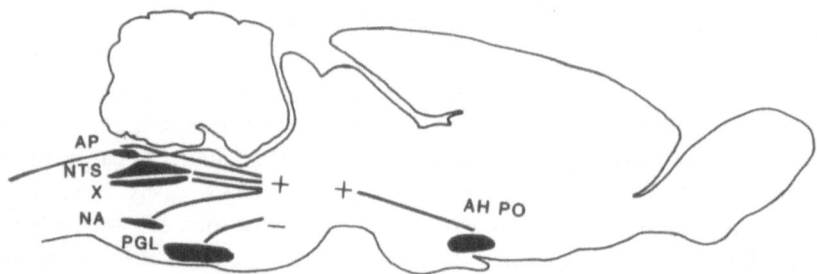

Figure 1. Parasaggital section of rat brain showing key cardiovascular control areas in fore and hind brain and the likely excitatory (+) or inhibitory (−) action of 5-HT on them. AP, area postrema: NTS, nucleus tractus solitarius; X, nucleus of the tenth cranial nerve; NA, nucleus ambiguus; PGL, nucleus paragigantocellularis lateralis; AHPO, anterior hypothalamus, preoptic region.

References

1. Dahlstrom A, Fuxe K (1965): Evidence for the existence of monoamine neurones in the central nervous system II. Experimentally induced changes in the intraneuronal amine levels of bulbospinal neurone systems. *Acta Physiol Scand* 64 (suppl. 247): 5−36.

2. Fuxe K (1965): Evidence for the existence of monoamine nerve terminals in the central nervous system. *Acta Physiol Scand* 64 (suppl. 247): 37—85.

3. Azmitia EC, Segal M (1978): An autoradiographic analysis of the differential ascending projections of the dorsal and median raphe nuclei in the rat. *J Comp Neurol* 179: 641—668.

4. Moore RY, Halaris AE, Jones BE (1978): Serotonin neurons of the mid brain raphe: Ascending projections. *J Comp Neurol* 180: 417—438.

5. Bowker RM, Westlund KN, Coulter JD (1981): Serotonergic projections to the spinal cord from the mid brain in the rat. An immunocytochemical and retrograde transport study. *Neurosci Lett* 24: 221—226.

6. Steinbusch HWM (1981): Distribution of serotonin immunoreactivity in the central nervous system of the rat — cell bodies and terminals. *Neurosci* 6: 557—618.

7. Pickel VM, Joh TH, Chan J, Beaudet A (1984): Serotonergic terminals: ultrastructure and synaptic interaction with catecholamine-containing neurons in the medial nuclei of the solitary tract. *J Comp Neurol* 225: 291—301.

8. Lanca AJ, van der Kroy D (1985): A serotonin containing pathway from the area postrema to the parabrachial nucleus in the rat. *Neuroscience* 14: 1117—1126.

9. Krnjevic K (1974): Chemical nature of synaptic transmission in vertebrates. *Physiol Rev* 54: 418—540.

10. Fozard JR (1984): Neuronal 5-HT receptors in the periphery. *Neuropharmacology* 23: 1473—1486.

11. Coote JH (1988): Organisation of cardiovascular neurones in the spinal cord. *Rev Physiol Biochem Pharmacol* 10: 147—285.

12. Smits JF, Struyker-Boudier HA (1976): Intrahypothalamic serotonin and cardiovascular control in rats. *Brain Res* III: 422—427.

13. Saavedra JM, Palkovits M, Browstein MJ, Axelrod J (1974): Serotonin distribution in the nuclei of the rat hypothalamus and preoptic region. *Brain Res* 77: 157—165.

14. Smits JF, van Essen H, Struyker-Boudier HA (1978): Serotonin mediated cardiovascular responses to electrical stimulation of the raphe nuclei in the rat. *Life Sci* 23: 173—178.

15. Kuhn DM, Wolf WA, Lovenberg W (1980): Pressor effects of electrical stimulation of the dorsal and median raphe nuclei in anaesthetised rats. *J Pharmac Exp Ther* 214: 403—409.

16. Robinson SE (1982): Interaction of the median raphe nucleus and hypothalamic serotonin with cholinergic agents and pressor responses in the rat. *J Pharmac Exp Ther* 223: 662—668.

17. Sukamoto T, Yamomoto T, Watanabe S, Ueki S (1984): Cardiovascular responses to centrally administered serotonin in conscious normotensive and spontaneously hypertensive rats. *Europ J Pharmacol* 100: 173—179.

18. Piper RD, Goadsby PJ (1985): Pressor response to electrical and chemical stimulation of nucleus raphe dorsalis in the cat. *Stroke* 16: 307—312.

19. Robinson SE, Austin MJF, Gibbens DM (1985): The role of serotonergic neurones in dorsal raphe, median raphe and anterior hypothalamic pressor mechanisms. *Neuropharmacology* 24: 51—58.

20. Robinson SE (1984): Cardiovascular effects of alpha-adrenergic agents in the dorsal raphe nucleus of the cat. *Brain Res* 295: 249—254.

21. Lambert GA, Friedman E, Gershon S (1975): Centrally mediated cardiovascular responses to 5-HT. *Life Sci* 17: 915—919.

22. Krstic MK, Djurkovic D (1976): Hypertension mediated by activation of the rat brain 5-hydroxytryptamine receptor sites. *Experientia* 32: 1187—1189.

23. Krstic MK, Djurkovic D (1980): Analysis of cardiovascular responses to central administration of 5-hydroxytryptamine in rats. *Neuropharmacology* 19: 455—463.

24. Krstic MK, Djurkovic D (1981): Comparison of the cardiovascular responses to intracerebroventricular administration of tryptamine, 5-hydroxytryptamine, tryptophan and 5-hydroxytryptophan in rats. *Arch Int Physiol Biochem* 89: 385—391.

25. Lambert GA, Friedman E, Buchweitz E, Gershon S, (1978): Involvement of 5-hydroxy-tryptamine in the central control of respiration, blood pressure and heart rate in the anaesthetised rat. *Neuropharmacology* 17: 807—813.

26. Dalton DW, Fortune DH, Tyers MB (1983): Central cardiovascular effects of 5-hydroxy-tryptamine in the conscious rat. *Brit J Pharmacol Proc* 78 (suppl. 1): 132P.

27. Dalton DW (1986): The cardiovascular effects of centrally administered 5-hydroxytrypta-mine in the conscious normotensive and hypertensive rat. *J Auton Pharmac* 6: 67—75.

28. Dalton DW (1987): An investigation of the central actions of 5.hydroxytryptamine on the cardiovascular system. *PhD Thesis CNAA Glaxo Group Research Ltd* Ware, Hertfordshire.

29. Coote JH, Dalton DW, Feniuk W, Humphrey PPA (1987): The central site of the sympatho-inhibitory action of 5-hydroxytryptamine in the cat. *Neuropharmacology* 26: 147—154.

30. Krstic MK, Djurkovic D (1987): Modification by physostigmine of the cardiovascular responses to intracerebroventricular administration of 5-hydroxytryptamine in rats. *Arch Int Physiol Biochem* 95: 153—158.

31. Bennaroch EE, Balda MS, Finkielman S, Nahmod VE (1983): Neurogenic hypertension after depletion of norepinephrine in anterior hypothalamus induced by 6-hydroxydopa-mine administration into the ventral pons: the role of serotonin. *Neuropharmacology* 22: 29—34.

32. Lovick TA (1987): Differential control of cardiac and vasomotor activity by neurones in nucleus paragigantocellularis lateralis in the cat. *J Physiol* 389: 23—35.

33. Guertzenstein PG, Silver A (1974): Fall in blood pressure produced from discrete regions of the ventral surface of the medulla by glycine and lesions. *J Physiol* 242: 489—503.

34. Dampney RAL, Goodchild AK, Robertson LG, Montgomery W (1982): Role of the ventrolateral medulla in vasomotor regulation: a correlative anatomical and physiological study. *Brain Res* 249: 223—235.

35. Howe PRC, Kuhn DM, Minson JB, Stead BH, Chalmers P (1983): Evidence for a bulbospinal serotonergic pressor pathway in the rat brain. *Brain Res* 270: 29—36.

36. Hilton SM, Marshall JM, Timms RJ (1983): Ventral medullary relay neurones in the pathway from the defence areas of the cat and their effects on blood pressure. *J Physiol* 345: 149—166.

37. Ross CA, Ruggiero DA, Park D, Joh A, Sved AF, Fernandez-Pardal J, Saavedra JM, Reis DJ (1984): Tonic vasomotor control by the rostral ventrolateral medulla: effect of electrical and chemical stimulation of the area containing C_1 adrenaline neurones on arterial blood pressure, heart rate and plasma catecholamines and vasopressin. *J Neurosci* 4: 474—494.

38. Guertzenstein PG (1973): Blood pressure effects obtained from drugs applied to the ventral surface of the brainstem. *J Physiol* 229: 395—408.

39. Wilette RN, Barcas PP, Krieger AJ, Sapru HN (1983): Vasopressor and depressor areas in the rat medulla: identification by microinjection of l-glutamate. *Neuropharmacology* 22: 1071—1079.

40. Dean C, Coote JH (1987): A ventromedullary relay involved in the hypothalamic and chemoreceptor activation of sympathetic postganglionic neurones to skeletal muscle, kidney and splanchnic area. *Brain Res* 377: 279—285.

41. McAllen RM (1986a): Location of neurones with cardiovascular and respiratory function at the ventral surface of the cats medulla. *Neuroscience* 18: 43—49.

42. Adrezik JA, Chan-Palay V, Palay SL (1981): The nucleus paragigantocellularis lateralis in the rat. Conformation and cytology. *Anatomy and Embryology* 161: 355—377.

43. Newman DB (1985): Distinguishing rat brainstem reticulospinal nuclei by their neuronal morphology. I Medullary nuclei. *J fur Hirnforschung* 26: 187—226.

44. Lovick TA (1988): Hypotensive action of 5-HT in the ventrolateral medulla of anaesthetised rats. *J Physiol* 412: 14P.

45. McAllen RM (1986): Action and specificity of ventral medullary vasopressor neurones in the cat. *Neuroscience* 18: 43—49.
46. Dampney RAL, McAllen RM (1986): Functional specificity of ventral medullary pre-sympathetic neurones in the cat. *J Physiol* 377, 58P.
47. Lovick TA (1988): Covergent afferent inputs to neurones in nucleus paragigantocellularis lateralis in the cat. *Brain Res* 456: 183—187.
48. Jordan D, Spyer KM, Writhington-Wray DJ, Wood LM (1986): Histochemical and electrophysiological identification of cardiac and pulmonary vagal preganglionic neurones in the cat. *J Physiol* 372, 87P.
49. Jordan D, Khalid MEM, Schniederman N, Spyer KM (1982): The location and properties of preganglionic vagal cardiomotor neurones in the rabbit. *Pflugers Arch* 395: 244—250.
50. Jordan D, Spyer KM (1987): Central neural mechanisms mediating respiratory-cardiovascular interactions, pp. 322—341 in: Taylor EW (ed), *Neurobiology of the cardio-respiratory system.* Manchester: University Press.
51. Jordan D, Izzo PN, Spyer KM, Rammage AG (1987): Pharmacological and immunocyto-chemical evidence that central 5-HT neurones participate in cardiac regulation in the cat. *Neurosci Lett* (suppl. 32) S12.
52. Bevan P, Pammage AG, Wouters W (1986): Investigation of the effects of DU 29373 on the cardiovascular system of the anaesthetised cat. *Brit J Pharmacol* 89, 506P.
53. Fozard JR, Mir AK, Middlemiss DN (1987): Cardiovascular response to 8-hydroxy-2-(di-n-Propylamino) Tetralin (8 OH DPAT) in the rat: Site of action and pharmacological analysis. *J Cardiovasc Pharmac* 9: 328—347.
54. Rammage AG, Fozard JR (1987): Evidence that the putative 5-HT$_{1A}$ agonists, 8 OH DPAT and ipsapirone, have a central hypotensive action that differs from that of clonidine in anaesthetised cats. *Europ J Pharmac* 138: 179—191.
55. Gradin K, Petterson A, Hechner T, Persson B (1985): Acute administration of 8-hydroxy-2-(di-n-Propylamino) Tetralin (8 OH DPAT), a selective 5-HT receptor agonist, causes a biphasic blood pressure response and bradycardia in the normotensive Sprague Dawley rat and in the spontaneously hypertensive rat. *J Neurol Trans* 62: 305—319.
56. Pazos A, Palacios JM (1985): Quantitative autoradiographic mapping of serotonin receptors in the rat brain. I. Serotonin-I receptors. *Brain Res* 346: 205—230.
57. Pazos A, Probst A, Palacios JM (1987): Serotonin receptors in the human brain III. Autoradiographic mapping of serotonin I receptors. *Neurosci* 21: 123—139.
58. Spyer KM (1981): Neural organisation and control of the baroreceptor reflex. *Rev Physiol Biochem Pharmacol* 88: 23—124.
59. Talman WT, Perrone MH, Scher P, Kwo S, Reis DJ (1981): Antagonism of the baroreceptor reflex by glutamate diethylester on antagonist to L-glutamate. *Brain Res* 217: 186—191.
60. Talman WT, Reis DJ (1981): Baroreceptor actions of SP microinjected into the nucleus tractus solitarii in rat: a consequence of local distortion. *Brain Res* 220: 402—407.
61. Basbaum AI, Clanton CH, Fields HL (1978): Three bulbospinal pathways from the rostral medulla of the cat: an autoradiographic study of pain modulating systems. *J Comp Neurol* 178: 567—574.
62. Laguzzi R, Reis DJ, Talman WT (1984): Modulation of cardiovascular and electrocor-tical activity through serotonergic mechanisms in the nucleus tractus solitarius of the rat. *Brain Res* 304: 321—328.
63. Wsniewski H, Olszewski J (1963): Vascular permeability in the area postrema and hypothalamus. *Neurology* 13: 885—894.
64. Klara PM, Briszee KR (1977): Ultrastructure of the feline area postrema. *J Comp Neurol* 171: 409—432.
65. Takeuchi Y, Sano Y (1983): Serotonin distribution in the circumventricular organs of the rat. *Anat Embryol* 167: 311—319.
66. Newton BW, Maley B, Traurig H (1985): The distribution of substance P, enkephalin,

and serotonin immunoreactivities in the area postrema of the rat and cat. *J Comp Neurol* 234: 87—104.

67. Barnes KL, Ferrario CM (1980): Characterisation of the sympathofacilitative area postrema pathway. *Clin Sci* 59: 255s—257s.
68. Joy MD, Lowe RD (1970): Evidence that the area postrema mediates the central cardiovascular response to Angiotensin II. *Nature* 228: 1303—1304.
69. Joy MD, (1971): The intramedullary connections of the area postrema involved in the central cardiovascular response to Angiotensin II. *Clin Sci* 41: 89—100.
70. Gildenberg PL, Ferrario CM, McCubbin JW (1973): Two sites of cardiovascular action of Angiotensin II in the brain of the dog. *Clin Sci* 44: 417—420.
71. Szilagyi JE, Ferrario CM (1981): Central opiate system modulation of the area postrema pressor pathway. *Hypertension* 3: 313—317.
72. Kosten T, Contreras RJ, Stetson PW, Ernest MJ (1983): Enhanced saline intake and decreased heart rate after area postrema ablations in rat. *Physiol Behav* 31: 777—785.
73. Carpenter DO, Briggs DB, Strominger N (1983): Responses of neurones of canine area postrema to neurotransmitters and peptides. *Cell Mol Biol* 3: 113—126.
74. Baum T, Shropshire AT (1975): Inhibition of efferent sympathetic nerve activity by 5-hydroxytryptophan and centrally administered 5-hydroxytryptamine. *Neuropharmacol* 14: 227—233.
75. Kircheim HR (1976): Systemic arterial baroreceptor reflexes. *Physiol rev* 56: 100—176.

XX. The role of 5-hydroxytryptamine in the regulation of sympathetic nerve discharge

ROBERT B. McCALL

1. Introduction

A large amount of evidence has accumulated to indicate that central serotonergic (5-hydroxytryptamine, 5-HT) neurons participate in the regulation of sympathetic nerve discharge (SND) and, therefore, blood pressure. Areas of the brain stem and spinal cord involved in vasomotor control are heavily innervated by 5-HT neurons [1, 2]. The area of the midline medulla that contains 5-HT neurons which project to autonomic nuclei corresponds to the classic medullary depressor region [3]. The close association between 5-HT descending neurons and midline sites that elicit vasodepressor responses when electrically stimulated has led to the conclusion that descending 5-HT medullospinal pathways inhibit sympathetic preganglionic neurons [4—7]. The findings that stimulation of presumed 5-HT-containing axons in the dorsolateral funiculus of the spinal cord inhibits sympathetic activity supports this hypothesis [8]. Early pharmacological studies based on the effects of 5-HT precursors and synthesis inhibitors support the concept that 5-HT neurons normally inhibit transmission in central sympathetic pathways. For example, administration of the 5-HT precursor 5-hydroxytryptophan results in a decrease in mean arterial blood pressure (MAP), heart rate (HR) and SND [9]. Furthermore, precursor administration produces a dose-dependent depression of spinal sympathetic reflexes. Taken together, these data suggest that central 5-HT neurons inhibit sympathetic neurons. However, a great deal of data generated in our laboratory suggests that 5-HT neurons excite rather than inhibit sympathetic neurons in the central nervous system. This chapter is intended to review this data with particular emphasis paid to the type of 5-HT receptor subtypes involved in the regulation of sympathetic neurons.

P.R. Saxena, D.I. Wallis, W. Wouters and P. Bevan (eds), Cardiovascular Pharmacology of 5-Hydroxytryptamine, pp. 271—283.

2. 5-HT neurons excite sympathetic nerve activity

In an early study in our laboratory we investigated the effects of the 5-HT antagonists methysergide, metergoline, cyproheptadine and cinanserin on MAP, HR and spontaneous SND [10]. We found that these compounds produced a dose-related decrease in MAP, HR and SND. The fact that these compounds reduced preganglionic as well as postganglionic sympathetic activity indicated that they acted in the central nervous system to produce their sympatholytic actions. The 5-HT antagonists failed to inhibit SND in animals which had been depleted of brain 5-HT by pretreatment with the 5-HT synthesis inhibitor p-chlorophenylalanine [10]. Similarly, methysergide had no affect on SND in animals in which the midline medulla (site of 5-HT cell bodies projecting to the cord) had been lesioned [11]. These data indicate that methysergide, metergoline, cyproheptadine and cinanserin reduced SND via their common ability to antagonize 5-HT receptors. Since these agents block the excitatory but not the inhibitory effects of microionto-phoretically applied 5-HT in the central nervous system [12], these data support the hypothesis that 5-HT neurons excite central sympathetic neurons.

3. Site of excitatory effects of 5-HT

One site at which this 5-HT excitatory interaction may occur is at the level of sympathetic preganglionic neurons (SPNs) located in the intermediolateral cell column of the spinal cord. In this regard, 5-HT neurons in the midline medulla (i.e. nucleus raphe (n.r.) obscurus, n.r. pallidus and n.r. magnus) heavily innervate SPNs [13, 14]. Therefore we initiated a study to determine the effects of microiontophoretically applied 5-HT on SPNs. We found that iontophoretic 5-HT consistently excited sympathetic preganglionic neurons [15]. This effect was blocked by either intravenous or iontophoretically applied methysergide or metergoline. These data suggest that 5-HT neurons excite SPNs and that the receptors mediating this excitation are sensitive to methysergide and metergoline. Interestingly, we found that the 5-HT antagonists decreased the spontaneous discharge rate of SPNs in intact cats but not in spinally transected animals. These data provide strong evidence to suggest that medullary 5-HT neurons provide a tonic excitatory input to SPNs and are necessary, at least in the anesthetized cat, to maintain the firing rate of these sympathetic neurons.

The above data suggests that medullospinal 5-HT neurons provide a tonic excitatory input to SPNs. The problem with this conclusion, however, is that electrical stimulation of the area of the midline medulla which contains these medullospinal 5-HT neurons typically elicits an inhibition of sympathetic nerve activity [3—7, 16]. In order to resolve these apparent contradictory findings, we initiated a study in which we electrically stimulated the midline medulla and searched for sites which elicited pressor responses as well as the more commonly observed depressor responses [16]. High frequency electrical stimulation of the midline area produced both pressor and depressor responses. Single shock stimulation elicited an excitatory evoked potential recorded from the inferior cardiac nerve. Conduction velocity in the descending medullospinal pathway was calculated to be 1.24 m/s. This value is consistent with it being mediated by small unmyelinated fibers such as 5-HT containing axons. Intravenous or intrathecal administration of the 5-HT antagonists methysergide or metergoline blocked the excitation of sympathetic activity evoked from medullary raphe nuclei. In contrast, these agents failed to alter the sympathoexcitatory response to electrical stimulation of lateral medulla pressor sites or the sympathoinhibitory response elicited by raphe stimulation. The 5-HT uptake inhibitor chlorimipramine increased the duration of the sympathoexcitatory response evoked from the raphe but not from the rostral ventrolateral medulla [16]. Finally, we demonstrated that the sympathoinhibitory response elicited by stimulation of the midline medulla was mediated by GABA [17]. The GABAergic inhibition occurs at the level of sympathoexcitatory medullospinal neurons located in the rostral ventrolateral medulla [18]. Taken together, these data indicate that 5-HT neurons provide a tonic excitatory input to neurons in the central nervous system involved in the regulation of sympathetic nerve activity.

4. Nature of 5-HT receptors involved

Although the data described above indicate that 5-HT neurons facilitate central sympathetic neurons, very little is known about the nature of the 5-HT receptors that mediate this excitatory interaction. Therefore, we initiated a study to investigate the effects of $5-HT_{1A}$, $5-HT_{1B}$ and $5-HT_2$ agonists and $5-HT_2$ antagonists on MAP, HR and SND [19]. In an early study in our laboratory we found that 5-methoxy-dimethyl-tryptamine and lisuride produced dose dependent decreases in MAP, HR and SND [10]. With the advent of 5-HT receptor subtype classification, these two compounds were found to be potent $5-HT_{1A}$ agonists. Therefore, we determined the effects of the selective $5-HT_{1A}$ agonist 8-hydroxydipropylamino-tetralin (8-OH-DPAT) on MAP, HR and SND. Figure 1 illustrates polygraph tracings of a typical response to intravenous administration of 8-OH-DPAT. The lowest dose of 8-OH-DPAT (10 μg/kg) produced a marked fall in arterial blood pressure and SND. In a similar fashion, HR declined, but the decrease was not as profound (Figure 1A). The onset of the reduction of MAP, HR and SND after 8-OH-DPAT was rapid (i.e. < 1 min) and reached a maximum within 5 min. Larger doses of 8-OH-DPAT resulted in an almost complete inhibition in SND and further declines in MAP and HR (Figure 1B). Figure 1C illustrates the dose-response relationship for the effects of 8-OH-DPAT on MAP, HR and inferior cardiac SND. Low doses of 8-OH-

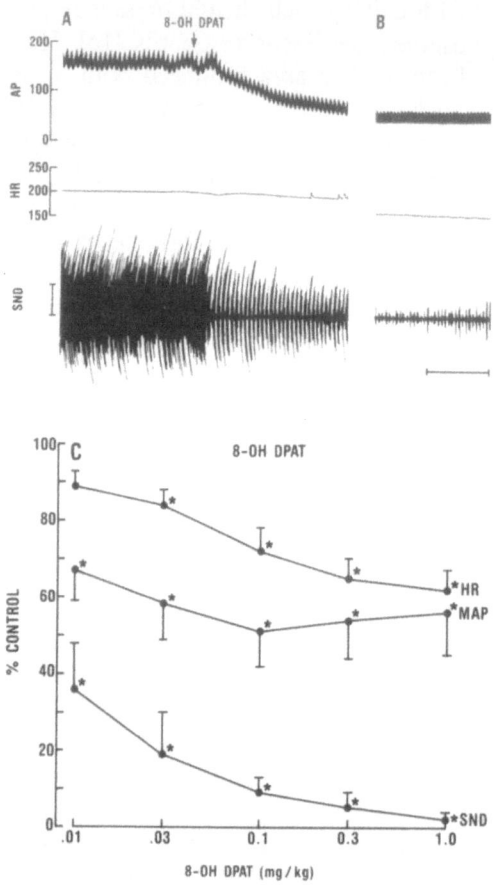

Figure 1. Effects of 8-OH-DPAT on arterial blood pressure (AP), heart rate (HR) and inferior cardiac SND. Panel A: 10 μg/kg, i.v. of 8-OH-DPAT administered at arrow reduces AP, HR and SND. Panel B: 10 min after 0.1 mg/kg, i.v. of 8-OH-DPAT. Panel C: dose-response curve illustrating effects of 8-OH-DPAT on MAP, HR and SND. Horizontal calibration is 1 min. Vertical calibration is 60 μV.

DPAT (0.01 mg/kg, i.v.) significantly reduced MAP and SND. Maximum reductions in MAP, HR and SND were 49, 38 and 96% of pretreatment values, respectively. Similarly, 8-OH-DPAT decreased SND recorded from the preganglionic splanchnic nerve indicating that the sympatholytic effect of 8-OH-DPAT is mediated in the central nervous system. Two observations indicate that the effects of 8-OH-DPAT resulted from the drug's 5-HT$_{1A}$ agonist properties. First, like 8-OH-DPAT, a second chemically distinct 5-HT$_{1A}$ agonist, p-aminophenyl-ethyl-m-trifluoromethylphenyl piperazine (PAPP), produced significant dose-related decreases in MAP, HR and SND [19]. Second, the 5-HT$_{1A}$ antagonist spiperone reversed the central sympatholytic effects produced by 8-OH-DPAT. Taken together, these data indicate that activation of 5-HT_{1A} receptors in the central nervous system leads to an inhibition of sympathetic nerve activity.

The effects of the 5-HT_{1B} agonists 1-[3-(trifluoromethyl)phenyl]-piperazine (TFMPP), 1-(3-chlorophenyl) piperazine (mCPP) and 1-(2-methoxyphenyl) piperazine (2-MPP) on MAP, HR and SND were also investigated [19]. Intravenous administration of these agents (0.01—1.0 mg/kg) had minimal effects of MAP and HR. The largest dose of these compounds all significantly increased SND. The most striking feature of the sympathetic effects of 5-HT_{1B} agonists was the huge variability in the response of SND. For example, TFMPP decreased SND by 75% in two animals while increasing activity by 144% in four animals. The inconsistent effects of 5-HT_{1B} agonists and their lack of efficacy suggest that 5-HT_{1B} receptors do not play an important role in the serotonergic regulation of sympathetic neurons.

We utilized the 5-HT_2 agonist 1-(2,5-dimethoxy-4-iodophenyl)-2-amino-propane (DOI) and the 5-HT_2 antagonists ketanserin and LY 53857 to investigate the role of 5-HT_2 receptors in the interactions between 5-HT and sympathetic neurons [19]. The effect of DOI on inferior cardiac SND is illustrated in Figure 2. Administration of a single dose of DOI (1 mg/kg) produced an increase in arterial blood pressure and a massive increase in SND (Figure 2A). MAP returned to pretreatment levels within twenty minutes but sympathetic nerve discharge remained elevated by an average of 938% in 5 experiments. Heart rate was initially depressed as the drug was administered but rapidly returned to pretreatment levels. The selective 5-HT_2 receptor antagonist ketanserin (1 mg/kg, i.v.) reversed the increase in sympathetic nerve discharge produced by DOI (Figure 2A, B; n = 3). Similarly, LY 53857 (1 mg/kg, i.v.) also reversed the sympathoexcitatory effect of DOI (Figure 2C; n = 5).

Figure 2 also illustrates the cumulative dose response effects of DOI on sympathetic nerve discharge alone and in animals pretreated with the selective 5-HT_2 receptor antagonists ketanserin (Figure 2A, B) or LY 53857 (Figure 2C). DOI (0.01—1.0 mg/kg) produced a dose related increase in spontaneous sympathetic nerve discharge (n = 9). DOI failed to increase sympathetic nerve discharge at all tested doses (0.01—1.0 mg/kg, i.v.) in animals pretreated with ketanserin (1 mg/kg, i.v., n = 5, Figure 2A). In contrast, DOI significantly increased sympathetic nerve discharge in animals pretreated with the alpha$_1$-adrenoceptor antagonist prazosin (1 mg/kg, i.v.). Like ketanserin, LY 53857 (1 mg/kg, i.v.) blocked the increase in sympathetic nerve discharge produced by DOI. These data indicate that DOI increases SND as a result of its 5-HT_2 receptor agonist properties.

Since DOI increases SND, it might be expected that the 5-HT_2 receptor antagonist ketanserin would decrease SND. Indeed, previous studies in our laboratory demonstrated that ketanserin acted centrally to inhibit SND [20]. In order to determine whether ketanserin inhibited SND as a result of its alpha$_1$-adrenoceptor or its 5-HT_2 receptor blocking properties, animals were pretreated with a large dose of prazosin and then given ketanserin. In this

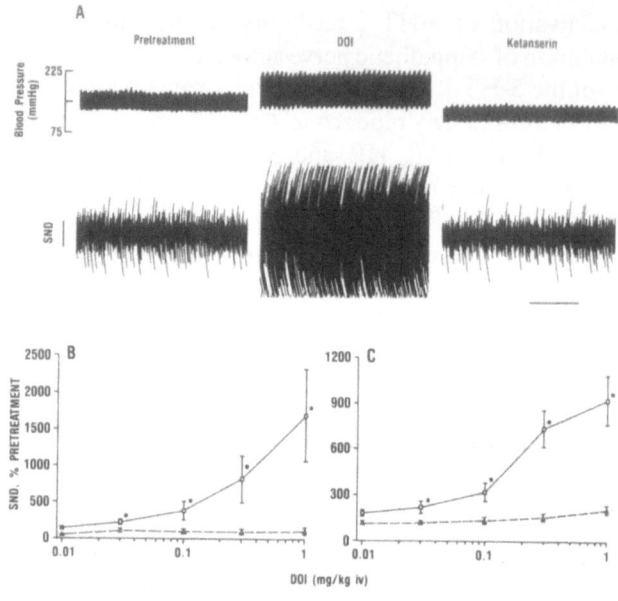

Figure 2. Panel A: Reversal of the sympathoexcitatory effect of DOI by ketanserin. Traces from top to bottom are blood pressure, heart rate and SND, respectively. Doses of DOI and ketanserin are 1 mg/kg i.v. Vertical calibration is 80 μV. Horizontal calibration is 1 min. Panels B and C: cumulative dose-response curve of DOI in the presence (squares) and absence (triangles) of a 1 mg/kg i.v. pretreatment dose of ketanserin (panel B) and LY 53857 (panel C).

regard we have previously shown that alpha$_1$-adrenoceptor antagonists (e.g. prazosin) act centrally to reduce SND [21]. We found that prazosin pretreatment completely prevented the central sympatholytic action of ketanserin [22]. These data suggest that the sympatholytic effect of ketanserin is a result of the ability of the drug to block alpha$_1$-adrenoceptors rather than 5-HT$_2$ receptors. In order to further test this hypothesis, we studied the effects of the highly selective 5-HT$_2$ antagonist LY 53857 on SND [22]. In contrast to ketanserin, LY 53857 (0.1–3.0 mg/kg, i.v.) failed to affect arterial blood pressure, heart rate or SND. These data provide strong evidence to indicate that blockade of 5-HT$_2$ receptors does not result in an inhibition of spontaneous SND. In addition, these data coupled with the observation that DOI increases SND via a 5-HT$_2$ receptor, suggest that the 5-HT$_2$ receptors which mediate the sympathoexcitatory effect of DOI do not normally receive a 5-HT input in the anesthetized cat.

As described in the beginning of this chapter, the role of 5-HT in the regulation of sympathetic nerve discharge and, therefore, blood pressure has long been a controversial subject. Many early pharmacoloical studies suggest that 5-HT increases sympathetic nerve discharge and blood pressure while other investigations have reached the opposite conclusion (see Kuhn [9]). We found that 5-HT$_{1A}$ agonists act centrally to inhibit sympathetic nerve discharge [19]. Similar observations have been made by Fozard and coworkers [23, 24]. As described above, activation of 5-HT$_2$ receptors increase sympathetic nerve discharge. Thus one subset of central nervous system 5-HT receptors (i.e. 5-HT$_{1A}$) can inhibit sympathetic nerve discharge while a second subset of receptors (i.e. 5-HT$_2$) can increase sympathetic nerve discharge. It is possible that the opposing effects of activation of 5-HT$_{1A}$ and 5-HT$_2$ receptors on sympathetic nerve discharge may help to explain much of the earlier controversial pharmacological data. Thus, the effect of administration of 5-HT precursors or 5-HT agonists would depend on the net activation of 5-HT$_{1A}$ and 5-HT$_2$ receptors.

5. Studies on the mechanism of the sympatholytic action of 8-OH-DPAT

The fact that 8-OH-DPAT inhibits SND indicates that activation of 5-HT$_{1A}$ receptors results in an inhibition of central sympathetic neurons. A large body of evidence exists to indicate that microiontophoretically applied 5-HT has a powerful inhibitory action of the firing rate of 5-HT neurons in dorsal raphe nucleus [12]. These studies suggest that receptor sites sensitive to 5-HT are located on 5-HT neurons. These receptors have been termed "autoreceptors" since they mediate the response of a 5-HT neuron to its own transmitter [12]. More recent studies suggest that the 5-HT "autoreceptor" may be identical to the 5-HT$_{1A}$ receptor [25]. Since our data supports the concept that medullary 5-HT neurons tonically excite SPNs, we hypothesized that 8-OH-DPAT produced its central sympatholytic action by inhibiting the firing of medullary 5-HT neurons and thereby disfacilitating SND. In order to test this hypothesis we initiated a study to record the extracellular discharges of 5-HT neurons located in n.r. obscurus and n.r. pallidus. Previous studies have attempted to electrophysiologically identify medullary 5-HT neurons using criteria such as: (1) axonal conduction velocity of less than 12 m/s [26, 27], 2) spontaneous discharge rates of less than 3 spikes/s [26, 27], 3) shape and duration of the action potential [28, 29], 4) regular discharge rate [28, 30] or 5) relative lack of sensitivity to LSD [29–31]. These criteria lack specificity and likely apply to the discharge of large numbers of neurons in the central nervous system. Therefore we used a more rigorous set of criteria fashioned after the discharge and pharmacologic characteristics of identified 5-HT neurons in the dorsal raphe nucleus [12, 32, 33] to identify medullary 5-HT neurons. Using extracellular recording techniques, we identified a group of midline medullary neurons which had characteristics that were nearly identical to those of dorsal raphe 5-HT neurons [34]. Several observations indicate that these neurons were medullary 5-HT neurons. First, these neurons fired in an extremely regular manner. Dorsal raphe 5-HT neurons are also characterized by an extremely regular discharge pattern [12, 33]. Second, the mean discharge rate of regularly firing medullary neurons was 1.2 ± 0.1 spikes/s. The small standard error indicates that there was very little variation in the discharge rate of these neurons. Similarly, dorsal raphe cells are characterized by their 1 spike/s discharge rate. Again, the variability in dorsal raphe 5-HT firing is very small [12]. Third, the spike duration of regularly firing medullary neurons and dorsal raphe 5-HT neurons is similar (i.e. 2 ms, [12, 35]). Fourth, the regularly firing medullary units did not receive a significant baroreceptor input. This is demonstrated by a lack of probability of discharging in a portion of the cardiac cycle, by a negative spike triggered average of inferior cardiac SND and by a lack of effect on the neuronal firing rate during an increase in blood pressure produced by occlusion of the descending aorta. Similarly, 5-HT neurons in the dorsal raphe do not receive a significant baroreceptor input [35]. Fifth, regularly firing medullary raphe neurons could be antidromically activated by electrical stimulation of the intermediolateral cell column of the spinal cord. Anatomically, it has been shown that medullary 5-HT neurons project to the intermediolateral cell column [2, 13, 14]. We found that the axonal conduction velocity of descending regularly firing neurons was 1.3 m/s. The axonal conduction velocity of dorsal raphe 5-HT neurons ranges from 0.3—1.5 m/s [32]. The slow conduction velocity of these neurons is consistent with the small diameter of unmyelinated 5-HT fibers. Finally dorsal raphe 5-HT neurons are extremely sensitive to the inhibitory effects of microiontophoretically applied 5-HT [12]. The inhibitory effect of 5-HT are thought to be mediated via a 5-HT autoreceptor [12]. We found that microiontophoretic application of 5-HT produced a marked inhibition in the firing of the regularly discharging medullary units [34]. The small ejecting currents required to produce the inhibition attest to the sensitivity of these neurons to and 5-HT. Taken together, these data suggest that regularly firing, 5-HT sensitive medullospinal neurons were 5-HT neurons.

In order to test our hypothesis that 8-OH-DPAT produced its central sympatholytic action by inhibiting the firing of medullary 5-HT neurons, we determined the effect of 8-OH-DPAT on the firing rate of medullary 5-HT neurons (Figure 3) [34]. Intravenous 8-OH-DPAT inhibited the discharges of medullary 5-HT neurons. A dose of 1 μg/kg of 8-OH-DPAT reduced the unitary firing by approximately 50%. A total of 2 μg/kg of 8-OH-DPAT typically completely inhibited these neurons (Figure 3a). Similarly, a dose of 1 μg/kg of 8-OH-DPAT reduces firing of dorsal raphe 5-HT neurons by 50%. 8-OH-DPAT was microiontophoretically applied in order to determine if the drug acted directly on 5-HT neurons. The rate histograms in Figure 3B characterize the response of regularly firing medullary raphe units to microiontophoretic application of 8-OH-DPAT and 5-HT. Microiontophoresis of 8-OH-DPAT and 5-HT consistently inhibited the discharges of 5-HT neurons. The inhibitory effect of 8-OH-DPAT was of long duration and the firing rate of the neuron failed to return to the original discharge rate. The ejecting currents of 8-OH-DPAT required to produce an inhibition of firing

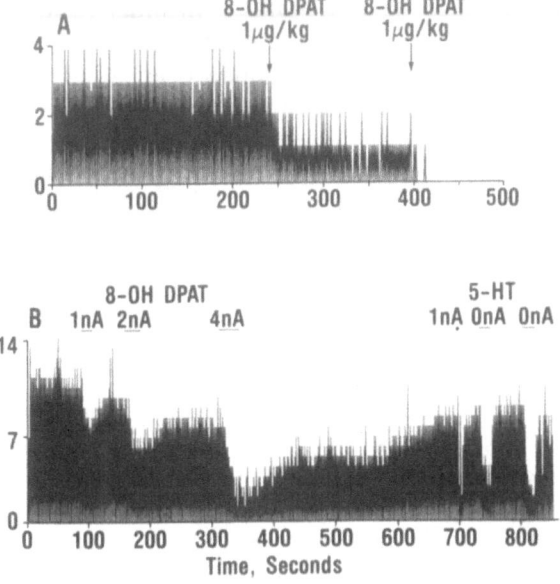

Figure 3. Panel A: Rate histogram illustrating the effects of intravenous 8-OH-DPAT on the firing rate of a medullary 5-HT neuron. Arrows mark injections. 4 ms bins. Panel B: Rate historgram depicting inhibitory effects of microiontophoretically applied 8-OH-DPAT and 5-HT.

were typically quite low (1—4 nA). Microiontophoretically applied 8-OH-DPAT inhibited every 5-HT neuron tested. 5-HT neurons responded to increasing iontophoretic 8-OH-DPAT ejecting currents with an increase in the maximum inhibition and a prolongation in the time to recovery (Figure 3B). The cell represented by the histogram in Figure 3B was also extremely sensitive to 5-HT, responding with an inhibition of firing following discontinuation of the retaining current (i.e. ejecting current 0 nA). All 5-HT neurons tested were inhibited by iontophoretic 5-HT. The largest ejecting current required to produce inhibition was 5 nA.

The above data indicate that 8-OH-DPAT inhibits the discharges of medullary 5-HT neurons which project to SPNs in the intermediolateral cell column of the spinal cord. This supports the hypothesis that 8-OH-DPAT acts centrally to inhibit SND by inhibiting 5-HT firing and thereby removing an excitatory input to SPNs. However, caution should be taken in arriving at this conclusion. We found that a dose of 1 μg/kg, i.v. of 8-OH-DPAT reduced 5-HT neuronal firing by 50%. A 2 μg/kg dose of the drug totally inhibited the discharges of these neurons. In contrast, the dose respone curve illustrated in Figure 1B shows that 10 μg/kg, i.v. of 8-OH-DPAT was required to reduce SND by 50%. SND was totally inhibited at doses of 8-OH-DPAT between 30 and 100 μg/kg. Thus 5-HT neurons are much more sensitive to the inhibitory effects of 8-OH-DPAT than is SND. These data suggests that inhibition of 5-HT neuronal firing does not contribute to the sympatholytic action of 8-OH-DPAT. In order to test this hypothesis more critically, 5-HT neuronal firing and inferior cardiac SND were simultaneously recorded and the inhibitory effect of 8-OH-DPAT was determined (n = 14). Figure 4 illustrates a representative experiment. The oscillographic traces of unitary activity (Figure 4, bottom trace) show that several neurons were found in the recording field. The large unit was identified as being a 5-HT neuron using the criteria described above. The lowest dose of 8-OH-DPAT (1 μg/kg, i.v.) reduced 5-HT neuronal firing by approximately 50% but had no obvious effects on SND. Increasing the dose of 8-OH-DPAT to a total of 2 μg/kg, i.v. resulted in an almost complete inhibition of 5-HT neuronal firing but had little affect on SND. SND and arterial blood pressure appeared to be obviously decreased by a cumulative dose of 10 μg/kg, i.v. and markedly affected by the 30 μg/kg, i.v. dose of 8-OH-DPAT. These data provide strong evidence to indicate that direct inhibition of medullospinal 5-HT neuronal firing is not sufficient to explain the central sympatholytic effects of 8-OH-DPAT. Rather, these data suggest that 8-OH-DPAT is acting postsynaptically to inhibit SND.

Recently, we have investigated the effects of 8-OH-DPAT on the firing rates of SPNs in the intermediolateral cell column and medullospinal sympathoexcitatory neurons located in the rostral ventrolateral medulla. We found that microiontophoretically applied 8-OH-DPAT failed to alter the firing rates of SPNs but blocked the excitatory effects of microiontophoretic 5-HT. Thus, 8-OH-DPAT acts as a 5-HT antagonist at the level of SPNs (unpublished observation). The importance of this action 8-OH-DPAT in the hypotensive action of the compound remains to be determined. In addition, we have found that intravenous 8-OH-DPAT inhibits the firing medul-

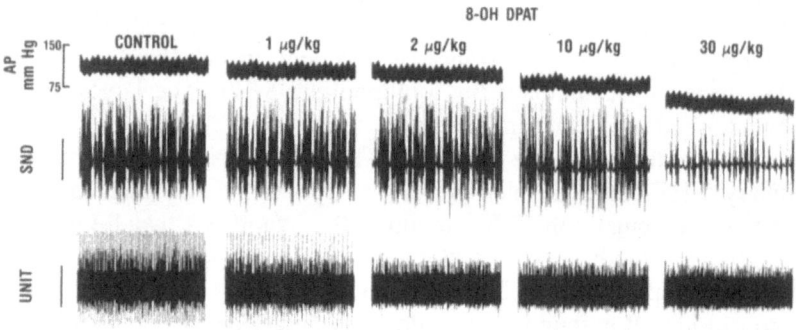

Figure 4. Effects of 8-OH-DPAT on arterial pressure (AP), sympathetic nerve discharge (SND) and medullary 5-HT neuronal firing (unit). Largest amplitude unit in recording field was determined to be a 5-HT neuron (lower trace). Low doses of 8-OH-DPAT (1—2 μg/kg, i.v.) markedly depressed the firing rate of the 5-HT neuron but had little effect on blood pressure or SND. Larger doses of 8-OH-DPAT (10—30 μg/kg, i.v.) were required to depress blood pressure and SND. Horizontal calibration is 1 min. Vertical calibration is 70 μV for SND and 50 μ V for unit.

lospinal sympathoexcitatory neurons located in the rostral ventrolateral medulla in a dose-related manner. The inhibition of sympathoexcitatory neuronal firing is directly correlated to the inhibition of sympathetic activity recorded from the inferior cardiac nerve (unpublished observations). These data, coupled with the observation that microinjection of 8-OH-DPAT into the rostral ventrolateral medulla lowers arterial blood pressure (Gillis, personal communication) suggests that 8-OH-DPAT may act postsynaptically on medullospinal sympathoexcitatory neurons in the rostral ventrolateral medulla to produce its hypotensive effect.

6. Conclusion

In summary, available data indicates that 5-HT neurons in the midline medulla provide a tonic excitatory input to SPNs located in the intermediolateral cell column of the spinal cord. The data is consistent with the idea that 5-HT is acting as a neuromodulator to set the level of excitability of SPNs rather than relaying sympathetic information over a functionally specific pathway from brain stem to spinal cord. In this regard, it appears that these 5-HT neurons do not receive significant inputs from baroreceptors or from other central sympathetic pathways. Activation of $5-HT_{1A}$ receptors leads to inhibition of SND while activation of $5-HT_2$ receptors results in an increase in SND. This observation may help to explain many of the early contradictory results regarding the role of 5-HT in cardiovascular regulation. Finally, the available data suggests that 8-OH-DPAT may be acting postsynaptically, possibly at the level of descending sympathoexcitatory neurons located in the rostral ventrolateral medulla, to produce its sympatholytic effects.

References

1. Fuxe K (1965): Evidence for the existence of monoamine neurons in the CNS. IV. The distribution of monoamine terminals in the CNS. *Acta Physiol Scand* 64 (suppl. 247): 38—85.
2. Bobillier P, Sequin S, Petitjean F, Salvert D, Touret M, Jouvet M (1976): The raphe nuclei of the cat brain stem: A topographical atlas of their efferent projections as revealed by autoradiography. *Brain Res* 113: 449—486.
3. Wang SC, Ranson SW (1939): Autonomic responses to electrical stimulation of the lower brain stem. *J Comp Neurol* 71: 437—455.
4. Cabot JB, Wild J, Cohen DN (1979): Raphe inhibition of sympathetic preganglionic neurons. *Science* 203: 184—186.
5. Coote JH, Macleod VH (1974): The influence of bulbospinal monoaminergic pathways on sympathetic nerve activity. *J Physiol* (London) 241: 453—475.
6. Gilbey MP, Coote JH, Macleod VH, Peterson DF (1981): Inhibition of sympathetic activity by stimulating in the raphe nuclei and the role of 5-hydroxytryptamine in this effect. *Brain Res* 226: 131—142.

7. Howe PRC (1985): Blood pressure control by neurotransmitters in the medulla oblongata and spinal cord. *J Auton Nerv Syst* 12: 95—115.

8. Coote JH, Macleod VH (1975): The spinal route of sympathoinhibitory pathways descending from the medulla. *Pflugers Arch* 359: 335—347.

9. Kuhn DM, Wolf WA, Lovenberg W (1980): Review of the role of the central serotonergic neuronal system in blood pressure. *Hypertension* 2: 243—255.

10. McCall RB, Humphrey SJ (1982): Involvement of serotonin in the central regulation of blood pressure: evidence for a facilitation effect on sympathetic nerve activity. *J Pharmacol exp Therap* 222: 94—102.

11. McCall RB, Harris LT (1987): Sympathetic alterations after midline medullary raphe lesions. *Am J Physiol* 253: R91—R107.

12. Aghajanian GK, Wang RY (1978): Physiology and pharmacology of central serotonergic neurons, pp. 171—183 in: Lipton MA, DiMascio A, Killam KF (eds), *Psychopharmacology: A Generation of Progress*. New York: Raven Press.

13. Loewy AD (1981): Raphe pallidus and raphe obscurus projections to the intermediolateral cell column in the rat. *Brain Res* 222: 129—133.

14. Loewy AD, McKellar S (1981): Serotonergic projections from the ventral medulla to the intermediolateral cell column in the rat. *Brain Res* 211: 146—152.

15. McCall RB (1983): Serotonergic excitation of sympathetic preganglionic neurons: a microiontophoretic study. *Brain Res* 289: 121—127.

16. McCall RB (1984): Evidence for a serotonergically mediated sympathoexcitatory response to stimulation of medullary raphe nuclei. *Brain Res* 311: 131—139.

17. McCall RB, Humphrey SJ (1985): Evidence for GABA mediation of sympathetic inhibition evoked from midline medullary depressor sites. *Brain Res* 339: 356—361.

18. McCall RB (1988): GABA-mediated inhibition of sympathoexcitatory neurons by midline medullary stimulation. *Am J Physiol* 225: in press.

19. McCall RB, Patel BN, Harris LT (1987): Effects of serotonin$_1$ and serotonin$_2$ receptor agonists and antagonists on blood pressure, heart rate and sympathetic nerve activity. *J Pharmacol exp Therap* 242: 1152—1159.

20. McCall RB, Schuette MR (1984): Evidence for the alpha-1 receptor-mediated central sympathoinhibitory action of ketanserin. *J Pharmacol exp Therap* 228: 704—710.

21. McCall RB, Humphrey SJ (1981): Evidence for a central depressor action of postsynaptic alpha-1 adrenergic antagonists. *J Auton Nerv Syst* 3: 9—23.

22. McCall RB, Harris LT (1987): Characterization of the central sympathoinhibitory action of ketanserin. *J Pharmacol exp Therap* 241: 736—740.

23. Fozard JR, Mir AK, Middlemiss DN (1987): The cardiovascular response to 8-hydroxy-2-(di-n-propylamino)tetralin (8-OH-DPAT) in the rat: site of action and pharmacological analysis. *J Cardiovasc Pharmacol* 9: 328—347.

24. Ramage AG, Fozard JR (1987): Evidence that the putative 5-HT^1_A receptor agonists, 8-OH-DPAT and isapirone, have a central hypotensive action that differs from that of clonidine in anaesthetized cats. *Europ J Pharmacol* 138: 179—191.

25. Verge D, Daval G, Patey A, Gozlan H, El Mestikaway S, Hamon M (1985): Presynaptic 5-HT autoreceptors on serotonergic cell bodies and/or dendrites but not terminals are of the 5-HT$_{1A}$ subtype. *European J Pharmacol* 113: 463—464.

26. Chiang CY, Pan ZZ (1985): Differential responses of serotonergic and non-serotonergic neurons in nucleus raphe magnus to systemic morphine in rats. *Brain Research* 337: 146—150.

27. Wei JB, Chiang CC (1986): Responses of serotonergic and non-serotonergic neurons in the rat nucleus raphe magnus to systemic lysergic acid diethylamide. *Neuroscience Research* 3: 268—273.

28. Heym J, Steinfels GF, Jacobs BL (1982): Activity of serotonin-containing neurons in the nucleus raphe pallidus of freely moving cats. *Brain Research* 251: 259—276.

29. Wessendorf MW, Anderson EG (1983): Single unit studies of identified bulbospinal serotonergic units. *Brain Research* 279: 93—103.

30. Heym J, Steinfels GF, Jacobs BL (1982): Medullary serotonergic neurons are insensitive to 5-MeODMT and LSD. *European J Pharmacol* 81: 677—680.
31. Jacobs BL, Heym J, Rasmussen K (1983): Raphe neurons: firing rate correlates with size of drug response. *European J Pharmacol* 90: 275—278.
32. Wang RY, Aghajanian GK (1977): Antidromically identified serotonergic neurons in the rat midbrain raphe: evidence for collateral inhibition. *Brain Research* 132: 186—193.
33. Wang RY, Aghajanian GK (1982): Correlative firing patterns of serotonergic neurons in rat dorsal raphe nucleus. *J Neuroscience* 2: 11—16.
34. McCall RB, Clement ME (1988): Identification of serotonergic and sympathetic neurons in medullary raphe nuclei. *Brain Research* 477: 172—182.
35. Morilak DA, Fornal C, Jacobs BL (1986): Single unit activity of noradrenergic neurons in locus coeruleus and serotonergic neurons in the nucleus raphe dorsalis of freely moving cats in relation to the cardiac cycle. *Brain Research* 399: 262—270.

XXI. 5-Hydroxytryptamine and related drugs and transmitter release from autonomic nerves in the cardiovascular system

M. GÖTHERT, K. FINK, G. MOLDERINGS and E. SCHLICKER

1. Introduction

Under in vivo conditions, 5-hydroxytryptamine (5-HT) and related drugs influence transmitter release from autonomic nerves in the cardiovascular system not only by acting on the sympathetic and parasympathetic nerve endings, but also by modifying ganglionic transmission [1] as well as central regulation of circulatory function [2, 3]. Within this framework, the present report will focus on effects of relevant drugs on the peripheral autonomic nerve endings, particularly those innervating cardiovascular tissues.

5-HT and related compounds produce both stimulatory and inhibitory effects on transmitter release and, as a rule, these effects are receptor-mediated; emphasis will be laid on such effects. The only exception which will be mentioned here is the receptor-independent 5-HT-induced noradrenaline (NA) release by a tyramine-like mechanism. Generally, effects of 5-HT and related drugs on transmitter release in cardiovascular tissue have been more extensively studied for noradrenergic than for cholinergic neurons.

2. Stimulation of transmitter release

2.1 *Noradrenergic neurons*

It is well established that 5-HT and other tryptamine derivatives can induce vasoconstriction or cardiac stimulation not only by acting postsynaptically but also by inducing release of NA from sympathetic nerve fibres in cardiovascular tissue. Such indirect sympathomimetic effects are mediated by two different mechanisms, one involving the neuronal uptake mechanism ("uptake$_1$") in a manner similar to tyramine and the other mediated by the 5-HT$_3$ receptor.

P.R. Saxena, D.I. Wallis, W. Wouters and P. Bevan (eds), Cardiovascular Pharmacology of 5-Hydroxytryptamine, pp. 285–294.
© 1990 *Kluwer Academic Publishers, Dordrecht* —

2.1.1 *"Tyramine-like" mechanism*

Since transport of 5-HT into the sympathetic nerve axon by the neuronal uptake mechanism and subsequent accumulation therein are prerequisites for the indirect sympathomimetic effect, a slow time course of NA release and, as a consequence, a slow time course of end organ response have been observed with 5-HT. High doses or concentrations of 5-HT are necessary to produce these effects. In many investigations NA was not measured directly, but the involvement of transmitter release was derived from the effects of appropriate pharmacological manipulations of end-organ responses. The 5-HT-induced cardiovascular responses can be abolished by: (1) antagonists of α-adrenoceptors (blood vessels) or β-adrenoceptors (heart), (2) relatively low doses/concentrations of neuronal uptake inhibitors, (3) depletion of neuronal NA stores or (4) surgical or chemical sympathectomy. On the other hand, the stimulant effect of 5-HT on NA release is resistant to: (1) omission of Ca^{2+} ions, (2) colchicine, which inhibits exocytosis, and (3) relatively low doses/concentrations of specific 5-HT (in particular, $5\text{-}HT_3$) receptor antagonists. By application of such pharmacological tools and of techniques for determination of end organ effects or by more direct evaluation of NA release (involving determination of radioactively labelled or endogenous NA), tyramine-like effects of 5-HT have been observed, e.g., in rat, dog, cat and human heart or blood vessels in vitro or in vivo [4, 5, 6, 7, 8].

Other hydroxylated tryptamine derivatives mimic 5-HT with respect to this type of indirect sympathomimetic effects. For instance, 6-hydroxytryptamine (6-HT) stimulates NA release in the perfused rabbit heart independently of 5-HT receptors, as suggested by the slow development of NA-releasing and positive chronotropic effects during continuous exposure to a constant 6-HT concentration [9]. The involvement of a tyramine-like mechanism is supported by the observations that desipramine abolished both the NA-releasing and positive chronotropic effects and, in contrast, pindolol only abolished the positive chronotropic response.

2.1.2 *Receptor-mediated stimulation*

That 5-HT itself induces positive chronotropic and inotropic effects in rabbit heart by an indirect sympathomimetic mechanism was already shown in 1960 by Trendelenburg [10] as well as Jacob and Poite-Bevierre [11]. Evidence for the involvement of a 5-HT receptor on rabbit cardiac sympathetic nerve terminals was presented more than 15 years later by Fozard and his coworkers [12, 13]; their conclusions were mainly based on determinations of the end-organ (positive chronotropic) responses to injection or infusion of 5-HT and other tryptamine derivatives (hearts perfused according to the Langendorff technique). Measurement of the overflow of endogenous noradrenaline into the perfusate provided further direct evidence for the suggested mechanisms [9, 14].

Important characteristics of this type of indirect sympathomimetic effect in the rabbit heart are: (1) the rapid onset of noradrenaline release and, consequently, of the end organ response, (2) its Ca^{2+}-dependence, (3) its blockade by colchicine, an inhibitor of exocytosis, (4) the rapid desensitization to 5-HT and some of its analogues, but not to tyramine, and (5) the failure of relatively low concentrations of desipramine (which attenuated the response to tyramine) to inhibit the effect of 5-HT [9, 12, 13, 14]. Furthermore, it is obvious that the NA-releasing and/or positive chronotropic response(s) to 5-HT and other 5-HT receptor agonists can be blocked by pharmacological tools suitable to disclose any indirect sympathomimetic effects irrespective of the underlying mechanism, namely β-adrenoceptor antagonists, pretreatment with reserpine or chemical sympathectomy by means of 6-hydroxydopamine [9, 12, 13, 14].

The pharmacological characterization of the presynaptic receptor assumed to be involved was first exclusively based on studies with agonists. Not only 5-HT but also, e.g., 5,6-dihydroxytryptamine (5,6-DHT), 5,7-dihydroxytryptamine (5,7-DHT), 7-hydroxytryptamine (7-HT), tryptamine (T) and N-methyl-5-hydroxytryptamine (N-CH$_3$-5-HT) concentration-dependently increase NA release and/or heart rate in response to bolus injection, whereas, e.g., 5-methoxytryptamine (5-OCH$_3$-T) and 5-methyltryptamine are ineffective [9, 13]. The relative potency order of the agonists (5-HT > 5,7-DHT > 5,6-DHT > T; 5-OCH$_3$-T ineffective) does not correspond to the pharmacological properties of 5-HT$_1$ or 5-HT$_2$ recognition sites. It should be noted that 2-methyl-5-hydroxytryptamine (2-CH$_3$-5-HT), which has a high affinity for 5-HT$_3$ binding sites [16, 17], is highly potent in eliciting tachycardia in the rabbit [18].

As already mentioned, rapid desensitization occurs in response to sustained presence of an agonist: continuous perfusion of rabbit hearts with medium containing 5-HT or 5,7-DHT produces a transient increase (maximum within the first 2 min of drug perfusion) in both NA release and heart rate (9, 14). When an indolethylamine such as 5-HT, 5,6-DHT, 7-HT or T is present in the perfusion fluid, the positive chronotropic effect of a 5-HT bolus is attenuated. The rank order of the compounds for their inhibitory potency is identical to that for their stimulant potency when applied as bolus. Excellent correlation exists between the desensitizing and stimulant potencies of the agonists (slope of the regression line close to 1) [9], suggesting that both effects are mediated by the same 5-HT receptor on the sympathetic nerve fibres.

It is of interest that the 5-HT-induced positive chronotropic effect can be blocked by general anaesthetics such as thiopental, halothane and diethyl ether at concentrations relevant to their anaesthetic effect and by rather low concentrations of ethanol [19]; the inhibition is not due to a postsynaptic site of action of these drugs. Their potencies in inhibiting 5-HT-induced tachycardia correlate with their lipophilic properties suggesting a hydrophobic interaction of the drugs with constituents of the neuronal cell membrane [19]. Another non-selective inhibitor of the 5-HT-induced NA release is mianserin [9].

The development of specific antagonists at the 5-HT receptor on the sympathetic nerve terminal was based on the observation that metoclopramide [20], (−)-cocaine and some cocain-related compounds [21] antagonized the [³H]NA—releasing and/or positive chronotropic response(s) to 5-HT. In search for more potent and selective derivatives of benzoic esters of tropine, the 5-HT₃ receptor antagonist MDL 72222 (1αH, 3α, 5αH-tropan-3-yl-3, 5-dichlorobenzoate) was synthesized which competitively antagonized the stimulant effect of 5-HT in the rabbit heart [22]. The receptor mediating the release of NA from rabbit cardiac sympathetic nerve terminals is therefore a 5-HT₃ receptor [see 23—25].

2.2 Cholinergic neurons

5-HT also seems to induce acetylcholine (ACh) release from postganglionic cholinergic nerves of the isolated rabbit heart; this effect is also blocked by MDL 72222 at concentrations similar to those antagonizing the stimulatory effect of 5-HT on NA release. This suggests that the cholinergic nerves are also endowed with stimulant 5-HT₃ receptors [1]. These receptors share with those on noradrenergic neurons the property to undergo rapid desensitization.

3. Inhibition of transmitter release

3.1 Noradrenergic neurons

Inhibition of electrically evoked [³H]NA release from the sympathetic nerves in an isolated blood vessel, namely the dog saphenous vein, was first described by McGrath [4]. Several groups of authors who used the same preparation confirmed and extended this observation [26, 27, 28, 29]. Thus, it was found that the inhibitory effect of 5-HT on [³H]NA release, as reflected by a decreased contractile response to transmural electrical stimulation [26, 27], is mimicked by methysergide (potency and maximum effect less than those of 5-HT), and is not antagonized by cyproheptadine or phentolamine [27]. In several experiments the end organ response has been used to indirectly determine effects of 5-HT receptor ligands on NA release. The extent of inhibition by 5-HT is inversely related to the frequency and number of electrical impulses applied and to the Ca^{2+} concentration in the super-fusion fluid [26]; these results are compatible with the idea that 5-HT decreases the availability of Ca^{2+} ions for stimulus-release coupling in the varicosities. Despite the ineffectiveness of the 5-HT receptor antagonists investigated in the above studies [4, 26, 27], the involvement of a 5-HT receptor was likely in view of, e.g., the high potency of 5-HT and the effectiveness of methysergide which posesses partial agonistic properties at certain 5-HT receptors [23]. Furthermore the existence of an inhibitory 5-HT receptor on the sympathetic nerve terminals was strongly supported by the findings that various tryptamine derivatives share with 5-HT the ability to inhibit NA release [28] and, above all, that the 5-HT receptor antagonist methiothepin counteracts the 5-HT-induced inhibition [29]. This antagonism was also observed in the dog coronary [30] and tibial arteries [31], the rat vena cava [8] and renal vascular bed [32] and the human saphenous vein [33]. A synopsis of the cardiovascular tissues and species in which such presynaptic inhibitory 5-HT receptors have so far been identified is given in Table 1.

What are the pharmacological properties of this receptor or, in other words, how can it be classified? In canine, rat and human blood vessels, the involvement of a "$5-HT_1$" receptor was derived from the observations that methiothepin, which blocks both $5-HT_1$ and $5-HT_2$ receptors, antagonizes the 5-HT-induced inhibition of NA release, but the selective $5-HT_2$ receptor antagonist ketanserin does not [8, 30, 32, 33]. Attempts to provide a more detailed classification were made in the rat vena cava and renal vascular bed and in the human saphenous vein.

In the rat vena cava, not only 5-HT but also the "$5-HT_1$" receptor

Table 1. Occurrence of inhibitory presynaptic 5-HT receptors on the sympathetic nerves of cardiovascular tissue.

Species and tissue investigated	References
Rat	
Iliac artery	[34]
Vena cava	[8, 35]
Renal vascular bed	[32]
Heart	[8, 36]
Guinea pig	
Atrium	[37, 38]
Dog	
Tibial artery	[4, 31]
Femoral arterial circulation	[39]
Saphenous vein	[4, 26, 29]
Coronary artery	[30]
Heart	[40, 41]
Pig	
Coronary artery	[42]
Man	
Saphenous vein	[33]

agonists, 5-carboxamidotryptamine (5-CT) and 5-methoxy-3(1,2,3,6-tetra-hydropyridine-4-yl)-1H indole (RU 24969) as well as 4 other non-selective 5-HT receptor agonists inhibited [³H]-NA release; their potencies were correlated with their affinities for 5-HT$_{1B}$ (but not 5-HT$_{1A}$, 5-HT$_{1C}$ and 5-HT$_2$) binding sites. The 5-HT$_{1A}$ receptor agonist ipsapirone and 8-hydroxy-2(di-n-propylamino)tetralin (8-OH-DPAT) were ineffective. These results strongly suggest that the receptor involved belongs to the 5-HT$_{1B}$ subclass. The results with the antagonists, although not providing much additional evidence, are compatible with this conclusion: besides methiothepin, metergoline and propranolol (Figure 1) also acted as antago-nists, whereas the 5-HT$_{1A}$ and 5-HT$_2$ receptor antagonist spiperone did not

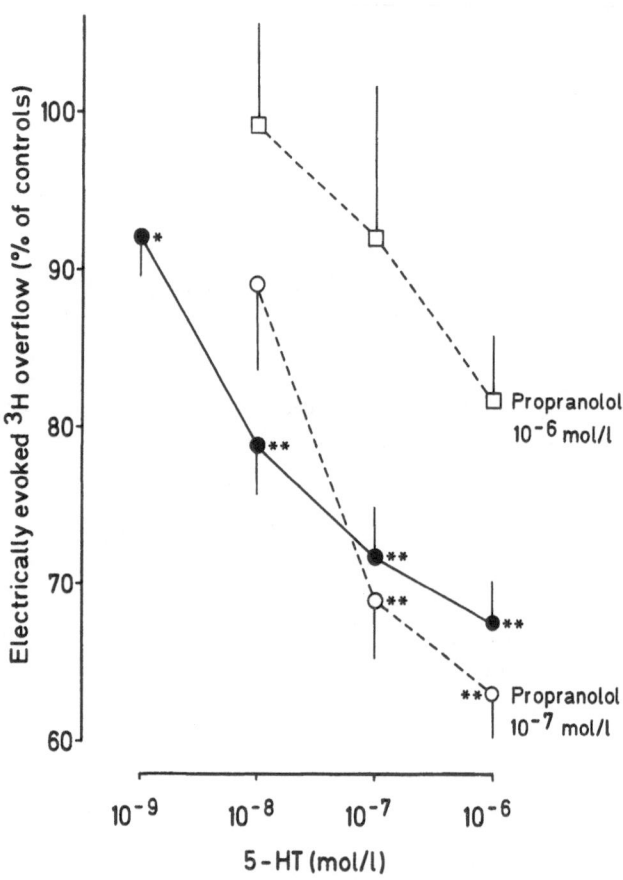

Figure 1. Inhibitory effect of 5-HT on the electrically (0.66 Hz) evoked [³H] overflow from the rat inferior vena cava preincubated with [³H]noradrenaline and interaction with propranolol. The veins were superfused with physiological salt solution. [³H] overflow was expressed as percentage of that in the respective control experiments. Means ± SEM of 4—9 experiments. *P < 0.05, **P < 0.025 (compared to the corresponding controls). For methodological details, see [35].

[35]. In contrast, the pharmacological properties of the presynaptic inhibitory 5-HT receptors in the perfused rat renal vascular bed do not conform to the criteria for the 5-HT_{1B} receptor, but they fit to the basic characteristics of the "5-HT_1" receptor "family": "5-HT_1" receptor agonists inhibited release and methiothepin and metergoline counteracted the effect of 5-HT. The ineffectiveness of propranolol, pindolol, cyanopindolol and mesulergine as antagonists excludes subclassification not only as a 5-HT_{1B} but also as a 5-HT_{1A} and 5-HT_{1C} receptor [32]. Rather, this pharmacological profile may resemble that of the recently defined 5-HT_{1D} binding site [25]. The presynaptic inhibitory 5-HT receptor in the human saphenous vein is responsive to 5-HT and 8-OH-DPAT (the latter in the low micromolar range), but not to ipsapirone. The agonist-induced inhibition of NA release is antagonized by methiothepin, but not propranolol or ketanserin. Therefore, the characteristics of this receptor restrict the classification to the "5-HT_1" receptor family without further differentiation [33].

The sympathetic nerve endings of the pig coronary artery seem to be endowed with an inhibitory 5-HT receptor as well, but with respect to its classification this receptor seems to be an exception to the rule inasmuch as it does not belong to the "5-HT_1" receptor class: 5-HT in the nanomolar range, 5-aminotryptamine, tryptamine and RU 24969 inhibit NA release, whereas 5-HT_{1A} receptor agonists (such as 8-OH-DPAT, ipsapirone, urapidil) and, surprisingly, the nonselective "5-HT_1" receptor agonist 5-CT do not. Since neither methiothepin nor ketanserin nor the 5-HT_3 receptor antagonist $(3\alpha$-tropanyl)-lH-indole-3-carboxylic acid ester (ICS 205-930) block the 5-HT-induced inhibition of NA release, an unknown 5-HT receptor class distinct from the 5-HT_1, 5-HT_2 and 5-HT_3 type may be involved [42]. Interestingly, such a 5-HT receptor is also involved in the positive chronotropic response to 5-HT in the anaesthetized pig [43].

Aggregating platelets may be assumed to be the physiological source of 5-HT for activation of inhibitory presynaptic 5-HT receptors in vivo. Accordingly, aggregating platelets were shown to inhibit [^{3}H]NA release in the canine saphenous vein and coronary artery; this effect is sensitive to blockade by methiothepin [29]. In vivo, exposure of the blood vessel wall and particularly of its sympathetic nerves may occur at sites of acute injury to the endothelium or of atherosclerotic disease. This may lead to accumulation of 5-HT in sympathetic nerve endings. In vitro, exposure of isolated blood vessels to 5-HT leads to its accumulation in the noradrenergic nerves and, subsequently, this 5-HT can be released in response to electrical stimulation [31, 44, 45]. Under these conditions, the presynaptic 5-HT receptor can function as an "autoreceptor" for the "false co-transmitter" 5-HT.

3.2 *Cholinergic neurons*

To our knowledge, an inhibitory effect of 5-HT on ACh release due to a presynaptic site of action on cholinergic neurons has not been shown in cardiovascular tissue, probably because of methodological problems. Since such data are available for enteric neurons, they will be briefly mentioned in this section. 5-HT [46], lysergide (LSD) or 8-OH-DPAT in the nanomolar concentration range [47] inhibit the electrically-evoked [^{3}H]ACh release in the myenteric plexus-longitudinal muscle preparation of guinea-pig ileum. Methiothepin and methysergide, but not ketanserin, counteract the effect of 5-HT. Since buspirone, spiperone and pindolol also act as antagonists at the receptors activated by 8-OH-DPAT, this receptor seems to belong to the 5-HT$_{1A}$ subclass.

4. Conclusions

The *excitatory* 5-HT receptors on the autonomic nerve endings belong to the 5-HT$_3$ receptor class. In general, the *inhibitory* 5-HT receptors on these nerve endings are of the "5-HT$_1$" category; however, there are species and tissue differences with respect to the receptor subtype. In the pig coronary artery, NA release appears to be inhibited by a "new" class of 5-HT receptor.

Acknowledgements

The work carried out in the authors' laboratory was supported by the Deutsche Forschungsgemeinschaft.

References

1. Fozard JR (1984): Neuronal 5-HT receptors in the periphery. *Neuropharmacology* 23: 1473—1486.
2. Kuhn DM, Wolf WA, Lovenberg W (1980): Review of the role of the central serotonergic neuronal system in blood pressure regulation. *Hypertension* 2: 243—255.
3. Wolf WA, Kuhn DM, Lovenberg W (1981): Pressor effects of dorsal raphe stimulation and intrahypothalamic application of serotonin in the spontaneously hypertensive rat. *Brain Res* 208: 192—197.
4. McGrath MA (1977): 5-Hydroxytryptamine and neurotransmitter release in canine blood vessels. Inhibition by low and augmentation by high concentrations. *Circ Res* 41: 428—435.
5. Humphrey PPA (1978). The effects of α-adrenoceptor antagonists on contractile responses to 5-hydroxytryptamine in dog saphenous vein. *Br J Pharmacol* 63: 671—675.
6. Marin J, Arias M, Salaices M. Sanchez CF, Recio LM (1981): Vasoconstrictor effects of serotonin in the isolated superior mesenteric artery of cat. *Gen Pharmacol* 12: 97—101.
7. Freeman WK, Rorie DK, Tyce GM (1981): Effects of 5-hydroxytryptamine on neuroeffector junction in human pulmonary artery. *J appl Physiol Respir Environ* 51: 693—698.
8. Göthert M, Schlicker E, Kollecker P (1986): Receptor mediated effects of serotonin and 5-methoxytryptamine on noradrenaline release in the rat vena cava and in the heart of the pithed rat. *Naunyn-Schmiedeberg's Arch Pharmacol* 332: 124—130.

9. Göthert M, Dührsen U (1979): Effects of 5-hydroxytryptamine and related compounds on the sympathetic nerves of the rabbit heart. *Naunyn-Schmiedeberg's Arch Pharmacol* 308: 9—18.
10. Trendelenburg U (1960): The action of histamine and 5-hydroxytryptamine on isolated mammalian atria. *J Pharmacol exp Ther* 130: 450—460.
11. Jacob J, Poite-Bevierre M (1960): Actions de la serotonine et de la benzyl-l-demethyl-2,5-serotonine sur le coeur isolé de lapin. *Arch int Pharmacodyn Ther* 127: 11—26.
12. Fozard JR, Mwaluko GMP (1976): Mechanism of the indirect sympathomimetic effect of 5-hydroxytryptamine on the isolated heart of the rabbit. *Br J Pharmacol* 57: 115—125.
13. Fozard JR, Mobarok Ali ATM (1978): Receptors for 5-hydroxytryptamine on the sympathetic nerves of the rabbit heart. *Naunyn-Schmiedeberg's Arch Pharmacol* 301: 223—235.
14. Göthert M, Klupp N (1978): Cardiovascular effects of neurotoxic indolethylamines. *Ann N Y Acad Sci* 305: 457—476.
15. Engel G, Göthert M, Hoyer D, Schlicker E, Hillenbrand K (1986): Identity of inhibitory presynaptic 5-hydroxytryptamine (5-HT) autoreceptors in the rat brain cortex with 5-HT$_{1B}$ binding sites. *Naunyn-Schmiedeberg's Arch Pharmacol* 332: 1—7.
16. Kilpatrick GJ, Jones BJ, Tyers MB (1987): Identification and distribution of 5-HT$_3$ receptors in brain using radioligand binding. *Nature* 330: 746—748.
17. Neijt HC, Karpf A, Schoeffter P, Engel G, Hoyer D (1988): Characterisation of 5-HT$_3$ recognition sites in membranes of NG 108—15 neuroblastoma-glioma cells with [^{3}H]ICS 205—930. *Naunyn-Schmiedeberg's Arch Pharmacol* 337: 493—499.
18. Richardson BP, Engel G, Donatsch P, Stadler PA (1985): Identification of serotonin M-receptor subtypes and their specific blockade by a new class of drugs. *Nature* 316: 126—131.
19. Göthert M, Dührsen U, Rieckesmann J-M (1979): Ethanol, anaesthetics and other lipophilic drugs preferentially inhibit 5-hydroxytryptamine- and acetylcholine-induced noradrenaline release from sympathetic nerves. *Arch int Pharmacodyn Ther* 242: 196—209.
20. Fozard JR, Mobarok Ali ATM (1978): Blockade of neuronal tryptamine receptors by metoclopramide. *European J Pharmacol* 49: 109—112.
21. Fozard JR, Mobarok Ali ATM, Newgrosh G (1979): Blockade of serotonin receptors on autonomic neurones by (−)-cocaine and some related compounds. *European J Pharmacol* 59: 195—210.
22. Fozard JR (1984): MDL 72222: a potent and highly selective antagonist at neuronal 5-hydroxytryptamine receptors. *Naunyn-Schmiedeberg's Arch Pharmacol* 326: 36—44.
23. Bradley PB, Engel G, Feniuk W, Fozard JR, Humphrey PPA, Middlemiss DN, Mylecharane EJ, Richardson BP, Saxena PR (1986): Proposals for the classification and nomenclature of functional receptors for 5-hydroxytryptamine. *Neuropharmacology* 25: 563—576.
24. Leff P, Martin G (1988): The classification of 5-hydroxytryptamine receptors. *Medicinal Research Reviews* 8: 187—202.
25. Peroutka SJ (1988): 5-Hydroxytryptamine receptor subtypes. *Ann Rev Neurosci* 11: 45—60.
26. Feniuk W, Humphrey PPA, Watts AD (1979): Presynaptic inhibitory action of 5-hydroxytryptamine in dog isolated saphenous vein. *Br J Pharmacol* 67: 247—254.
27. Watts AD, Feniuk W, Humphrey PPA (1981): A prejunctional action of 5-hydroxytryptamine and methysergide on noradrenergic nerves in dog isolated saphenous vein. *J Pharm Pharmacol* 33: 515—520.
28. Engel G, Göthert M, Müller-Schweinitzer E, Schlicker E, Sistonen L, Stadler PA (1983): Evidence for common pharmacological properties of [^{3}H]5-hydroxytryptamine binding sites, presynaptic 5-hydroxytryptamine autoreceptors in CNS and inhibitory presynaptic 5-hydroxytryptamine receptors on sympathetic nerves. *Naunyn-Schmiedeberg's Arch Pharmacol* 324: 116—124.

29. Lorenz RR, Vanhoutte PM (1985): Prejunctional adrenergic inhibition by aggregating platelets in canine blood vessels. *Am J Physiol* 249: H685—H689.

30. Cohen RA (1985): Serotonergic prejunctional inhibition of canine coronary adrenergic nerves. *J Pharmacol Exp Ther* 235: 76—80.

31. Cohen RA (1987): Inhibition of adrenergic neurotransmission in canine tibial artery after exposure to 5-hydroxytryptamine in vitro. *J Pharmacol Exp Ther* 242: 493—499.

32. Charlton KG, Bond RA, Clarke DE (1986): An inhibitory prejunctional 5-HT$_1$-like receptor in the isolated perfused rat kidney. Apparent distinction from the 5-HT$_{1A}$, 5-HT$_{1B}$ and 5-HT$_{1C}$ subtypes. *Naunyn-Schmiedeberg's Arch Pharmacol* 332: 8—15.

33. Göthert M, Kollecker P, Rohm N, Zerkowski HR (1986): Inhibitory presynaptic 5-hydroxytryptamine (5-HT) receptors on the sympathetic nerves of the human saphenous vein. *Naunyn-Schmiedeberg's Arch Pharmacol* 332: 317—323.

34. Schlicker E, Göthert M (1987): Noradrenaline release and its modulation via presynaptic serotonin receptors in blood vessels of spontaneously hypertensive rats. *J Cardiovasc Pharmacol* 10 (Suppl. 4): 141—143.

35. Molderings GJ, Fink K, Schlicker E, Göthert M (1987): Inhibition of noradrenaline release via presynaptic 5-HT$_{1B}$ receptors of the rat vena cava. *Naunyn-Schmiedeberg's Arch Pharmacol* 336: 245—250.

36. Docherty JR (1988): Investigations of cardiovascular 5-hydroxytryptamine receptor subtypes in the rat. *Naunyn-Schmiedeberg's Arch Pharmacol* 337: 1—8.

37. Adler-Graschinsky E (1983): Dual presynaptic effects of 5-hydroxytryptamine on peripheral noradrenergic synapses. *J Auton Pharmacol* 3: 303—315.

38. Adler-Graschinsky E, Butta NV, Elgoyhen AB (1986): Serotonin uptake inhibitors and the prejunctional effects of serotonin on peripheral sympathetic nerves. *Life Sciences* 39: 61—68.

39. Phillips CA, Mylecharane EJ, Shaw J (1985): Mechanisms involved in the vasodilator action of 5-hydroxytryptamine in the dog femoral arterial circulation in vivo. *European J Pharmacol* 113: 325—334.

40. Martinez AA, Lokhandwala MF (1980): Evidence for a presynaptic inhibitory action of 5-hydroxytryptamine on sympathetic neurotransmission to the myocardium. *European J Pharmacol* 63: 303—311.

41. Kimura T, Satoh S (1983): Presynaptic inhibition by serotonin of cardiac sympathetic transmission in dogs. *Clin Exp Pharmacol Physiol* 10: 535—542.

42. Molderings GJ, Göthert M, Fink K, Roth E, Schlicker E (1989): Inhibition of noradrenaline release in the pig coronary artery via a novel serotonin receptor. *Eur J Pharmacol* 164: 213—222.

43. Bom AH, Duncker DJ, Saxena PR, Verdouw PD (1988): 5-Hydroxytryptamine-induced tachycardia in the pig: possible involvement of a new type of 5-HT receptor. *Br J Pharmacol* 93: 663—671.

44. Verbeuren TJ, Jordaens FH, Herman AG (1983): Accumulation and release of [^{3}H]-5-hydroxytryptamine in saphenous veins and cerebral arteries of the dog. *J Pharmacol Exp Ther* 226: 579—588.

45. Saito A, Lee TJ-F (1987): Serotonin as an alternative transmitter in sympathetic nerves of large cerebral arteries of the rabbit. *Circ Res* 60: 220—228.

46. Kilbinger H, Pfeuffer-Friedrich I (1985): Two types of receptors for 5-hydroxytryptamine on the cholinergic nerves of the guinea-pig myenteric plexus. *Br J Pharmacol* 85: 529—539.

47. Fozard JR, Kilbinger H (1985): 8-OH-DPAT inhibits transmitter release from guinea-pig enteric cholinergic neurones by activating 5-HT$_{1A}$ receptors. *Br J Pharmacol* 86, 601P.

XXII. Receptors for 5-hydroxytryptamine in the cardiovascular system

MARLENE L. COHEN

1. Introduction

5-Hydroxytryptamine (5-HT; serotonin) receptor characterization has revealed three broad classes of receptors: $5\text{-}HT_1$, $5\text{-}HT_2$, and $5\text{-}HT_3$ [1, 2]. At least four subtypes of the $5\text{-}HT_1$ receptor exist: $5\text{-}HT_{1A}$, $5\text{-}HT_{1B}$, $5\text{-}HT_{1C}$ and $5\text{-}HT_{1D}$. The suggestion has been made that $5\text{-}HT_3$ receptors may also be heterogeneous; however, general consensus in this regard has not been achieved. Although the precise number of 5-HT receptors is controversial (due to limitations and specificity of drugs used to study these receptors), it is clear that many of the receptors identified in brain membrane binding studies also exist within the cardiovascular system.

5-HT exerts marked effects throughout the cardiovascular system with diverse effects being observed in cardiac tissue, blood vessels, and platelets. The diverse effects of 5-HT may be attributed to both direct and indirect effects and its interaction with multiple receptors. Furthermore, in cardiac tissue and blood vessels, 5-HT may exert opposing effects, e.g. both increases and decreases in heart rate and both contraction and relaxation of blood vessels have been demonstrated, again effects mediated by different receptor mechanisms. For some responses, multiple 5-HT receptors may mediate the same pharmacological effect. Several specific agonists and antagonists have been utilized to study these responses and to characterize the receptors involved.

2. 5-HT receptors in the heart

2.1 Receptors mediating bradycardia

The most prominent effect of 5-HT in cardiac tissue involves modulation of heart rate although 5-HT may exert modest effects on myocardial contractility [3, 4]. 5-HT can induce a transient dose-dependent bradycardia due

P.R. Saxena, D.I. Wallis, W. Wouters and P. Bevan (eds), Cardiovascular Pharmacology of 5-Hydroxytryptamine, pp. 295–302.
© 1990 *Kluwer Academic Publishers, Dordrecht* –

to activation of 5-HT$_3$ receptors on afferent nerves in cardiac muscle. Activation of this reflex response (the von Bezold Jarisch reflex) occurs within seconds of intravenous administration of serotonin with heart rate returning toward control values within one minute. The transient bradycardia produced by serotonin can be antagonized by potent 5-HT$_3$ receptor antagonists (Figure 1) such as ICS 205930 [5], GR38032F [6], and zacopride [7]. Because 5-HT-induced bradycardia results from activation of acetylcholine release, anticholinergic agents such as atropine will also block this effect (Figure 1).

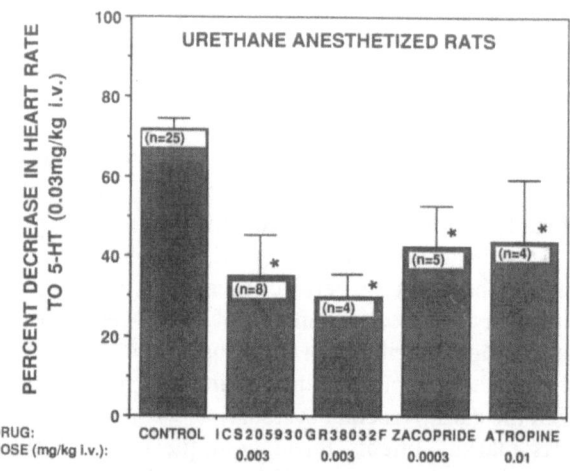

Figure 1. Effect of ICS-205930, GR38032F, zacopride and atropine to antagonize serotonin (0.03 mg/kg i.v.)-induced bradycardia in urethane anesthetized rats. 5-HT was injected into the femoral vein of anesthetized rats resulting in a transient bradycardia. When 5-HT-induced bradycardia returned to control values (within 5 minutes) the antagonist was administered intravenously and heart rate was measured 15 minutes after ICS 205930, zacopride and atropine or 5 minutes after GR38032F. Bars represent mean values and vertical lines the standard error of the mean for the number of tissues indicated in parentheses. Asterisks indicate those values that differ significantly (P < 0.05) from control bradycardia.

Activation of the von Bezold-Jarisch reflex has been shown to occur during myocardial ischemia or infarction in cats [8], dogs [9], and humans [10] and most recently, after thrombolysis with streptokinase in dogs [11]. Several mechanical manipulations and mediators may activate this reflex, and the precise role, if any, for 5-HT in the initiation of the reflex under physiological or pathological conditions remains to be established. Thus, the physiological importance of activation of the von Bezold Jarisch reflex is unclear and additional studies will be required to determine if serotonin plays a role in the activation of this reflex clinically.

2.2 *Receptors mediating tachycardia*

When the von Bezold Jarisch reflex is inoperative or overridden, 5-HT may produce tachycardia. Depending on the species and the preparation utilized, tachycardia to 5-HT may be mediated via several serotonergic and/or adrenergic receptor mechanisms. Tachycardia can result from direct activation of 5-HT$_1$-like [12], 5-HT$_2$ [13], and 5-HT$_3$ [14] cardiac receptors, in addition to an indirect effect involving release of noradrenaline either from the adrenal gland or adrenergic nerves [15]. Some studies suggest that 5-HT-induced tachycardia may also result from activation of a receptor not yet characterized [16, 17].

In the conscious instrumented dog (Wilson, H. C. and Cohen, M. L., unpublished) tachycardic responses have been observed to 5-HT, to the 5-HT$_{1A}$ and 5-HT$_{1B}$ receptor agonist, 5-carboxyamidotryptamine, and to the 5-HT$_3$ receptor agonist, 2-methyl 5-HT (Figure 2). To a lessor extent, the 5-HT$_2$ receptor agonist, α-methyl 5-HT also modestly increased heart rate in the conscious dog (Figure 2). These data support the contention that even in the same preparation, multiple receptors and/or mechanisms may be involved in 5-HT-induced tachycardia.

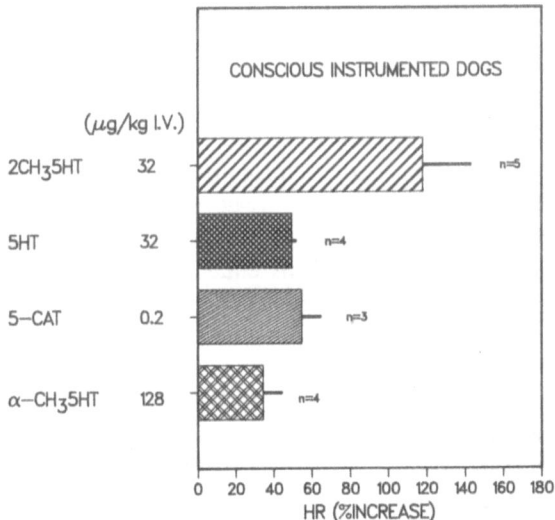

Figure 2. Effect of 5-HT, 2-methyl 5-HT (2-CH$_3$ 5-HT), 5-carboxamidotryptamine (5-CAT) and alpha-methyl 5-HT (α CH$_3$ 5-HT) on heart rate in conscious dogs after intravenous administration (Wilson, H. C. and Cohen, M. L., manuscript in preparation). Heart rate was measured in conscious dogs with a precalibrated Konigsberg implantable pressure transducer (7 mm) positioned into the left ventricle. For all agonists, heart rate responses were transient with values returning to or below control heart rates within one minute after intravenous administration of agonists. Bars represent mean values and lines represent standard error of the mean for the number of animals indicated.

3. 5-HT receptors in blood vessels

3.1 Receptors mediating contraction

In addition to pronounced effects on cardiac rate, perhaps the most studied effects of serotonin are on vascular reactivity. 5-HT is a potent contractile agonist of blood vessels and in many vascular beds, this effect is mediated by activation of 5-HT_2 receptors with a resultant increase in phosphoinositide turnover (for review see 18).

Although 5-HT_2 receptors are involved in contractile responses to 5-HT in many blood vessels, in some tissues, such as cerebral arteries, contraction to 5-HT was not potently or competitively antagonized by 5-HT_2 receptor antagonists [22, 23]. Some believe that the receptors mediating contraction to 5-HT in certain blood vessels may be similar to 5-HT_{1A} binding sites [24, 25]. The ability to detect some blockade of 5-HT contractile responses in cerebral vessels with 5-HT_2 receptor antagonists [22, 26] may reflect the minimal presence of this receptor in some arteries. Studies in animal [27] and human [28] blood vessels have provided evidence for the existence of at least two 5-HT receptors that may be responsible for 5-HT-induced contractions. Thus, in certain blood vessels, contractile responses to 5-HT may involve activation of more than one receptor type.

3.2 Receptors mediating relaxation

In addition to potent vasoconstrictor properties, 5-HT may vasodilate some vascular beds. Relaxation of vascular tissue produced by 5-HT may result from (1) a direct effect on smooth muscle [29], (2) an indirect effect to release vasodilating substances such as endothelium derived relaxing factor (EDRF) [30] or prostaglandin derivatives [31], or (3) inhibition of neurotransmission [Table 6 in 18]. No evidence has been obtained to suggest that 5-HT_2 receptor antagonists can block 5-HT-induced vascular relaxation. In contrast, agonists that show high affinity at 5-HT_1 binding sites and non-selective antagonists have been shown to mimic and antagonize, respectively, the vasodilating responses to 5-HT [32, 33]. Saxena and colleagues [34] have recently demonstrated a vasorelaxant effect of 5-HT in porcine skin and ear that was attenuated by the 5-HT_3 receptor antagonist, MDL72222. Thus, pending confirmation, 5-HT_3 receptors may also be involved in 5-HT-mediated vascular relaxation in some tissues.

3.3 Receptors mediating increases in vascular permeability

5-HT can increase microvascular permeability, an effect most studied in the rat. This effect of serotonin to enhance vascular permeability has been demonstrated using cutaneous blood vessels [35], mesenteric blood vessels [36], and blood vessels in the foot pad [37]. 5-HT is approximately 100-fold more potent than histamine in inducing increases in cutaneous vascular permeability in rats [38]. 5-HT$_2$ receptor antagonists can block increases in vascular permeability produced by 5-HT in rats [38, 39]. In fact, LY53857, a 5-HT$_2$ receptor antagonist, markedly blocked cutaneous dye extravasation produced by intradermal injection of serotonin and blocked edema formed by intradermal injection of 5-HT in the foot pad of rats (Figure 3). The possibility that other receptors may be involved in this response has not been investigated in detail.

4. 5-HT receptors on platelets

In contrast to the multiple receptors in cardiac and vascular tissue, only 5-HT$_2$ receptors have been identified on platelets. 5-HT$_2$ receptor antagonists blocked 5-HT-induced amplification of platelet aggregation (40), providing evidence that the 5-HT receptor involved in platelet aggregation is indeed a

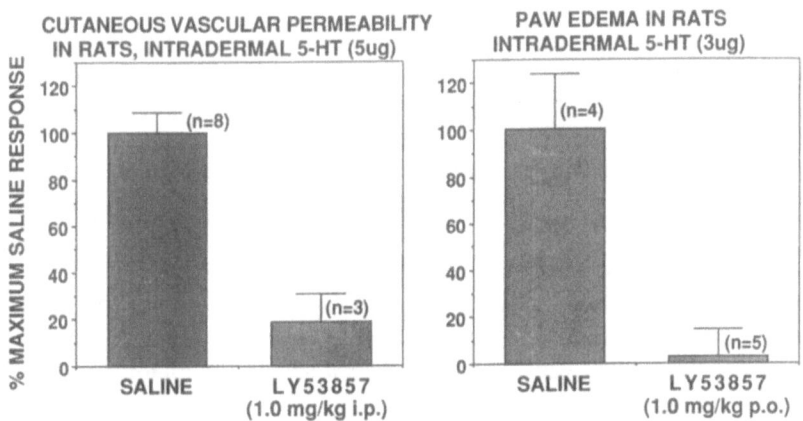

Figure 3. Effect of the 5-HT$_2$ receptor antagonist, LY53857, to antagonize increases in vascular permeability produced by intradermal injection of 5-HT into the skin (left) and into the paw (right). Cutaneous vascular permeability was determined by the amount of dye extravasation occurring at the site of intradermal serotonin administration in animals pretreated with Evans Blue dye (35 mg/kg i.v.) given two minutes before serotonin. LY53857 (1.0 mg/kg i.p.) was administered 15 minutes before intradermal serotonin. Animals were sacrificed 30 minutes after intradermal serotonin and dye extravasation determined in the skin patch after extraction, spectrophotometrically.

Paw edema was evaluated in rats receiving 5-HT intradermally in the foot pad by means of calipers measuring thickness of the paw, 45 minutes after intradermal 5-HT administration. LY53857 (1.0 mg/kg po) was administered 60 minutes prior to intradermal challenge with serotonin in the foot pad. Bars are mean values and vertical lines represent the standard error of the mean for the number of tissues indicated in parenthesis. In both studies, the effect of LY53857 was highly significant (P < 0.05).

5-HT$_2$ receptor. These receptors mediate a shape change in platelets and activation of 5-HT$_2$ receptors can amplify aggregation produced by other platelet aggregating agents such at ADP, adrenaline and collagen. The ability of 5-HT to amplify platelet aggregation produced by other aggregating agents may be associated with activtion of 5-HT$_2$ receptor-mediated phosphoinositide turnover (41).

Platelets may be critical to the effects of 5-HT on the cardiovascular system because 5-HT is found in high concentration in platelets from virtually all species. Upon platelet aggregation, 5-HT, along with other mediators, is released and may provide one primary source of 5-HT for interaction with cardiovascular tissues.

5. Clinical significance

5-HT has been suggested to play a role in several cardiovascular diseases including hypertension, peripheral vascular disease, atherosclerosis, thrombosis, and migraine. The involvement of 5-HT in each of these disease states or in the actions of drugs used to treat the diseases has not been unequivocally established to date. Establishment of a definitive role for 5-HT in cardiovascular disease will be aided by the development of highly selective and potent agonists and antagonists at each of the 5-HT receptor sites and the demonstration of clinical utility for such agents in specific cardiovascular diseases.

Thus, 5-HT and drugs that modify serotonergic function may influence the cardiovascular system by mechanisms that affect one or more of the receptors on the heart, blood vessels or platelets. In addition, it is important to remember that modification of central serotonergic function, alteration in platelet aggregability, fragility and vascular wall interactions, and enhancement of vascular (as may occur with endothelial cell damage) or cardiac sensitivity to serotonin will also play a critical role in the total involvement of 5-HT in cardiovascular disease.

References

1. Bradley PB, Engel G, Feniuk W, Fozard JR, Humphrey PPA, Middlemiss DN, Mylecharane EJ, Richardson BP, Saxena PR (1986): Proposals for the classification and nomenclature of functional receptors for 5-hydroxytryptamine. *Neuropharmacol* 25: 563—576.
2. Humphrey PPA, Richardson BP (1988): 5-HT receptor classification: A current view based on a workshop debate, (in press) in: Mylecharane E, Angus J, De La Lande I, Humphrey PPA (eds), *Serotonin*. Basingstoke, England: Macmillan Press.
3. Buccino RA, Covell JW, Sonnenblick EH, Braunwald E (1967): Effects of serotonin on the contractile state of the myocardium. *Am J Physiol* 213: 483—486.
4. Sakai K, Akima M (1979): An analysis of the stimulant effects of 5-hydroxytryptamine on isolated, blood-perfused rat heart. *Eur J Pharmacol* 55: 421—424.

5. Richardson BP, Engel G, Donatsch P, Stadler PA (1985): Identification of serotonin M-receptor subtypes and their specific blockade by a new class of drugs. *Nature* 316: 126—131.

6. Brittain RT, Butler A, Coates IM, Fortune DM, Hagan R, Hill JM, Humber DC, Humphrey PPA, Ireland SJ, Jack D, Jordan CC, Oxford A, Straughan DW, Tyers MB (1987): GR38032F, a novel selective 5-HT₃ receptor antagonist. *Br J Pharmacol* 90: 87P.

7. Smith WW, Sancilio LF, Owera-Atepo JB, Naylor RJ, Lambert L (1988): Zacopride, a potent 5-HT₃ antagonist. *J Pharm Pharmacol* 40: 301—302.

8. Thoren PN (1973): Evidence for a depressor reflex elicited from left ventricular receptors during occlusion of one coronary artery in the cat. *Acta Physiol Scand* 88: 23—34.

9. Toubes DB, Brody MJ (1970): Inhibition of reflex vasoconstriction after experimental coronary embolization of the dog. *Circ Res* 27: 211—224.

10. Ahmed SS, Gupta RC, Branceto RR (1978): Significance of nausea and vomiting during acute myocardial infarction. *Am Heart J* 93: 671.

11. Koren G, Weiss AT, Ben-David Y, Hasin Y, Luria MH, Gotsman MS (1986): Bradycardia and hypotension following reperfusion with streptokinase (Bezold-Jarisch reflex): A sign of coronary thrombolysis and myocardial salvage. *Am Heart J* 112: 468.

12. Saxena PR, Mylecharane EJ, Heiligers J (1985): Analysis of the heart rate effects of 5-hydroxytryptamine in the cat; mediation of tachycardia by 5-HT₁-like receptors. *Naunyn-Schmiedeberg's Arch. Pharmacol* 330: 121—129.

13. Saxena PR, Lawang A (1985): A comparison of cardiovascular and smooth muscle effects of 5-hydroxytryptamine and 5-carboxamidotryptamine, a selective agonist of 5-HT₁ receptors. *Arch int Pharmacodyn* 227: 235—252.

14. Fozard JR (1984): MDL 72222: a potent and highly selective antagonist at neuronal 5-hydroxytryptamine receptors. *Naunyn-Schmiedeberg's Arch Pharmacol* 326: 36—44.

15. Feniuk W, Hare J, Humphrey PPA (1981): An analysis of the mechanism of 5-hydroxy-tryptamine-induced vasopressor responses in ganglion-blocked anaesthetized dogs. *J Pharm Pharmacol* 33: 155—160.

16. Bom AH, Duncker DJ, Verdouw PD, Saxena PR (1986): 5-hydroxytryptamine-induced tachycardia in the pig: mediation by a new type of 5-hydroxytryptamine receptor? *Pharm Weekbl Sci* 8: 270.

17. Kaumann AJ (1985): Two classes of myocardial 5-hydroxytryptamine receptors that are neither 5-HT₁ nor 5-HT₂. *J Cardiovasc Pharmacol* 7: S76—S78.

18. Cohen ML Serotonin receptors in vascular smooth muscle, in: Sanders E (ed), *The serotonin receptors*. New Jersey: Bush Human Press Inc.

19. Roth BL, Nakaki T, Chuang D-M, Costa E (1984): Aortic recognition sites for serotonin (5-HT) are coupled to phospholipase C and modulate phosphatidylinositol turnover. *Neuropharmacol* 23: 1225—1335.

20. Cohen ML, Wittenauer LA (1987): Serotonin receptor activation of phosphoinositide turnover in uterine, fundal, vascular and tracheal smooth muscle. *J Cardiovas Pharmacol* 10: 176—181.

21. Kaumann AJ, Frenken M (1985): A paradox: the 5-HT₂-receptor antagonist ketanserin restores the 5-HT-induced contraction depressed by methysergide in large coronary arteries of calf. *Naunyn-Schmiedeberg's Arch Pharmacol* 328: 295—300.

22. Cohen ML, Colbert WE (1986): Relationship between receptors mediating serotonin (5-HT) contractions in the canine basilar artery to 5-HT₁, 5-HT₂ and rat stomach fundus 5-HT receptors. *J Pharmacol Exp Ther* 237: 713—718.

23. Peroutka SJ, Noguchi M, Tolner DJ, Allen GS (1983): Serotonin-induced contraction of canine basilar artery: mediation by 5-HT₁ receptors. *Brain Res* 259: 327—330.

24. Taylor EW, Duckles SP, Nelson DL (1986): Dissociation constants of serotonin agonists in the canine basilar artery correlate to K_i values at the 5-HT$_{1A}$ binding site. *J Pharmacol Exp Ther* 236: 118—125.

25. Peroutka SJ, Huang S, Allen GS (1986): Canine basilar artery contractions mediated by 5-hydroxytryptamine$_{1A}$ receptors. *J Pharmacol Exp Ther* 237: 901—906.
26. Muller-Schweinitzer E, Engel G (1983): Evidence for mediation by 5-HT$_2$ receptors of 5-hydroxytryptamine-induced contraction of canine basilar artery. *Naunyn-Schmiedeberg's Arch Pharmacol* 324: 287—292.
27. Frenken M, Kaumann AJ (1985): Ketanserin causes surmountable antagonism of 5-hydroxytryptamine-induced contractions of large coronary arteries of dog. *Naunyn-Schmiedeberg's Arch Pharmacol* 328: 301—303.
28. Docherty JR, Hyland L (1986): An examination of 5-hydroxytryptamine receptors in human saphenous vein. *Br J Pharmacol* 89: 77—81.
29. Trevethick MA, Feniuk W, Humphrey PPA (1984): 5-hydroxytryptamine-induced relaxation of neonatal porcine vena cava *in vitro*. *Life Sci* 35: 477—486.
30. Luscher TF, Vanhoutte PM (1986): Endothelium-dependent responses to platelets and serotonin in spontaneously hypertensive rats. *Hypertension* 8: II-55-II-60.
31. Hirafuji M, Akiyama Y, Ogura Y (1987): Receptor-mediated stimulation of aortic prostacyclin release by 5-hydroxytryptamine. *Eur J Pharmacol* 143: 259—265.
32. Trevethick MA, Feniuk W, Humphrey PPA (1986): 5-Carboxamidotryptamine: A potent agonist mediating relaxation and elevation of cyclic AMP in the isolated neonatal porcine vena cava. *Life Sci* 38: 1521—1528.
33. Feniuk W, Humphrey PPA, Watts AD (1983): 5-Hydroxytryptamine-induced relaxation of isolated mammalian smooth muscle. *Eur J Pharmacol* 96: 71—78.
34. Saxena PR, Duncker DJ, Bom AH, Heiligers J, Verdouw, PD (1986): Effects of MDL 72222 and methiothepin on carotid vascular responses to 5-hydroxytryptamine in the pig: Evidence for the presence of "5-hydroxytryptamine$_1$-like" receptors. *Naunyn-Schmiedeberg's Arch Pharmacol* 333: 198—204.
35. Katayama S, Shionoya H, Ohtake S (1978): A new method for extraction of extravasated dye in the skin and the influence of fasting stress on passive cutaneous anaphylaxis in guinea pigs and rats. *Microbiol Immunol* 22(2): 89—101.
36. De Clerck F, Van Gorp L, Beetens J, Reneman RS (1985): Platelet-mediated vascular permeability in the rat: a predominant role of 5-hydroxytryptamine. *Thrombosis Res* 38: 321—339.
37. Doepfner W, Cerletti A (1958): Comparison of lysergic acid derivatives and antihistamines as inhibitors of the edema provoked in the rat's paw by serotonin. *Int Arch Allergy* 12: 89—97.
38. Cohen ML, Schenck K (in press): Effect of LY53857, a selective 5-HT$_2$ receptor antagonist on 5-HT-induced increases in cutaneous vascular permeability in rats. *Life Sci*.
39. Awouters F, Niemegeers CJE, Janssen PAJ (1981): Inhibitors of mast cell-mediated shock in the rat: Relationship to histamine and serotonin antagonism. *Drug Develop Res* 1: 107—114.
40. De Clerck F, Xhonneux B, Leysen J, Janssen PAJ (1984): Evidence for functional 5-HT$_2$ receptor sites on human blood platelets. *Biochem Pharmacol* 33: 2807—2811.
41. Chaffoy de Courcelles D, Roevens P, Van Belle H, De Clerck F (1987): The synergistic effect of serotonin and epinephrine on the human platelet at the level of signal transduction. *FEBS Letters* 219: 283—288.

XXIII. Altered responses to 5-hydroxytryptamine in hypertension and other cardiovascular disorders

J. M. VAN NUETEN, W. J. JANSSENS and P. A. J JANSSEN

1. Introduction

5-Hydroxytryptamine (5-HT; serotonin) can either cause vasodilatation or vasoconstriction with resulting increases in blood flow and decreases in blood pressure or vice versa [1]. This complexity can be explained by the interaction of the monoamine with different receptors within the vascular wall. On the one hand, activation of endothelial receptors by 5-HT will cause the release of a short-lived vasodilatator substance (EDRF: endothelium derived relaxing factor) and activation of 5-HT receptors on the adrenergic nerve endings will result in a decreased liberation of noradrenaline [2—7]. The receptors involved in these actions of 5-HT leading to vasodilatation belong to the 5-HT$_1$-like type [4, 7—9]. On the other hand, 5-HT can cause vasoconstriction by activation of 5-HT$_2$ receptors on the vascular smooth muscle cells [10—12]. Whether a particular vascular bed will respond to 5-HT with a vasodilatation or a vasoconstriction will ultimately depend upon a balance between factors which determine which of the two receptor systems can play a dominating role. It is the aim of this chapter to specifically review the evidence of pathological changes favouring the 5-HT$_2$ receptor mediated vasoconstriction.

2. Vasoconstrictor responses to endogenous 5-HT: role of the endothelium

The major source of 5-HT available to the vascular wall are aggregating blood platelets which can contract isolated blood vessels in vitro [13—18]. These contractions are caused to a major extent by the release of endogenous 5-HT since ketanserin, a 5-HT$_2$ receptor antagonist, can prevent them [12, 14—17, 19]. To a certain extent, they are also mediated by an enhancing effect of 5-HT on the vasoconstrictor action of thromboxane A$_2$ [14]. During exposure of vascular tissue to aggregating platelets, ketanserin may even unmask a vasodilator effect which is mediated by the endothelium and can be

P.R. Saxena, D.I. Wallis, W. Wouters and P. Bevan (eds), Cardiovascular Pharmacology of 5-Hydroxytryptamine, pp. 303—310.
© 1990 *Kluwer Academic Publishers, Dordrecht —*

explained by an interaction of 5-HT with $5-HT_1$-like receptors [3—5, 19]. Thus, it is not surprising that aggregating blood platelets, as well as exogenous 5-HT, cause more pronounced vasoconstriction if the endothelium is absent (Figure 1) [4, 5, 11, 12, 20]. Dysfunction of the endothelium can therefore be an important factor contributing to an enhanced vasoconstrictor response to 5-HT as described in atherosclerotic rabbit blood vessels during acute hypertension, in canine coronary arteries or in coronary arteries of pigs after re-endothelialisation [21—23].

Furthermore, it has also been shown in particular strains of hypertensive rats that the endothelium may release a contractile factor [24] which may lead to an enhanced vasoconstrictor response to 5-HT.

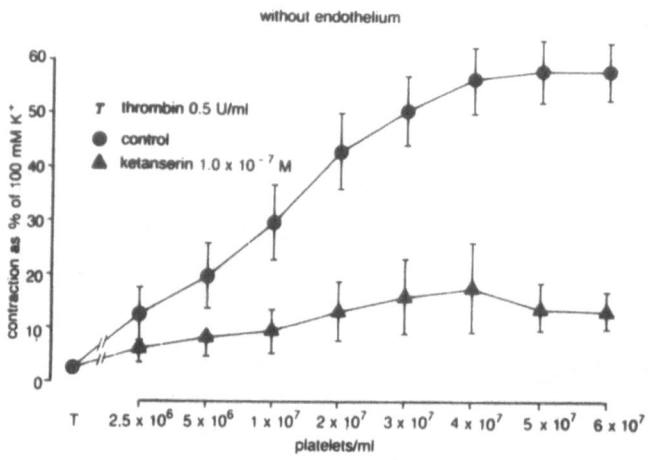

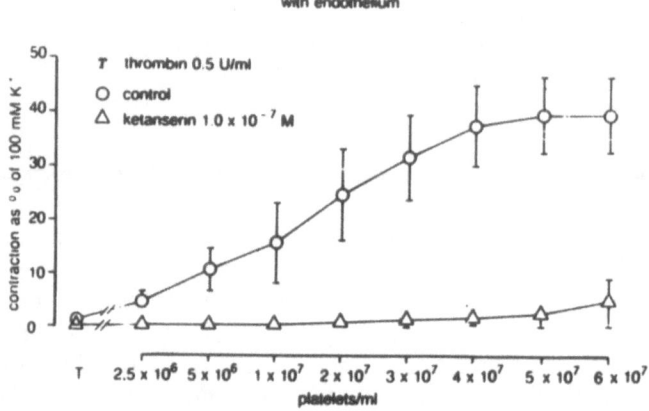

Figure 1. Contraction of isolated rabbit pulmonary arteries, evoked by increasing amounts of aggregating rat platelets, are augmented in the absence of endothelium and inhibited by ketanserin.

3. Indirect vasoconstrictor effects of 5-HT (amplification)

In addition to its direct vasoconstrictor effects, 5-HT augments ("amplifies") the vasoconstrictor effects of other neurohumoral mediators such as nor-adrenaline, angiotensin II, histamine, prostaglandin $F_{2\alpha}$ and thromboxane A_2. This was observed in a variety of isolated vascular tissues and beds, including human blood vessels. It also has been reported in vivo in various species, including the human [19, 25—28]. Amplification has been demonstrated with endogenous 5-HT and noradrenaline released from aggregating platelets and adrenergic nerve endings, respectively. It can be inhibited by 5-HT receptor antagonists, such as ketanserin, indicating that amplification is mediated by $5\text{-}HT_2$ receptors [5, 11, 12, 19]. This amplifying effect can also be observed (Figure 2) using aggregating blood platelets, despite the release of possible vasodilator substances such as ADP [15] and it is also operational during adrenergic nerve stimulation in certain blood vessels despite possible pre-junctional inhibitory effects of 5-HT or other platelet-derived materials (Figure 2) [29].

5-HT also potentiates the pressor effect of noradrenaline in dogs, cats and

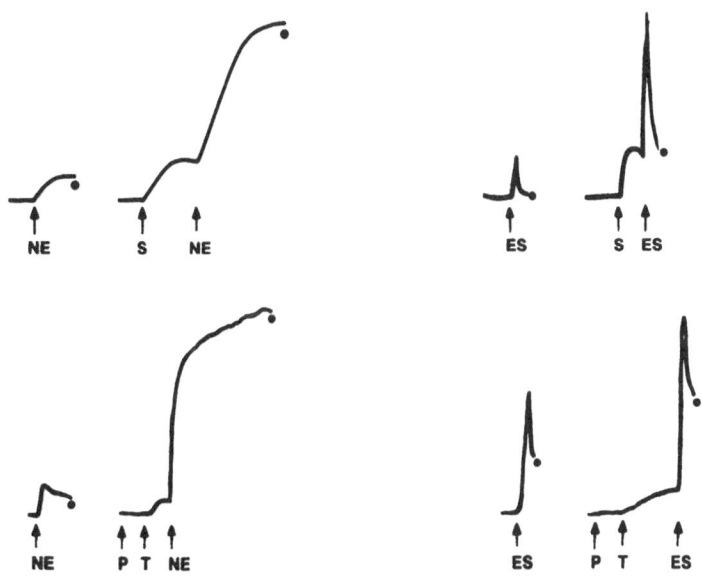

S : Serotonin ; NE : Norepinephrine ; ES : Electrical Stimulation ; P : Platelets ; T : Thrombin ; ● : Washout ;

Figure 2. Amplification in isolated rabbit femoral arteries. Small amounts of exogenous 5-HT (S: 3×10^{-8} M) or of rat platelets (P; 2.5×10^6/ml) activated with thrombin (T; 0.5 N.I.H. Units/ml) potentiate the contractile response to exogenous noradrenaline (NE: 5.9×10^{-9} M) or to endogenous noradrenaline released by electrical stimulation of the periarterial sympathetic nerves (ES; 16 Hz, 0.5 msec, 9 V). ●, washout.

sheep. Most likely this is due to amplification by 5-HT of the vasoconstrictor effect of the catecholamine observed in a number of species, including humans. The amplifying effect of 5-HT on noradrenaline-induced vasoconstrictions was confirmed in a study on anaesthetized rabbits [30].

3.1 Age

Blood vessels taken from different animal species become more sensitive for the direct contractile effect of 5-HT with increasing age [17, 31, 32]. In kidneys from 6 month old Wistar rats and spontaneously hypertensive rats, the amplifying effect of 5-HT in noradrenaline-induced vasoconstriction is enhanced when compared to kidneys from 2 month old rats [33]. It has also been shown that vascular tissues from aged rats are much less susceptible to tachyphylaxis for both the direct and the amplifying vasoconstrictor effect of 5-HT [33, 34]. Old age may thus be a predisposing factor leading to enhanced 5-HT_2 receptor-mediated vasoconstriction.

3.2 Hypertension

Increased vasoconstriction to 5-HT has been observed in hypertensive animals and man and isolated vascular preparations taken from hypertensive animals are more sensitive to the vasoconstrictor action of the monoamine [27, 33–40]. It has also been observed in portal hypertensive rats [41]. The amplifying effect of 5-HT on noradrenaline-induced vasoconstrictor in vitro or pressor in vivo responses is more pronounced in hypertensive animals [27, 29]. In the renal bed of normotensive and hypertensive animals such a difference was, however, not observed [33]. Some evidence suggests that dysfunction of the endothelium may be responsible for the increased responsiveness to 5-HT during hypertension [22, 24]. It has also been suggested that the loss of prejunctional inhibitory effects of 5-HT may contribute to an increased responsiveness to adrenergic nerve stimulation in the presence of 5-HT [29].

3.3 Atherosclerosis

In aortas from atherosclerotic rabbits the vasoconstrictor effect of 5-HT is augmented when compared to control animals, which may be related to a decreased effectiveness of the endothelium-derived relaxing factors to cause relaxation [21]. In normal monkeys a vasodilator action of 5-HT is observed in the hindlimb, which is changed into vasoconstriction in atherosclerotic monkeys [42]. This may be due to a loss of effect of the endothelium-derived relaxing factor, but it cannot be excluded that the prejunctional inhibitory action of 5-HT on the adrenergic nerves is also reduced. In these atherosclerotic animals, the 5-HT-induced exaggerated vasoconstriction is inhibited by 5-HT$_2$ receptor antagonists [43].

3.4 Other cardiovascular diseases

It has been shown that coronary arteries from patients suffering from cardiac disease contract more to 5-HT, noradrenaline and histamine than those from individuals who died from other causes [44]. This finding, together with observations on digital arteries of sclerodermic patients [45] and varicose saphenous vein obtained after surgery [46], also points to an increased vasoconstrictor effect of 5-HT. This may be indicative of preponderance of 5-HT$_2$ receptors in a number of human cardiovascular diseases.

4. Conclusions

5-HT causes vasoconstriction by direct effects and amplification of the

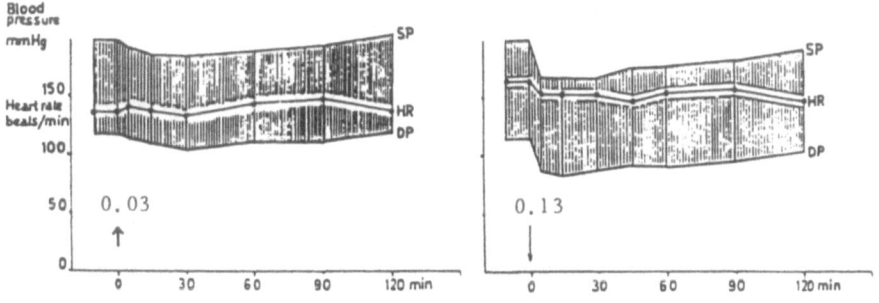

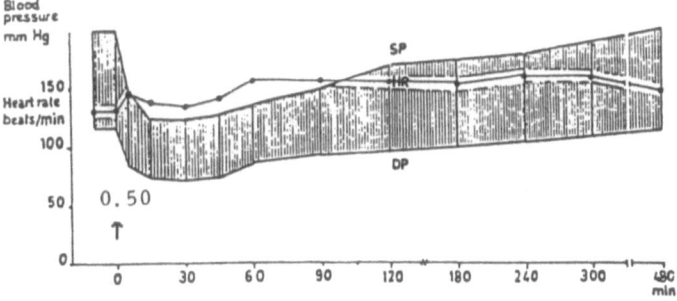

Figure 3. Ketanserin (I.V.) dose-dependently decreases systolic (SP) and diastolic (DP) blood pressure in old hypertensive dogs without modifying heart rate (HR; ●——●); mean values from n: 4[12, with permission].

response to other agonists. The direct and amplifying vasoconstrictor effects are mediated by 5-HT$_2$ receptors. These effects of 5-HT can be enhanced in a number of cardiovascular diseases (e.g. hypertension, atherosclerosis), particularly at old age. This may explain the more pronounced antihypertensive effect of ketanserin in animals (Figure 3) and patients [12].

Acknowledgements

The authors wish to thank, L. Geentjens, L. Leijssen and J. Kuyps for skilful secretarial assistance.

References

1. Page IH (1954): Serotonin (5-hydroxytryptamine). *Physiol Rev* 34: 563—588.
2. Furchgott RF (1983): Role of the endothelium in responses of vascular smooth muscle. *Circ Res* 53: 557—573.
3. Cocks RM, Angus JA (1983): Endothelium-dependent relaxation of coronary arteries by noradrenaline and serotonin. *Nature* (Lond) 305: 627—630.
4. Cohen RA, Shepherd JT, Vanhoutte PM (1983): 5-Hydroxytryptamine can mediate endothelium-dependent relaxation of coronary arteries. *Am J Physiol* 245: H1077—H1080.
5. Vanhoutte PM (1987): Endothelium and the control of vascular tissue. *NIPS* 2: 18—22.
6. McGrath MA (1977): 5-Hydroxytryptamine and neurotransmitter release in canine blood vessels. *Circ Res* 41: 428—435.
7. Cohen RA (1985): Serotonergic prejunctional inhibition of canine coronary adrenergic nerves. *J Pharmacol Exp Ther* 235: 76—80.
8. Houston DS, Shepherd JT, Vanhoutte PM (1985): Adenine nucleotides, serotonin and endothelium-dependent relaxations to platelets. *Am J Physiol* 248: H389—H395.
9. Engel G, Göthert M, Müller-Schweinitzer E, Schlicker E, Sistonen L, Stadler PA (1983): Evidence for common pharmacological properties of [^{3}H]5-hydroxytryptamine binding sites, presynaptic 5-hydroxytryptamine autoreceptors in CNS and inhibitory presynaptic 5-hydroxytryptamine receptors on sympathetic nerves. *Naunyn Schmiedeberg's Arch Pharmacol* 324: 116—124.
10. Van Nueten JM, Leysen JE, De Clerck F, Vanhoutte PM (1984): Serotonergic receptor subtypes and vascular reactivity. *J Cardiovasc Pharmacol* 6: S564—S574.
11. Van Nueten JM, Janssens WJ, Vanhoutte PM (1985): Serotonin and vascular reactivity. *Pharmacol Res Commun* 17: 585—608.
12. Van Nueten JM, Janssen PAJ, Symoens J, Janssens WJ, Heykants J, De Clerck F, Leysen JE, Vancauteren H, Vanhoutte PM (1987): Ketanserin, pp. 1—56 in: Scriabine A (ed.), *New Cardiovascular Drugs.* New York: Raven Press.
13. Starling LM, Bouillin DJ, Grahame-Smith DG, Adams CBT, Gye RS (1975): Responses of isolated human basilar arteries to 5-hydroxytryptamine, noradrenaline, serum, platelets, and erythrocytes. *J Neurol Neurosurg Psychiatry* 38: 650—656.
14. De Clerck F, Van Nueten JM (1982): Platelet-mediated vascular contractions: inhibition of the serotonergic component by ketanserin. *Thromb Res* 27: 713—727.
15. Cohen RA, Shepherd JT, Vanhoutte PM (1983): Inhibitory role of the endothelium in response of isolated coronary arteries to platelets. *Science* 221: 273—274.
16. McGoon MD, Vanhoutte PM (1984): Aggregating platelets contract isolated canine pulmonary arteries by releasing 5-hydroxytryptamine. *J Clin Invest* 74: 828—833.
17. Vanhoutte PM (1985): Peripheral serotonergic receptors and hypertension, pp. 123—

133 in: Vanhoutte PM (ed.), *Serotonin and the Cardiovascular System*. New York: Raven Press.

18. Vanhoutte PM, Houston DS (1985): Platelets, endothelium and vasospasm. *Circulation* 72: 728—734.
19. Van Nueten JM, Janssen PAJ, Van Beek J, Xhonneux R, Verbeuren TJ, Vanhoutte PM (1981): Vascular effects of ketanserin (R 41 468), a novel antagonist of 5-HT$_2$ serotonergic receptors. *J Pharmacol Exp Ther* 218: 217—230.
20. Garland CJ (1985): Endothelial cells and the electrical and mechanical responses of the rabbit coronary artery to 5-hydroxytryptamine. *J Pharmacol Exp Ther* 233: 158—162.
21. Verbeuren TJ, Jordaens FH, Zonnekeyn LL, Van Hove CE, Coene MC, Herman AG (1986): Effect of hypercholesterolemia on vascular reactivity in the rabbit. 1. Endothelium-dependent and endothelium-independent contractions and relaxations in isolated arteries of control and hypercholesterolemic rabbits. *Circ Res* 58: 552—564.
22. Lamping KG, Dole WP (1987): Acute hypertension selectively potentiates constrictor responses of large coronary arteries to serotonin by altering endothelial function in vivo. *Circ Res* 61: 904—913.
23. Shimokawa H, Aarhus LL, Vanhoutte PM (1987): Porcine coronary arteries with regenerated endothelium have a reduced endothelium-dependent responsiveness to aggregating platelets and serotonin. *Circ Res* 61: 256—270.
24. Lüscher TF, Vanhoutte PM (1986): Endothelium-dependent responses to platelets and serotonin in spontaneously hypertensive rats. *Hypertension* 8: II.55—II.60.
25. de la Lande IS, Cannell VA, Waterson JG (1966): The interaction of serotonin and noradrenaline on the perfused artery. *Br J Pharmacol Chemother* 28: 255—272.
26. Van Nueten JM, Janssen PAJ, De Ridder W, Vanhoutte PM (1982): Interaction between 5-hydroxytryptamine and other vasoconstrictor substances in the isolated femoral artery of the rabbit: effect of ketanserin (R 41 468). *Eur J Pharmacol* 77: 281—287.
27. Myers JH, Mecca TE, Webb RC (1985): Direct and sensitizing effects of serotonin agonists and antagonists on vascular smooth muscle. *J Cardiovasc Pharmacol* 7 (suppl. 7): S44—S48.
28. Scroop GC, Walsh JA (1968): interactions between angiotensin, noradrenaline and serotonin on the peripheral blood vessels in man. *Aust J Exp Biol Med Sci* 46: 573—580.
29. Kubo T, Su C (1983): Effects of serotonin and some other neurohumoral agents on adrenergic neurotransmission in spontaneously hypertensive rat vasculature. *Clin Exp Hypertens* (A) 5: 1501—1510.
30. Van Nueten JM, Janssens WJ, Xhonneux R, Janssen PAJ (1988): Interaction between S$_2$-serotonergic and α_1-adrenergic receptor activities at vascular sites. *J Cardiovasc Pharmacol* 11 (suppl. 1): S10—S15.
31. Toda N, Hayashi S (1979): Age-dependent alteration in the response of isolated rabbit basilar arteries to vasoactive agents. *J Pharmacol Exp Ther* 211: 716—721.
32. Toda N, Bian K, Inoue S (1987): Age-related changes in the response to vasoconstrictor and dilator agents in isolated beagle coronary arteries. *Naunyn Schmiedebergs Arch Pharmacol* 336: 359—364.
33. Janssens WJ, Van Nueten JM (1986): The direct and amplifying effects of serotonin are increased with age in the isolated perfused kidney of wistar and spontaneously hypertensive rats. *Naunyn Schmiedebergs Arch Pharmacol* 334: 327—332.
34. De Mey C, Vanhoutte PM (1981): Effect of age and spontaneous hypertension on the tachyphylaxis to 5-hydroxytryptamine and angiotensin II in the isolated rat kidney. *Hypertension* 3: 718—724.
35. Doyle EA, Fraser JRE, Marshall RJ (1959): Reactivity of forearm vessels to vasoconstrictor substances in hypertensive and normotensive subjects. *Clin Sci* 18: 441—454.
36. McGregor DD, Smirk FH (1970): Vascular responses to 5-hydroxytryptamine in genetic and renal hypertensive rats. *Am J Physiol* 219: 687—690.
37. Haeusler G, Finch L (1972): Vascular reactivity to 5-hydroxytryptamine and hypertension in the rat. *Naunyn Schmiedebergs Arch Pharmacol* 272: 101—116.

38. Collis MG, Vanhoutte PM (1977): Vascular reactivity of isolated perfused kidneys from male and female spontaneously hypertensive rats. *Circ Res* 41: 759—767.
39. Webb RC (1982): Increased vascular sensitivity to serotonin and methysergide in hypertension in rats. *Clin Sci* 63: 73s—75s
40. Mecca TE, Mitchell J, Bohr DF, Webb RC (1985): Effects of serotonin antagonists on blood pressure in mineralocorticoid hypertensive sheep. *J Cardiovasc Pharmacol* 7: 660—665.
41. Cummings SA, Groszmann RJ, Kaumann AJ (1986): Hypersensitivity of mesenteric veins to 5-hydroxytryptamine-and ketanserin-induced reduction of portal pressure in portal hypertensive rats. *Br J Pharmacol* 89: 501—513.
42. Heistad DD, Armstrong ML, Marcus ML, Piegors DJ, Mark AL (1984): Augmented responses to vasoconstrictor stimuli in hypercholesterolemic and atherosclerotic monkeys. *Circ Res* 54: 711—718.
43. Heistad DD, Armstrong ML, Marcus ML, Piegors DJ, Mark AL (1986): Potentiation of vasoconstrictor responses to serotonin in the limb of atherosclerotic monkeys. *J Hypertension* 4: S17—S21.
44. Kalsner S, Richards R (1984): Coronary arteries of cardiac patients are hyperreactive and contain stores of amines: a mechanism for coronary spasm. *Science* 223: 1435—1437.
45. Winkelmann RK, Goldyne ME, Linscheid RL (1976): Hypersensitivity of scleroderma cutaneous vascular smooth muscle to 5-hydroxytryptamine. *Br J Dermatol* 95: 51—56.
46. Van Nueten JM, Janssens WJ (1986): Augmentation of vasoconstrictor responses to serotonin by acute and chronic factors: inhibition by ketanserin. *J Hypertension* 4 (suppl. 1): S55—S59.

XXIV. 5-Hydroxytryptamine receptor antagonists as antihypertensive drugs

PRAMOD R. SAXENA

1. Introduction

Though 5-hydroxytryptamine (5-HT) exerts powerful pharmacological effects on the heart and blood vessels [1, 2], the physiological role of 5-HT in cardiovascular regulation is not clear. The effect of 5-HT on arterial blood pressure is triphasic [3] and consists mainly of an initial short-lasting depressor phase due to the Von Bezold-Jarisch reflex mediated by 5-HT$_3$ receptors [4—7], followed by a 5-HT$_2$ receptor-mediated hypertensive phase [5, 6, 8], and a late, long-lasting, hypotensive phase mediated by 5-HT$_1$-like receptor stimulation [see 9]. It is, therefore, obvious that only antagonists at 5-HT$_2$ receptors may be expected to have an antihypertensive effect in the event that these receptors are involved in the pathophysiology of hypertension.

2. Antihypertensive effects of 5-HT receptor antagonists

Amongst the antagonists of 5-HT only ketanserin has so far been shown to have an undisputed antihypertensive effect in both animals and man. The mechanism of the antihypertensive effect of ketanserin is still under debate [see 10—12] and probably involves several factors (Figure 1; [9]), such as the blockade of 5-HT$_2$ receptor- or α_1-adrenoceptor-mediated vasoconstriction, combined blockade of α_1-adrenoceptors and 5-HT$_2$ receptor-mediated amplification of noradrenaline vasoconstriction, inhibition of central vasomotor loci, and a 'direct' vasodilatation.

2.1 Blockade of 5-HT$_2$ receptor-mediated vasoconstriction

Since ketanserin possesses a high antagonistic activity against 5-HT-induced vasoconstriction (mediated by 5-HT$_2$ receptors) and unmasks the vasodilator effects of 5-HT [10, 12—15], many investigators concluded that the

P.R. Saxena, D.I. Wallis, W. Wouters and P. Bevan (eds), Cardiovascular Pharmacology of 5-Hydroxytryptamine, pp. 311—318.
© 1990 *Kluwer Academic Publishers, Dordrecht* —

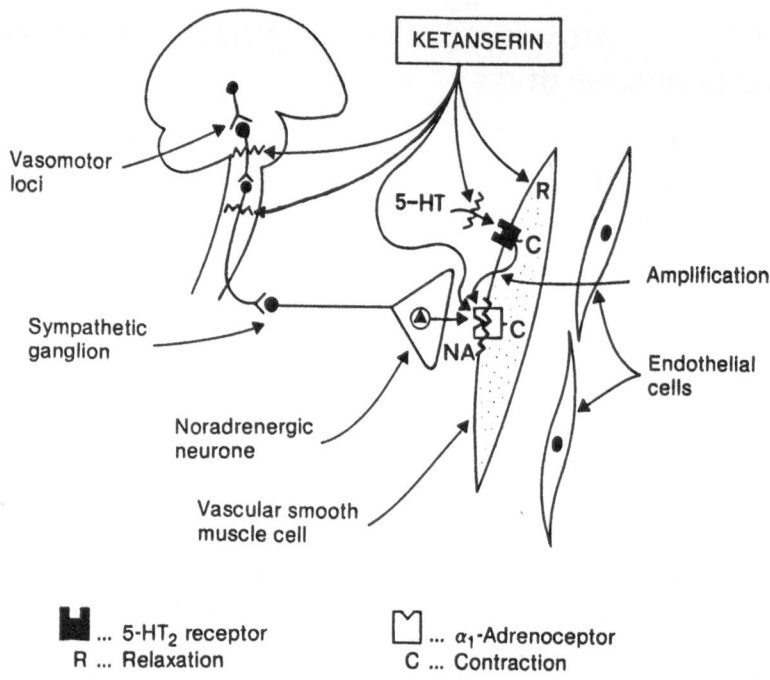

Figure 1. The possible sites and mechanisms of antihypertensive action exerted by ketanserin. NA, noradrenaline. From [9].

antihypertensive effect of ketanserin is mainly related to 5-HT$_2$ receptor blockade [13, 16, 17]. The above conclusion is not valid for several reasons. Firstly, though some abnormalities in the metabolism of 5-HT may exist in hypertension [18], 5-HT is present in very low concentrations in the plasma and there is little convincing evidence to suggest a major role for 5-HT$_2$ receptors in the development or maintenance of hypertension. Secondly, though not often realized, the vasodilator effect of 5-HT on resistance vessels is much more marked than its vasoconstrictor response. Thirdly, there is a poor correlation between 5-HT$_2$ receptor antagonism and the antihypertensive potential of a number of drugs [19, 20]. And lastly, several highly selective 5-HT$_2$ antagonists — LY 53857 [19], ritanserin [15, 21, 22], 2-(2-dimethylamino-2-methylpropylthio)-3-phenylquinoline hydrochloride (ICI 170809 [23]) — do not seem to be effective as antihypertensive agents.

2.2 α_1-Adrenoceptor blockade

It is well known that ketanserin has an appreciable α_1-adrenoceptor blocking activity. In experimental animals this effect is observed at doses which, though higher than needed for 5-HT$_2$ receptor antagonism, show antihypertensive activity [10, 24—26] and there is a remarkable similarity in the systemic and regional haemodynamic profiles of ketanserin and prazosin in hypertensive rabbits [10, 26]. In normal volunteers and hypertensive subjects also, distinct (though perhaps weaker than prazosin) α_1-adrenoceptor antagonism has been demonstrated with ketanserin after acute, but particularly chronic, administration [15, 27—30]. It should, however, be recalled that acute administration of ketanserin can lower blood pressure for a short time in hypertensive subjects without concomitant α_1-adrenoceptor blockade [16, 31] or in normotensive subjects with autonomic insufficiency [31].

Recently, some compounds, e.g. irindalone [32] and 4-{3-[3-(4-(4-fluorobezoyl)-1-piperidinyl)-propoxy]-4-methoxyphenyl}-1-pyrrolidone (ZK 33.839) [33], have been described which, like ketanserin, antagonize responses mediated by both 5-HT_2 receptors and α_1-adrenoceptors. These compounds also decrease arterial blood pressure in hypertensive animals.

2.3   Combind blockade of α_1-adrenoceptors and 5-HT_2 receptor-mediated amplification of noradrenaline response

Since at levels giving similar antihypertensive effects ketanserin may be weaker than prazosin as an α_1-adrenoceptor antagonist and since ritanserin and LY 53857 are devoid of antihypertensive properties, Van Nueten et al. [13] suggest that a combination of 5-HT_2 receptor (responsible for the potentiation of noradrenaline-induced vasoconstriction) and α_1-adrenoceptor blockade is involved in the antihypertensive action of ketanserin. Some evidence for this is provided by the observation that ritanserin, which has no effect against phenylephrine-induced vasoconstriction, potentiates the hypotensive action of prazosin and phentolamine [14, 34].

2.4   Inhibition of central vasomotor loci

Contrary to initial suggestions, ketanserin does seem to enter into the CNS as it causes sedation and electroencephalographic changes in humans [27, 35]. The drug also interferes with central cardiovascular control mechanisms. Thus, ketanserin-induced hypotension: (a) is accompanied by a decrease in sympathetic nerve discharges after i.v. administration to baroreceptor denervated [36] or innervated [37] cats and spontaneously hypertensive rats [38]; (b) can be observed after intracarotid [39], intravertebral [22] or intrathecal [40] administration in animals; (c) is associated with suppression of centrally integrated pressor responses (carotid occlusion and nicotine) in dogs after low i.v. doses that do not affect peripheral sympathetic transmission [41]; (d) is exerted without clear changes in baroreceptor sensitivity [11]; and (e) is not accompanied by sustained reflex increases in heart rate [10, 16, 24—26, 38, 42] or plasma renin and catecholamine levels [38, 42] in both hypertensive animals and humans; such changes would be expected with a drug lowering blood pressure via peripheral vasodilatation only.

The receptors mediating the central antihypertensive action are not clearly delineated. The mixed 5-HT$_1$ and 5-HT$_2$ receptor antagonist methysergide, which may function as a partial agonist at some 5-HT$_1$-like receptors [43], reduces blood pressure, heart rate, pressor responses to bilateral carotid occlusion, and sympathetic nerve activity [37, 44], but the other highly selective 5-HT$_2$ receptor antagonists, LY 53857 [15, 37] and ritanserin [21, 22], do not exhibit hypotensive activity. Since ketanserin (see above), prazosin [36] or phentolamine [40], all of which block α_1-adrenoceptors, but not corynanthine or rauwolscine [22], which preferably antagonize α_2-adrenoceptors, show central hypotensive activity, a blockade of α_1-adrenoceptors may be responsible for antihypertensive action. Further investigation is, however, required to establish the exact role of 5-HT$_2$ and/or α_1-adrenoceptors in the antihypertensive activity of ketanserin as well as in the central regulation of cardiovascular activity.

2.5 'Direct' vasodilatation

In renal hypertensive rabbits, ketanserin produces a biphasic hypotensive effect, consisting of a short-lasting but pronounced phase and a longer-lasting but more moderate phase [10]. Since the initial hypotensive response persists after blockade of autonomic ganglia by hexamethonium, this phase of ketanserin's effect seems to be due to a 'direct' vasodilatation [10] that may play some role in the acute antihypertensive action of the drug. Indeed, this property of ketanserin may explain the moderate hypotensive effect observed in normotensive subjects with autonomic insufficiency [31].

3. Clinical effects of 5-HT receptor antagonists

Among the 5-HT receptor antagonists only ketanserin, which blocks 5-HT$_2$ receptors but also has other properties (see above), has been shown to lower arterial blood pressure in hypertensive patients [see 12]. Acute administration of ketanserin (10 mg, i.v.) lowers both systolic and diastolic pressures with only small increases in heart rate and cardiac output showing that the drug mainly decreases total peripheral resistance. It does not consistently lower pressure in patients with uncontrolled hypertension and, therefore, is not suitable for use in hypertensive emergencies, except perhaps for hypertensive episodes during or after coronary artery bypass surgery or in carcinoid syndrome [12].

Long term use of ketanserin in several placebo-controlled trials has established the antihypertensive effect of the drug. The magnitude of the depressor effect of ketanserin is comparable to that of β-adrenoceptor antagonists or diuretics with which it shows an additive (not synergistic) effect. Several studies indicate that the antihypertensive effect of ketanserin is more marked in patients over 60 years of age [12]. It may, however, be pointed out that ketanserin may not be unique in this respect because, with increasing age and arterial calcification, the wall to lumen ratio is altered and other vasodilator agents may also show an age-related hyper-effectiveness in hypertension.

The side effects of ketanserin (drowsiness, sleepiness, lack of concentration and lightheadedness) are usually mild and disappear after a few days. In early studies using high doses (60 mg or more) side effects, mainly drowsiness, fatigue, dizziness and headache, were often noted. In addition, ketanserin seems to prolong the Q-Tc interval, particularly in patients who have low blood potassium levels or are also receiving antiarrhythmics [12].

The exact place of ketanserin in the therapy of hypertension is not yet clear. More extensive use of the drug, as is expected after its marketing in several countries, will determine its value in comparison with other drugs in the treatment of hypertension.

4. Conclusions

5-HT elicits a triphasic blood pressure response, consisting of an initial transient hypotension (5-HT$_3$ receptor mediated), a middle hypertension (5-HT$_2$ receptor mediated) and, finally, a long-lasting hypotension (5-HT$_1$ receptor mediated). Therefore, it may be argued that antihypertensive drug therapy can be achieved via selective blockade of 5-HT$_2$ receptors. However, of the various antagonists of 5-HT$_2$ receptors, arterial blood pressure is lowered by ketanserin and some other newer drugs which have other properties such as α_1-adrenoceptor antagonism, central inhibition of sympathetic activity and/or 'direct' vasodilatation. Thus, it is doubtful that 5-HT$_2$ receptor antagonism plays a primary role in the antihypertensive action of such drugs. Early clinical experience with ketanserin seems to suggest that its antihypertensive effect is equivalent to that of β-adrenoceptor antagonists or thiazide diuretics and is apparently more marked in elderly patients. Clinical data with ketanserin is so far limited and, therefore, its correct place in the antihypertensive regimen is yet to be determined.

Acknowledgements

We are grateful to the *Journal of Cardiovascular Pharmacology* for the use of Figure 1 [9].

References

1. Saxena PR (1986): Nature of the 5-hydroxytryptamine receptors in mammalian heart. *Prog Pharmacol* 6: 173—185.
2. Cohen ML (1989): Receptors for 5-hydroxytryptamine in the cardiovascular system. Ch. XXII, This book.
3. Page IH (1957): Cardiovascular actions of serotonin (5-hydroxytryptamine), pp. 93—108 in: Lewis GP (ed), *5-Hydroxytryptamine*. London: Pergamon Press.
4. Fozard JR (1984): MDL 72222: a potent and highly selective antagonist at neuronal 5-HT receptors. *Naunyn Schmiedebergs Arch Pharmacol* 326: 36—44.
5. Kalkman HO, Engel G, Hoyer D (1984): Three distinct types of serotonergic receptors mediate the triphasic blood pressure response to serotonin in rats. *J Hypertens* 6 (suppl. 2): S421—S428.
6. Saxena PR, Lawang A (1985): A comparison of cardiovascular and smooth muscle effects of 5-hydroxytryptamine and 5-carboxamidotryptamine, a selective agonist of 5-HT$_1$-like receptors. *Arc Int Pharmacodyn Ther* 227: 235—252.
7. Saxena PR, Mylecharane EJ, Heiligers J (1985): Analysis of the heart rate effects of 5-hydroxytryptamine in the cat; mediation by 5-HT$_1$-like receptors. *Naunyn Schmiedebergs Arch Pharmacol* 330: 121—129.
8. Leysen JE, De Chaffoy De Courcelles D, De Clerck F, Niemegeers CJE, Van Nueten JM (1984): Serotonin-S$_2$ receptor binding sites and functional correlates. *Neuropharmacology* 23: 1493—1501.
9. Saxena PR, Bolt GR, Dhasmana KM (1987): Serotonin agonists and antagonists in experimental hypertension. *J Cardiovasc Pharmacol* 10 (suppl. 3): S12—S18.
10. Bolt GR, Saxena PR (1985): Cardiovascular profile and hypotensive mechanism of ketanserin in the rabbit. *Hypertension* 7: 499—506.
11. Vanhoutte PM, Ball SG, Berdeaux A, Cohen ML, Hedner T, McCall R, Ramage AG, Reimann IH, Richer C, Saxena PR, Schalekamp MADH, Struyker-Boudier HAJ, Symoens J, Van Nueten JM, Van Zwieten PA (1986): Mechanism of action of ketanserin in hypertension. *Trends Pharmacol Sci* 7: 58—59.
12. Vanhoutte PM, Amery A, Birkenhäger W, Breckenridge A, Bühler F, Distler A, Dormandy J, Doyle A, Frohlich E, Hansson L, Hedner T, Hollenberg N, Jensen H-E, Lund-Johansen P, Meyer P, Opie L, Robertson I, Safar M, Schalekamp M, Symoens J, Trap-Jensen J, Zanchetti A (1988): Serotonergic mechanisms in hypertension: Focus on the effects of ketanserin. *Hypertension* 11: 111—133.
13. Van Nueten JM, Schuurkes JAJ, De Ridder WJE, Kuyps JJMD, Janssens WJ (1986): Comparative pharmacological profile of ritanserin and ketanserin. *Drug Dev Res* 8: 187—195.
14. Van Nueten JM, Xhonneux R, Janssens WJ, Schuurkes JAJ, Janssen PAJ (1988): Interaction between S$_2$-serotonergic and alpha$_1$-adrenergic receptors and control of blood pressure, (in press) in: Vanhoutte PM (ed), *Mechanism of Vasodilatation*. New York: Raven Press.
15. Blauw GJ, van Brummelen P, Chang PC, Van Zwieten PA (1988): Regional vascular effects of serotonin and ketanserin in young, healthy subjects. *Hypertension* 11: 256—263.
16. Wenting GJ, Man in't Veld AJ, Woittiez AJJ, Boomsma F, Schalekamp MADH (1982): Haemodynamic effects of ketanserin, a selective 5-hydroxytryptamine (serotonin) receptor antagonist, in essential hypertension. *Clin Sci* 63: 435S—438S.
17. Janssen PAJ (1985): Pharmacology of potent and selective S$_2$-serotonergic antagonists. *J Cardiovasc Pharmacol* 7 (suppl. 7): S2—S11.
18. Symoens J, Vanhoutte PM (1985): The role of serotonin in blood pressure regulation, pp. 141—164 in: Smith JAR, Watkins J (eds), *Care of the postoperative patient*. London: Butterworth.

19. Cohen ML, Fuller RW, Kurz KD (1983): LY 53857, a selective new potent serotonergic (5-HT$_2$) receptor antagonist, does not lower blood pressure in the spontaneously hypertensive rat. *J Pharmacol Exp Ther* 227: 327—332.

20. Kalkman HO, Harms YM, Van Gelderen EM, Batink HD, Timmermans PBMWM, Van Zwieten PA (1983) Hypotensive activity of serotonin antagonists; correlation with α_1-adrenoceptor and serotonin receptor blockade. *Life Sci* 32: 1499—1505.

21. Hosie J, Stott DJ, Robertson JIS, Ball SG (1987): Does acute serotenergic type-2 antagonism reduce blood pressure? Comparative effects of single doses of ritanserin and ketanserin in essential hypertension. *J Cardiovasc Pharmacol* 10 (suppl. 3): S86—S88.

22. Van Zwieten PA, Mathy MJ, Boddeke HWGM, Doods HN (1987): Central hypotensive activity of ketanserin in cats. *J Cardiovasc Pharmacol* 10 (suppl 3): S54—S58.

23. Blackburn TP, Haworth SJ, Jessup CL, Morton PB, Williams C (1989): ICI 170809, A selective 5-hydroxytryptamine antagonist, inhibits human platelet aggregation *in vitro* and *ex vivo*. Ch. XXXX, This book.

24. Fozard JR (1982): Mechanism of the hypotensive effect of ketanserin. *J Cardiovasc Pharmacol* 4: 829—838.

25. Kalkman HO, Timmermans PBMWM, Van Zwieten PA (1982): Characterization of the antihypertensive properties of ketanserin (R41468) in rats. *J Pharmacol Exp Ther* 222: 227—231.

26. Wright CE, Angus JA (1983): Haemodynamic response to ketanserin in rabbits with page hypertension: Comparison with prazosin *J Hypertension* 1: 183—190.

27. Reimann IW, Frohlich JC (1983): Mechanism of antihypertensive action of ketanserin in man. *Br Med J* 287: 381—383.

28. Fagard R, Fioli R, Lijnen P, Staessen J, Moeman E, De Schaepdryver A, Amery A (1984): Haemodynamic and humoral responses to chronic ketanserin treatment in essential hypertension. *Br Heart J* 51: 149—156.

29. Casiglia E, Gava R, Semplicini A, Nicolin P, Pessina AC (1986): The mechanism of the antihypertensive effects of ketanserin: a comparison with metoprolol. *Br J Clin Pharmacol* 22: 751—752.

30. Berdeaux A, Edouard A, Samii K, Giudicelli JF (1987): Ketanserin and the arterial baroreceptor reflex in normotensive subjects. *Eur J Clin Pharmacol* 32: 27—33.

31. Wenting GJ, Woittiez AJJ, Man in't Veld AJ, Schalekamp MADH (1984): 5-HT, alpha-adrenoceptors, and blood pressure; effects of ketanserin in essential hypertension and autonomic insufficiency. *Hypertension* 6: 100—109.

32. Dragsted N, Boeck V (1988): Cardiovascular effects of irindalone, a novel 5-HT$_2$ antagonist with antihypertensive activity (Abstr P43). International Congress on Cardiovascular Pharmacology of 5-HT, Oct 4—7, Amsterdam.

33. Schröder G, Beckmann R, Müller B, Schulz BG, Stock G (1988): Pharmacological profile of ZK 33.839, a new 5-HT$_2$/α_1-antagonist (Abstr P38). International Congress on Cardiovascular Pharmacology of 5-HT, Oct 4—7, Amsterdam.

34. Van der Starre PJA (1988): Ketanserin and hypertension in cardiac surgery. Thesis, State University of Limburg, Maastricht, The Netherlands.

35. Herrmann WM, Baumgartner P (1986): Combined pharmaco-EEG and pharmacopsychological study to estimate CNS effects of ketanserin in hypertensive patients. *Neuropsychobiology* 16: 47—56.

36. McCall RB, Schuette MR (1984): Evidence for an alpha-1 receptor-mediated central sympathoinhibitory action of ketanserin. *J Pharmacol Exp Ther* 228: 704—710.

37. Ramage AG (1985): The effects of ketanserin, methysergide and LY 53857 on sympathetic nerve activity. *Eur J Pharmacol* 113: 295—303.

38. Hedner T, Pettersson A, Gradin K, Persson B (1986): Peripheral serotonergic mechansims in cardiovascular regulation in the spontaneously hypertensive rat. *J Hypertension* 4 (suppl. 3): S223—S225.

39. Copeland IW, Bentley GA (1985): A possible central action of prazosin and ketanserin to cause hypotension. *J Cardiovasc Pharmacol* 7: 822—825.

40. Dhasmana KM, Banerjee AK, Saxena PR (1989): The effects of intrathecal ketanserin and phentolamine on heart rate and arterial blood pressure in the rat. Ch. XXX, This book.
41. Phillips CA, Mylecharane EJ, Markus JK, Shaw J (1985): Hypotensive actions of ketanserin in dogs: involvement of a centrally mediated inhibition of sympathetic vascular tone. *Eur J Pharmacol* 111: 319—327.
42. Woittiez AJJ, Wenting GJ, Van der Meiracker AH, Ritsma Van Eck HJ, Man in't Veld AJ, Zantvoort FA, Schalekamp MADH (1986): Chronic effect of ketanserin in mild to moderate essential hypertension. *Hypertension* 8: 167—173.
43. Bradley PB, Engel G, Feniuk W, Fozard JR, Humphrey PPA, Middlemiss DN, Mylecharane EJ, Richardson B, Saxena PR (1986): Proposals for the classification and nomenclature of functional receptors for 5-hydroxytryptamine. *Neuropharmacology* 25: 563—575.
44. Antonaccio MJ, Taylor DJ (1977): Reduction in blood pressure, sympathetic nerve discharge and centrally evoked pressor responses by methysergide in anaesthetized cats. *Eur J Pharmacol* 42: 331—338.

XXV. Ketanserin in hypertension and vasospastic disease: mechanism of action

MAARTEN A. D. H. SCHALEKAMP and GERT-JAN WENTING

1. Introduction

5-Hydroxytryptamine (5-HT; serotonin) has fascinated and confused scientists since its discovery some 40 years ago. The monoamine, released from aggregating blood platelets, has been implicated in the peripheral control of vascular tone and in the pathogenesis of hypertension and peripheral vascular disorders. Its exact role, however, has remained elusive [1]. Exogenous 5-HT causes either contraction or relaxation of vascular smooth musle depending on blood vessel type, monoamine concentration, presence of intact endothelium and experimental conditions [2]. Most isolated large blood vessels, arteries as well as veins, are constricted by 5-HT whereas arterioles may be dilated. In addition, 5-HT markedly potentiates the constrictor effects of other agonists including noradrenaline. Local factors such as hypoxia and low temperature also contribute to the vasoconstrictor effect of 5-HT. This constrictor effect is mediated by 5-HT_2 receptors on vascular smooth musle [3—5].

Ketanserin is a selective 5-HT_2 receptor antagonist. Whereas this drug has virtually no affinity for 5-HT_1 receptors, it binds to alpha_1-adrenergic receptors. Unlike many other 5-HT antagonists, ketanserin has no partial agonist activity [6].

2. Haemodynamic profile of ketanserin

2.1 Hypertension

Acute haemodynamic effects of ketanserin (10 mg i.v.) in subjects with uncomplicated hypertension are a 10—20% decrease in systolic and diastolic systemic arterial pressure, a small decrease in right atrial pressure, pulmonary arterial and pulmonary capillary wedge pressures and a small transient increase in heart rate and cardiac output. The fall in systemic arterial

P.R. Saxena, D.I. Wallis, W. Wouters and P. Bevan (eds), *Cardiovascular Pharmacology of 5-Hydroxytryptamine*, pp. 319—327.
© 1990 *Kluwer Academic Publishers, Dordrecht* —

pressure is caused by a fall in total peripheral resistance. The rise in heart rate is accompanied by a rise in plasma noradrenaline probably due to baroreflex mediated sympathetic stimulation [7, 8]. The haemodynamic profile is that of vasodilator drug that has its main action on the arterioles with some additional action on capacitance vessels. Studies on regional haemodynamics in subjects with hypertension demonstrated vasodilatation in the fingers, the forearm, the leg and the kidney.

Ketanserin, 20 or 40 mg twice a day orally, has been demonstrated to lower blood pressure effectively in subjects with hypertension. Its effect on standing blood pressure is similar to that on supine pressure. During chronic treatment there are no significant effects on heart rate and cardiac output. Plasma noradrenaline is unaltered [9, 10].

2.2 Raynaud's phenomenon

In patients suffering from this disorder we found that systemic i.v. adminis-tration of 10 mg ketanserin caused the digital skin temperature to rise from 24.2 $\pm$ 0.8°C at an ambient temperature of 22—24°C to 31.5 $\pm$ 0.7°C (mean $\pm$ SEM, $p < 0.01$, n = 11). Finger blood flow measured by semicontinuous venous occlusion plethysmography, rose from 7.8 $\pm$ 0.7 to 27 $\pm$ 2.2 ml/min per 100 g tissue ($p < 0.001$).

3. Mechanism of action of ketanserin

The profile of ketanserin's haemodynamic actions is similar to that of the postsynaptic alpha$_1$-adrenergic receptor antagonist prazosin. Prazosin is also considered to act on both arteriolar and venous tone, and the drug is effective in hypertension and in some patients with Raynaud's phenomenon. It is therefore possible that the blood pressure lowering action of ketanserin is due to alpha$_1$ blockade rather than 5-HT$_2$ blockade. To address this point we tried to answer the following questions. First, does ketanserin in therapeutic doses antagonize vascular responses to 5-HT? Second, is ketanserin capable of lowering blood pressure indepently of alpha$_1$-adrenergic blockade? Third, are the pressor responses to bolus injections of the alpha$_1$-adrenergic receptor agonist phenylephrine altered by ketanserin? Finally, are the haemodynamic effects of ketanserin modified by pretreat-ment with prazosin?

3.1 5-HT receptor blockade

In six men with essential hypertension the effect of ketanserin on 5-HT induced venoconstriction was studied. A 22 gauge polyethylene cathether was inserted into a dorsal hand vein and connected to a pressure transducer. Saline was infused into this vein at a constant rate of 55 ml/hour. Then incremental doses of serotonin and noradrenaline (bolus injections) were added to the infusate and the rise and fall in pressure were recorded in time. The area under the curve was taken as a measure of the venous response. Systemic administration of ketanserin (10 mg i.v.) significantly reduced the 5-HT induced contraction of the hand vein, but had no effect on the responses of these veins to noradrenaline (Figure 1 and 2).

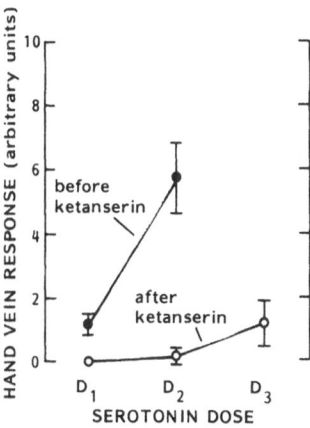

Figure 1. Constrictor responses of hand vein to serotonin in six patients with essential hypertension before and during ketanserin infusion.

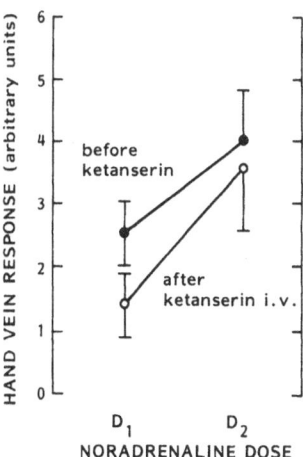

Figure 2. Constrictor responses of hand vein to noradrenaline in six patients with essential hypertension before and during ketanserin infusion.

3.2 *Effects in autonomic insufficiency*

That ketanserin can lower blood pressure independently of alpha₁-adrenergic blockade was substantiated in four patients with chronic autonomic insufficiency. All patients had combined efferent sympathetic and parasympathetic lesions of the baroreflex arc and they were suffering from incapacitating orthostatic hypotension. Plasma noradrenaline was abnormally low and was, like heart rate, unresponsive to head-up tilting. Phentolamine (20 mg i.v.) had no effect on blood pressure and heart rate in these patients which confirmed the presence of an efferent sympathetic lesion. Even so, ketanserin (10 mg i.v.) had a distinct hypotensive effect (Figure 3).

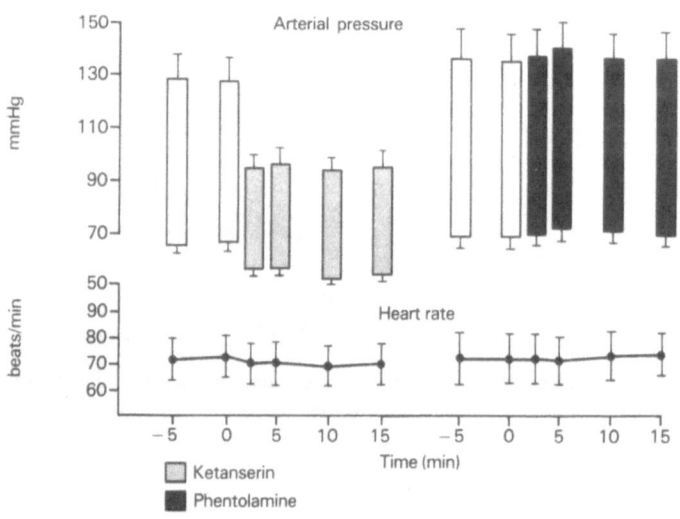

Figure 3. Effects of ketanserin (10 mg i.v.) and phentolamine (20 mg i.v.) on arterial pressure and heart rate in 4 patients with autonomic insufficiency.

3.3 *Effects on responses to phenylephrine*

In seven subjects with hypertension bolus injections of phenylephrine (25, 50, 100 and 200 ug), which were given in random order, were flushed into the circulation through a cannula in an antecubital vein, before and during ketanserin infusion (loading dose 10 mg, sustaining infusion 2 mg/hour i.v.). The changes in mean arterial pressure and heart rate were not modified by ketanserin (Figure 4). This contrasted with the shift of the dose-response curve to the right observed after treatment with prazosin. Thus as compared with prazosin, ketanserin does not seem to be a potent competetive antagonist on alpha₁-adrenergic receptors, at least not in the dose we have

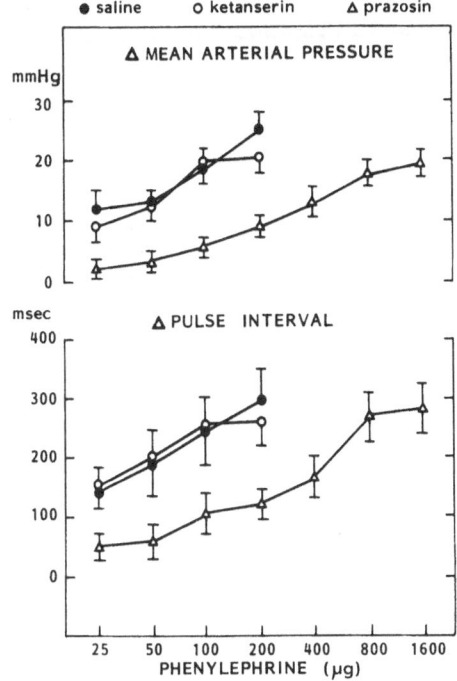

Figure 4. Dose-response curves for phenylephrine in seven patients with essential hypertension before (black circles) and during (open circles) ketanserin infusion. In five patients, phenylephrine injections were also given after treatment with prazosin (open triangles) (From Wenting et coll. 1984; with permission of the American Heart Association Inc.).

used. A slight but significant reduction of the pressor response to phenylephrine and to the selective alpha$_1$-adrenergic receptor agonist methoxamine has been observed during oral treatment of normotensive and hypertensive subjects with therapeutic doses of ketanserin [11, 12]. Methoxamine is more specific for vascular alpha$_1$-adrenergic receptors than phenylephrine. Although the vasopressor action of phenylephrine is due mainly to direct activation of alpha$_1$-receptors on vascular smooth muscle, it also has a tyramine like action resulting in the displacement of norepinephrine from adrenergic nerves and therefore can cause stimulation of beta- and alpha$_2$-adrenergic receptors as well. Thus methoxamine may be more suitable than phenylephrine from studying the importance of alpha$_1$-adrenoceptors in the action of ketanserin. In practice however, the tyramine-like effect of phenylephrine appears to be of little importance. Indeed, the pressor responses to bolus injections of doses of phenylephrine that are used in human studies are completely blocked by clinically effective amounts of the selective alpha$_1$-adrenergic receptor antagonist prazosin. Ketanserin unlike prazosin causes no parallel shift of the dose response curve to methoxamine. As a matter of fact it only affects the highest of the three doses of methoxamine studied [11, 13]. These data provide little evidence that ketanserin acts as an alpha$_1$-adrenergic receptor antagonist in man.

3.4   *Effects in subjects pretreated with prazosin*

Fourteen subjects with hypertension, in whom the effects of a first dose of ketanserin (10 mg i.v.) had been followed, were randomly assigned to two treatment modalities. Eight patients were treated with prazosin (4 mg three times a day) for one week and six patients were treated with furosemide (40 mg once daily) for one week. The response of blood pressure to both treatment modalities was more or less equal. The blood pressure response to a second dose of ketanserin (10 mg i.v.) was blunted by pretreatment with prazosin but not with furosemide (Figure 5). Therefore, it is possible that a certain degree of endogenous tone on vascular alpha$_1$-adrenergic receptors is required for ketanserin to exert its full antihypertensive action. This is in accordance with the contention that 5-HT$_2$-receptor stimulation is capable of amplifying the pressor response to endogenous noradrenaline.

In patients with Raynaud's phenomenon pretreatment with prazosin did not effect basal digital skin temperature. The rise in digital skin temperature after injection of ketanserin was comparable to the response to ketanserin

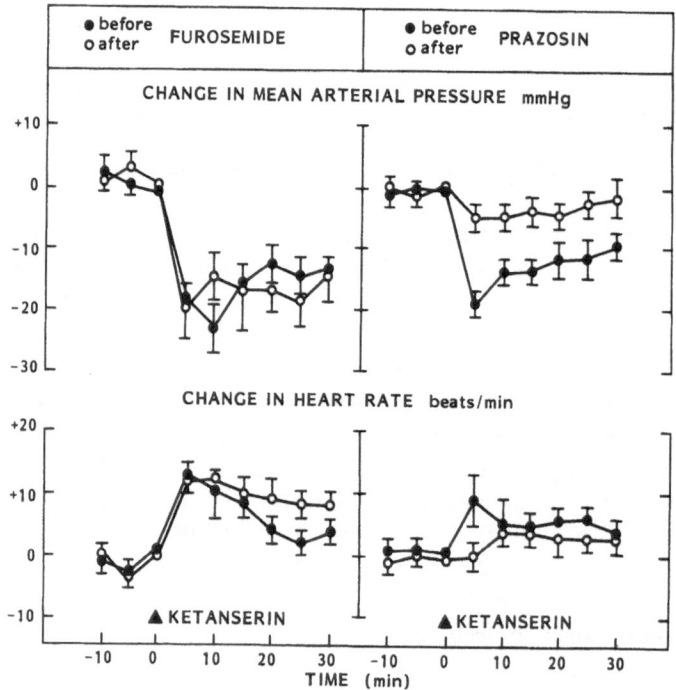

Figure 5. Effects of pretreatment with furosemide or prazosin on the antihypertensive action of ketanserin (10 mg i.v.). Mean arterial pressure was 114 ± 8 mmHg in 8 patients who were to be treated with prazosin and 116 ± 6 mmHg in the 6 patients to be treated with furosemide. After 1 week of treatment, mean arterial pressure was 103 ± 6 mmHg in the prazosin group and 102 ± 4 mmHg in the furosemide group (From Wenting et coll, 1984; with permission of the American Heart Association).

without pretreatment with prazosin (Figure 6). Thus, the increase of digital blood flow after ketanserin probably does not depend on an important interaction of the drug with digital alpha$_1$-adrenergic receptors.

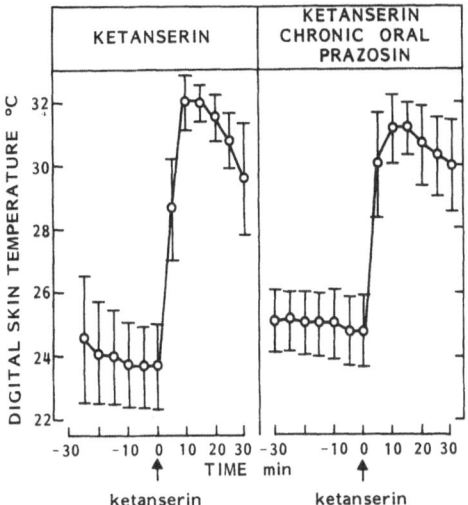

Figure 6. Effect of ketanserin on digital skin temperature in 7 patients with Raynaud's phenomenon before (left panel) and after pretreatment with prazosin (4 mg three times daily for at least three weeks).

3.5 *Central effects*

Experiments in rats, cats and dogs suggest that a centrally mediated inhibition of sympathetic nerve activity contributes to the hypotensive action of ketanserin (14). However, the receptors mediating these responses are not clearly delineated. Since ketanserin and prazosin, but *not* ritanserin which is a highly selective 5-HT$_2$ receptor antagonist and penetrates the brain more than ketanserin, show hypotensive activity (15), it could be that blockade of central alpha$_1$-adrenoceptors somehow is involved in these responses. In humans, however, we found no evidence that ketanserin suppressed the central adrenergic system. The sensitivity of the baroreflex was not affected by the drug (8) and levels of circulating catecholamines were not altered during chronic administration (9).

4. Conclusions

It appears that in humans acute administration of the 5-HT$_2$ receptor antagonist ketanserin is capable of causing vasodilatation independently of alpha$_1$-adrenergic receptor blockade. On the other hand a certain degree of alpha$_1$-adrenergic tone may be required for ketanserin to exert its full blood pressure lowering effect in subjects with hypertension. The drug also lowers blood pressure during chronic administration and it does so at a dose that causes less alpha$_1$-blockade than an equipotent (in terms of blood pressure response) dose of prazosin. Although the profile of ketanserin's haemodynamic effects resembles that of prazosin, an important difference appears to be that the venous action of prazosin is stronger; orthostatic hypotension is a well known side effect of prazosin treatment and this is rarely seen with ketanserin. The data collected for ketanserin, together with recent evidence [15, 16] that 5-HT$_2$ receptor antagonist with less affinity for alpha$_1$-adrenergic receptors do not lower blood pressure in animals and in man, suggest that the long term antihypertensive effect of ketanserin is caused by vascular 5-HT$_2$ receptor blockade combined with antagonism on vascular alpha$_1$-receptors. Until now there is little evidence that a central action of ketanserin is an important mechanism for explaining its antihypertensive activity.

References

1. Page IH (1968): *Serotonin*. Chicago: Year Book Medical Publishers.
2. Vanhoutte PM, Luescher TF (1986): Serotonin and the blood vessel wall. *J Hypertens* (suppl. 1) 4: S29—S35.
3. Leysen JE, Awouters F, Kennis L, Laduron PM, Vandenberk J, Janssen PAJ (1981): Receptor binding profile of R 41468, a novel antagonist at 5-HT$_2$ receptors. *Life Sci* 28: 1015—1022.
4. Cohen ML, Fuller RW, Wiley KS (1981): Evidence for 5-HT$_2$ receptors mediating contraction in vascular smooth muscle. *J Pharmacol Exp Ther* 218: 421—425.
5. Janssen PAJ (1983): 5-HT$_2$ receptor blockade to study serotonin-induced pathology. *Trends Pharmacol Sci* 4: 198—206.
6. Van Nueten JM, Janssen PAJ, Van Beek J, Xhonneux R, Verbeuren TJ, Vanhoutte PM (1981): Vascular effects of ketanserin (R 41468), a novel antagonist of 5-HT$_2$ serotonergic receptors. *J Pharmacol Exp Ther* 218: 217—230.
7. Wenting GJ, Man in 't Veld AJ, Woittiez AJ, Boomsma F, Schalenkamp MADH (1982): Treatment of hypertension with ketanserin, a new selective 5-HT$_2$ receptor antagonist. *Br Med J* 284: 537—539.
8. Wenting GJ, Woittiez AJ, Man in 't Veld AJ, Schalenkamp MADH: 5-HT, alpha-adrenoceptors and blood pressure. Effects of ketanserin in essential hypertension and autonomic insufficiency. *Hypertension* 6: 100—109.
9. Woittiez AJ, Wenting GJ, Van den Meiracker AJ, Ritsema van Eck HJ, Man in 't Veld AJ, Zantvoort FA, Schalenkamp MADH (1986): Chronic effect of ketanserin in mild to moderate essential hypertension. *Hypertension* 8: 167—173.
10. Vanhoutte PM, Amery AA, Birkenhager WH, Breckenridge A et al. (1988): Serotonergic mechanisms in hypertension. Focus on the effects of ketanserin. *Hypertension* 11: 111—133.
11. Reimann IW, Frolich JC (1983): Mechanism of antihypertensive action of ketanserin in man. *Br Med J* 287: 381—383.
12. Zabludowski JR, Zoccali C, Isles CG, Murray GD, Robertson JIS, Inglis GC, Fraser R, Ball SG (1984): Effect of the 5-hydroxytryptamine type 2 receptor antagonist, ketanserin,

on blood pressure, the renin-angiotensin system and sympatho-adrenal function in patients with essential hypertension. *Br J Clin Pharmacol* 17: 309—316.

13. Fagard R, Fioli R, Lijnen P, Staessen J, Moerman E, De Schaepdrijver A, Amery A (1984): Haemodynamic and humoral responses to chronic ketanserin treatment in essential hypertension. *Br Heart J* 51: 149—156.

14. Saxena PR (1989): 5-Hydroxytryptamine antagonists as antihypertensive drugs. This book.

15. Hosie J, Stott DJ, Robertson JIS, Ball SG (1987): Does acute serotonergic type-2 antagonism reduce blood pressure? Comparative effects of single doses of ritanserin and ketanserin in essential hypertension. *J Cardiovasc Pharmacol* (suppl. 3) 10: S86—S88.

16. Ramage AG (1985): The effects of ketanserin, methysergide and LY 53857 on sympathetic nerve activity. *Eur J Pharmacol* 113: 295—303.

XXVI. Renin secretion and 5-hydroxytryptamine

WILLIAM F. GANONG, M. D.

1. Introduction

A chance observation that intravenous 5-hydroxytryptophan (5-HTP) increased plasma renin activity (PRA) in dogs led us to a detailed study of the role of 5-hydroxytryptamine (5-HT) in the central nervous system in the regulation of renin secretion.

The essential components of the circulating renin-angiotensin system [see 1] are summarized in Figure 1. Renin is an acid protease secreted by the juxtaglomerular cells of the kidneys. It acts in the blood stream on angiotensinogen, a glycoprotein secreted by the liver, to release the decapeptide angiotensin I from the N terminal end of the angiotensinogen molecule. Angiotensin converting enzyme, a dipeptidyl carboxypeptidase, then releases histidyl-leucine from the C terminal end of angiotensin I to form the active octapeptide, angiotensin II (AII). AII is metabolized to biologically inactive fragments by a variety of different peptidases.

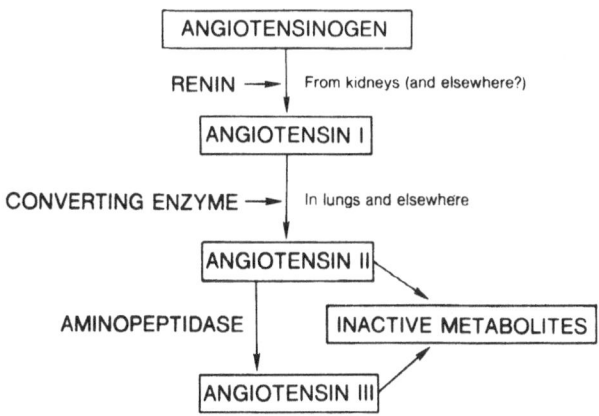

Figure 1. The circulating renin angiotensin system. From [1].

P.R. Saxena, D.I. Wallis, W. Wouters and P. Bevan (eds), Cardiovascular Pharmacology of 5-Hydroxytryptamine, pp. 329—337.
© 1990 *Kluwer Academic Publishers, Dordrecht —*

The main factors that regulate renin secretion [see 1] are summarized in Figure 2. The secretion of renin by the juxtaglomerular cells appears to be inhibited by stretch, and secretion increases as intrarenal arterial pressure falls and stretch decreases through the operation of this "intrarenal baroreceptor mechanism". Secretion is also inversely proportional to the rate of transport of sodium and chloride across the macula densa, a group of "sensory" cells at the start of the distal convuluted tuble which bring about changes in renin secretion in response to alterations in the composition of the urine. Various peptides affect renin secretion, and in particular, angiotensin II and vasopressin inhibit and vasoactive intestinal peptide (VIP) stimulates secretion. However, one of the most important regulators of renin secretion is the sympathetic nervous system. The stimulatory effect of sympathetic discharge is produced by noradrenaline released by the postganglionic sympathetic nerves that innervate the juxtaglomerular cells, primarily via a direct action on β_1-adrenoceptors on the surface of the juxtaglomerular cells. Circulating noradrenaline and adrenaline also affect renin secretion, but probably to a lesser degree.

2. Pharmacological experiments in dogs

Our initial experiments, carried out in pentobarbital anesthetized dogs,

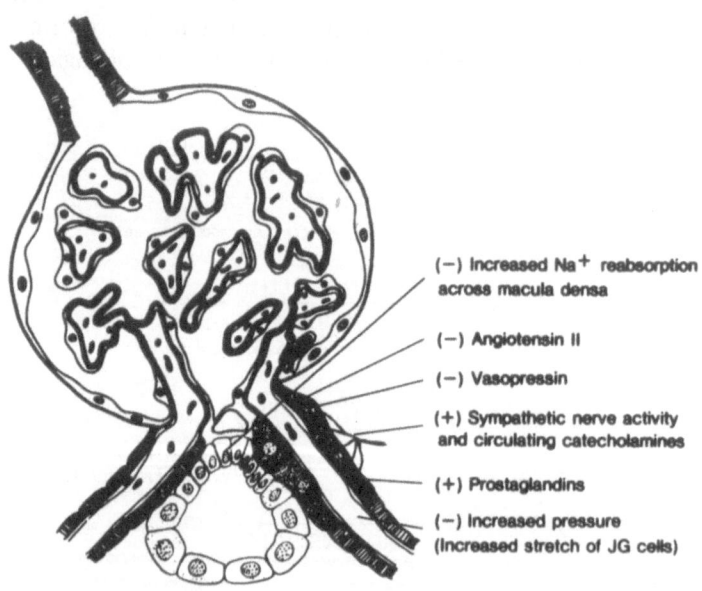

(−) Increased Na+ reabsorption across macula densa

(−) Angiotensin II

(−) Vasopressin

(+) Sympathetic nerve activity and circulating catecholamines

(+) Prostaglandins

(−) Increased pressure (Increased stretch of JG cells)

Figure 2. Principal factors involved in the regulation of renin recretion. +, stimulation; −, inhibition. From [1].

showed that 5-HTP stimulated renin secretion via the sympathetic nervous system; renal denervation abolished the 5-HTP response [2]. However, the increase was not associated with a significant change in blood pressure, indicating that it was due to selective stimulation of neural pathways regulating renin secretion, rather than diffuse sympathetic discharge. It is also significant, but probably not surprising, that the amount of renin released was not large enough to raise blood pressure. We previously observed that with stimuli producing mass sympathetic discharge in dogs, the magnitude of the pressor response was little changed when increased renin secretion was prevented by renal denervation [3].

Since noradrenaline and adrenaline affect renin secretion and 5-HTP is known to release catecholamines [4], we investigated the effect of tryptophan on renin secretion. This amino acid, which is only 5-hydroxylated in 5-HT-producing cells, also increased PRA. The 5-HT uptake inhibitor zimeldine also increased PRA (unpublished observations). Furthermore, we tested the effect of metergoline on the response to 5-HTP and tryptophan, and found that this 5-HT receptor blocking drug prevented the increase in PRA produced by both compounds. Thus, the response appears to be due to release of 5-HT rather than catecholamines.

The next question we addressed was the site of the 5-HT release that affected renin secretion. Carbidopa, which blocks 5-HT synthesis by inhibiting 5-HTP decarboxylase but does not cross the blood brain barrier to any degree, potentiated rather than inhibited the increase in PRA produced by systemic injection of 5-HTP. However, when benserazide was administered in a dose reported to inhibit central as well as peripheral 5-HTP decarboxylase [5], the PRA response to systemically administered 5-HTP was abolished. Thus, the data in the dog indicate that the site of the discharge that increases renin secretion is the CNS.

3. Pharmacological experiments in rats

To explore the role of 5-HT further, we switched from anesthetized dogs to unanesthetized rats. In experiments carried out by Van de Kar and others, we made extensive use of parachloramphetamine (PCA), a compound which eventually produces 5-HT depletion, but initially causes release of 5-HT [6]. In rats, we found [7] that PCA produced a dose-dependent increase in PRA (Figure 3). This compound also raises blood pressure, and the effect of the acutely increased pressure on the kidney via the intrarenal baroreceptor mechanism may explain the failure of PRA to increase 30 min after administration of the drug. However, PCA is markedly elevated 60 min after administration, and this increase is mediated by 5-HT because it is prevented if 5-HT is depleted by administration of parachlorophenylalanine.

To determine if in the rat, as in the dog, the site of the 5-HT release triggering increased renin secretion is in the brain, we administered 5,7-

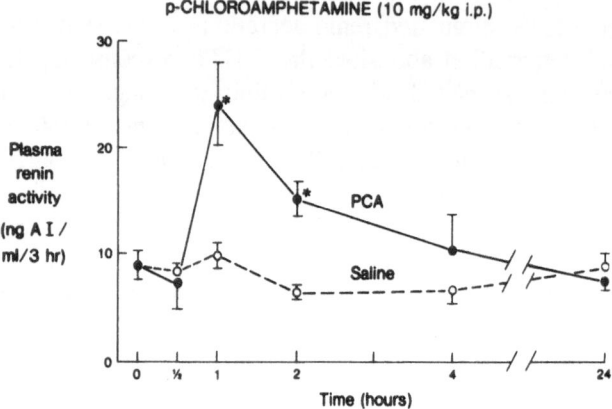

Figure 3. Time course of the effect of PCA on plasma renin activity in rats. From [7].

dihydroxytryptamine intraventricularly. The destruction of serotonergic neurons by this technique inhibited the PRA response to PCA. To determine which of the serotonergic neurons were involved, selective lesions in the various raphe nuclei were made by microinjection of 5, 7-dihydroxytrypta-mine. The neurochemical lesions of the dorsal raphe nucleus inhibited the PRA response to PCA; lesions of the medial and pontine raphe nuclei had no effect [8]. In subsequent experiments, we found that electrolytic lesions of the dorsal raphe nucleus had the same effect [9].

Our research has focused on the pathways by which serotonergic neurons in the dorsal raphe nucleus affect renin secretion, and we have done little research on the type of 5-HT receptors involved in the response. In addition, with the exception of our early experiments with metergoline in dogs and parachlorophenylalanine in rats, we have not explored the effects of 5-HT depleting or blocking drugs. However, Lorens and Van de Kar [10] found that fenfluramine and the 5-HT agonist MK-212 increased PRA, and that these increases were blocked by the 5-HT$_2$ receptor blocking drug LY53857. At low doses, the 5-HT$_{1A}$ agonists 8-OH-DPAT and ipsapirone did not increase PRA. Our results with metergoline are also consistent with the hypothesis that the effects of 5-HT on renin secretion are mediated by 5-HT$_2$ receptors.

4. Neural pathways

To determine whether PCA in the rat, like 5-HTP in the dog, affected renin secretion by way of the sympathetic nervous system, we tested the effect of β-adrenergic blockade. This blocks the final common sympathetic path, since sympathetic effects on renin secretion are mediated primarily by β_1-adreno-ceptors on the juxtaglomerular cells. The 1-isomer of propranolol produced a complete blockade of the PRA response [11]. In control rats, injection of the d-isomer, which has much less β-adrenoceptor blocking activity, failed to reduce the response. To avoid the criticism that propranolol might be acting centrally rather than peripherally to produce the inhibition, we also tested sotalol, a β-adrenoceptor blocking drug which does not penetrate the brain. It also inhibited the PRA response to PCA. In addition, we found that while ganglionic blockade with chlorisondamine increased renin secretion by itself, probably because it lowered blood pressure, administrationn of PCA after chlorisondamine failed to produce any further increase in PRA. The juxtaglomerular cells were capable of additional increases in renin secretion in these rats because administration of the β-adrenoceptor agonist isoprenaline after chlorisondamine produced a large additional increase in PRA. Thus, our data indicate that the PRA response to PCA in the rat is mainly, if not entirely, due to increased sympathetic discharge.

We have also explored the pathway by which the serotonergic neurons in the dorsal raphe nucleus produce increased renin secretion. One of the sites to which the dorsal raphe projects is the hypothalamus, and we found that large lesions of the mediobasal hypothalamus inhibited the PRA response to PCA [12]. So did knife cuts in the posterior hypothalamus, which interrupted the serotonergic fibers and produced a sharp decline in the 5-HT content of the mediobasal hypothalamus. Control knife cuts in the anterior hypothalamus had no effect.

Thus, lesions of the dorsal raphe nucleus and the mediobasal hypothalamus inhibit the PRA response to PCA (Figure 4). However, the mediobasal hypothalamus is a large area. Consequently, we began to explore which of the specific nuclei in this general area mediated the serotonergic response. Subsequently, the effects of bilateral electrolytic lesions of the dorsomeidal, paraventricular, and ventromedial nuclei were investigated [9, 13]. Dorsomedial lesions had no effect, but paraventricular lesions inhibited the response. However, paraventricular lesions reduced plasma angiotensinogen. The usual way to determine PRA is to incubate plasma and determine the amount of

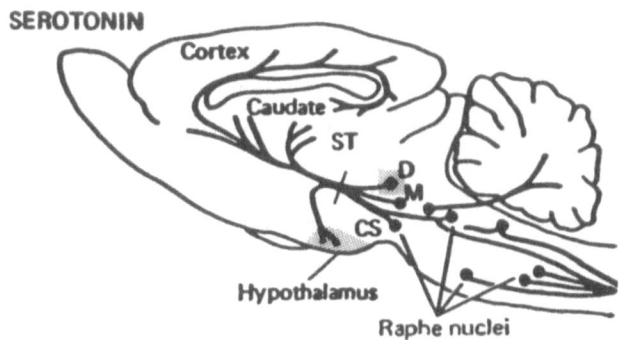

Figure 4. Lesions which inhibit the increase in PRA poduced by PCA, projected on a sagittal section of the brain of the rat. The sites of the lesions are shaded.

angiotensin I generated. This generation depends on the amount of angiotensinogen as well as the amount of renin in the sample [14]. If angiotensinogen is reduced, the amount of angiotensin I generated is reduced even if the amount of renin is normal. This can be overcome, of course, by adding excess exogenous angiotensinogen and measuring plasma renin concentration (PRC) rather than PRA. With this modification, the PRC response to PCA was not reduced to as great a degree as the PRA response, but it was still inhibited to a statistically significant degree [9]. The results with ventromedial lesions were also of considerable interest. These lesions did not effect plasma angiotensinogen, but they inhibited the PRA response to PCA. Thus, the serotonergic fibers involved in the renin response project from the dorsal raphe nucleus to the region of the paraventricular and ventromedial nuclei. A finer resolution of their exact location in this area will require additional research. In addition, we do not as yet know the pathway from the hypothalamus to the preganglionic sympathetic neurons in the thoracic spinal cord that are the orgin of the renal sympathetic output.

Although a side issue in the context of this review, the explanation of the decrease in circulating angiotensinogen produced by paraventricular lesions is an interesting topic to which we are currently devoting considerable attention. A neuroendocrine pathway seems likely, since angiotensinogen secretion is known to be regulated by adrenocortical, thyroid, and gonadal hormones [14], and the hypothalamus controls anterior pituitary secretion of the tropic hormones that regulate the secretion of the adrenals, thyroid, and glands.

5. Physiological implications

What is the physiological role of the brain serotonergic system in the regulation of renin secretion? To explore this question, we have studied three additional stimuli that were selected because they increase renin secretion in very different ways. They are the psychological stimulus of immobilization, the gravitational stimulus of head-up tilt, and the volume stimulus of sodium depletion. Each of these stimuli has been standardized in rats. The PRA responses to immobilization and head-up tilt are mediated by the nervous system, and both are mediated sympathetically, since they are blocked by propranolol [15]. The role of the nervous system in the renin response to sodium depletion is more controversial, but the bulk of the evidence indicates that although nonneural factors contribute when the depletion is marked, the initial increase in renin secretion produced by restricting dietary sodium intake is neurally mediated [see 16]. Since anesthetics also increase renin secretion by a mechanism that is uneffected by sympathetic blockade [see 17], we also investigated the effects of anesthesia produced by inactin (5-sec-butyl-5-ethyl-2-thiobarbituric acid).

The results of our investigations are summarized in Table 1. As mentioned

Table 1. Effect of lesions on the renin response to various stimuli.

		Increase in PRA produced by			
Lesions	PCA	Immobilization	Head-up tilt	Low Na$^+$ diet	Inactin anesthesia
Dorsal Raphe nucleus	−	+	+	+	+
Ventromedial nuclei	−	−	−	−	+

+, normal. −, inhibited.

above, the PRA response to PCA was abolished by dorsal raphe and ventromedial lesions. The response to inactin anesthesia was unaffected by lesions in either location, indicating that the lesions did not affect the responsiveness of the renin-angiotensin system. However, the ventromedial lesions abolished the renin response to the other three stimuli, whereas dorsal raphe lesions had no effect. These results indicate that the ventromedial nuclei play an important role in the brain control of renin secretion. However, the serotonergic fibers in the dorsal raphe nucleus do not mediate the response to immobilization, tilt, and sodium depletion.

On the other hand, Van de Kar and his associates explored the role of the serotonergic system using what is probably a more complex psychological stress than immobilization [18]. They placed rats in a special cage and exposed them briefly to unavoidable foot shock on each of three consecutive days. On the fourth day, the rats were placed in the same cage, but instead of receiving shocks, they were removed and sacrified. There was a marked increase in PRA which was absent in rats with dorsal raphe lesions. This suggests that the serotonergic fibers may mediate renin responses to some psychological stimuli. However, additional research is clearly needed to define the exact role of brain serotonergic fibers in the regulation of renin secretion.

6. Conclusions

A series of experiments in dogs and rats indicate that discharge of serotonergic neurons in the central nervous system leads to increased secretion of renin from the kidneys. At least in dogs, this effect appears to be selective, and not associated with mass sympathetic discharge. In rats, the neurons that are involved are in the dorsal raphe nucleus, and appear to exert their effects by way of 5-HT$_2$ receptors. The neurons project to the region of the paraventricular and ventromedial nuclei of the hypothalamus, and the final pathway to the kidneys is sympathetic. However, the connection between the hypothalamus and the sympathetic output to the kidneys is presently unknown. This system may mediate the increases in renin secretion produced by some psychological stimuli, although other neural stimuli exert their effects in other ways.

Acknowlegements

Research in the author's laboratory that is discussed in this review was supported by USPHS grant HL29714, NASA grant NAG 2-434, and the Smokeless Tobacco Research Council.

References

1. Ganong WF (1989): *Review of Medical Physiology*, 14th ed. Norwalk, CT/San Mateo, CA: Appleton and Lange.
2. Zimmermann H, Ganong WF (1980): Pharmacological evidence that stimulation of central serotonergic pathways increases renin secretion. *Neuroendocrinology* 30: 101—107.
3. Passo SS, Assaykeen T, Otsuka K, Wise BL, Goldfien A, Ganong WF (1971): Effect of stimulation of the medulla oblongata on renin secretion in dogs. *Neuroendocrinology* 7: 1—10.
4. Ng LKY, Chase TN, Colburn RW, Kopin IJ (1972): Release of (3H) dopamine by L-5 hydroxytryptophan. *Brain Res* 45: 499—505.
5. Bartholini G, Pletscher A (1969): Effect of various decarboxylase inhibitors on the cerebral metabolism of dihydroxyphenylalanine. *J Pharm Pharmac* 21: 323—324.
6. Trulson ME, Jacobs BL (1976): Behavioral evidence for the rapid release of CNS serotonin by PCA and fenfluramine. *Eur J Pharmacol* 36: 149—154.
7. Van de Kar LD, Wilkinson CW, Ganong WF (1981): Pharmacological evidence for a role of brain serotonin in the maintenance of plasma renin activity in unanesthethized rats. *J Pharmacol Exp Therap* 219: 85—90.
8. Van de Kar LD, Wilkinson CW, Skrobik Y, Brownfield MS, Ganong WF (1982): Evidence that serotonergic neurons in the dorsal raphe nucleus exert a stimulatory effect on the secretion of renin but not of corticosterone. *Brain Research* 235: 233—243.
9. Gotoh E, Murakami K, Bahnson TD, Ganong WF (1987): Role of brain serotonergic pathways and the hypothalamus in the regulation of renin secretion. *Am J Physiol* 253: R179—R185.
10. Lorens SA, Van de Kar LD (1987): Differential effects of serotonin (5-HT$_{1A}$ and 5-HT$_2$) agonists and antagonists on renin and corticosterone secretion. *Neuroendocrinology* 45: 305—310.
11. Alper RH, Ganong WF (1984): Pharmacological evidence that the sympathetic nervous system mediates the increase in renin secretion produced by para-chloroamphetamine. *Neuropharmacology* 23: 1237—1240.
12. Karteszi M, Van de Kar LD, Makara G, Stark E, Ganong WF (1982): Evidence that the mediobasal hypothalamus is involved in serotonergic stimulation of renin secretion. *Neuroendocrinology* 34: 323—326.
13. Gotoh E, Golin RMA, Ganong WF (1988): Relation of the ventromedial nuclei of the hypothalamus to the regulation of renin secretion. *Neuroendocrinology* 47: 518—522.
14. Menard J, Bouhnik J, Clauser E, Richoux JP, Corvol P (1983): Biochemistry and regulation of angiotensinogen. *Clin Exper Hyper — Theory and Practice* A5: 1005—1019.

15. Golin RMA, Gotoh E, Said SI, Ganong WF (1988): Pharmacological evidence that the sympathetic nervous system mediates the increase in renin secretion produced by immobilization and head-up tilt in rats. *Neuropharmacology* 27: 1209–1213.
16. Ganong WF, Barbieri C (1982): Neuroendocrine components in the regulation of renin secretion, pp. 231–262 in: Ganong WF, Martini L (eds), *Frontiers in Neuroendocrinology*, Volume 7. New York: Raven Press.
17. Keeton TK, Campbell WB (1984): Control of renin release and its alterations by drugs, pp. 65–118 in: Antonaccio M (ed), *Cardiovascular Pharmacology, 2nd edition*. New York: Raven Press.
18. Van de Kar LD, Lorens FA, McWilliams CR, Kunimoto K, Urban JH, Bethea CL (1984): Role of midbrain raphe in stress-induced renin and prolactin secretion. *Brain Research* 311: 333–341.

XXVII. Acute and long-term effects of 5-hydroxytryptamine in isolated renal arteries in vitro

J. G. R. DE MEY, M. P. UITENDAAL, H. C. M. BOONEN and
M. J. J. F. VRIJDAG

1. Introduction

Acute changes in vascular function are brought about by changes in the contractile reactivity of vascular smooth muscle. In chronic modulation of vascular function structural alterations of the vascular wall can participate as well (for review, see [1]). Similarly, the responsiveness of the arterial wall to lumenal injury in vivo consists of vasoconstriction and subsequent migration and proliferation of arterial smooth muscle cells (for review, see [2]). The exact relationship between fast responses such as constriction and the slower structural alterations is however unclear.

Since aggregating platelets can release both vasoconstrictor and mitogenic substances [3], we evaluated in the present study (i) whether 5-hydroxytryptamine (5-HT) induces proliferation of arterial smooth muscle cells and (ii) how contractile responses to 5-HT are affected by exposure of the arterial wall to serum derived mitogens. The experiments were performed in isolated arterial segments in tissue culture to facilitate recording of mechanical reactivity.

2. Material and methods

The experiments were performed on segments of renal arteries that had been isolated from 20 week old male Wistar-Kyoto rats, chemically sympathectomized with 6-hydroxydopamine and mechanically denuded of endothelium. To record contractile reactivity, arterial segments were mounted horizontally between a displacement device and an isometric force transducer in an organ chamber with Krebs-Ringer bicarbonate (KRB) solution that was aerated with 95% O_2–5% CO_2 and maintained at 37°C [4]. Prior to experimentation, the preparations were stretched to their optimal lumen diameter for mechanical performance by stepwise stretching and intermittent exposure to high potassium KRB (KRB in which NaCl was replaced by KCl). The

P.R. Saxena, D.I. Wallis, W. Wouters and P. Bevan (eds), Cardiovascular Pharmacology of
5-Hydroxytryptamine, pp. 339–342.
© 1990 Kluwer Academic Publishers, Dordrecht —

experiments which included recording of responses to high potassium (K^+), phenylephrine (PHE) and 5-HT were terminated by exposing the preparations to periodate-lysine paraformaldehyde fixative. Measurements of contractile reactivity were performed either acutely after isolation of the arterial segments or after up to 2 weeks of tissue culture.

To tissue culture arterial segments, they were suspended on a mounting support (outer diameter 0.9 mm) in Dulbecco's minimal Eagle's modified medium (DMEM) which unless specifically mentioned was supplemented with 20% fetal calf whole blood serum (FCS) [5, 6]. In part of the experiments 10 μM 5-HT or 1 μM ketanserin was added to the culture medium. To estimate the extent of DNA-synthesis during tissue culture, 20 μM of the thymidine analogue 5-bromodeoxyuridine (BrdUrd) was included in the culture medium for 6 days. BrdUrd labeling indices for the media of the arterial preparations were obtained following immunohistochemistry on cross sections [5, 6].

3. Results

In freshly isolated renal artery segments, 5-HT and PHE induced concentration-dependent contractions; sensitivity and maximal responses to the indolamine and catecholamine were comparable (Figure 1). 1 μM ketanserin, but not 1 μM prazosin, abolished contractile response to 5-HT.

DMEM induced a small contractile response (15 $\pm$ 1% of the response to 125 mM K^+), which was increased concentration-dependently when the medium was supplemented with FCS, a classical but undefined source of

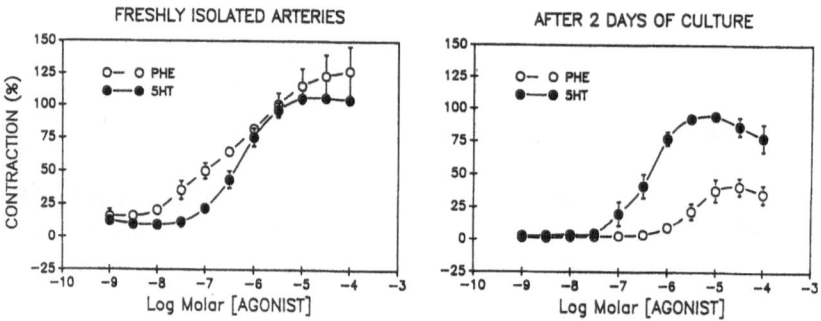

Figure 1. Effect of tissue culture on contractile responses to phenylephrine (O —— O) and 5-HT (● —— ●) in sympathectomized and de-endothelialized renal artery segments of the rat. Cumulative concentration response curves for the agonists were constructed in arterial preparations that had been stretched to their optimal lumen diameter. Data were expressed as percent of the contractile response to 125 mM KCl and are shown as mean $\pm$ SEM (n = 6). Left: freshly isolated preparations (100% = 4.7 $\pm$ 0.7 mN/mm); right: arterial preparations that had been maintained for 2 days in tissue culture in DMEM culture medium supplemented with 20% fetal calf serum (100% = 4.1 $\pm$ 0.7 mN/mm).

growth factors. The strong contractile response to 20% FCS (DMEM plus 20% FCS induced a contraction that averaged $126 \pm 4\%$ of the response to 125 mM K$^+$) was not affected by 1 μM prazosin but abolished by 1 μM ketanserin.

To judge from BrdUrd labeling indices, tissue culture in DMEM for 6 days induced DNA-synthesis in $24 \pm 4\%$ of the medial cells. This was not significantly affected by the presence of 10 μM 5-HT ($27 \pm 4\%$). Tissue culture in the presence of 20% FCS stimulated DNA-synthesis to a much larger extent ($79 \pm 9\%$). This was not significantly affected by the presence of 1 μM ketanserin ($85 \pm 6\%$).

In arterial segments that had been maintained in tissue culture in the presence of 20% FCS, 125 mM K$^+$ induced a contraction that averaged 88 ± 6, 64 ± 7 and $14 \pm 4\%$ of that in freshly isolated preparations after 2, 6 and 14 days of culture, respectively. The sensitivity of arterial preparations for the contractile effect of 5-HT and their maximal responsiveness to the indolamine (relative to the maximal response to K$^+$) were not affected by up to 2 weeks of culture. Sensitivity and responsiveness to PHE on the other hand were drastically reduced within 2 days of culture (Figure 1).

4. Discussion

To judge from inhibitory effects of ketanserin, but not prazosin, acute contractile responses to both 5-HT and FCS in sympathectomized and deendothelialized renal arteries were mediated by 5-HT$_2$ receptors on arterial smooth muscle cells [7]. Long-term exposure of arterial segments to FCS did not affect their contractile responses to 5-HT. This suggests that unlike the resistance part of the renal vasculature [8] the renal muscular artery does not display tachyphylaxis to the contractile effect of 5-HT.

Tissue culture of arterial segments in serum-free conditions resulted in a significant but low level of DNA-synthesis in the arterial media. This was not affected by the presence of a high concentration of 5-HT. FCS on the other hand stimulated DNA-synthesis in arterial segments in tissue culture. While ketanserin abolished the contractile effect of FCS, it did not affect stimulation of DNA-synthesis by FCS. Consequently, long-term stimulation of 5-HT$_2$ receptors or of contraction in general did not induce intra-arterial proliferation of smooth muscle cells and did not contribute to mitogenic effects of FCS.

After a lag time of at least 2 days, tissue culture of renal artery segments induced a progressive decrease in contractile responses to high potassium. The mechanisms involved in this decrease remain unclear in the present study. They could include modulation of the phenotype of arterial smooth muscle cells from contractile to synthetic prior or subsequent to entry into the cell cycle [12]. The evolution of contractile response to 5-HT during tissue culture paralleled that of responses to the non-receptor mediated stimulus, potassium. Responses to PHE on the other hand were readily decreased in tissue culture. The relevance of the latter pharmacological change when arterial smooth muscle is exposed to mitogenic stimuli merits further investigation. It seems however likely that 5-HT can participate in the responsiveness of the arterial wall to both acute and chronic conditions of platelet activation. Under these conditions contractile responses to 5-HT could persist during proliferative responses within the arterial wall to platelet-derived growth factors. 5-HT and the contraction it elicits would however not contribute to structural changes of the arterial wall in response to arterial injury and platelet aggregation in vivo.

5. Conclusions

In isolated arterial smooth muscle 5-HT$_2$ receptor stimulation does not induce cellular proliferation or participate in proliferative responses to serum. Unlike contractile responses to α_1-adrenoceptor stimulation, those to 5-HT$_2$ receptor stimulation are not affected by proliferating conditions.

Acknowledgement

This study was supported by an established investigatorship from the Royal Dutch Academy of Sciences to Jo De Mey.

References

1. Folkow B (1982): Physiological aspects of primary hypertension. *Physiol Rev* 62: 347–504.
2. Schwartz SM, Campbell GR, Campbell JH (1986): Replication of smooth muscle cells in vascular disease. *Circ Res* 58: 427–444.
3. Ross R, Glomset JA (1976): The pathogenesis of atherosclerosis. *New Engl J Med* 295: 369–380.
4. De Mey JGR, Defreyn G, Lenaers A, Calderon P, Roba J (1987): Arterial reactivity, blood pressure, and plasma levels of atrial natriuretic peptides in normotensive and hypertensive rats: effects of acute and chronic administration of atriopeptin III. *J Cardiovasc Pharmacol* 9: 525–535.
5. Fingerle J, Kraft T (1987): The induction of smooth muscle cell proliferation in vitro using an organ culture system. *Int Angiol* 6: 65–72.
6. De Mey JGR, Uitendaal MJ, Boonen HCM, Vrijdag MJJE, Daemen MJAP (1989): Acute and long-term effects of tissue culture on contractile reactivity in renal arteries of the rat. *Circ Res* (in press).
7. Van Nueten JM, Janssen PAJ, Van Beek J, Xhonneux R, Verbeuren TJ, Vanhoutte PM (1981): Vascular effects of ketanserin (R41468), a novel antagonist of 5-HT$_2$ serotonergic receptors. *J Pharmacol Exp Ther* 218: 217–230.
8. De Mey C, Vanhoutte PM (1981): Effect of age and spontaneous hypertension on the tachyphylaxis to 5-hydroxytryptamine and angiotensin II in the isolated rat kidney. *Hypertension* 3: 718–724.

XXVIII. Ventrolateral medullary pressor area: site of hypotensive and sympatho-inhibitory effects of (±) 8-OH-DPAT in anaesthetized dogs

MICHEL LAUBIE, MADELEINE DROUILLAT, HUBERT DABIRÉ, CLAUDIE CHERQUI and HENRI SCHMITT

1. Introduction

The central $5\text{-}HT_{1A}$ agonist, 8-OH-DPAT has been reported to produce dose-related decreases in blood pressure and heart rate in anaesthetized rats [1, 3]. The hypotensive effect of 8-OH-DPAT appears to be due to a central sympatho-inhibitory effect [4, 5] and these effects are antagonized by spiperone [5], metergoline [3] and (-) pindolol [6] indicating that the decrease in sympathetic tone produced by 8-OH-DPAT is probably due to the stimulation of central $5\text{-}HT_{1A}$ receptors. The propose of the present work was mainly to localize the sites of action of 8-OH-DPAT in the CNS.

2. Materials and methods

Mougrel dogs of either sex weighing 9—11 kg were anaesthetized with pentobarbital sodium (30 mg/kg, i.v.) and paralyzed with gallamine triethiodide (5 mg/kg i.v.). Artificial ventilation was provided with a Bird Mark VII respirator. Arterial blood pressure was recorded with a Statham P23 Db transducer from a catheter introduced into the aorta via the femoral artery. The renal sympathetic activity was recorded from branches of the left renal nerve plexus as described previously [7]. Injections into the vertebral artery were performed using a catheter inserted into this artery. Intracisternal injections were performed through the muscles of the neck. Microinjections into the medullary tissue (nucleus tractus solitarii, ventrolateral pressor area, medullary raphe nuclei) were performed with a glass micropipette as previously described [7]. The volume injected was 0.2 to 0.4 μl/site.

3. Results

8-OH-DPAT (0.1 to 3 μg/kg) injected into the vertebral artery in intact

P.R. Saxena, D.I. Wallis, W. Wouters and P. Bevan (eds), Cardiovascular Pharmacology of 5-Hydroxytryptamine, pp. 343—346.
© 1990 *Kluwer Academic Publishers, Dordrecht* —

anaesthetized dogs produced a dose-dependent reduction in blood pressure, heart rate and renal sympathetic nerve activity. 8-OH-DPAT (0.1 to 6 μg/kg) injected into the vertebral artery in baroreceptor-denervated dogs and in catecholamine depleted dogs also reduced the rate of sympathetic discharge. The sympatho-inhibitory effects of 8-OH-DPAT (3 μg/kg) were prevented by methiothepin (0.2 mg/kg) or ($\pm$) pindolol (0.2 mg/kg). In addition methiothepin reversed the central sympatho-inhibitory effects of 8-OH-DPAT.

Bilateral microinjections of 8-OH-DPAT (1 μg/site) within the area of the nucleus tractus solitarii or microinjections of 8-OH-DPAT into the medullary raphe nuclei failed to alter blood pressure, heart rate or renal sympathetic nerve activity in intact anaesthetized dogs.

In the ventrolateral medulla, 8-OH-DPAT was injected in the dog into the clonidine sensitive sites, 4.0—4.5 mm rostral to the middle rootlets of the XIIth nerve and 4.5—5 mm lateral to the midline. Bilateral microinjection (1 μg) into this area, 0.5 mm beneath the ventral surface produced a rapid decrease in mean blood pressure from 130 $\pm$ 3 to 106 $\pm$ 7 mmHg, heart rate from 139 $\pm$ 6 to 116 $\pm$ 10 beats/min and renal sympathetic nerve activity from 42 $\pm$ 7 to 4 $\pm$ 3 NU, 5 min after injection (n = 6). These effects were long lasting (2 h, n = 3) and subsequent microinjection of methiothepin (10 μg) failed to reverse blood pressure, heart rate and the rate of sympathetic nerve discharge (n = 3).

In subsequent experiments, the dose of 8-OH-DPAT was reduced and 0.2 μg 8-OH-DPAT (0.2 μg) into the ventrolateral pressor area also reduced blood pressure, heart rate and renal sympathetic nerve activity. Subsequent bilateral microinjection of methiothepin (10 μg), which by itself had no effect, reversed the effects of 8-OH-DPAT. No cardiovascular or neural effects were produced by microinjections of vehicle 0.2—0.4 μl, n = 5) in this area.

4. Discussion

The medulla oblongata is probably the site of the sympatho-inhibitory effect of 8-OH-DPAT. Indeed, injection of 8-OH-DPAT into the vertebral artery produced a dose-dependent decrease in renal sympathetic nerve activity. Similar results were obtained after administration of the drug into the cisterna magna.

8-OH-DPAT injected into the vertebral artery reduced the renal sympathetic nerve activity in catecholamine depleted dogs indicating that the presence of central catecholamines was not a prerequisite for the central cardiovascular affects of 8-OH-DPAT. Depletion of brain serotonin by p-chlorophenylalanine also fails to alter the hypotensive of 8-OH-DPAT in spontaneous hypertensive rats [2]. These results indicate that the central sympatho-inhibitory effect of 8-OH-DPAT is not mediated by an action at 5-HT autoreceptors.

In the rostal ventrolateral medulla, 5-HT — sensitive cells are found near the ventral surface and in lateral areas in and around the ventral aspect of the retrofacial nucleus. This region corresponds to the ventrolateral pressor area. Bilateral microinjections of 8-OH-DPAT in this area in the dog, identified by microinjections of 1-glutamate and clonidine, produced a rapid decrease in blood pressure, heart rate and in renal sympathetic activity. These effects were reversed by subsequent microinjections of methiothepin indicating the involvement of putative $5\text{-}HT_{1A}$ receptors in the ventrolateral medullary pressor area.

5. Conclusions

The stimulation of $5\text{-}HT_{1A}$ receptor located into the ventrolateral pressor area appears to be involved in the central sympatho-inhibitory effects of 8-OH-DPAT.

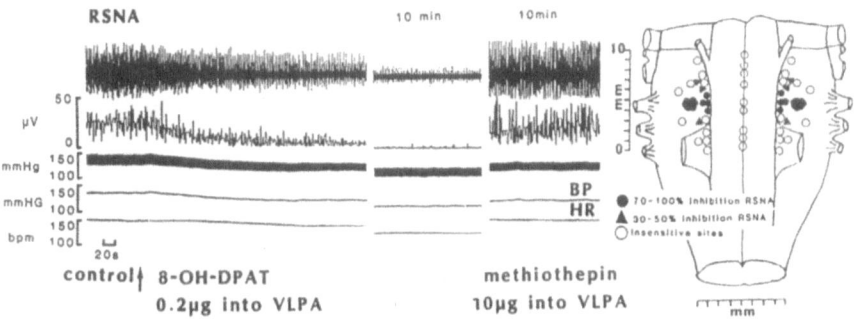

Figure 1. Effects of a bilateral microinjection of 8-OH-DPAT (0.2 μg/site) into the ventrolateral medullary pressor area on blood pressure (BP), heart rate (HR) and renal sympathetic nerve activity (RSNA, calibrated in μV/s.). Methiothepin 10 μg/site) was injected into the same site, 10 min. after 8-OH-DPAT-. Ventral view of the dog brainstem showing the microinjections sites of 8-OH-DPAT. ● 70—100% inhibition of renal sympathetic activity; ▲ 30—50% inhibition; ○ insensitive sites.

References

1. Gradin K, Petterson A, Hedner T, Persson B (1985): Acute administration of 8-hydroxy-2-(di-n-propylamino) tetralin (8-OH-DPAT), a selective 5-HT receptor agonist, causes a biphasic blood pressure response and a bradycardia in the normotensive Sprague-Dawley rat in the spontaneously hypertensive rat. *J Neural Transm* 62: 305.
2. Fozard JR, Mir AK, Middlemiss DN (1987): Cardiovascular response to 8-hydroxy-2-

(di-n-propylamino) tetralin (8-OH-DPAT) in the rat. Site of action and pharmacological analysis. *J Cardiovasc Pharmacol* 9: 328.

3. Dabire H, Cherqui C, Fournier B, Schmitt H (1987): Comparison of effects of some 5-HT$_1$ agonists on blood pressure and heart rate of normotensive anaesthetized rats. *European J Pharmacol* 140: 259.

4. Ramage AG, Fozard JR (1987): Evidence that the putative 5-HT$_{1A}$ receptor agonists, 8-OH-DPAT and ipsapirone, have a central hypotensive action that differs from that of clonidine in anaesthetized cats. *European J Pharmacol* 138: 179.

5. McCall RB, Patel BN, Harris LT (1987): Effects of serotonin$_1$ and serotonin$_2$ receptor agonists and antagonists on blood pressure, heart rate and sympathetic nerve activity. *J Pharmacol Exp Ther* 242: 1152.

6. Doods NH, Boddeke WG, Kalkman HD, Hoyer D, Mathy MJ, Van Zwieten PA (1988): Central 5-HT$_{1A}$ receptors and the mechanism of the central hypotensive effect of (+) 8-OH-DPAT, DP-5-CT, R28935 and urapidil. *J Cardiovasc Pharm* 11: 432.

7. Laubie M, Schmitt H (1988): Brainstem mechanism in the modulation of the sympathetic baroreflex by piperoxan. *European J Pharmacol* 148: 143.

XXIX. Evidence that spiperone reverses the additional sympathoinhibitory action of urapidil in anaesthetised, prazosin-pretreated cats

ANDREW G. RAMAGE

1. Introduction

Urapidil is a novel antihypertensive agent which lowers blood pressure by decreasing total peripheral resistance and also reduces central sympathetic outflow [1—3]. As urapidil blocks α_1-adrenoceptors, this profile of action is what would be expected from such a drug. However, many authors have been unable to relate the central sympathoinhibitory effect of urapidil to its α_1-adrenoceptor blocking action [3]. It has been suggested that urapidil could also be acting on 5-HT_{1A} receptors [3] and the ability of urapidil to bind to these receptors [4] supports such a hypothesis, However, using the intravertebral route of administration [5] (giving drugs via the vertebral artery) (−)pindolol, which attenuated the hypotensive action of several putative 5-HT_{1A} receptor agonists, did not influence the hypotensive response to urapidil. This suggests that the central hypotensive action of urapidil is not related to an agonist action at 5-HT_{1A} receptors but it is possible that the α_1-adrenoceptor antagonist action of urapidil is masking this inhibition, and/ or (−) pindolol may not be the 'ideal' antagonist. The present experiments were designed to overcome these problems by, first, pretreating the animals with a large dose of prazosin to ensure complete α_1-adrenoceptor blockade and by using spiperone as the antagonist as spiperone has been reported to reverse the sympathoinhibitory action of 8-OH-DPAT [6].

2. Methods

Experiments were performed on 9 male adult cats anaesthetised with a mixture of α-chloralose (70 mg kg^{-1}) and pentobarbitone sodium (12 mg). The animals were artificially ventilated using positive pressure after paralysis with vecuronium bromide (200 μk kg^{-1}). Simultaneous recordings of blood pressure, heart rate, femoral arterial flow (from which conductance is

P.R. Saxena, D.I. Wallis, W. Wouters and P. Bevan (eds), Cardiovascular Pharmacology of 5-Hydroxytryptamine, pp. 347—350.
© 1990 *Kluwer Academic Publishers, Dordrecht —*

derived), cardiac, splanchnic and renal nerve activity were made as previously described [7]. Nerve activity was quantified by rectifying and integrating the signal above background noise over 5s. Activity was tested to ensure that it was under baroreceptor modulation also as previously described. Following these tests the above variables were recorded for 20 min before injection of prazosin (0.75 mg kg^{-1}) followed 10 min later by a second injection of prazosin (0.25 mg kg^{-1}). Urapidil (0.75 mg kg^{-1}) was injected 5 min later followed 7 min later by 3 separate injections of spiperone (1 mg kg^{-1}) at 2—3 min intervals. Two types of control were carried out, one in which urapidil was substituted by 0.04 M lactic acid and the other in which spiperone was replaced by its vehicle alone (0.4 M lactic acid plus 10% 1 M bicarbonate).

3. Results

Ten minutes after the first injection and 5 min after the second injection of prazosin the changes from baseline values (mean ± s.e.; n = 9) were respectively: mean blood pressure −42 ± 5 and −43 ± 5 mmHg; heart rate −7 ± 5 and −11 ± 7 beats min^{-1}, femoral arterial conductance +63 ± 12 and +63 ± 13 (x10^{-3}) ml mmHg^{-1} min^{-1}, cardiac nerve activity +14 ± 21 and +1 ± 23%, splanchnic nerve activity +6 ± 13 and −7 ± 11% and renal nerve activity +7 ± 11 and −5 ± 9%.

In 3 of these experiments urapidil caused a further mean decrease from prazosin pretreated levels in mean blood pressure of −7 mmHg, heat rate −90 beats min^{-1}, femoral arterial conductance −13 (x10^{-3}) ml mmHg^{-1} min^{-1}, cardiac nerve activity −96%, splanchnic nerve activity −61% and renal nerve activity −55%. Spiperone injections caused dose related reversal of these decreases towards the prazosin pretreated levels which were, by 3 min after the third injection: mean blood pressure −3mmHg, heart rate −40 beats min^{-1}, cardiac nerve activity −8%, splanchnic nerve activity +32% and renal nerve activity −14%. Femoral arterial conductance increased by +40 (x10^{-3}) ml mmHg^{-1} min^{-1} after the first injection of spiperone. Subsequent injections spiperone had little further effect on femoral arterial conductance. A trace from one these experiments is shown in Figure 1.

In another 3 experiments vehicle alone had little effect on the prazosin pretreated levels. However spiperone injections caused a dose related decrease in mean blood pressure reaching −24mmHg and heart rate of −22 beats min^{-1}. This was associated with a further increase of 18 (x10^{-3}) ml mmHg^{-1} min^{-1} in femoral arterial conductance while only cardiac nerve activity increased by 20%. These latter changes being near maximum after the first injection of spiperone. In the other 3 control experiments 'spiperone vehicle' had little effect of the changes caused by urapidil on prazosin pretreated levels.

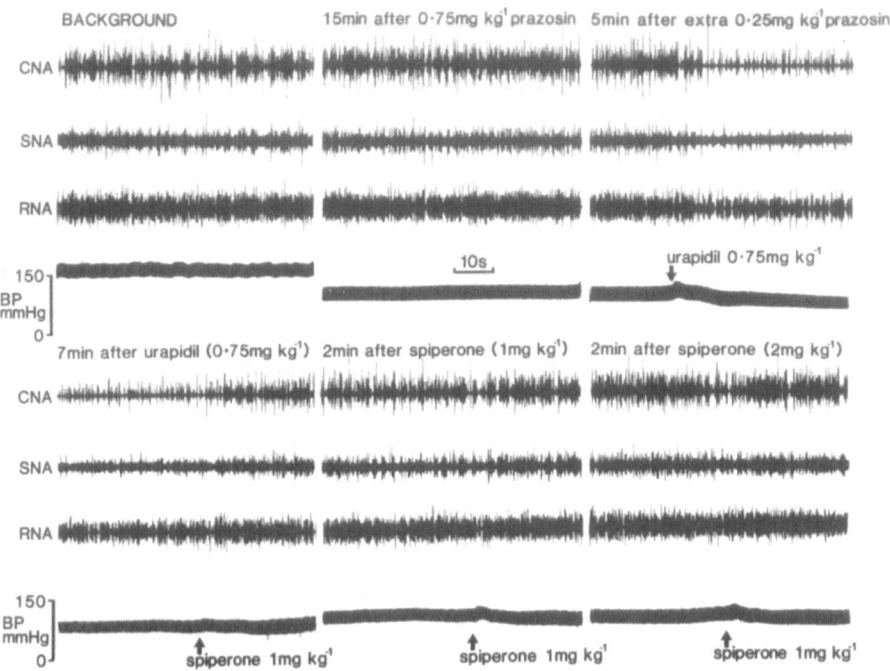

Figure 1. A record showing the effects of prazosin followed by subsequent injections of urapidil and spiperone on cardiac (CNA), splanchnic (SNA), renal (RNA) nerve activity and arterial blood pressure in an anaesthetised cat.

4. Discussion

The results of this investigation demonstrate that urapidil has a sympathoin-hibitory action and a bradycardiac effect in prazosin-pretreated anaesthetised cats. This 'additional' sympathoinhibitory action of urapidil can be reversed by spiperone. Furthermore, this reversal by spiperone is not due to a physio-logical but to a pharmacological antagonist action. Both spiperone and urapidil bind to 5-HT_{1A} receptors [4, 8, 9] and the sympathoinhibitory action of 8-OH-DPAT is reversed by spiperone [6]. Therefore, these present results strongly indicate that the additional sympathoinhibitory action of urapidil is due to activation of 5-HT_{1A} receptors. The site at which urapidil stimulates these 5-HT_{1A} receptors to cause this additional sympathoinhibitory action has been suggested to be the lateral reticular nucleus in the brainstem [10].

5. Conclusions

Urapidil decreases heart rate and blood pressure in prazosin-treated anaesthetised cats by acting on central 5-HT_{1A} receptors.

Acknowledgements

I wish to thank Mr. S. Wilkinson for technical assistance and Byk Gulden Pharmazeutika for financial support.

References

1. Schoetensack W, Bischler P, Ditterman E Ch, Steinijans V (1977): Tierexperimentelle Untersuchungen uber den Einfluss des Antihypertensivums Urapidil auf den Kreislauf und die Kreislaufregulation. *Arzneim Forsch Drug Res* 27: 1908—1919.
2. Sanders KH, Jurna I (1985): Effects of urapidil, clonidine, prazosin and propranolol on autonomic nerve activity and heart rate in anaesthetised rat and cat. *Eur J Pharmac* 110: 181—190.
3. Ramage AG (1986): A comparison of the effects of doxazosin and alfuzosin with those of urapidil on preganglionic sympathetic nerve activity in anaesthetised cats. *Eur J Pharmac* 129: 307—314.
4. Fozard JR, Mir AK (1987): Are 5-HT receptors involved in the hypotensive effects of urapidil? *Br J Pharmac* 90: 24P.
5. Doods HN, Boddeke WG, Kalkman HD, Hoyer D, Mathy MJ, Van Zwieten PA (1988): Central 5-HT$_{1A}$ receptors and the mechanism of the central hypotensive effect of (+) 8-OH-DPAT, DP-5-CT, R28935 and urapidil. *J Cardiovasc Pharmac* 11: 432—438.
6. McCall RB, Patel BN, Harris LT (1987): Effects of serotonin$_1$ and serotonin$_2$ receptor agonists and antagonists on blood pressure, heart rate and sympathetic nerve activity. *J Pharmac Exp Ther* 242: 1152—1159.
7. Ramage AG (1988): Are drugs that act both on serotonin receptors and α_1-adrenoceptors more potent hypotensive agents than those that act only on α_1-adrenoceptors? *J Cardiovasc Pharmac* 11 (suppl. 1): S30—S34.
8. Leysen JE (1985): Serotonergic binding sites, pp. 43—62 in: Vanhoutte PM (ed), *Serotonin and the Cardiovascular System.* New York: Raven Press.
9. Gillis RA, Kellar KJ, Quest JA, Namath IJ, Martino-Barrows A, Hill K, Gratti PJ, Dretchen K (1988): Experimental studies on the Neurocardiovascular effects of urapidil. *Drugs* 35 (Suppl. 6): 20—33.
10. Groß G, Hanft G, Kolassa N (1987): Urapidil and some analogues with hypotensive properties show high affinity for 5-hydroxytryptamine (5-HT) binding sites of the 5-HT$_{1A}$ subtype and for α_1-adrenoceptor binding sites. *Naunyn-Schmiedebergs Arch Pharmac* 336: 597—601.

XXX. The effects of intrathecal ketanserin and phentolamine on heart rate and arterial blood pressure in the rat

K. MOHAN DHASMANA, AJAY K. BANERJEE and
PRAMOD R. SAXENA

1. Introduction

Ketanserin lowers arterial blood pressure in both animals and humans, but the mechanism of its antihypertensive action is in debate [see 1]. In general, it is now accepted that ketanserin, at least partly, lowers blood pressure by α_1-adrenoceptor blockade [2—4]. However, additional mechanisms, such as the blockade of 5-HT$_2$ receptor-mediated amplification of the vasoconstrictor action of noradrenaline by 5-hydroxytryptamine (5-HT) [see 5], direct vaso-dilatation [4] and a CNS action [6—8], have also recently been implicated. In this investigation the effects of intrathecal administration of ketanserin and phentolamine on arterial blood pressure and heart rate in normotensive anaesthetized rats have been studied.

2. Methods

Wistar rats of either sex (250—350 g) were anaesthetized with halothane (1—2%), nitrous oxide and oxygen (2:1) and put on positive pressure venti-lation. Muscle paralysis was achieved with an i.v. infusion of pancuronium bromide (90 μg.kg^{-1}.hr^{-1}). Arterial blood pressure and heart rate were recorded on a model 7 Grass polygraph. Subsequently, a polyethylene tube (o.d. 0.61 mm, length 14 cm, volume 10 μl) was placed into the subarach-noid space via the cisterna magna [9]. After baseline measurements, physio-logical saline (10 μl; n = 7) and ketanserin tartrate (n = 7) or phentolamine hydrochloride (n = 8) in doses of 50, 100 or 200 μg.kg^{-1} (dissolved in saline; volume not exceeding 10 μl) were injected into the subarachnoid space.

The effects of saline and each drug dose was observed for at least 30 min and the next dose was given following recovery of heart rate and blood pressure effects. The extent to which peripheral leakage of the drugs caused consequent α_1-adrenoceptor blockade was checked by observing the pressor

P.R. Saxena, D.I. Wallis, W. Wouters and P. Bevan (eds), Cardiovascular Pharmacology of 5-Hydroxytryptamine, pp. 351—354.
© 1990 *Kluwer Academic Publishers, Dordrecht* —

responses to phenylephrine (5 μg.kg^{-1}, i.v.) before and 5 min after each dose of the two drugs.

3. Results

3.1 *Blood pressure and heart rate responses*

Intrathecal injection of ketanserin as well as phentolamine, but not of saline, decreased arterial blood pressure and heart rate dose-dependently. Recovery was observed within 30 min (Table 1).

3.2 *Pressor responses to phenylephrine*

The pressor responses to phenylephrine (5 μg.kg^{-1}, i.v.) before and after the three doses (50, 100 and 200 μg.kg^{-1}) of ketanserin were 32 $\pm$ 4, 39 $\pm$ 5, 40 $\pm$ 3 and 39 $\pm$ 3 mmHg, respectively. Such responses in the phentolamine group were 32 $\pm$ 2, 32 $\pm$ 1, 44 $\pm$ 5 and 39 $\pm$ 6 mmHg, respectively. The responses to phenylephrine were not significantly affected by the two drugs.

4. Discussion

Both ketanserin and phentolamine decreased arterial blood pressure and heart rate in a dose-dependent manner after intrathecal administration. These effects were observed without any change in the pressor responses to i.v. phenylephrine and, therefore, the drugs seem to lower blood pressure and heart rate by reducing the activity of preganglionic sympathetic nerve fibres at their origin in the spinal cord. These findings are in agreement with earlier reports that i.v. injections of ketanserin and phentolamine decrease sympathetic neural discharges [6] and that ketanserin inhibits centrally-elicited pressor responses [7]. Since both ketanserin and phentolamine block α_1-adrenoceptors, but only ketanserin antagonizes 5-HT$_2$ receptors, it is suggested that a blockade of spinal α_1-adrenoceptors, and not 5-HT$_2$ receptors, mediates the hypotensive and bradycardiac effects of ketanserin and phentolamine.

5. Conclusions

Ketanserin and phentolamine may decrease arterial blood pressure and heart rate by acting within the spinal cord, probably by antagonizing α_1-adrenoceptors.

Table 1. Effects of intrathecal injections of saline (n = 7), ketanserin (n = 7) and phentolamine (n = 8) on blood pressure and heart rate in anaesthetized rats.

Substance (μg/kg)	Minutes after administration of substances							
	0	1	2	3	5	10	20	30
Blood pressure (mmHg)								
Saline (10 μl)	129 ± 3	131 ± 3	131 ± 4	134 ± 5	134 ± 5	129 ± 3	131 ± 3	129 ± 3
Ketanserin (50)	124 ± 5	104 ± 10*	100 ± 11*	109 ± 9*	111 ± 8*	121 ± 4	120 ± 6	119 ± 6
Ketanserin (100)	116 ± 6	77 ± 6*	79 ± 8*	91 ± 8*	100 ± 7*	115 ± 3	119 ± 5	119 ± 5
Ketanserin (200)	123 ± 4	78 ± 6*	91 ± 6*	98 ± 6*	102 ± 3*	113 ± 3*	116 ± 4	117 ± 4
Phentolamine (50)	133 ± 3	126 ± 5	113 ± 7*	101 ± 7*	97 ± 8*	111 ± 10*	119 ± 9	124 ± 8
Phentolamine (100)	135 ± 4	102 ± 13	80 ± 7*	76 ± 7*	68 ± 6*	82 ± 9*	107 ± 6*	112 ± 6*
Phentolamine (200)	115 ± 6	93 ± 9*	77 ± 3*	76 ± 5*	73 ± 3*	83 ± 7*	93 ± 8	101 ± 5
Heart rate (beats.min^{-1})								
Saline (10 μl)	426 ± 13	426 ± 13	429 ± 14	429 ± 14	431 ± 15	429 ± 14	431 ± 15	430 ± 14
Ketanserin (50)	421 ± 20	399 ± 24*	379 ± 26*	374 ± 32*	381 ± 29*	393 ± 24*	413 ± 20	411 ± 19
Ketanserin (100)	414 ± 17	376 ± 21*	356 ± 20*	350 ± 18*	354 ± 19*	371 ± 18*	400 ± 13	411 ± 13
Ketanserin (200)	413 ± 15	350 ± 30*	328 ± 21*	325 ± 19*	332 ± 19*	332 ± 25*	368 ± 24*	400 ± 15
Phentolamine (50)	430 ± 10	426 ± 8	415 ± 10	408 ± 10*	390 ± 17*	395 ± 23	405 ± 17	424 ± 11
Phentolamine (100)	432 ± 12	415 ± 14*	401 ± 12*	391 ± 10*	374 ± 9*	370 ± 18*	397 ± 11*	400 ± 13
Phentolamine (200)	403 ± 6	392 ± 8*	368 ± 14*	360 ± 17*	353 ± 21	355 ± 24	362 ± 22	372 ± 27

Data in means ±¡SEM. *, P < 0.05 vs respective control value.

References

1. Saxena PR, Bolt GR, Dhasmana KM (1987): Serotonin agonists and antagonists in experimental hypertension. *J Cardiovasc Pharmacol* 10 (suppl. 3): S12—S18.
2. Fozard JR (1982): Mechanism of the hypotensive effect of ketanserin. *J Cardiovasc Pharmacol* 4: 829—838.
3. Kalkman HO, Timmermans PBMWM, Van Zwieten PA (1982): Characterization of the antihypertensive properties of ketanserin (R 41486) in rats. *J Pharmacol Exp Ther* 22: 227—231.
4. Bolt GR, Saxena PR (1985): Cardiovascular profile and hypotensive mechanism of ketanserin in the rabbit. *Hypertension* 7: 499—506.
5. Vanhoutte PM, Amery A, Birkenhäger W, Breckenridge A, Bühler F, Distler A, Dormandy J, Doyle A, Frohlich E, Hansson L, Hedner T, Hollenberg N, Jensen H-E, Lund-Johansen P, Meyer P, Opie L, Robertson I, Safar M, Schalekamp M, Symoens J, Trap-Jensen J, Zanchetti A (1988): Serotonergic mechanisms in hypertension: Focus on the effects of ketanserin. *Hypertension* 11: 111—133.
6. McCall RB, Schuette MR (1984): Evidence for an alpha-1 receptor-mediated central sympathoinhibitory action of ketanserin. *J Pharmacol Exp Ther* 228: 704—710.
7. Mylecharane EJ, Phillips CA, Markus JK, Show J (1985): Evidence for a central component to the hypotensive action of ketanserin in the dog. *J Cardiovasc Pharmacol* 7: 514—516.
8. Van Zwieten PA, Mathy MJ, Boddeke HWGM, Doods HN (1987): Central hypotensive activity of ketanserin in cats. *J Cardiovasc Pharmacol* 10 (suppl. 3): S54—S58.
9. Yaksh TL, Rudy TA (1976): Chronic catheterization of the spinal subarachnoid space. *Physiol Behav* 17: 1031—1036.

XXXI. Early clinical experience with flesinoxan, a new selective 5-HT$_{1A}$ receptor agonist

DE VOOGD, J. M. and PRAGER, G.

1. Introduction

Flesinoxan hydrochloride has been shown in pharmacological experiments to be a potent and selective 5-HT$_{1A}$ receptor agonist with centrally-mediated antihypertensive properties. Flesinoxan lowers blood pressure in various species, and the effect lasts for more than four hours after a single administration [1]. The cardiovascular profile of the compound includes a reduction of total peripheral resistance, a small, vagally mediated decrease in heart rate, little or no effect on cardiac output, no direct negative inotropic effect and strong renal vasodilatation. Further, no orthostatic hypotension or tachyphylaxis has been found [1, 2]. In the investigation reported here flesinoxan has been studied in normotensive and hypertensive human subjects. Special attention was paid to cardiovascular parameters, safety, tolerability, psychometric performance and pharmacokinetics of the drug after single and repeated doses.

2. Materials and methods

2.1 Healthy normotensive volunteers

In nine studies, 85 healthy volunteers received one or more administrations of oral flesinoxan in a single dose between 0.05—2.2 mg, and 32 volunteers received the compound in repeated doses (0.3—4.8 mg per day) for a week. Six studies were placebo-controlled. Assessments included frequent (7—13) measurements of blood pressure (BP) and heart rate (HR), supine and erect, on each study day. Psychometric tests and visual analogue scales were done three times each study day. Side-effects could be reported any time.

P.R. Saxena, D.I. Wallis, W. Wouters and P. Bevan (eds), Cardiovascular Pharmacology of 5-Hydroxytryptamine, pp. 355—359.
© 1990 *Kluwer Academic Publishers, Dordrecht* —

2.2 Hypertensive patients

Following the experience in normotensive subjects, a small study in patients with essential hypertension was performed to assess the acute effects of four *single* doses of flesinoxan versus placebo on HR and BP. This study was double-blind with a cross-over design. Twelve patients with a mean sitting DBP of > 95 mmHg at entry, after at least three weeks wash-out period, were included in the study. No other antihypertensive medication was allowed. Six patients received 0.8 and 1.0 mg flesinoxan and placebo (Group 1), six others received 0.6 and 1.6 mg flesinoxan and placebo (Group 2).

Assessments were the same as in the volunteer studies, but with the addition of frequent ECGs and echocardiography. For the statistical analysis, the results of the HR and BP were summarized over the 24 hours treatment period and analysed using a Randomization test. The resulting P-values indicate whether or not the treatments are different from each other, but not the direction of the difference.

3. Results

3.1 Healthy normotensive volunteers

Single doses of about 1.0 mg and onwards showed pharmacological activity. Both systolic blood pressure (SBP) and diastolic blood pressure (DBP) decreased by about 10 mmHg. The effects after a single dose lasted for 8–12 hours. Effects on heart rate were variable. No clear orthostatic hypotension has been observed.

The side-effect profile seen consistently in healthy volunteers after a *single* dose is shown in Table 1. Side-effects were usually reported 2 to 4 hours after dosing. Dizziness was especially reported in standing position. There was no direct relationship to lowering of blood pressure. The side-effect pro-

Table 1. Side-effects seen after single doses in healthy volunteers. Data represent percentage of subjects per dose range. n = total number of subjects within a dose range group.

	Placebo	Flesinoxan		
	n = 42	0.05–0.6 mg n = 44	0.8–1.2 mg n = 48	1.8–2.2 mg n = 32
Asthenia	26	11	31	63
Dizziness	5	7	63	56
Nausea	2	2	17	38
Vomiting	0	0	21	13
Paleness	0	0	17	13

file seen after *repeated* dosing was comparable to the single dose profile. However, the side-effects disappeared rapidly within 48 hours, even when the dosing was increased in that time period.

Further notable results in healthy volunteers were an acute diuretic effect, no influence on psychomotor performance, no behavioural changes, and no effects on laboratory parameters. Plasma drug level analysis indicated that flesinoxan has a high bioavailability and an elimination half-life of about 8 hours. The peak plasma level is reached in about one hour after oral administration.

3.2 Hypertensive patients

3.2.1 Group 1.
There was a statistically significant difference among the treatment sessions for supine and erect DBP (P = 0.022 and 0.044). The SBP was not significantly different. The drop in BP in both active sessions was maximal at one to two hours after dosing, and was about 8 mmHg larger than after placebo. HR remained virtually unchanged. The effects of the two flesinoxan doses were not clearly different from each other. The effects of the drug on blood pressure in supine position are shown in Figure 1.

3.2.2 Group 2.
There was a statistically significant difference among the treatment sessions for SBP and DBP, both in erect and supine position (P = 0.011 and 0.022).

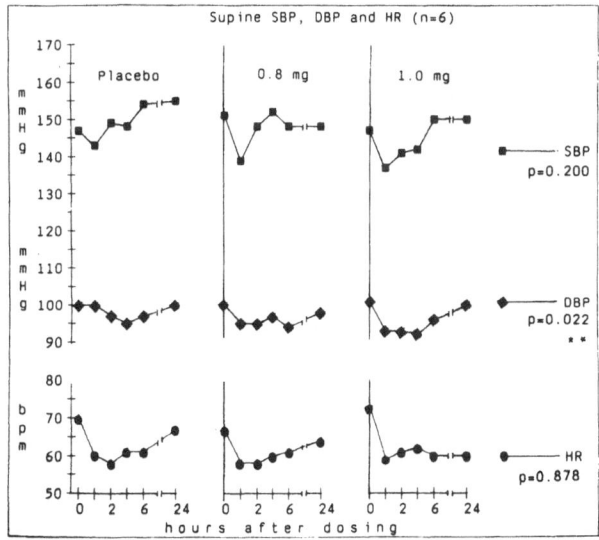

Figure 1. Effects of flesinoxan (0.8 and 1.0 mg) on supine systolic (SBP) and diastolic (DBP) blood pressure and on heart rate (HR). Data represent the mean of six subjects. *, p < 0.05; **, p < 0.01.

In the 0.6 mg group, the drop in supine BP from baseline was 11/4 mmHg larger than following placebo; in the 1.6 mg group the drop was 17/9 mmHg larger than following placebo. For erect BP, these values were in the same range. The decreases were dose dependent. The maximal decrease was seen one hour after dosing and lasted for at least six hours. After 24 hours, the effects had disappeared. The HR decreased in the active group compared to placebo. The supine values almost reached statistical significance ($P = 0.056$). The maximal drop occurred about one to two hours after dosing. The effects of the drug on supine blood pressure are shown in Figure 2.

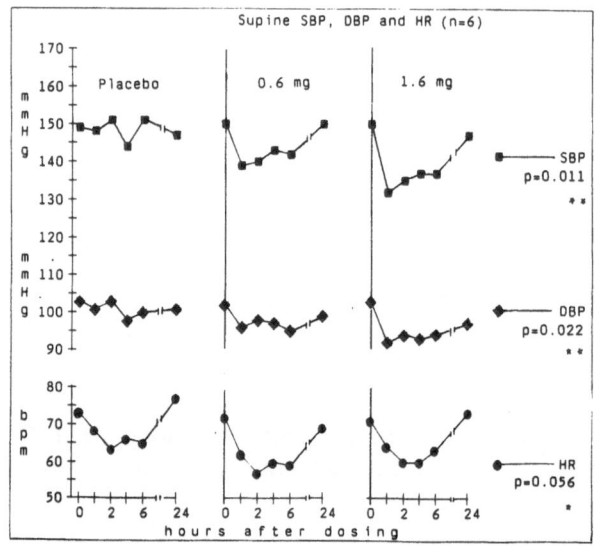

Figure 2. Effects of flesinoxan (0.6 and 1.6 mg) on supine systolic (SBP) and diastolic (DBP) blood pressure and on heart rate (HR). Data represent the mean of six subjects. *, $p < 0.05$; **, $p < 0.01$.

Side-effects were reported by all twelve patients when receiving flesinoxan, but not when receiving placebo, see Table 2. The duration and severity increased with increasing doses. The symptoms usually started in the first two hours after dosing, and lasted from several minutes to up to some hours. Dizziness was mostly reported whilst standing. There were no differences between placebo and active treatment in echocardiography, ECGs or laboratory variables.

4. Discussion

In normotensive volunteers, BP and HR were modestly reduced by flesinoxan in doses from about 1.0 mg and onwards. There were no differences in the erect and supine blood pressure values.

Table 2. Side-effects seen after single doses in hypertensive patients. Data represent number of patients per dose. n = total number of patients within a dose group.

	Placebo	Flesinoxan			
	n = 12	0.6 mg n = 6	0.8 mg n = 6	1.0 mg n = 6	1.6 mg n = 6
Dizziness	0	5	4	4	6
Nausea	0	1	2	3	4
Vomiting	0	0	0	1	2
Paleness	0	2	3	2	2

In the 12 hypertensive patients, flesinoxan lowered blood pressure at all dose levels studied, reaching statistical significance in DBP, and partly in SBP. Overall, the drop in DBP was dose dependent. No postural changes were observed.

Effects on HR were less marked, but in hypertensive patients a moderate bradycardia was seen in one group. Reflex tachycardia, as often seen with vasodilating agents, was never observed.

The side-effects reported by the healthy volunteers and patients were uncomfortable, but tolerable and appeared to be dose dependent. The mechanism of action of the side-effects is at present unclear, but the nausea and vomiting are probably of central origin. The dizziness and paleness were often reported whilst standing, suggesting a relationship with the peripheral cardiovascular changes. In all other measured parameters, flesinoxan appeared to be safe.

5. Conclusion

The results of the healthy volunteers studies and the small patient study, suggests that flesinoxan, a new selective 5-HT$_{1A}$ agonist lowers blood pressure. At the moment trials with repeated dosing are running in patients with hypertension to further define the profile of this interesting new compound.

References

1. Hartog J, Wouters W (1988): Flesinoxan hydrochloride. *Drugs of the future* 13: 31—33.
2. Wouters W, Hartog J, Bevan P (1988): Flesinoxan. *Cardiovasc. Drug Reviews* 6: 71—83.

Coronary and Peripheral Vascular Diseases

XXXII. Coronary circulation and 5-hydroxytryptamine

JAMES A. ANGUS, ARCHER BROUGHTON, THOMAS M. COCKS and CHRISTINE E. WRIGHT

1. Introduction

Coronary vasospasm or Prinzmetal's variant angina [1] is probably caused by a variety of substances that arise from aggregating platelets, from nerve varicosities or from different cells within the wall itself. It may not however, be simply a matter of identifying some pathological constrictor substance. The vascular reactivity, defined here by the "sensitivity" of the artery to the substance (conveniently taken as the EC_{50}) and by the "range" or magnitude (E_{max}) of the contraction may have changed considerably in patients with angina pectoris.

Definitive information on the role of serotonin (5-hydroxytryptamine; 5-HT) in variant angina is not yet available. The measurement of changes in plasma 5-HT levels has not been useful because platelets are readily damaged during blood sampling. A clearer cause and effect relationship between 5-HT and angina must await the discovery of a specific 5-HT receptor antagonist that would prevent or terminate an episode of coronary vasospasm. Nevertheless, 5-HT remains an attractive candidate because it is stored in high concentrations in platelets and is readily released when platelets aggregate on only the slightest damaged intimal surface [2]. In addition, 5-HT is a powerful constrictor of large arteries; a response that is amplified by other autacoids released from platelets such as thromboxane A_2 [3, 4]. Clinically, ergometrine (ergonovine), is a 5-HT receptor agonist [5, 6] and has been used to diagnose variant angina in patients by inducing spasm often at the site of a small atheromatous lesion [7].

In this review we will consider the reactivity of the coronary vasculature to 5-HT under experimental conditions where (i) the perfusion pressure is lowered and (ii) where the architecture of the wall is altered by loss of endothelium or atherosclerosis. We will explore the classification of the coronary 5-HT receptors.

P.R. Saxena, D.I. Wallis, W. Wouters and P. Bevan (eds), Cardiovascular Pharmacology of 5-Hydroxytryptamine, pp. 363—378.

2. Coronary perfusion pressure

Of fundamental importance for the degree of active constriction of large artery by any substance is the opposing transmural or distending pressure. We developed an *in situ* model of a blood perfused left anterior descending (LAD) coronary artery of the greyhound dog under controlled conditions of flow and perfusion pressure [8, 9] (Figure 1). Heparinised blood was pumped from the femoral artery of an anaesthetized support dog into the proximal

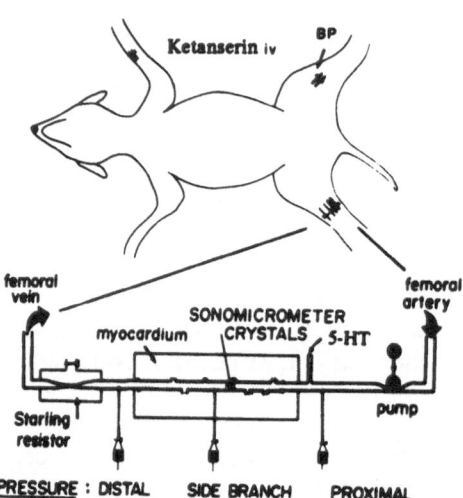

Figure 1. Schematic diagram of the support dog and perfusion in situ of the left anterior descending coronary artery of a separate greyhound dog heart. 5-HT was infused into the coronary proximal to the sonomicrometer crystals. Ketanserin was given as bolus injections (0.1, 0.3 or 1 mg/kg) to the support dog. (Reprinted from [8] with permission of Am. J. Cardiology.)

LAD. About 5 cm distally, the blood was withdrawn through a Starling resistor (to control distal resistance) and returned to the support dog via a femoral vein. In the perfused coronary artery, the external diameter was recorded by a pair of sonomicrometer crystals. The pressure in this perfused segment was measured at the proximal cannula, at a side branch close to the sonomicrometer crystals, and at the distal cannula. Large clamps were placed 1 cm either side of the LAD in the longitudinal direction to prevent myocardial perfusion. The side branch pressure (SBP) was altered in 1 minute stages from 30-150-30 mmHg by changing the external pressure in the Starling resistor. The relationship between SBP and external diameter was hyperbolic and there was some hysteresis on the return leg (Figure 2). Taking the measurement of external and internal diameter and lumen area as 100%, at a SBP of 90 mmHg, intracoronary infusions of 5-HT lowered these

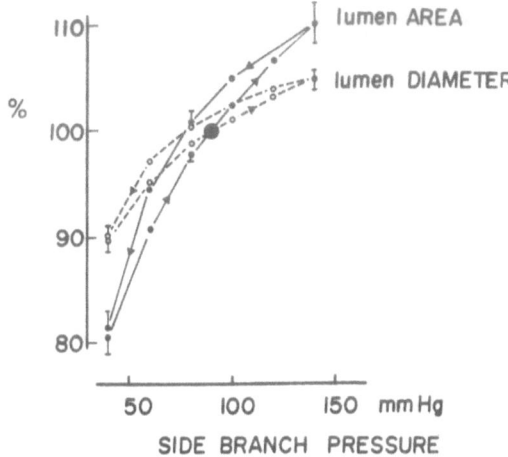

Figure 2. Effect of alterations in side branch perfusion pressure on the resting lumen area and diameter of 10 dog coronary arteries perfused under condition of constant flow as in Figure 1. Error bars are ± 1 SEM. The circle indicates the value taken as 100% at 90 mmHg perfusion pressure. (Reprinted from [8] with permission of Am. J. Cardiol.)

three parameters in a concentration dependent manner (Figures 3, 4). Repeating the experiment at a passive perfusion pressure in the side branch of 60 mmHg did not alter the sensitivity (EC_{50}) of 5-HT but increased the range of the fall in the three dimensions when compared with the resting values at 90 mmHg (Figure 4).

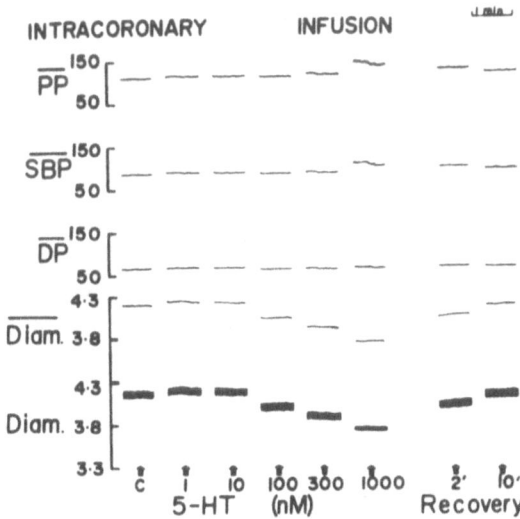

Figure 3. Chart records of haemodynamic changes during intra-coronary infusion of 5-HT into the preparation described in Figure 1. C = control; $\overline{PP}$ = mean proximal pressure; $\overline{SBP}$ = mean side branch pressure; $\overline{DP}$ = distal pressure all in mmHg; $\overline{Diam}$ and Diam = mean and phasic external diameter (in mm). (Reprinted from [8] with permission of Am. J. Cardiol.)

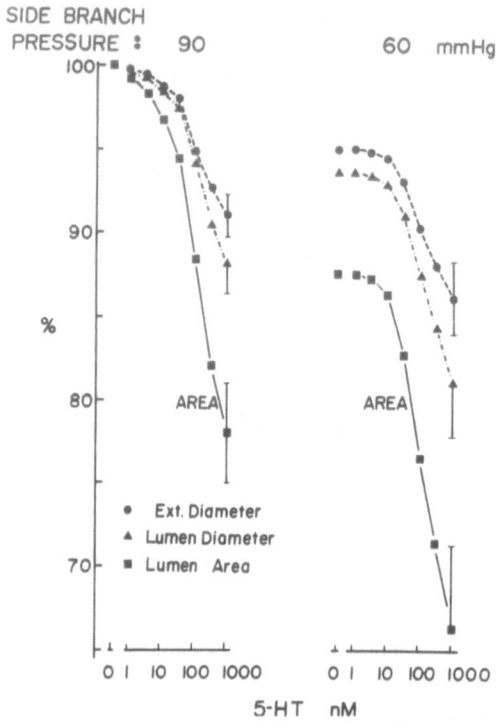

Figure 4. Effect of alterations in perfusion pressure (90 or 60 mmHg) on external diameter, lumen diameter and lumen area in 10 arteries during the intra-coronary infusion of 5-HT. Both curves were completed in each artery. (Reprinted from [8] with permission of Am. J. Cardiol.)

These experiments highlight the effect of a combination of a low perfusion pressure and the direct vasoconstriction of 5-HT on the large coronary artery. Such a scenario may be the explanation of recurrent nocturnal pain that wakes patients with variant angina from sleep (13 of 17 patients with pain at rest [10]). Here the lower systemic blood pressure during sleep presumably combined with some constrictor stimulus may cause sufficient reduction in large coronary artery diameter and blood flow to induce angina.

In the dog large coronary artery the greatest reduction in lumen diameter was about 20% in response to 5-HT and low perfusion pressure (Figure 4). This decrease in diameter would not normally be "critical", i.e. associated with reduction in blood flow. In the diagnosis of variant angina, patients often showed coronary vasospasm in response to ergometrine i.e. at the site of a small atheromatous lesion [7, 11]. We therefore sought to quantify the relationship between a change in geometry of the lumen by atherosclerosis and the reactivity to 5-HT.

3. Geometry of the artery wall and atherosclerosis

In atherosclerosis there may be two factors that will alter the reactivity of the large coronary artery to 5-HT or other stimuli. First, the bulk of the lesion would encroach upon the lumen area to effectively reduce the *available* lumen area (free of lesion) for blood flow. In this case, even normal contraction of the artery wall smooth muscle cells (10—15%) may be sufficient to cause a critical stenosis. Second, the atherosclerosis may not only cause a passive encroachment of the lumen but also cause a change in the reactivity of the smooth muscle cells. The latter can only be evaluated in vitro where the isometric contractile force can be measured under steady-state conditions independently of changes to the lumen geometry.

We fed rabbits a normal pellet diet (N) or one enriched with 1% cholesterol (C) for 16—20 weeks before removing a 2 mm segment of the large left main coronary artery and a small side branch on the left ventricle wall. These vessels were mounted on 40 μm diameter wires in a Mulvany double myograph for measurement of isometric wall force [12, 13]. After normalization, concentration response curves were constructed to K^+, 5-HT and histamine. The large arteries (901 ± 74 μm i.d.) from 8 N rabbits contracted poorly to 5-HT (0.01—3 μM). The increase in isometric force was less than 16% of the maximum force E_{max} obtained with K^+ (50 mM) de-polarising solution. In large arteries (1113 $\pm$ 84 μm i.d.) from 10 cholesterol fed rabbits, the maximum contraction to 5-HT was 51.4% of the E_{max} to K^+ (Figure 5, top) indicating a greater contraction range in C arteries without any increase in sensitivity. This enhanced response to 5-HT seemed to be receptor specific since no such change was observed for histamine. We also applied an additional 10 mM K^+ (K_{10}^+) to partially depolarise the cell membrane and enhance the reactivity to 5-HT. Both groups showed a marked increase in the range of contraction to 5-HT but the N arteries were still markedly less reactive than C arteries (Figure 5, bottom). In both normal and K_{10}^+ Krebs' solution, very little contraction was observed to 5-HT in either the N (252 ± 18 μm i.d., n = 7) or C (252 $\pm$ 27 μm i.d., n = 11) small coronary arteries consistent with the general view that 5-HT is pri-marily a large artery spasmogen. At the end of each experiment the arteries were fixed and prepared for light microscopy. The vessels were cut trans-versely into 29 μm thick segments and the average lesion area calculated with a projecting microscope and digiplot programme. The average lesion area for 10 large arteries was 69.7% with 25.8% lesion free circumference. For the small arteries from 11 rabbits the lesion area was 33.3% and lesion free circumference was 51%. These data support the findings from human coronary vessels that atherosclerosis is mainly confined to the larger arteries. With this morphological knowledge, we calculated the fall in the free lumen area that would have occurred in vivo in the large arteries if the 5-HT had been allowed to shorten the smooth muscle cells rather than increase the isometric wall tension. Thus, the normal arteries without lesion had a

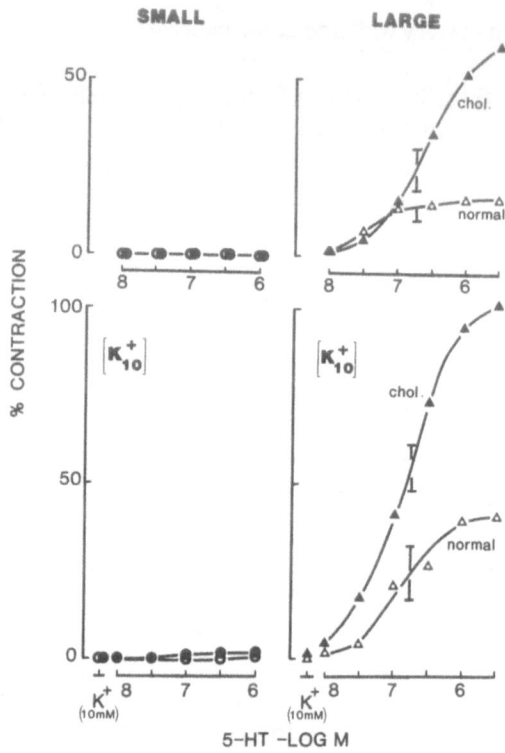

Figure 5. Concentration response curves to 5-HT in large and small coronary arteries of rabbits fed normal or cholesterol 1% enriched diet (chol.). Top, normal K^+; bottom, K^+ 10 mM; n > 8 in each case (Angus, unpublished).

calculated maximum fall in lumen area of 30% in response to 5-HT (Figure 6). In contrast, the atherosclerotic vessels, assuming a concentric lesion of 70% of lumen area, only had 30% free lumen area at rest. This free lumen area was abolished ("spasm") at a concentration of 5-HT just above 0.1 μM (Figure 6).

These studies suggest that the experimental atherosclerosis had apparently increased the contractility (E_{max}) of the large coronary arteries to 5-HT, probably by a receptor specific mechanism. We were unable to find any increase in sensitivity (lower EC_{50}) to 5-HT in C arteries in contrast to reports in rabbit aorta [14], or in coronary arteries from Watanabe rabbits with familial hypercholesterolemia [15]. The enhanced contraction to a given concentration of 5-HT observed in our isometric studies and the implications when combined with lumen encroachment calculated from morphology underline the concern for the potential role for 5-HT in angina pectoris.

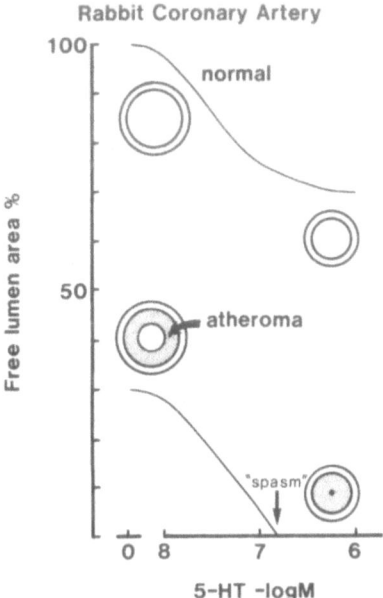

Figure 6. Theoretical diagram of the change in free lumen area (%) (control = 100%) during the contraction of the smooth muscle to 5-HT in large coronary arteries from rabbits on normal diet or fed a 1% cholesterol intake.

4. Loss of endothelium

The discovery by Furchgott and Zawadzki [16] that a number of vasodilator substances could release EDRF (endothelium-derived relaxing factor, now thought to be nitric oxide, NO) in many large arteries, prompted us to ask whether two coronary vasoconstrictor substances, noradrenaline and 5-HT might have a dual effect on the artery wall [17, 18]. They may release EDRF that would tend to relax the underlying smooth muscle but also contract the smooth muscle through appropriate receptors. This is a plausible explanation for the marked increase in range and increase in sensitivity to 5-HT and noradrenaline observed in dog and pig large coronary artery rings when the endothelium was removed [17]. More direct evidence for the release of EDRF by 5-HT was the relaxation of a precontracted pig coronary artery ring in the presence of ketanserin and only with intact endothelium (Figure 7). This phenomenon of 5-HT-induced large coronary artery relaxation has been demonstrated in anaesthetized and conscious dogs [19, 20]. 5-HT released from aggregating platelets will also relax dog isolated coronary arteries but only when the endothelium is intact [21].

This demonstration of an endothelium-dependent relaxation to 5-HT in coronary arteries implies that any loss of endothelial cells not only encourages platelet aggregation but renders the artery wall more reactive to the

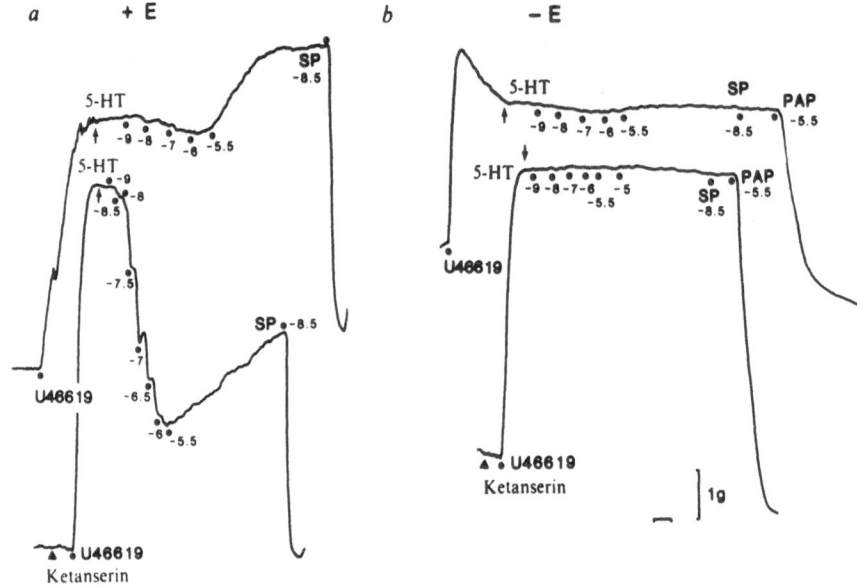

Figure 7. Chart records of 5-HT causing an endothelium-dependent relaxation of precontracted (U46619) pig isolated circumflex coronary artery in the presence of ketanserin (3 μM). Substance P (SP) relaxed the rings only in the presence of endothelium (+E) while papaverine (PAP) still relaxed the arteries in the absence of endothelium (−E). (Reprinted from [17] with permission of Macmillan Magazines Ltd.)

constrictor action of 5-HT. Acute loss of endothelial cells can occur in vivo. This has been shown experimentally by scanning electron microscopy in dog coronary arteries when the artery was only partially constricted to a level that did not substantially lower blood flow [22].

Atherosclerotic lesions contain a thickened neo-intima with macrophage-derived foam cells, and synthetic state smooth muscle cells covered with a layer of endothelium. Presumably EDRF, when released, would need to penetrate this neo-intima to relax the medial smooth muscle cells. In rabbit large coronary artery we found atherosclerosis produced a marked loss of relaxation sensitivity to acetylcholine and substance P. Both are endothelium dependent relaxants; presumably EDRF was thus unable to penetrate the atherosclerotic neo-intima. By contrast, there was no change in reactivity to glyceryl trinitrate [23]. Similar studies with atherosclerotic rabbit aorta have indicated a relatively normal EDRF release from the lumen on bioassay but a loss of relaxant activity that was correlated with the extent of the atherosclerosis [23, 24]. Thus the enhanced constrictor reactivity to 5-HT that we observed in atherosclerotic rabbit coronary artery may in part reflect a loss of EDRF (Figure 5).

5. Flow resistance in coronary disease

We have identified above, mechanisms that may alter the structure of the artery and local substances that will alter the contractility of the smooth muscle cells. How might these factors alter resistance to blood flow? Consider the resistance to blood flow is 2 units in a theoretical artery of wall thickness to internal radius ratio of 1:6 at rest under zero tone (Figure 8). Under physiological conditions 5-HT may cause the smooth muscle cells to shorten 10%. This would lower the internal circumference and raise the flow resistance (R) to 3.6 units as the radius (r) falls ($R \propto 1/r^4$) (Topline, Figure 8). Loss or damage of endothelium would abolish the dilator actions of EDRF and prostacyclin, and may induce the synthesis of the newly dis-covered constrictor peptide endothelin (Et) [26]. These factors would effec-tively increase the active contraction to 15% of resting length and raise flow resistance to 5 units. In arteries where there is lumen encroachment of 50% from atherosclerosis or medial hypertrophy, the 10% or 15% shortening of smooth muscle leads to 34 or 136 units of resistance (Figure 8, bottom line). These simple calculations confirm that arteries with any geometric alterations such as lumen encroachment are necessarily more "reactive" to any stimulus in terms of blood flow control even though the myocyte responds to a

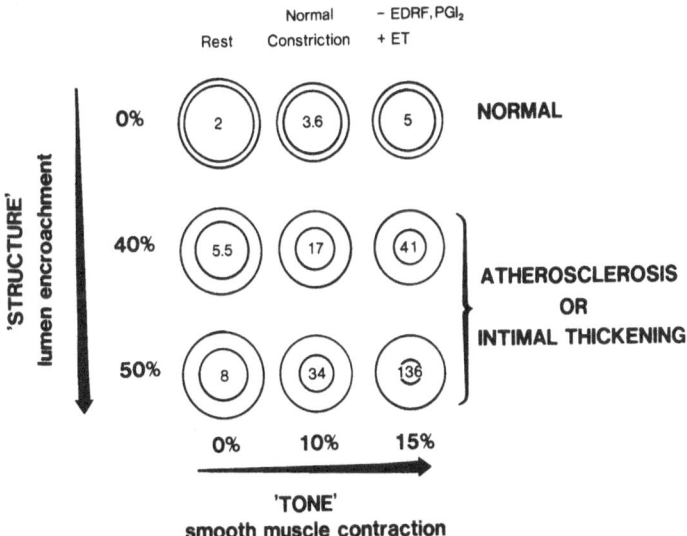

Figure 8. Theoretical representations of the cross-section of an artery at normal tone (left column) with 10% smooth muscle cell contraction (middle column) and 15% contraction (right column). The figures in the lumen are the flow resistance units ($R \propto 1/r^4$). The same contraction changes in an artery with structural changes that lower the lumen area by 40% or 50% are shown in the middle row and lower row respectively. This analysis emphasises the important role of structural changes in vascular reactivity. (Reprinted from [27] with permis-sion of ADIS Press Ltd.)

constrictor stimulus quite normally. If the contractility of the smooth muscle cell does alter in *addition* to these geometric changes in structure, the scene could be set for "vasospasm".

6. 5-HT receptors in the coronary circulation

6.1 *Large coronary arteries*

Potentially, there are 3 distinct sites on the wall of coronary arteries where 5-HT may act — the endothelium to release EDRF, the smooth muscle cell to cause either relaxation or contraction and sympathetic nerve varicosities to alter transmitter release.

6.1.1 *Endothelium*
There may be two distinct $5-HT_1$-like receptor subtypes that mediate relaxation that are different in location; one on the endothelial cell and one on the smooth muscle cell. The endothelial cell receptor on dog and pig coronary arteries that presumably releases EDRF is blocked by methysergide [21] and methiothepin [28] but is not antagonised by ketanserin [17]. If results from endothelium-dependent relaxation response to 5-HT in rabbit external jugular vein can be extrapolated to the coronary artery, then (i) this receptor is not blocked by MDL 72222; (ii) 5-carboxamidotryptamine has a lower affinity than α-methyl 5-HT for this receptor and (iii) spirerone is inactive [29].

6.1.2 *Smooth muscle cell — contraction*
In early experiments in dog isolated coronary artery we found that ketanserin behaved as an unsurmountable, non-competitive antagonist [30]. Similar results were found in the blood perfused dog large coronary artery pre-paration in situ (Figure 9). To complicate the issue, ketanserin behaves as a silent competitive antagonist in calf large coronary artery [31] in dog gastrosplenic, internal carotid and basilar arteries [32]. The anomalous behaviour of ketanserin in dog large coronary artery was not due to EDRF release nor to uptake of 5-HT into the vessel wall [33]. Another interesting finding was that methysergide, a competitive but partial agonist in dog coronary artery [3] was an unsurmountable 5-HT receptor antagonist in calf coronary arteries [31]. Kaumann [31] has put forward a model of allosteric regulation of the $5-HT_2$ receptors with possible modulation by endogenous substances. He has evidence for the allosteric regulation of $5-HT_2$ receptors in calf coronary [31] guinea pig trachea [34] and rat tail artery [35].

An additional complication could be that $5-HT_2$ receptors are not the only subtype of receptor that mediate contraction in large coronary arteries. Recent evidence suggests that in human large coronary artery rings, the compound GR 43175, a selective $5-HT_1$-like receptor agonist that contracts

DOG   CORONARY   ARTERY

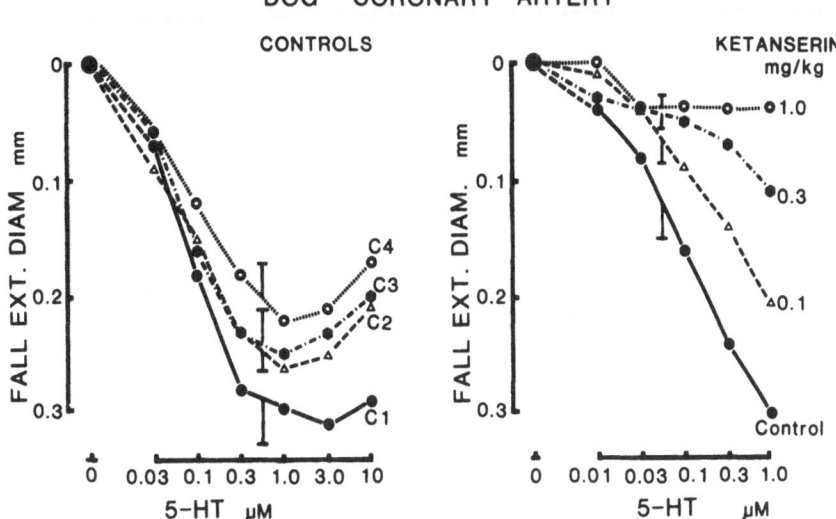

Figure 9. Mean falls in the external diameter of dog large coronary artery perfused with blood from a support dog in response to local infusions of 5-HT (see Figure 1). *Left*: responses from 5 dogs where the 5-HT curve was constructed 4 times $C_1 - C_4$) allowing 30 min between curves. *Right*: in a second group of 5 dogs 5-HT curves were repeated after 0, 0.1, 0.3 or 1.0 mg/kg ketanserin given intravenously to the support dog 30 minutes prior to constructing the 5-HT concentration-response curve. Error bars are average SEM from two-way analysis of variance (see [47]). (Angus, unpublished)

the dog [36], rabbit [37] and human [38] saphenous vein, has weak agonist activity [39]. The maximum contraction of GR 43175 was only 29% of that to 5-HT and was unaffected by ketanserin (1 μM) or MDL 72222 (1 μM). Methiothepin (0.1 μM) behaved as a surmountable antagonist shifting the sensitivity (EC_{50}) by 10 fold [39].

6.1.3   *Smooth muscle cell — relaxation*
In contrast with the endothelial cell $5\text{-}HT_1$-like receptor, the myocytes have another $5\text{-}HT_1$-like receptor that mediates relaxation (independently of the presence of endothelium) by raising c-AMP, where 5-CT has high affinity, α-methyl 5-HT is inactive and spiperone is an antagonist. A similar profile of tryptamine agonist activity was observed in pentobarbitone anaesthetized rats suggesting that the hypotension in response to 5-CT in vivo may be predominantly endothelium-independent [40].

6.1.4   *Nerve terminal*
5-HT released from platelets can accumulate in, and be released from sympathetic nerve varicosities of dog large coronary arteries in vitro [41]. In addition, 5-HT can inhibit release of transmitter noradrenaline by a pre-junctional receptor mechanism in this tissue [42]. The classification of this

5-HT receptor is unclear at present but bears some similar features to the loosely defined 5-HT$_1$-like receptors.

With this short summary of the subtypes of 5-HT receptors in the coronary artery it is not surprising that ketanserin was ineffective in treating variant angina in man [43, 44]. One explanation is that 5-HT is not involved. Alternatively, the constrictor action of 5-HT may be mediated through non 5-HT$_2$ receptors. Interestingly, Kaumann has suggested that an allosteric interaction of ketanserin with the 5-HT$_2$ receptor could explain the documented clinical case of coronary spasm induced by ketanserin treatment [44].

6.2 Small coronary arteries — relaxation

Cambridge and Chapple [45] recently reported that intra-left atrial injections of 5-HT and tryptamine analogues caused dose-dependent increases in coronary blood flow in the presence of ketanserin and MDL 72222 in anaesthetized dogs. The rank order of potency of the tryptamine analogues was consistent with an action at 5-HT$_1$-like receptors located on the coronary smooth muscle as observed in the rabbit jugular vein [40]. In agreement with the in vivo reports, we found that 5-CT ($0.01-1$ μM) could relax K$^+$ contracted small arteries (190 μm i.d.) removed from dog left ventricle and suspended in a myograph. Unlike the large conduit coronary arteries of most species, the small coronary arteries of the rabbit do not contract to 5-HT (see Figure 5).

Similary, in small coronary arteries removed from human right atrial appendage, 5-HT generally (10 out of 14) caused less than 10% of the maximum contraction obtained with K$^+$ depolarisation (K$^+$, 124 mM). However, in arteries from 4 patients, 5-HT concentration-response curves could be generated with a markedly variable range of contration (Figures 10, 11). The classification of this receptor is presently unknown. These preliminary human studies probably indicate the variability of the number and/or the subtype of 5-HT receptors on human small coronary vessels.

7. Conclusions

Prinzmetal's variant angina pectoris or vasospasm may be triggered by the local release of 5-HT or another autacoid from platelet aggregation. Experimental evidence supports two mechanisms that may contribute to coronary vasospasm, (i) a change in the geometry of the wall from atherosclerosis or perfusion pressure and (ii) a change in the contractile response of the vascular smooth muscle cell. This change in vascular smooth muscle reactivity may be caused by either an intrinsic receptor specific change in maximum contraction or from the loss of a dilator substance such as EDRF. The receptors for 5-HT on the coronary artery are currently classified as 5-HT$_1$-like, releasing EDRF from the endothelium and a distinct 5-HT$_1$-like receptor that directly relaxes the myocyte. In addition, there are 5-HT$_2$

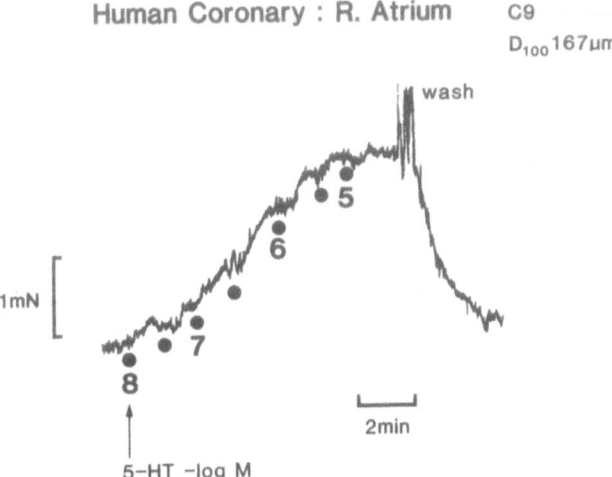

Figure 10. Chart record of the contraction of a human isolated small coronary artery removed from the right atrial appendage in response to 5-HT (Experiment number C9). The internal diameter of the vessel segment was 167 μm (D_{100}). (Angus and Broughton, unpublished)

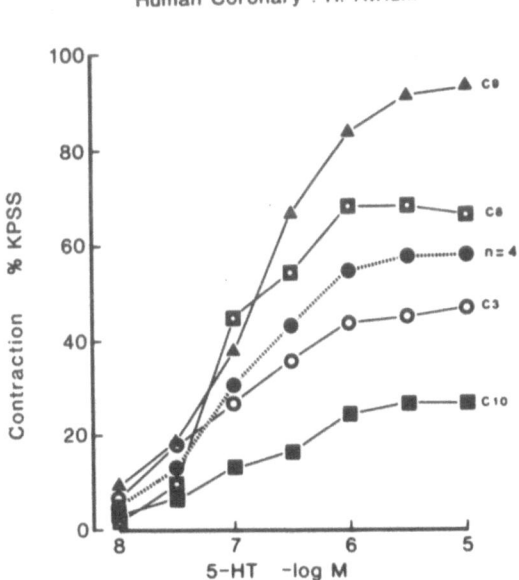

Figure 11. Concentration-response curves for 5-HT in 4 human isolated small coronary arteries (coded C_3, C_8, C_9, C_{10}) removed from the right atrial appendage. Contractions are expressed as percentage of the maximum contraction to K^+ (125 mM), termed KPSS, in each artery. The internal diameters ranged from 117 μm to 200 μm. (Angus and Broughton, unpublished).

receptors and possibly another receptor subtype that contract the vessel. The 5-HT$_2$ receptor antagonist ketanserin is an unsurmountable, non-competitive antagonist in dog and human large coronary artery.

There is a need for additional work in human large and small coronary arteries to identify the site and receptors for 5-HT involved in myocyte contractility and its interaction with the endothelium. There is still no acceptable 5-HT antagonist for use clinically to evaluate the role of 5-HT in coronary artery disease.

Acknowledgements

This work was supported by an Institute grant from the National Health and Medical Research Council and the National Heart Foundation of Australia. We thank Clara Chan for typing the manuscript.

References

1. Prinzmetal M, Kennamer R, Merliss R, Wada T, Bor N (1959): Angina pectoris. 1. A variant form of angina pectoris. *Am J Med* 27: 375—388.
2. Oates JA, Hawiger J, Ross R (1985): Preface to *Interaction of platelets with the vessel wall*. Bethesda: *Am Physiol Soc*
3. De Clerk F, Van Neuten JM (1982): Platelet-mediated vascular contractions: Inhibition of the serotonergic component by ketanserin. *Thromb Res* 27: 713—27.
4. Mullane KM, Bradley G, Moncada S (1982): The interactions of platelet-derived mediators on isolated canine coronary arteries. *Eur J Pharmacol* 84: 115—118.
5. Brazenor RM, Angus JA (1981): Ergometrine contracts isolated canine coronary arteries by a serotonergic mechanism: no role for alpha-adrenoceptors. *J Pharmacol Exp Ther* 218: 530—536.
6. Müller-Schweinitzer E (1980): The mechanism of ergometrine-induced coronary arterial spasm: In vitro studies on canine arteries. *J Cardiovasc Pharmacol* 2: 645—655.
7. Higgings CB, Wexler L, Silverman JF, Hayden WG, Anderson WL, Schroeder JH (1976): Spontaneously and pharmacologically provoked coronary arterial spasm in Prinzmetal variant angina. *Radiology* 119: 521—527.
8. Angus JA, Brazenor RM, Le Duc MA (1983): Responses of dog large coronary arteries to constrictor and dilator substances: Implications for the cause and treatment of variant angina pectoris. *Am J Cardiol* 52: 52A—60A.
9. Angus JA, Brazenor RM, Le Duc MA (1982): Verapamil: a selective antagonist of constrictor substances in dog coronary artery: Implications for variant angina. *Clin Exp Pharmacol Physiol Suppl* 6: 15—28.
10. Richmond DR. (1979): Results of treatment with verapamil in patients with coronary artery spasm, pp. 94—106 in: Kelly DT (ed), *Variant Angina, Diagnosis and Treatment*. Sydney, Australia: Hogbin Poole.
11. MacAlpin RN (1980): Relation of coronary arterial spasm to sites of organic stenosis. *Am J Cardiol* 46: 143—153.
12. Mulvany M, Halpern W (1977): Contractile properties of small arterial resistance vessels in spontaneously hypertensive and normotensive rats. *Circ Res* 41: 19—26.
13. Angus JA, Broughton A, Mulvany M (1988): Role of α-adrenoceptors in constrictor

responses of rat, guinea-pig and rabbit small arteries to neural activation. *J Physiol* 403: 495—510.

14. Henry PD, Yokoyama J (1980): Supersensitivity of atherosclerotic rabbit aorta to ergonovine. Mediation by a serotonergic mechanism. *J Clin Invest* 66: 306—313.

15. Yokoyama M, Akita H, Mizutani T, Fukazaki H, Watanabe Y (1983): Hyperactivity of coronary arterial smooth muscle in response to ergonovine from rabbits with hereditary hyperlipidemia. *Circ Res* 53: 63—71.

16. Furchgott RF, Zawadzki JV (1980): The obligatory role of endothelial cells in the relaxation of arterial smooth muscle by acetylcholine. *Nature* 288: 373—376.

17. Cocks TM, Angus JA (1983): Endothelium-dependent relaxation of coronary arteries by noradrenaline and serotonin. Nature 305: 627—630.

18. Angus JA, Cocks TM (1989): Endothelium-derived relaxing factor. *Pharmacol Ther* 41: 303—351.

19. Lamping KG, Marcus ML, Dole WP (1985). Removal of the endothelium potentiates canine large coronary artery constrictor responses to 5-hydroxytryptamine in vivo. *Circ Res* 57: 46—54.

20. Chu A, Cobb FR (1987): Vasoactive effects of serotonin on proximal coronary arteries in awake dogs. *Circ Res* 61 (suppl. II): II81—II87.

21. Cohen RA, Shepherd JT, Vanhoutte PM (1983): 5-hydroxytryptamine can mediate endothelium-dependent relaxation of coronary arteries. *Am J Physiol* 245: H1077—H1080.

22. Gertz SD, Uretsy G, Wajnberg RS, Navat N, Gotsman MS (1981): Endothelial cell damage and thrombus formation after partial arterial constriction: Relevance to the role of coronary arterial spasm in the pathogenesis of myocardial infarction. *Circulation* 63: 476—486.

23. Angus JA, Wright CE, Cocks TM (1989): Vascular actions of serotonin in large and small arteries are amplified by loss of endothelium, atherosclerosis and hypertension, (in press) in: Mylecharane E, Angus JA, De La Lande IS, Humphrey P (eds), *Serotonin*. London: Macmillan Press.

24. Verbeuren TJ, Jordaens FH, Zonnekeyn LL, Van Hove CE, Coene M—C, Herman AG (1986): Effect of hypercholesterolemia on vascular reactivity in the rabbit. 1. Endothelium-dependent and endothelium-independent contractions and relaxations in isolated arteries of control and hypercholesterolemic rabbits. *Cirs Res* 58: 552—564.

25. Chappell SP, Lewis MJ, Henderson AH (1987): Effect of lipid feeding on endothelium-dependent relaxation in rabbit aortic preparations. *Cardiovasc Res* 21: 34—38.

26. Yanigasawa M, Kurihara H, Kimura S, Tomobe H, Kobayashi M, Mitsui Y, Yazaki Y, Goto K, Masaki T (1988): A novel potent vasoconstrictor peptide produced by vascular endothelial cells. *Nature* 332: 411—415.

27. Angus JA, Cocks TM (1989): Endothelial cell function and blood vessel reactivity. *Current Therapeutics* (in press).

28. Houston DS, Shepherd JT, Vanhoutte TM (1985): Adenine nucleotides, serotonin and endothelium-dependent relaxations to platelets. *Am J Physiol* 248: H389—H395.

29. Leff P, Martin GR, Morse JM (1987): Differential classification of vascular smooth muscle and endothelial cell 5-HT receptors by use of tryptamine analogues. *Br J Pharmacol* 91: 321—331.

30. Brazenor RM, Angus JA (1982): Actions of serotonin antagonists on dog coronary artery. *Eur J Pharmacol* 81: 569—576.

31. Kaumann AJ, Frenken M (1985): A paradox: the 5-HT$_2$ receptor antagonist ketanserin restores the 5-HT-induced contraction depressed by methysergide in large coronary arteries of calf. *Naunyn-Schmiedeberg's Arch Pharmacol* 328: 295—300.

32. Van Nueten JM, Janssen PAJ, Van Beek J, Xhonneux R, Verbeuren TJ, Vanhoutte PM (1981): Vascular effects of ketanserin R41468, a novel antagonist of 5-HT$_2$ serotonergic receptors. *J Pharmacol Exp Ther* 218: 217—230.

33. Cohen RA (1986): Contractions of isolated canine coronary arteries resistant to S_2 serotonergic blockade. *J Pharmacol Exp Ther* 237: 548—552.

34. Lemoine H, Kaumann AJ (1986): Allosteric properties of 5-HT$_2$ receptors in tracheal smooth muscle. *Naunyn-Schmiedeberg's Arch Pharmacol* 333: 91—97.

35. Frenken M, Kaumann AJ (1987): Allosteric properties of the 5-HT$_2$ receptor system of the rat tail artery. *Naunyn-Schmiedeberg's Arch Pharmacol* 335: 359—366.

36. Feniuk W, Humphrey PPA, Perren MJ, Watts AD (1985): A comparison of 5-hydroxy-tryptamine receptors mediating contraction in rabbit aorta and dog saphenous vein: evidence for different receptor types obtained by use of selective agonists and antagonists. *Br J Pharmacol* 86: 697—704.

37. Martin GR, Leff P, MacLennan SJ, Dougall I (1988): Three types of 5-HT$_1$-like receptors recognised by tryptamine affinity and efficacy fingerprints. *Br J Pharmacol* 95: 626P.

38. Chester A, Arneklo-Nobin B, Bodelsson M, Martin G, Tadjkarinni S, Törnebrandt K, Yacoub M (1988): Characterization of 5-HT receptors in human saphenous vein. Cardiovascular Pharmacology of 5-HT, Amsterdam, October 1988, Abstract p. 57.

39. Chester A, Martin GR, Bodelsson M, Arneklo-Nobin B, Törnebrandt K, Martin JF, Yacoub M (1988): Evidence for 5-HT$_1$-like and 5-HT receptors mediating contraction of human epicardial coronary arteries. Cardiovascular Pharmacology of 5-HT, Amsterdam, October 1988, Abstract p. 54.

40. Martin GR, Leff P, Cambridge D, Barrett VJ (1987): Comparative analysis of two types of 5-hydroxytryptamine receptor mediating vasorelaxation: Differential classification using tryptamines. *Naunyn-Schmiedeberg's Arch Pharmacol* 336: 365—373.

41. Cohen RA (1985): Platelet-induced neurogenic coronary contractions due to accumulation of the false neurotransmitter 5-hydroxytryptamine. *J Clin Invest* 75: 286—292.

42. Cohen RA (1985): Serotonergic prejunctional inhibition of canine coronary adrenergic nerves. *J Pharmacol Exp Ther* 235: 76—80.

43. De Caterina R, Carpeggiani C, L'Abbate A (1984): A double-blind, placebo-controlled study of ketanserin in patients with Prinzmetal's angina. Evidence against a role for serotonin in the genesis of coronary vasospasm. *Circulation* 69: 889—894.

44. Freedman SB, Chierchia S, Rodriguex-Plaza L, Burgiardini R, Smith G, Maseri A (1984): Ergonovine-induced myocardial ischaemia: No role for serotonergic receptors? *Circulation* 70: 178—183.

45. Cambridge D, Chapple DJ (1988): Characterisation of the coronary vascular response to 5-HT in vivo using tryptamine analogues. Cardiovascular Pharmacology of 5-HT, Amsterdam, October 1988, Abstract p. 56.

XXXIII. The endothelium and the role of 5-hydroxytryptamine in vascular disease

PAUL M. VANHOUTTE

1. Introduction

The vascular actions of 5-hydroxytryptamine (5-HT), originally named serotonin [1], remain difficult to understand, as it causes varying responses depending on the isolated blood vessel or vascular bed studied, or the experimental conditions imposed. The present essay will summarize some of the experiments performed in the author's laboratory suggesting that the presence of the endothelium helps to determine if the monoamine causes constriction or dilatation of blood vessels. In particular, the emerging role of endothelium-derived vasoactive factors in the mediation of the vascular effects of 5-HT will be addressed. For details and original references not cited here the reader is referred to several earlier reviews on related topics [2—17].

In the following discussion, it will be assumed that the 5-HT which plays the major role in modulating peripheral vascular responses originates from aggregating platelets. Obviously, in addition, in certain blood vessels serotonergic neurones also may be a source of 5-HT [18—20], as may endothelial cells themselves [21, 22]. It should be emphasized that its action on the endothelium is only one of the mechanisms by which 5-HT can evoke dilatation (Figure 1) or constriction (Figure 2) of blood vessels.

2. Endothelium-dependent relaxations to 5-HT

2.1 *The phenomenon and the receptors involved*

The ability of 5-HT to evoke endothelium-dependent relaxations was demonstrated first and repeatedly confirmed in isolated coronary arteries [23—27]. The response is concentration-dependent (Figure 3) and can be antagonized by methysergide, methiothepin and metergoline, but not by cyanopindolol, ketanserin or MDL 72222; it cannot be mimicked by 8-OH

P.R. Saxena, D.I. Wallis, W. Wouters and P. Bevan (eds), Cardiovascular Pharmacology of 5-Hydroxytryptamine, pp. 379—389.
© 1990 *Kluwer Academic Publishers, Dordrecht* —

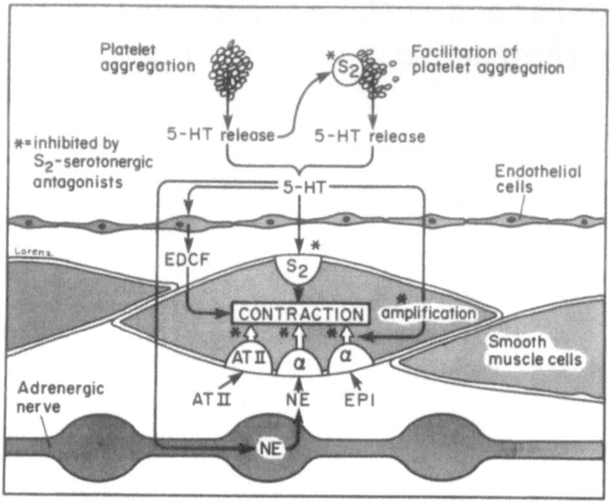

380   *P. M. Vanhoutte*

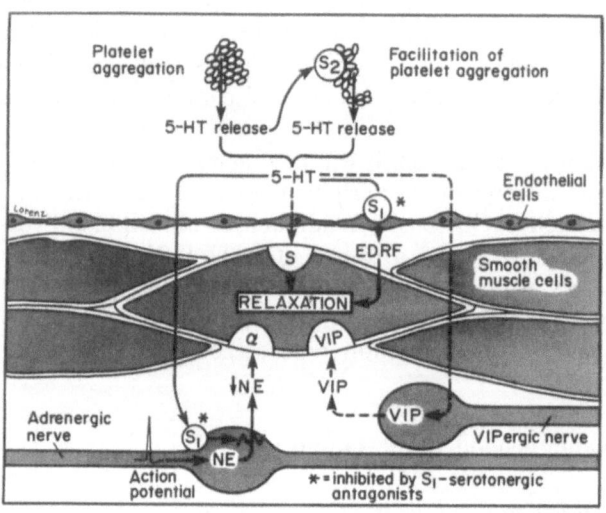

Figure 1. Direct and indirect vasoconstrictor effects of 5-HT. α, α-adrenoceptor; AT II, angiotensin II; EDCF, endothelium-derived contracting factor(s); EPI, epinephrine; NE, noradrenaline; 5-HT$_2$, 5-HT$_2$ receptor (from [14], by permission).

Figure 2. Direct and indirect vasodilator effects of 5-HT, α, α-adrenoceptor; NE, noradrenaline; 5-HT$_1$, 5-HT$_1$-like receptors; VIP, vasoactive intestinal polypeptide; EDRF, endothelium-derived relaxing factor(s); jagged line, inhibition of adrenergic neurotransmission (from [14], by permission).

DPAT [24—28]. Hence, it must be mediated by a 5-HT$_1$-like, but not 5-HT$_{1A}$, receptor on the endothelial cells [28]. When studies are performed

With endothelium

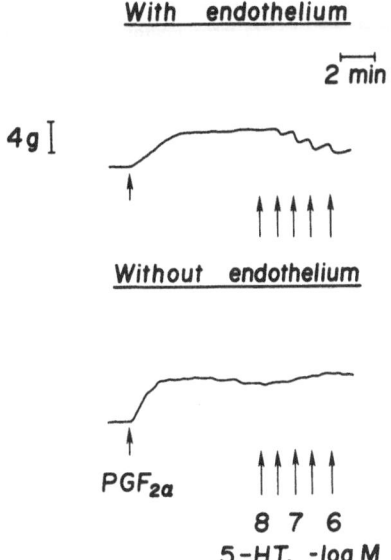

Without endothelium

Figure 3. Example of isometric tension recordings in a pair of rings from the same coronary artery with (upper) and without (lower) endothelium. Rings were contracted with prostaglandin F_{2a} (2×10^{-6} M); when the contractions had stabilized, 5-HT ($10^{-8} - 10^{-6}$ M) was added cumulatively in half-log increments (from [24], by permission).

on rings of isolated arteries suspended in organ chambers it may be necessary to block 5-HT_2 receptors on the vascular smooth muscle to demonstrate convincingly the endothelium-dependent relaxation [27]. However, in perfused coronary arteries, if 5-HT is given extra- and intraluminally, the vasodilator response originating in the endothelium is strong enough to inhibit the contractions due to the direct action of the monoamine on the vascular smooth muscle (Figure 4; [24]).

2.2 Cellular mechanisms

As for a variety of substances causing endothelium-dependent relaxation, the endothelium-dependent relaxations to 5-HT can be attributed to the release by the endothelial cells of a powerful vasodilator substance, endothelium-derived relaxing factor(s) (EDRF; [8, 29]). The factor(s), presumably nitric oxide [30—32], causes relaxation by activation of guanylate cyclase in the smooth muscle, leading to accumulation of cyclic GMP. To judge from experiments in the porcine coronary artery, the coupling between the 5-HT_1-like endothelial receptors and the release of endothelium-derived relaxing factor involves a G_i protein, which mediates the inhibitory effects of receptors on adenylate cyclase. This conclusion is derived from the observation that pertussis toxin, an inactivator of the G_i protein [33—35] markedly

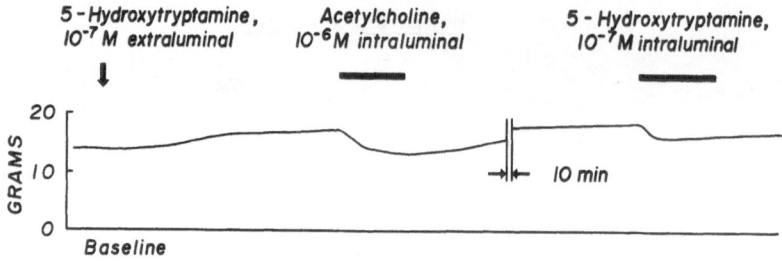

Figure 4. In an isolated, perfused canine coronary artery with intact endothelium, 5-HT caused contraction if given extraluminally (left), but relaxation if given intraluminally (right). The inhibitory response to acetylcholine (middle), demonstrates the presence of endothelial cells (from [5], by permission).

reduces the endothelium-dependent relaxations evoked by 5-HT (Figure 5); this is also the case for the alpha$_2$-adrenoceptor agonist UK 14,304 (Figure 5) but not for bradykinin [36].

2.3 *Physiological role*

It appears that a balance between the endothelium-dependent relaxing effect of 5-HT and the direct activation of the smooth muscle cells in the favor of the former probably contributes to the protective role of the endothelium in preventing unwanted platelet-aggregation and the resulting vasospasm

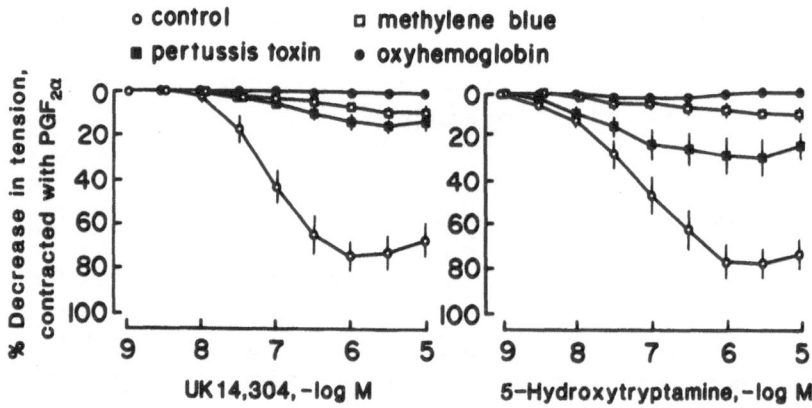

Figure 5. Influence of pertussis toxin (100 ng/ml), methylene blue (10^{-5} M), or oxyhemoglobin (10^{-5} M) on the endothelium-dependent relaxations produced by the alpha$_2$-adrenoceptor agonist, UK 14,304 (10^{-9} to 10^{-5} M) (left) and by 5-HT (10^{-9} to 10^{-5} M) in porcine coronary arteries. Arterial rings were contracted with prostaglandin F$_{2\alpha}$ (2×10^{-6} M), and responses are expressed as percentage relaxation of the contraction (presented as means ± S.E.M.). Symbols: O, control; ■, pertussis toxin (100 ng/ml); □, methylene blue (10^{-5} M); ●, oxyhemoglobin (10^{-5} M) (from [36], by permission).

(Figure 6; [2–17]). Any traumatic interruption of the endothelial lining would remove the considerable braking effect of endothelium-derived relaxing factor(s) on the underlying vascular smooth muscle, and allow the full vasoconstrictor response to 5-HT (and other activators such as thromboxane A_2) released from the platelets aggregating at the site of endothelial lesion; this, of course, contributes to the vascular phase of hemostasis (Figure 6).

2.4   Pathological conditions

Blunting of endothelium-dependent relaxations to 5-HT may be a very early sign of vascular disease. This is suggested by the finding that, four weeks after mechanical removal of the endothelium in situ, and despite recovery of a full endothelial lining, endothelium-dependent relaxations to 5-HT (and hence to

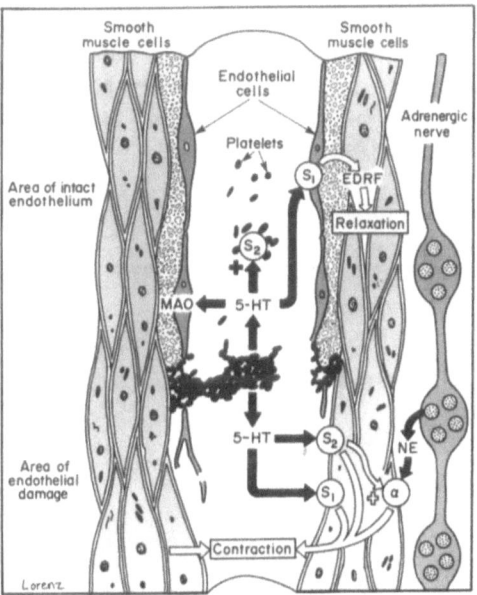

Figure 6. Possible roles of 5-HT in hemostasis. 5-HT released from aggregating platelet amplifies further platelet aggregation; it is, however, avidly taken up and cleared from plasma by unaggregated platelets. If the endothelium is intact, 5-HT is also taken up and degraded by monoamine oxidase (MAO). Endothelial cells of some vessels can release endothelium-derived relaxing factor (EDRF) in response to 5-HT and other platelet products. If the fragile endothelium is damaged during trauma, and 5-HT gains access to the underlying smooth muscle, it causes contraction directly (the receptor subtype depending on the blood vessel) and amplifies contraction to other vasoconstrictors such as noradrenaline (NE). Thus, the absence of endothelium favors not only platelet aggregation but also vasospasm and hence control of blood loss [S_1 = 5-HT$_1$- like receptor; S_2 = 5-HT$_2$ receptor; α = α-adrenoceptor; + = amplification) (from [10], by permission).

aggregating platelets), are greatly reduced (Figure 7; [27]). The loss of responsiveness to 5-HT is maintained for several months after the endothelial injury [37]. At the site of a previous traumatic removal of the coronary endothelium repeated vasoconstrictor episodes, accompanied by signs of myocardial ischemia can be evoked by the intracoronary injection of 5-HT (Shimokawa and Vanhoutte, unpublished observations). Hence, a previous injury to the endothelium may become a predisposing factor for the occurrence of vasospasm, and this despite the presence of regenerated endothelium.

The loss in responsiveness to 5-HT is accompanied by a similar reduction in the ability of the alpha$_2$-adrenoceptor agonist UK 14,304 to induce endothelium-dependent relaxations while the response to bradykinin is preserved; in arteries covered with such regenerated endothelium, pertussis toxin no longer inhibits the relaxations to 5-HT (or UK 14,304) [38]. Hence it is likely that the reduced endothelium-dependent relaxation to 5-HT represents a selective loss of the G$_i$-protein linked to the release of endothelium-derived relaxing factor. Cultured porcine endothelial cells also lose the ability to respond to 5-HT (and UK 14,304) [39]. Thus, dysfunction of the G$_i$-protein, and the resulting impairment of certain endothelium-dependent relaxations may be a characteristic of endothelial regrowth.

The loss in endothelium-dependent relaxations following endothelium-denudation can be exacerbated if the animals are fed a high cholesterol diet

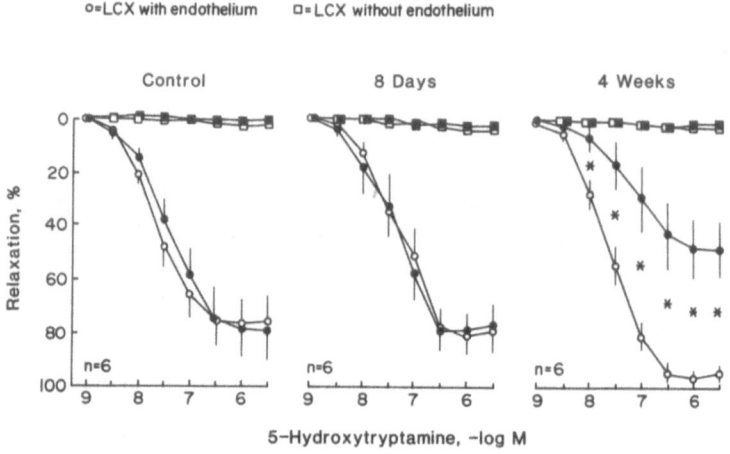

Figure 7. Cumulative concentration-response curves to 5-HT in rings with and without endothelium during contractions to prostaglandin F$_{2\alpha}$ (2×10^{-6} M) under control conditions (left), 8 days (middle), and 4 weeks (right) after endothelial denudation. All rings were treated with indomethacin (10^{-5} M) and ketanserin (10^{-6} M). LAD is left anterior descending coronary artery; LCX is left circumflex coronary artery. *Denotes a statistically significant difference between rings with endothelium of left anterior descending and left circumflex coronary arteries (from [27], by permission).

and the sites of denudation become atherosclerotic. This helps to explain the reports that vasoconstrictor responses to the monoamine are augmented considerably in atherosclerotic blood vessels [40—44].

2.5 *Influence of diet*

Chronic intake of increased amounts of cholesterol blunts moderately endothelium-dependent relaxations to 5-HT [45] and accelerates the occurrence of atherosclerosis. Conversely, chronic intake of cod liver oil (Figure 8; [46]) or of the ω_3-unsaturated acids that it contains [47] potentiates endothelium-dependent relaxations to 5-HT. A reassuring finding is that chronic intake of cod liver oil prevents the reduction of the response due to hypercholesterolemia, and considerably reduces that resulting from an atherosclerotic lesion [45].

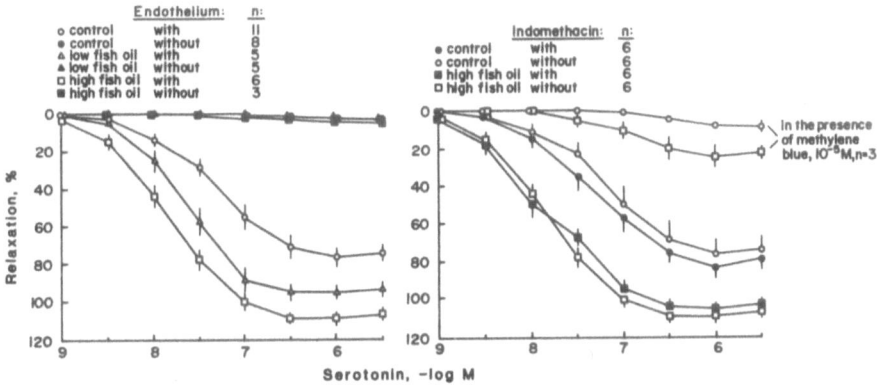

Figure 8. Cumulative concentration-response curves to 5-HT (serotonin) during contractions evoked by prostaglandin F_{2a} (2×10^{-6} M) in the presence of ketanserin (10^{-6} M) in coronary arteries taken from control pigs or pigs treated with cod liver oil. The relaxation responses are expressed as percent decrease in tension of the contraction evoked by prostaglandin F_{2a}. Data shown as means ± SEM. Left: relaxations in the three different groups. Right: Relaxations in control and high fish oil groups under control conditions and in the presence of indomethacin (to inhibit production of prostacyclin) or methylene blue (to inhibit guanylate cyclase) (from [46], by permission).

3. Endothelium-dependent contractions to 5-HT

A number of stimuli and vasoactive substances can cause endothelium-dependent contractions which have been attributed to the release of at least two different endothelium-derived contracting factors (EDCF; [see 12, 48, 49]). Endothelium-dependent increases in tension have been obtained with

5-HT, but so far only in isolated blood vessels taken from pathological models. This is the case for the aorta of the spontaneously hypertensive rat (Figure 9; [50]), and the coronary artery of the pig, both after regeneration of the endothelium or induction of atherosclerosis (Figure 10; [27, 45]). The

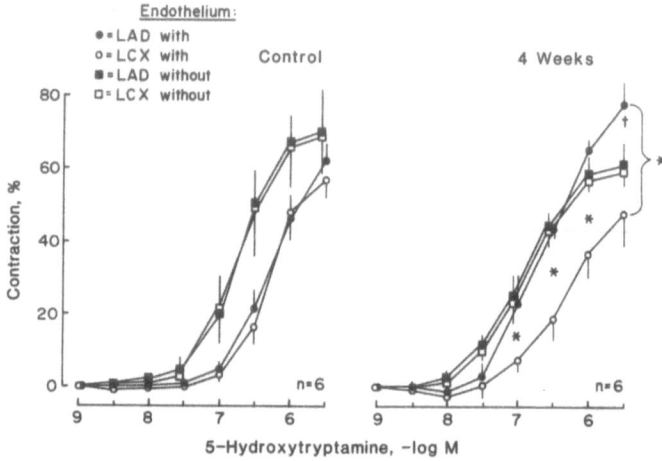

Figure 9. Responses to 5-HT in aortic rings (with and without endothelium) from spontaneously hypertensive rats (SHR) contracted with prostaglandin $F_{2\alpha}(PGF_{2\alpha})$. Data shown as means ± S.E.M. Asterisks denote statistically significant differences between rings with and without endothelium (from [50], by permission).

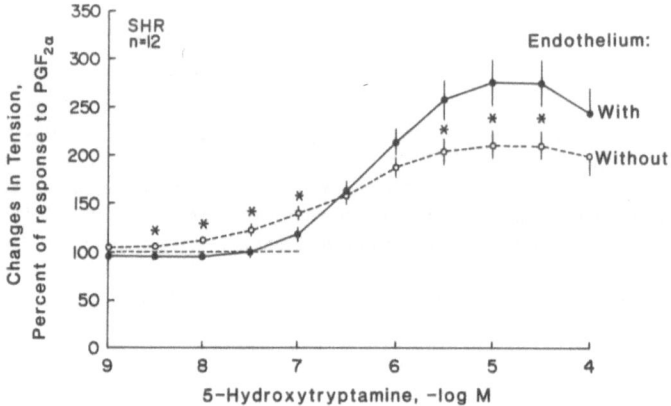

Figure 10. Cumulative concentration-response curves to 5-HT in quiescent rings under control conditions (left) and 4 weeks after endothelial denudation (right). LAD is left anterior descending coronary artery; LCX is left circumflex coronary artery. *Denotes a statistically significant difference between left anterior descending and left circumflex coronary arteries. † denotes a statistically significant difference between rings with and without endothelium of the left anterior descending coronary artery (from [27], by permission).

receptors involved in the contractions and the cellular mechanism underlying them, and the nature of the contracting factor released are unknown.

4. Conclusion

5-HT can activate 5-HT_1-like receptors on endothelial cells, particularly in coronary arteries; this, by means of a Gi-protein mediated process, leads to the release of endothelium-derived relaxing factor(s), and relaxation of the underlying smooth muscle. The endothelium-dependent relaxation to 5-HT probably contributes to the protective role of the endothelium to prevent intraluminal platelet-aggregation and coagulation. It seems that after injury of the endothelium, and despite regeneration of endothelial cells, these cells lose the ability to react to 5-HT, presumably because of a selective dysfunction of the G_i-protein-mediated response. Under pathological conditions, the endothelium becomes more capable of releasing endothelium-derived contracting factor(s) in response to 5-HT. The reduced ability to release endothelium-derived relaxing factor and/or the increased propensity to secrete endothelium-derived contracting factor(s) favor vasoconstrictor (vasospastic) response to the monoamine [17].

Acknowledgements

The author would like to thank Mrs. Cindy Camrud for secretarial assistance and Mr. Robert Lorenz for preparation of the illustrations.

References

1. Page IH (1954): Serotonin (5-hydroxytryptamine). *Physiol Rev* 34: 563—588.
2. Vanhoutte PM (1983): 5-hydroxytryptamine and vascular disease. *Fed Proc* 42: 233—237.
3. Vanhoutte PM, Cohen RA, Van Nueten JM (1984): Serotonin and arterial vessels *J Cardiovasc Pharmacol* 6: S421—S428.
4. Cohen RA, Vanhoutte PM (1985): Platelets, serotonin, and endothelial cells, pp. 105—112 in: Vanhoutte PM (ed), *Serotonin and the Cardiovascular System*. New York: Raven Press.
5. Vanhoutte PM (1985): Peripheral serotonergic receptors and hypertension. pp. 123—134 in: Vanhoutte PM (ed), *Serotonin and the Cardiovascular System*. New York: Raven Press.
6. Vanhoutte PM, Houston DS (1985): Platelets, endothelium and vasospasm. *Circulation* 72: 728—734.
7. Vanhoutte PM, Luscher TF (1989): Serotonin and the blood vessel wall. *J Hypertension* (in press).
8. Vanhoutte PM, Rubanyi GM, Miller VM, Houston DS (1986): Modulation of vascular smooth muscle contraction by the endothelium. *Ann Rev Physiol* 48: 307—320.

9. Vanhoutte PM (1986): Could the absense or malfunction of vascular endothelium precipitate the occurrence of vasospasm? *J Mol Cell Cardiol* 18: 679—689.
10. Houston DS, Vanhoutte PM (1986): Serotonin and the vascular system. Role in health and disease and implications for therapy. *Drugs* 3: 149—163.
11. Vanhoutte PM (1987): Serotonin and the vascular wall. *Int J Cardiol* 14: 189—203.
12. Vanhoutte PM (1987): Endothelium and the control of vascular tissue. *News in Physiol Sci* 2: 18—22.
13. Houston DS, Vanhoutte PM (1988): Platelets and endothelium-dependent responses. Chapter 21, pp. 425—449 in: Vanhoutte PM (ed), *Endothelium-Derived Vasoactive Factors*. Clifton, NJ: The Humana Press.
14. Vanhoutte PM (1987): Cardiovascular effects of serotonin. *J Cardiovasc Pharmacol* 10: (Suppl. 3): S8—S11.
15. Vanhoutte PM, Luscher TF (1987): Vascular endothelium and hypertension. *J Cardiovasc Pharm* 10 (Suppl. 4), S19—S24.
16. Vanhoutte Paul M (1987): State of the Art Lecture: Endothelium and responsiveness of vascular smooth muscle. *J Hypertension* (Suppl. 5) 5: S115—S120.
17. Vanhoutte PM (1988): The endothelium-modulator of vascular smooth-muscle tone. *New England Journal of Medicine* 319: 512—513, August 25.
18. Griffith SG, Lincoln J, Burnstock G (1982): Serotonin as a neurotransmitter in cerebral arteries. *Brain Res* 247: 388—392.
19. Edvinsson L, Degueurce A, Duverger D, Mackenzie ET, Scatton B (1983): Central serotonergic nerves project to the pial vessels of the brain. *Nature* 306: 55—57.
20. Marco EJ, Balfagon G, Salaices M, Sanchez-Ferrer CF, Marin J (1985): Serotonergic innervation of cat cerebral arteries. *Brain Research* 338: 137—139.
21. Burnstock G (1987): Mechanisms of interaction of peptide and nonpeptide vascular neurotransmitter systems. *J Cardiovasc Pharmacol* 10 (Suppl. 12): S74—S81.
22. Loesch A, Burnstock G (1988): Ultrastructural localization of serotonin and substance P in vascular endothelial cells of rat femoral and mesenteric arteries. *Anat Embryol* 178: 137—142.
23. Cocks TM, Angus JA (1983): Endothelium-dependent relaxation of coronary arteries by noradrenaline and serotonin. *Nature* 305: 627—630.
24. Cohen RA, Shepherd JT, Vanhoutte PM (1983): 5-Hydroxytryptamine can mediate endothelium-dependent relaxation of coronary arteries. *Am J Physiol* 245: H1077—H1080.
25. Cohen RA, Shepherd JT, Vanhoutte PM (1984): Endothelium and asymmetrical responses of the coronary arterial wall. *Am J Physiol*. 247: H403—H408.
26. Houston DS, Shepherd JT, Vanhoutte PM (1985): Adenine nucleo-tides, serotonin and endothelium-dependent relaxations to platelets. *Am J Physiol* 248: H389—H395.
27. Shimokawa H, Aarhus AA, Vanhoutte PM (1987): Porcine coronary arteries with regenerated endothelium have a reduced endothelium-dependent responsiveness to aggregating platelets and serotonin. *Circ Res* 61: 256—270.
28. Houston DS, Vanhoutte PM (1988): Comparison of serotonergic receptor subtypes on the smooth muscle and endothelium of the canine coronary artery. *JPET* 244: 1—10.
29. Furchgott RF (1981): The requirement for endothelial cells in the relaxation of arteries by acetylcholine and some other vasodilators. *Trends Pharmacol Sci* 2: 173—176.
30. Furchgott RF (1988): Studies on relaxation of rabbit aorta by sodium nitrite: the basis for the proposal that the acid-activatable inhibitory factor from bovine retractor penis is inorganic nitrite and the endothelium-derived relaxing factor is nitric oxide, pp. 401—405 in: Vanhoutte PM (ed), *Vasodilatation*. NY: Raven Press.
31. Ignarro LJ, Byrns RE, Berga GM, Wood KS (1987): Endothelium-derived relaxing factor from pulmonary artery and vein possesses pharmacological and chemical properties identical to those of nitric oxide radical. *Circ Res* 61: 866—879.
32. Palmer RMJ, Ferrige AG, Moncada S (1987): The release of nitric oxide by vascular endothelial cells accounts for the activity of EDRF. *Nature* 327: 524—526.

33. Rodbell M (1985): Programmable messengers: a new theory of hormone action. *Trends in Biochem Sci* 7: 461—464.
34. Dohlman HG, Caron MG, Lefkowitz RJ (1987): A family of receptors coupled to guanine regulatory proteins. *Biochem* 26: 2657—2664.
35. Dolphin AC (1987): Nucleotide binding proteins in signal transduction in health and disease. *Trends in Neurosci* 10: 53—57.
36. Flavahan NA, Shimokawa H, Vanhoutte PM (1989): Pertussis toxin inhibits endothelium-dependent relaxations to certain agonists in porcine coronary arteries. *J Physiol* 408: 549—560.
37. Shimokawa H, Vanhoutte PM: Natural course of the impairment of endothelium-dependent relaxations after balloon endothelium-removal in porcine coronary arteries. *Circ* in press.
38. Shimokawa H, Flavahan NA, Vanhoutte PM: Impaired Gi protein function may account for endothelial dysfunction in regenerated state and in hypercholesterolemia. *Circ* in press.
39. Boulanger C, Hendrickson H, Lorenz RR, Vanhoutte PM: Release of different relaxing factors by cultured porcine endothelial cells. *Circ Res* in press.
40. Yokoyama M, Akita H, Mizutani T, Fukuzaki H, Watanabe Y (1983): Hyperreactivity of coronary arterial smooth muscles in response to ergonovine from rabbits with hereditary hyperlipidemia *Circ Res* 53: 63—71.
41. Henry PD, Yokoyama M (1980): Supersensitivity of atherosclerotic rabit aorta to ergonovine. Mediation by a serotonergic mechanism. *J Clin Invest* 66: 306—313.
42. Heric E, Tackett RL (1985): Altered vascular reactivity in the rabbit during hypercholesterolemia. *Pharmacol* 31: 72—81.
43. Kawachi Y, Tomoike H, Maruoka Y, Kikuchi Y, Araki H, Ishii Y, Tanaka K, Nakamura M (1984): Selective hypercontraction caused by ergonovine in the canine coronary artery under conditions of induced atherosclerosis. *Circ* 69: 441—450.
44. Heistad DD, Armstrong ML, Marcus ML, Piegors DJ, Mark AL (1984): Augmented responses to vasoconstrictor stimuli in hypercholesteolemic and atherosclerotic monkeys. *Circ Res* 54: 711—718.
45. Shimokawa H, Vanhoutte PM (1988): Dietary cod-liver oil improves endothelium-dependent responses in hypercholesterolemic and atherosclerotic porcine coronary arteries. *Circ* 78: 1421—1430.
46. Shimokawa H, Lam JYT, Chesebro JH, Bowie EJW, Vanhoutte PM (1987): Effects of dietary supplementation with cod-liver oil on endothelium-dependent responses in porcine coronary arteries. *Circ* 76(No. 4): 898—905.
47. Shimokawa H, Vanhoutte PM: Dietary ω_3 fatty acids and endothelium-dependent relaxations in porcine coronary arteries. *Amer J Physiol*, in press.
48. Vanhoutte PM (1987): Endothelium-dependent contractions in arteries and veins. *Blood Vessels*, 24: 141—144.
49. Vanhoutte PM (1988): Endothelium-dependent contractions in veins and arteries, Chapter 2 pp. 27—39 in: Vanhoutte PM (ed), *Relaxing and Contracting Factors; Biological and Clinical Research.* Clifton, NJ: The Humana Press.
50. Luscher TF, Vanhoutte PM (1986): Endothelium-dependent responses to platelets and serotonin in spontaneously hypertensive rats. *Hypertension* 8 (Suppl. II): II-55—II-60.

XXXIV. Vascular pharmacology of 5-hydroxytryptamine in humans

GERARD J. BLAUW, PETER VAN BRUMMELEN and
PIETER A. VAN ZWIETEN

1. Introduction

Forty years after its discovery the role of 5-hydroxytryptamine (5-HT) in the regulation of vascular tone in man still remains rather obscure. Soon after synthetic 5-HT became available it was shown that this monoamine influences vascular tone in a complex manner. Depending on the type of blood vessel and species investigated, as well as on the dose and route of administration, 5-HT was able to induce either vasodilatation or vasoconstriction [1, 2].

So far, most of our present knowledge of the mechanisms underlying the cardiovascular effects of 5-HT is based on experiments performed in vitro and in laboratory animals, whereas relatively few experimental data in humans are available. In view of considerable species differences in the vascular response to 5-HT, it was considered mandatory to test whether the findings from animal experiments also hold true in humans. For these reasons we have performed experiments in the forearm to study regional vascular effects of 5-HT and 5-HT receptor antagonists in man. The results of these experiments will be discussed in the context of the prevailing views on vascular 5-HT receptors.

2. Regional arterial and venous responses to 5-HT in humans

In 1955 it was shown by Roddie and co-workers [3] that an i.a. infusion of 5-HT in doses of 4 and 16 μg/min in the human forearm elicited arterial constriction, which was preceded by an initial transient increase in forearm blood flow (FBF). This haemodynamic effect was accompanied by an increase in volume and by erythema of the forearm and hand. When lower doses of 5-HT were infused only the initial transient dilatator response was observed [3]. The volume increase and the erythema were explained by a

P.R. Saxena, D.I. Wallis, W. Wouters and P. Bevan (eds), Cardiovascular Pharmacology of
5-Hydroxytryptamine, pp. 391–399.
© 1990 Kluwer Academic Publishers, Dordrecht —

simultaneous vasodilatation of the skin vessels and venoconstriction. Bock et al. [4], demonstrated that i.a. injections of 5-HT in the forearm induced an increase in muscle blood flow and a decrease of skin blood flow. At higher doses the increase in FBF was attenuated. Using the 5-HT antagonists BOL 148 [5] and methysergide [6] it was shown that the arterial constrictor response to 5-HT could be reversed and the venoconstriction attenuated.

Recently, we have further explored the regional arterial and venous responses to 5-HT in the human forearm. 5-HT was administered as single consecutive infusions into the brachial artery in doses of 0.1—80 ng/kg/min. Each infusion lasted 8—10 minutes with intervals of 30 minutes. Forearm blood flow was measured by computerized R-wave triggered venous occlusion plethysmography [7]. During some infusions the venous effect of 5-HT was also measured using determination of maximum venous outflow by venous occlusion plethysmography. Heart rate and i.a. blood pressure were recorded continuously. In all of the experiments only minor and inconsistent changes in heart rate and blood pressure were observed, excluding any important systemic haemodynamic effects of the drugs in the doses used.

In experiments in young healthy subjects it was confirmed that i.a. infusions of 5-HT induced a complex biphasic vascular response consisting of an initial rapid transient increase in FBF, followed by a persistent net arterial dilatation at lower doses (1.0—10 ng/kg/min), and an arterial constriction only at the high dose of 80 ng/kg/min [8]. Based on these experiments a dose-reponse curve was constructed (Figure 1), showing a

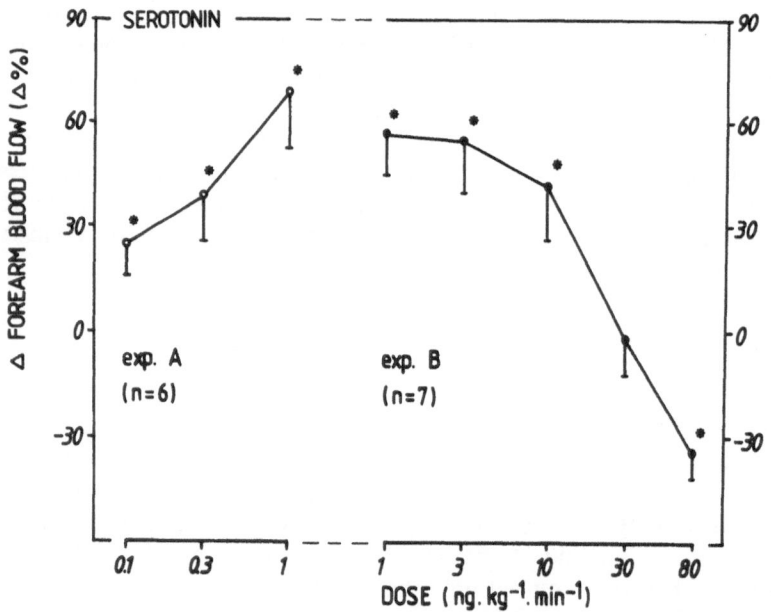

Figure 1. Mean percent changes in forearm blood flow (±SEM) induced by intra-arterial infusions of 5-HT. (From [8] with permission).

maximal dilatator response at the dose of 1 ng/kg/min. The *calculated* plasma levels of 5-HT during the infusions of the vasodilatator doses were 2—20 nM, which is in the range of the reported physiological levels of 5-HT [9]. At the highest dose of 80 ng/kg/min 5-HT elicited a vasoconstriction predominantly in the venous bed [10].

The abovementioned studies were performed in young healthy subjects. Since there is experimental evidence that the vascular responses to 5-HT are age-dependent [11, 12] it may well be that the results are different in older subjects. Therefore we also studied the arterial and venous vascular responses to 5-HT in the forearm of older healthy subjects (aged 50—69 years), but from this study no evidence was obtained that the vascular response to 5-HT is age-related in man [10]. In summary these results clearly demonstrate that 5-HT acts predominantly as a vasodilatator in the forearm of both young and older healthy subjects, and that very high ("pharmacological") doses are needed to induce vasoconstriction. The possible mechanisms underlying these complex vascular effects of 5-HT will be discussed below.

3. Interaction of 5-HT with other transmitters

From experiments performed in vitro and in laboratory animals evidence has been obtained that low doses of 5-HT amplify the constrictor reponses to other transmitters [13—15], suggesting that at low doses 5-HT would be able to increase vascular tone via an indirect mechanism. However, low vasodilatator doses of 5-HT (0.1 and 1 ng/kg/min) appeared not to amplify the constrictor responses to i.a. infused norepinephrine, tyramine, and angiotensine II [16]. These results are in accordance with previous findings by Scroop and Walsh [17], and raise doubt whether in vivo the amplifying effect of 5-HT is of any physiological importance in the regulation of vascular tone in a human vascular bed [17].

4. Demonstration of vascular 5-HT$_2$ receptors in humans

Since the introduction of ketanserin as a selective 5-HT$_2$ receptor antagonist [18], 5-HT$_2$ receptors have been identified in various types of smooth muscles, as well as on platelets and neurons [19]. In the vascular system 5-HT$_2$ receptors mediating vasoconstriction are mainly found in large conducting arteries and veins, but there is also evidence that they are present in the resistance vessels [18, 20, 21].

In isolated human saphenous vein preparations 5-HT evoked vascular constriction is, at least partly, mediated by 5-HT$_2$ receptor activation [22, 23]. Using the selective 5-HT$_2$ receptor antagonists ketanserin [18] and ritanserin [24] as pharmacological tools, in the vascular bed of the human forearm we have demonstrated in vivo that the 5-HT$_2$ receptor is involved in the vascular response to i.a. infused 5-HT. It was shown that both ketanserin and ritanserin reversed the arterial constriction induced by a high dose of 5-HT (80 ng/kg/min), thus providing evidence that the 5-HT induced arterial constriction is triggered by $5-HT_2$ receptor stimulation [8, 10]. Similar results were found for the 5-HT induced venoconstriction in the forearm, which could also be attenuated by ritanserin [10].

In other experiments the regional haemodynamic responses to ketanserin and ritanserin were studied. I.a. infusion of ketanserin in the human forearm elicited a dose-dependent vasodilatation, whereas ritanserin did not influence FBF (Table I). These results can be explained by the fact that ketanserin not only possesses affinity for $5-HT_2$ receptors but also for α_1-adrenoceptors [25], whereas ritanserin is devoid of α_1-adrenoceptor affinity [24]. Accordingly, ketanserin effectively antagonized the constrictor responses to the selective α_1-adrenoreceptor agonist methoxamine and the indirect sympathomimetic drug tyramine, whereas ritanserin did not influence the effect of methoxamine [8, 10]. The observation that ritanserin does not induce a dose-dependent vascular relaxation provides evidence that $5-HT_2$ receptors are not tonically active under basal conditions, and also raises serious doubts whether 5-HT is involved at all in maintaining peripheral basal vascular tone in man [8, 10, 16]. Moreover, such a role of 5-HT seems most unlikely because of the very low concentrations (~ 2 nM) of circulating plasma (free) 5-HT [9].

5. Vascular "$5-HT_1$-like" receptors

Since the nature of the $5-HT_1$ binding sites appears to be most heterogenous and because the functional correlates of these binding sites are still under investigation, it has been proposed to classify them tentatively as "$5-HT_1$-like" receptors [19].

Table 1. Percent change in forearm blood flow (FBF) induced by intra-arterial infusions of ketanserin and ritanserin.

Infusion (ng/kg/min)	ΔFBF $\pm$ SEM (%)	p	n
Ketanserin 5	8 $\pm$ 5	NS	13
Ketanserin 15	19 $\pm$ 4	<0.05	7
Ketanserin 50	46 $\pm$ 7	<0.01	13
Ketanserin 125	69 $\pm$ 9	<0.05	6
Ritanserin 5	1 $\pm$ 3	NS	6
Ritanserin 15	8 $\pm$ 6	NS	6
Ritanserin 50	11 $\pm$ 6	NS	12
Ritanserin 150	2 $\pm$ 2	NS	6
Ritanserin 500	7 $\pm$ 3	NS	6

In experiments performed with isolated blood vessels, it has been shown that 5-HT, like other neurohumoral transmitters, elicits relaxation of vascular smooth muscles in the presence of the intact endothelium, whereas a constrictor response was observed when the endothelium had been removed [26, 27]. Since this 5-HT induced endothelium dependent vasodilatation could not be attenuated by ketanserin, a "5-HT$_1$-like" receptor seems to be involved in mediating the release of an Endothelium Dependent Relaxant Factor (EDRF) by 5-HT [28]. At present, there is convincing evidence that EDRF plays an essential role in the vasodilatator response to numerous vasoactive agents, including those released from activated platelets like 5-HT, thrombin and ADP [27, 29, 30]. This has led to the concept that the intact endothelium protects the circulation against unwanted intraluminal platelet aggregation and vascular constriction by increasing blood flow [30]. The finding that in the forearm of healthy subjects i.a. infusions of low doses of 5-HT increased FBF [8] is in accordance with this hypothesis. However, so far there is no direct evidence that a "5-HT$_1$-like" receptor is involved in this dilatator response to 5-HT in man. Conversely, we have recently provided evidence that a 5-HT$_3$ receptor plays a role in the 5-HT induced biphasic vasodilatation [31] (see below).

Another mechanism by which low doses of 5-HT can induce vascular relaxation is the presynaptic inhibition of the release of norepinephrine from sympathetic nerve terminals [32, 33], but so far there is no direct evidence that this mechanism is present in humans. However, indirectly evidence has been provided that the vascular response to 5-HT occurs independently of the sympathetic nervous system [6], indicating that the presynaptic inhibitory effects of 5-HT, if present, is unlikely to be of physiological importance in man.

6. Evidence for the role of a 5-HT$_3$ receptor in the peripheral vascular response to 5-HT in humans

So far 5-HT$_3$ receptors are mainly identified on autonomic and sensory nerve fibers, evoking neuronal depolarization on activation [34]. From studies in the porcine carotid vascular bed evidence has been obtained that, in addition to a "5-HT$_1$-like" receptor, a 5-HT$_3$ receptor might be involved in the vasodilatator response to 5-HT [35]. Recently we have shown that in the human forearm the 5-HT induced biphasic vasodilatation could be abolished by concomitant infusion of the 5-HT$_3$ antagonist ICS 205—930, suggesting the involvement of a 5-HT$_3$ receptor (Figure 2). Since atropine had no effect on the dilatator response to 5-HT it could be excluded that release of acetylcholine from cholinergic nerve terminals was involved [31]. Based on the available evidence, it seems that the 5-HT$_3$ receptor is located on sensory neurons, evoking an axon-reflex [31].

I.a. infusions of ICS 205—930 did not influence FBF, indicating that the

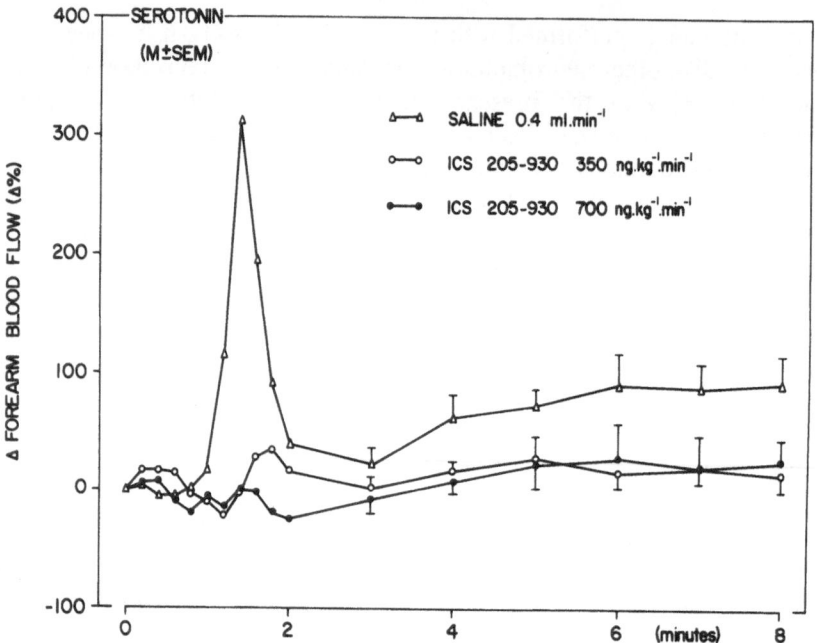

Figure 2. Mean percent changes in forearm blood flow ($\pm$ SEM) induced by simultaneous infusion of 5-HT 1 ng/kg/min with saline, and 5-HT with two doses of the selective 5-HT$_3$ antagonist ICS 205–930. (From [31] with permission).

5-HT$_3$ receptors are not tonically active under basal conditions [31]. Accordingly, experiments with MDL 72222 in humans [36] and pigs [35] did not influence the haemodynamic variables measured.

7. Conclusions: physiological role of 5-HT in the peripheral vascular system

The only relevant source of 5-HT in the peripheral vascular system are apparently the platelets, from which it is released during aggregation and it seems doubtful whether the plasma levels of free 5-HT present under physiological conditions have any influence on vascular tone. Our finding that blockade of vascular 5-HT$_2$ and 5-HT$_3$ receptors does not influence forearm blood flow in healthy volunteers supports this view.

An important role of 5-HT in the vascular system appears to be the facilitation of clotting and haemostasis at sites of blood vessel damage by inducing regional vasoconstriction and by inducing platelet aggregation [30, 37]. Both phenomena are mediated by 5-HT$_2$ receptor stimulation [19]. The finding that in man 5-HT$_2$ receptor mediated vasoconstriction is observed only at very high doses of 5-HT [8] supports the view that this occurs only at sites where 5-HT is liberated from activated platelets. The vascular relaxation induced by low doses of 5-HT in man, may reflect a biological defense mechanism against unwanted intraluminal platelet aggregation. There is convincing experimental evidence that the intact endothelium plays an important role in mediating this dilatator response to 5-HT. However so far there is no direct evidence that this is also the case in humans.

References

1. Page IH (1952): The vascular action of natural serotonin, 5- and 7-hydroxytryptamine and tryptamine. *J Pharmacol Exp Ther* 105: 58—73.
2. Page IH, McCubbin JW (1956): Arterial Response to infused serotonin in normotensive dogs, cats, hypertensive dogs and man. *Am J Physiol* 184: 265—270.
3. Roddie IC, Shepherd JT, Whelan RF (1955): The action of 5-hydroxtryptamine on the blood vessels of the human hand and forearm. *Brit J Pharmacol* 10: 445—450.
4. Bock KD, Dengler H, Kuhn HM, Matthes K (1957): Die wirkung von 5-hydroxytryptamin auf blutdruk, haut- und muskeldurchblutung des menschen. *Arch exper Path Pharmakol* 230: 257—273.
5. Glover WE, Marshall RJ, Whelan RF (1957): The antagonsim of the vascular effects of 5-hydroxytryptamine by BOL 148 and sodium salicylate in the human subject. *Brit J Pharmacol* 12: 498—503.
6. Walsh JA (1967): Antagonism by methysergide of vascular effects of 5-hydroxytryptamine in man. *Br J Pharmac Chemother* 30: 518—530.
7. Chang PC, Verlinde R, Bruning T, Van Brummelen P (1988): A microcomputer-based, R-wave triggered system for hemodynamic measurements in the forearm. *Comput Biol Med* 18: 157—163.
8. Blauw GJ, Van Brummelen P, Chang PC, Vermeij P, Van Zwieten PA (1988): Regional vascular effects of serotonin and ketanserin in young, healthy subjects. *Hypertension* 11: 256—263.
9. Anderson GM, Feibel FC, Cohen DJ (1987): Determination of serotonin in whole blood, platelet-rich plasma, platelet-poor plasma and plasma ultrafiltrate. *Life Sci* 40: 1063—1070.
10. Blauw GJ, Van Brummelen P, Chang PC, Vermeij P, Van Zwieten PA (1988): The arterial and venous effects of serotonin in the forearm of healthy subjects is not age-related. *J Cardivasc Pharmacol* 36 (suppl. 1): 74—77.
11. Cohen ML, Berkowitz BA (1976): Vascular contraction: Effect of age and extracellular calcium. *Blood Vessels* 13: 139—154.
12. De Mey C, Vanhoutte PM (1981): Effect of age and spontaneous hypertension on the tachyphylaxis to 5-hydroxytryptamine and angiotensin II in the isolated rat kidney. *Hypertension* 3: 718—724.
13. De La Lande IS, Cannel VA, Waterson JG (1966): The interaction of serotonin and noradrenaline on the perfused artery. *Br J Pharmac Chemother* 28: 255—272.
14. Van Nueten JM, Janssen PAJ, De Ridder W, Vanhoutte PM (1982): Interaction between 5-hydroxytryptamine and other vasoconstrictor substances in the isolated femoral artery of the rabbit; effect of ketanserin (R 41—468). *Eur J Pharmacol* 77: 281—287.
15. Lüscher TF, Vanhoutte PM (1988): Are there interactions between S_2-serotonergic and α_1-adrenergic receptors in isolated canine arteries? *J Cardiovasc Pharmacol* 11 (suppl 1): S16—S21.
16. Blauw GJ, Van Brummelen P, Chang PC, Vermeij P, Van Zwieten PA (1988): Direct and indirect vascular effects of serotonin in man [abstract]. *Br J clin Pharmac* 25: 629P—630P.

17. Scroop GC, Walsh JA (1968): Interactions between angiotensin, noradrenaline and serotonin on peripheral blood vessels in man. *Aust J exp Biol med Sci* 46: 573—580.

18. Van Nueten JM, Leysen JE, Van Beek J, Xhonneux R, Verbeuren TJ, Vanhoutte PM (1981): Vascular effects of ketanserin (R 41 468), a novel antagonist of 5-HT$_2$ serotonergic receptors. *J Pharmacol Exp Ther* 218: 217—230.

19. Bradley PB, Engel G, Feniuk W, Fozard JR, Humphrey PPA, Middlemiss DN, Mylecharane EJ, Ridchardson BP, Saxena PR (1986): Proposals for the classification and nomenclature of functional receptors for 5-hydroxytryptamine. *Neuropharmacol* 1986; 25: 563—576.

20. Saxena PR, Verdouw PD (1982): Redistribution by 5-hydroxytryptamine of carotid arterial blood at the expense of arteriovenous anastomotic blood flow. *J Physiol* 332: 501—520.

21. Reneman RS, Bollinger A (1986): Vascular and microvascular effects of serotonin. Some conclusive remarks. *Prog appl Microcirc* 10: 83—86.

22. Müller-Schweinitzer E (1984): Alpha-adrenoceptors, 5-hydroxytryptamine receptors and the action of dihydroergotamine in human venous preparations obtained during saphenectomy procedures for varicose veins. *Naunyn-Schmiedeberg's Arch Pharmacol* 327: 299—303.

23. Docherty JR, Hyland L (1986): An examination of 5-hydroxytryptamine receptors in human saphenous vein. *Br J Pharmac* 89: 77—81.

24. Leysen JE, Gommeren W, Van Gompel P, Janssen PFM, Laduron PM (1985): Receptor binding properties in vitro and in vivo of ritanserin. A very potent and long acting serotonin-S$_2$ antagonist. *Mol Pharmacol* 27: 600—611.

25. Kalkman HO, Timmermans PBMWM, Van Zwieten PA (1982): Characterization of the antihypertensive properties of ketanserin (R 41 468) in rats. *J Pharmacol Exp Ther* 222: 227—231.

26. Cocks TM, Angus JA (1983): Endothelium-dependent relaxation of coronary arteries by noradrenaline and serotonin. *Nature* 305: 627—630.

27. Peach MJ, Loeb AL, Singer HA, Saye J (1985): Endothelium-derived relaxing factor. *Hypertension* 7 (suppl I): I94—I100.

28. Cohen RA, Vanhoutte PM (1985): Platelets, serotonin, and endothelial cells, p. 105—112 in: Vanhoutte PM (ed), *Serotonin and the cardiovascular system*. New York: Raven Press.

29. Furchott RF, Jothianandan D, Cherry PD (1984): Endothelium-dependent responses: The last three years. *Biblthca cardiol* 38: 1—15.

30. Lüscher TF, Vanhoutte PM (1988): Endothelium-dependent reponses in human blood vessels. *Trends Pharmacol Sci* 9: 181—184.

31. Blauw GJ, Van Brummelen P, Van Zwieten PA (1988): Serotonin induced vasodilatation in the human forearm is antagonized by the selective 5-HT$_3$ receptor antagonist ICS 205—930. *Life Sci* 43: 1441—1449.

32. McGrath MA (1977): 5-Hydroxytryptamine and neurotransmitter release in canine blood vessels: inhibition by low and augmentation by concentrations. *Circ Res* 41: 428—435.

33. Engel G, Göthert M, Müller-Schweinitzer E, Schlicker E, Sistonen L, Stadler PA (1983): Evidence for common pharmacological properties of [^{3}H]5-hydroxytryptamine binding sites, presynaptic 5-hydroxyptamine autoreceptors in CNS and inhibitory 5-hydroxtryptamine receptors on sympathetic nerves. *Naunyn-Schmiedeberg's Arch Pharmacol* 324: 116—142.

34. Fozard JR (1984): Neuronal 5-HT receptors in the periphery. *Neuropharmacol* 23: 1473—1486.

35. Saxena PR, Duncker DJ, Bom AH, Heiligers J, Verdouw PD (1986): Effects of MDL 72222 and methiothepin on carotid vascular responses to 5-hydroxytryptamine in the pig: Evidence for the presence of "5-hydroxytryptamine$_1$-like" receptors. *Naunyn-Schmiedeberg's Arch Pharmacol* 333: 198—204.

36. Orwin JM, Fozard JR (1986): Blockade of the flare response to intradermal 5-hydroxy-

tryptamine in man by MDL 72.222, a selective antagonist at neuronal 5-hydroxytrypta-mine receptors. *Eur J Pharmacol* 30: 209—212.
37. Houston DS, Vanhoutte PM (1986): Serotonin and the vascular system. Role in health and disease, and implications for therapy. *Drugs* 31: 149—163.

XXXV. Ketanserin in the treatment of septic shock

AREND J. J. WOITTIEZ, JOT WOLTHUIS and LEO VAN BERGEIJK

1. Introduction

Septic shock is characterized by high output failure, systemic hypotension and decreased peripheral perfusion, eventually leading to multiple organ failure and death. The acute respiratory failure following septic shock is accompanied by pulmonary hypertension, bronchoconstriction and an increase in pulmonary shunt fraction. Serotonin, released from entrapped platelets, could be one of the mediators, involved in the cascade, leading to organ failure [1]. To study this role of serotonin, we administered ketanserin to patients with septic shock.

2. Patients and methods

Eleven patients, 5 male and 6 female, 56 ± 6 year (mean ± SEM) old, were enrolled in the study, after confirming the diagnosis of septic shock. Septic shock was defined according to the following criteria: (1) mean arterial pressure < 80 mmHg, (2) oliguria < 0.5 ml/kg/min, (3) leucocytosis > $15 \times 10^9/l$, (4), hypo-or hyperthermia, (5) no signs of heart failure; that is pulmonary capillary wedge pressure < 15 mmHg (Swan Ganz catheter), (6) delta T (core temperature minus skin temperature) > 7 °C and (7) a positive blood culture or a proven infective focus.

Four patients suffered from pneumonia, 3 from pancreatitis, 3 from peritonitis and 1 patient from endocarditis.

Routine support was given by means of antibiotics, mechanical ventilation (n = 9), fluid challenge guided by arterial pressure (intra-arterial) and ventricular filling pressures (Swan Ganz catheter) and by dopamine infusion (5–10 μg/kg/min). After stabilizing the patients, ketanserin (10 mg, i.v.) was injected and the effects on systemic arterial pressure, heart rate, pulmonary arterial pressure, right atrial pressure, pulmonary capillary wedge pressure, cardiac output (thermodilution method), diuresis and temperature were

P.R. Saxena, D.I. Wallis, W. Wouters and P. Bevan (eds), Cardiovascular Pharmacology of 5-Hydroxytryptamine, pp. 401–404.
© 1990 *Kluwer Academic Publishers, Dordrecht* –

followed for 2 hours. In 6 patients we registered the effects of ketanserin infusion (2mg/hr) for another 6 hours.

Total peripheral resistance, pulmonary vasculair resistance and pulmonary shunt fraction (Qs/Qt) were calculated according to well known formulas, using a bed-side computer [2].

3. Results

Ketanserin decreased arterial pressure with 8 mmHg 30 minutes after injection ($p < 0.05$). After 2 and after 8 hours blood pressure returned to baseline level (Figure 1). Heart rate decreased and remained below baseline level. Cardiac output and total peripheral resistance did not change consistently.

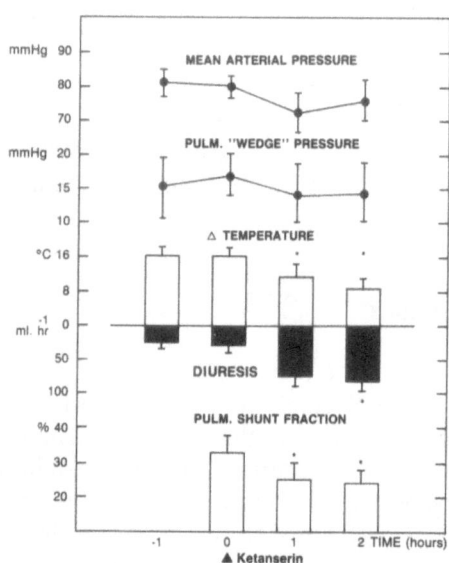

Figure 1. The effects of ketanserin (10 mg i.v.) on several parameters, as measured in septic shock patients.

Pulmonal artery pressure fell in the first hour due to a decrease in pulmonary vascular resistance, whereas cardiac filling pressures did not change (Figure 2).

The peripheral temperature was increased after two hours, while the central temperature did not change; thus the delta T decreased to 11.0 ± 2.3 °C. This effect was maintained also after infusion, delta T further decreased to 9.3 ± 1.8 °C after 8 hours.

A similar pattern could be demonstrated for the diuresis. (Figure 1). The

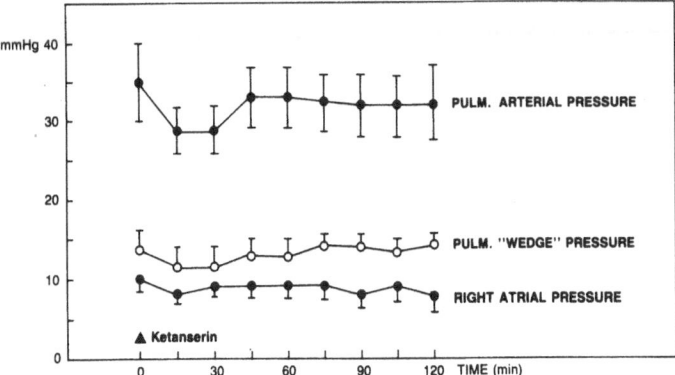

Figure 2. The effects of ketanserin (10 mg i.v.) on the central pressures in 11 patients with septic shock.

decrease in pulmonary artery pressure was followed by a fall in pulmonary shunt fraction from $33 \pm 5\%$ to $24 \pm 4\%$ after 2 and 8 hours ($p < 0.05$).

4. Discussion

Our data demonstrate that ketanserin has favourable effects in patients suffering from septic shock. Ketanserin caused no sharp fall in the systemic arterial pressure; so it can be given safely to patients with lowered blood pressure c.q. patients in shock. Perhaps a more pronounced hypotensive effect was counteracted by fluid repletion and inotropic support by dopamine, though the decrease in heart rate suggest only a moderate effect on the heamodynamics.

In contrast with other vasodilators ketanserin does not increase pulmonary shunt fraction, moreover a distinct decrease could be demonstrated. This is in agreement with earlier reports [3]. Though we did not examine the mechanism, it is likely that ketanserin decreases shunting by a combined pulmonary vasodilatation and bronchodilatation, without altering ventilation-perfusion relationships [4].

Despite stable blood pressures and central pressures ketanserin increased the urinary flow. Renal vasodilatation could be a plausible explanation, though direct tubular effects cannot be ruled out [5]. The rise in skin temperature supports the view that ketanserin may restore peripheral perfusion.

5. Conclusions

Administration of ketanserin in patients with septic shock may have favourable effects, in terms of restoring peripheral perfusion (in skin and kidney) and decreasing pulmonary shunt fraction, without detremental influence on blood pressure.

References

1. Sibbald W, Peters S, Lindsay RM (1980): Serotonin and pulmonary hypertension in human septic ARDS. *Crit Care Med* 8: 490—494.
2. Schoemaker W (1987): Relation of oxygen transport patterns to the pathophysiology and therapy of shock states. *Int Care Med* 13: 230—244.
3. Huval WV, Lelcuk S, Shepro D, Hechtman HB (1984): Role of serotonin in patients with acute respiratory failure. *Ann Surg* 200: 166—172.
4. Radermacher P, Huet Y, Pluskwa F, Herigault R, Mal H, Teisseire B, Lemaire F (1988): Comparison of ketanserin and sodium nitroprusside in patients with severe ARDS. *Anesthesiology* 68: 152—157.
5. Wenting GJ, Man in 't Veld AJ, Woittiez AJJ, Boomsma F, Schalekamp MADH (1982): Treatment of hypertension with ketanserin, a new selective 5-HT$_2$ receptor antagonist. *Br Med J* 284: 537—539.

Migraine

XXXVI. 5-Hydroxytryptamine and migraine

PRAMOD R. SAXENA

1. Introduction

Migraine is regarded as an episodic syndrome characterised by usually unilateral headache, nausea, vomiting and photophobia, sometimes preceded by certain premonitory aura symptoms. Despite a large number of investigations over the years, the multifactorial pathogenesis of migraine still remains ill understood. However, amongst a host of biogenic substances implicated in the pathophysiology of migraine, none seems to have a better claim than 5-hydroxytryptamine (5-HT) [1—6].

2. Endogenous 5-HT in migraine

2.1 Urinary excretion of 5-hydroxyindole acetic acid (5-HIAA)

Sicuteri's group provided the first link between 5-HT and migraine by reporting that the urinary execretion of 5-HIAA, the main metabolite of 5-HT, increases during migraine attacks [7]. These findings were confirmed by others, but such changes are observed in only about 50% of patients [2, 8, 9].

2.2 Platelet, whole blood and plasma 5-HT

Curran et al. [8] and, subsequently, many others (for references, see Anthony [2]) showed that both platelet 5-HT (control values usually around 3—4 nmol/10^6 platelets) and whole blood 5-HT (control values between 500 and 1200 nM) decrease during migraine attacks by 15 to 40%. This decrease is preceded by a transient rise. Experiments involving cross incubation of platelets and plasma obtained during migraine attacks and in headache-free periods point to the appearance of a 5-HT-releasing factor, the nature of

P.R. Saxena, D.I. Wallis, W. Wouters and P. Bevan (eds), Cardiovascular Pharmacology of 5-Hydroxytryptamine, pp. 407—416.
© 1990 *Kluwer Academic Publishers, Dordrecht —*

which has still to be properly elucidated [1, 2]. Recently, Ferrari et al. [10] have found that reduction in platelet 5-HT during attacks is noticed in common migraine (migraine without aura) but not in classic migraine (migraine with aura) patients.

The concentration of 5-HT in platelet-poor plasma has been reported to either decrease [11] or increase [10] during migraine attacks. Ferrari et al. [10] have found that the basal levels (headache-free period) of plasma 5-HT in both classic (13.1 nM) and common (12.2 nM) migraine patients are less than in healthy volunteers (30.1 nM) and suggested that the turnover of 5-HT may be enhanced between migraine attacks. It must, however, be pointed out that less than 1% of blood 5-HT is present in platelet-poor plasma and, therefore, plasma 5-HT concentration can be affected by platelet behaviour during the separation process.

2.3 *Influence of reserpine, fenfluramine and zimelidine*

Intramuscular injections of reserpine precipitate migraine-like headaches within 4–6 hours in migraine patients. These headaches, as well as spontaneous migraine headaches, can be relieved by intravenous administration of 5-HT [1, 12]. Fenfluramine, another drug which releases 5-HT, can also trigger headaches in migraineurs [13]. Similar observations have been made with the selective 5-HT uptake-blocker, zimelidine. However, with continued use of zimelidine the frequency of migraine attacks decreases, presumably due to an increase in plasma 5-HT concentration [14].

2.4 *5-HT release or depletion more important?*

The above findings strongly implicate that 5-HT is involved in the pathophysiology of migraine, though one may still argue whether it is the release or depletion of endogenous 5-HT that is actually responsible. In almost all investigations dealing with the measurements of 5-HT in migraine, the comparisons have been made between single values obtained at a certain time during attack-free and headache periods; it would have been far better, though very much more difficult, to perform serial measurements at shorter intervals. Despite this shortcoming, the beneficial effects of 5-HT, zimelidine (chronic use) and methysergide (a partial agonist at 5-HT receptors) and the poor effectiveness of 5-HT receptor antagonists, e.g. cyproheptadine, ketanserin and ICS 205-930, in migraine (see below), together with a lack of any marked increase in the incidence of migraine in carcinoid patients [15], do suggest that, at least in some patients, migraine may be considered as a 'low 5-HT syndrome' following depletion of endogenous 5-HT. However, it remains possible that 5-HT in the blood may be less important than that at neurovascular terminals [16—18].

3. Pharmacology and physiology of 5-HT in relation to migraine

3.1 *5-HT receptors*

The functional responses to 5-HT are mediated by three main receptor types — 5-HT$_1$-like (agonist: 5-carboxamidotryptamine; antagonist: methiothepin), 5-HT$_2$ (agonist: α-methyl-5-HT; antagonist: ketanserin) and 5-HT$_3$ (agonist: 2-methyl-5-HT; antagonist: MDL 72222) [19, 20]. Only 5-HT$_2$ and 5-HT$_3$ receptors have so far been well characterised using selective antagonists. No such compound is yet available for 5-HT$_1$-like receptors; methiothepin also blocks 5-HT$_2$ receptors. The 5-HT$_1$-like receptors, having a nanomolar affinity for 5-HT, are heterogeneous in nature but the exact association with the 5-HT$_1$ binding site subtypes is still unclear (Table 1 [21]).

3.2 *Central and peripheral neuronal effects of 5-HT*

5-HT seems to be involved in the transmission of pain sensation. The nociceptive afferents synapse with dorsal horn cells, and spinothalamic projection fibres synapse in the periaquaductal gray region of the spinal cord. The pain transmission from nociceptive afferents can be inhibited by serotonergic fibres descending from the nucleus raphe magnus [6]. Since this inhibitory response is not blocked by 5-HT$_2$ receptor antagonists, Richardson et al. [3] suggested that this receptor could be 5-HT$_1$-like in nature. Further, it is postulated that 5-HT$_3$ receptors serve as 'transducers' for painful stimuli originating from blood vessels (for example, due to putative changes in the activity of raphe neurons) and the resulting peripheral nociceptive input is then transmitted via afferent fibres to the dorsal horn cells [3, 6, 22]. However, there is no solid evidence yet that antimigraine drugs interfere with central nociceptive transmission and, except perhaps MDL 72222 [22, 23], the other 5-HT$_3$ receptor antagonists have not been found effective in migraine therapy (see below).

3.3 *Cephalovascular effects of 5-HT*

Isolated cerebral and extracerebral cephalic vessels usually contract in response to 5-HT. The 5-HT-induced contraction of large 'conducting' arteries is often mediated via 5-HT$_2$ receptors, but in several cephalic vessels 5-HT$_1$-like receptors, seemingly unrelated to the subtypes of 5-HT$_1$ binding sites described so far (Table 1), are involved in addition to or in place of 5-HT$_2$ receptors [21, 24—26].

In vivo, 5-HT redistributes carotid arterial blood flow (which remains either unchanged or decreases) in favour of extracerebral cephalic tissues (particularly the skin and ears) at the expense of the fraction shunted via

Table 1. Putative subtypes of 5-HT$_1$-like receptors.

Receptor subtype	Agonists	Antagonists	Binding site	Second messenger	Functional responses
5-HT$_{1A}$	5-CT, 8-OH-DPAT, 5-HT, RU 24969	Cyanopindolol, Methysergide[a], Methiothepin[a]	5-HT$_{1A}$	AC, K$^+$-channel, PI	Behavioral changes, centrally evoked hypotensive response.
5-HT$_{1B}$	RU 24969, 5-CT, 5-HT	Cyanopindolol, Methiothepin, Methysergide	5-HT$_{1B}$	Negative coupling to AC	Autorceptor in the rat brain.
5-HT$_{1C}$[b]	5-HT	Mesulergine, Methiothepin, Methysergide	5-HT$_{1C}$	PIte-specific PLA-C	Not yet convincingly demonstrated.
5-HT$_{1D}$	5-CT, 5-HT	Methiothepin	5-HT$_{1D}$	Negative coupling to AC	Not yet convincingly demonstrated.
5-HT$_{1x}$[c]	5-CT, 5-HT, AH25086[d], GR43175, 8-OH-DPAT, RU 24969	Methiothepin, Methysergide[e]	Not yet found[f]	Not yet known	Contraction of cephalic arteries (basilar, pial) and arteriovenous anastomoses in the carotid region, decrease of neuronal noradrenaline release.
5-HT$_{1y}$[c]	5-CT, 5-HT	Methiothepin, Methysergide	Not yet found[f]	Not yet known	Vascular smooth muscle relaxation, hypotension, tachycardia in the cat.

[a], Non-selective antagonist (also blocks 5-HT$_2$ receptors); [b], Shows little difference from the 5-HT$_2$ receptor; [c], The receptor subtype is as yet unnamed and this name has been put for convenience here to distinguish between the two unnamed 5-HT$_1$-like receptors; [d], Ligand binding profile is not yet reported; [e], Partial agonist; [f], Does not correlate with 5-HT$_{1A}$, 5-HT$_{1B}$, 5-HT$_{1C}$ or 5-HT$_{1D}$ binding sites. AC, adenyl cyclase; AH25086, 3-aminoethyl-N-methyl-1H-indole-5-methane carboxamide; 5-CT, 5-Carboxamido-tryptamine; GR43175, 3-[2-dimethylamino]ethyl-N-methyl-1H-indole-5-methane sulphonamide; 8-OH-DPAT, 8-hydroxy-2-(di-n-propylamino) tetralin; PI, phosphatidylinositol; PIte, phosphoinositide; PLA-C, phospholipase C; RU 24969, 5-methoxy-3(1,2,3,6-tetrahydropyridin-4-yl) 1H indole. From Saxena and Ferrari [21].

cephalic arteriovenous anastomoses [27]. These effects of 5-HT, being mimicked by 5-carboxamidotryptamine and blocked by methiothepin but not by ketanserin, are mediated by 5-HT$_1$-like receptors (Table 2 [26]). Table 2 further shows that some agonists (methysergide, BEA 1654, 8-OH-DPAT, GR43175) constrict arteriovenous anastomoses without eliciting much arteriolar vasodilatation, suggesting that the 5-HT$_1$-like receptors on arteriovenous anastomoses (5-HT$_{1x}$ subtype of 5-HT$_1$-like receptors) and arterioles (5-HT$_{1y}$ subtype of 5-HT$_1$-like receptors) are heterogeneous (Table 1). The constriction of arteriovenous anastomoses by 8-OH-DPAT tempts one to classify the 5-HT$_1$-like receptors on arteriovenous anastomoses as belonging

Table 2. 5-HT receptors and drug effect on arterioles and arteriovenous anastomoses (AVAs) in the porcine carotid artery bed.

Drug	Arterioles	AVAs	Antagonism by	Resistance to	Receptor type
5-HT	ᐨᐨᐨᐨ	++++	Methiothepin	Cyproheptadine, Ketanserin, WAL 1307, MDL 72222	$5\text{-}HT_1$-like
5-CT	ᐨᐨᐨᐨ	++++		Cyproheptadine	$5\text{-}HT_1$-like
Methysergide	−	+++			$5\text{-}HT_1$-like
BEA 1654	−−	+++		Ketanserin	$5\text{-}HT_1$-like
GR43175[a]	0	++++			$5\text{-}HT_1$-like
AH25086[a]	0	++++			$5\text{-}HT_1$-like
8-OH-DPAT	−	++++	Methiothepin	Ketanserin	$5\text{-}HT_1$-like
Ipsapirone	0	0			
Ergotamine	0	++++		Methiothepin	Not known

−, dilatation, +, contraction; 0, no or little effect. The number of − and + indicate the magnitude of effect. [a], Data in the cat. Based on Saxena et al. [26].

to the $5\text{-}HT_{1A}$ subtype, but ipsapirone, which also exhibits high affinity for $5\text{-}HT_{1A}$ recognition sites, proved inactive [28]. Lastly, it may be noted that the effect of ergotamine on arteriovenous anastomoses, being unaffected by methiothepin, is mediated by neither $5\text{-}HT_1$-like nor $5\text{-}HT_2$ receptors [29].

The cephalovascular pharmacology of 5-HT − constriction of large extracerebral arteries and arteriovenous anastomoses and dilatation of arterioles − may suggest a role for 5-HT in the distribution of arterial blood flow. There is evidence for the presence of 5-HT neurons and/or co-localization of 5-HT in some cephalovascular sympathetic neurons [18] and plasma 5-HT concentrations may reach values as high as 300 nM [26]. Thus, following a decrease in endogenous 5-HT activity during migraine attacks (see above), large arteries and arteriovenous anastomoses may dilate excessively (see below).

4. Vascular changes in migraine

There can be no doubt that migraine is associated with changes in cephalic (cerebral and non-cerebral) circulation; the doubts, however, concern the cause and nature of such changes. In a majority of migraine patients with 'aura', cerebral blood flow decreases but in 'classical' migraine patients both decreases and increases in cerebral blood flow have been reported [30, 31]. In the non-cerebral cephalic circulation (scalp and dura), vasodilatation and increased pulsations are observed principally on the side of migraine head-ache [30, 32], but the idea of simple arteriolar vasodilatation is paradoxical to the facial pallor and laxity of tissues usually noticed during headache. To resolve this paradox Heyck [33] suggested that arterial blood is directly shunted to the venous side due to dilatation of cephalic arteriovenous anastomoses present in the skin (cheeks, lips, forehead, nose and ears), nasal mucosa, eyes and dura mater [5, 34, 35].

5. 5-HT receptor profile of antimigraine drugs

The 5-HT receptor profile of a number of new and established antimigraine drugs is presented in Table 3 [36]. With respect to 5-HT_1-like receptors, it is obvious that selective agonists at the 5-HT_{1x} subtype mediating contractions of extracerebral cephalic arteries and arteriovenous anastomoses are effective in the treatment of acute migraine attacks (AH25086 and GR43175) [37–39]. These drugs do not penetrate into the central nervous system and, therefore, it seems likely that the site of antimigraine action is extracerebral cephalic vasculature. The same appears to be true for ergotamine though the drug fails to stimulate 5-HT_1-like receptors [29]. Since, in addition, ergotamine (oral bioavailability 5%) does not readily penetrate into the central nervous system [40], it is doubtful that its antimigraine action is due to stimulation of putative spinal 5-HT_1-like receptors interfering with pain transmission via primary nociceptive afferents [3, 6].

Some antimigraine drugs are 5-HT_2 receptor antagonists (methysergide, pizotifen), but several other antagonists at 5-HT_2 and/or 5-HT_1-like recep-

Table 3. Profile of potential and proven antimigraine drugs in relation to 5-HT_1-like receptors.

Antimigraine Drug	5-HT_1-like Receptor	5-HT_2 Receptor	5-HT_3 Receptor	Penetration into the CNS
AH25086	Agonist[a]	Inactive	Inactive	Poor or none
GR43175	Agonist[a]	Inactive	Inactive	Poor or none
Methysergide	Partial[a,b]	Antagonist[c]	Inactive	Possibly yes
Ergotamine	Inactive	Antagonist	Inactive	Poor or none
Dihydroergotamine	?	Antagonist	Inactive	?
Pizotifen	Inactive	Antagonist	Inactive	Possibly yes
Propranolol	Antagonist[d]	Inactive	Inactive	Rapid
MDL 72222	Inactive	Inactive	Antagonist[e]	?

CNS, Central nervous system; [a], Partial agonist action is selective on 5-HT_1-like receptors mediating the contraction of cephalic arteries and arteriovenous anastomoses; [b], Antagonists of 5-HT_1-like receptors (methiothepin, metergoline) have no antimigraine activity; [c], Many other 5-HT_2 antagonists (ketanserin, ritanserin, cyproheptadine) have not proved very effective in migraine therapy; [d], Weak antagonism; other antimigraine β-adrenoceptor antagonists (atenolol, timolol) have little affinity for 5-HT_1-like receptors; [e], ICS 205-930 and probably some other antagonists at 5-HT_3 receptors are not very effective in migraine. From Saxena [36].

tors (ketanserin, ritanserin, cyproheptadine, mianserin, methiothepin, meter-goline) are not known to be particularly effective in migraine therapy. Therefore, it appears that the constriction of extracerebral cephalic (dural and scalp) vessels by methysergide (partial agonism at 5-HT_1-like receptors) and the antidepressant action by pizotifen are more important than the 5-HT_2 receptor antagonism for their therapeutic action in migraine.

The idea that 5-HT_3 receptors play a crucial role in pain transduction in migraine by depolarizing nociceptive primary afferents on cephalic vessels was advocated by Fozard [21]. This suggestion seemed to be initially supported by the effectiveness of a 5-HT_3 receptor antagonist, MDL 72222, in aborting acute migraine attacks [21, 22]. However, another 5-HT_3 receptor antagonist, ICS 205-930, has proved ineffective in the treatment of acute migraine attacks [41]. Moreover, several newer 5-HT_3 receptor antagonists have been in clinical trial for sometime [4], but none of them has so far been reported of value in migraine.

6. Concluding remarks

Migraine attacks are associated with increased urinary excretion of 5-HIAA and there is a decrease, following an initial rise, in platelet and whole blood 5-HT during migraine attacks. This decrease in platelet 5-HT may be due to a 5-HT-releasing factor, the nature of which has still to be properly elucidated. Furthermore, intramuscular injections of reserpine precipitate migraine-like symptoms in migraine patients and intravenous administration of 5-HT relieves reserpine-induced and spontaneous headaches. These observations suggest that, at least in some patients, migraine headache may be considered as a 'low 5-HT syndrome'.

The craniovascular effects of 5-HT include constriction of large arteries (via 5-HT_2 receptors), dilatation of arterioles and closure of arteriovenous anastomoses (both via 5-HT_1-like receptors). Therefore, a reduction of blood 5-HT (particularly in view of a nanomolar affinity of 5-HT for 5-HT_1-like receptors) and/or neurovascular 5-HT activity may result in a combination of arterial dilatation, arteriolar constriction and an opening of arteriovenous anastomoses. Indeed, several drugs effective against acute migraine attacks, including ergotamine and selective 5-HT_1 agonists, constrict cephalic arteries and arteriovenous anastomoses.

The clinical effectiveness of the recently described 5-HT_1-like agonists (AH25086 and GR43175) against the headache, as well as the nausea, vomiting and photophobia during acute migraine attacks, and the selectivity of their pharmacological effects (constriction of the cephalic arteries and arteriovenous anastomoses, lack of penetration into the CNS, and the absence of antinociceptive effects, even after intrathecal administration) strongly suggest that one of the essential features of the headache phase of migraine is dilatation in the extracerebral cranial (dural and scalp) vasculature. This, in turn, can stimulate perivascular sensory afferents of the fifth cranial nerve to cause headache and, possibly, nausea, vomiting and photophobia via putative neurons to the chemoreceptor trigger zone and hypothalamus. Neurogenic inflammation via retrograde release of vasoactive neuropeptides as well as local ischaemia due to arteriovenous shunting may accentuate pain sensation (Figure 1).

Lastly, the analysis of the effects of antimigraine drugs on 5-HT receptors supports the view that, within the bounds of serotonergic mechanisms, antimigraine activity mainly depends upon agonism at the $5\text{-}HT_1$-like receptor subtype that mediates cephalovascular contraction. The antagonism at $5\text{-}HT_2$ or $5\text{-}HT_3$ receptors does not seem to be essential for antimigraine action.

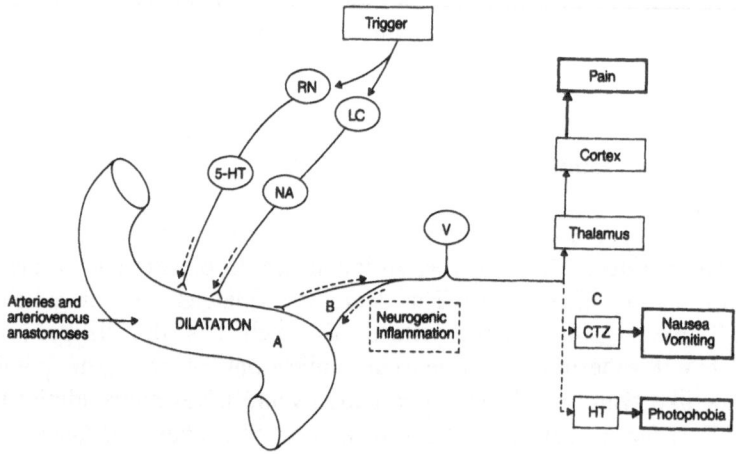

Figure 1. Putative sites of action of $5\text{-}HT_1$-like agonists in migraine (A—C). Changes in the activity of raphe nuclei (RN), with their 5-HT containing neurons and the locus ceruleus (LC), with its noradrenaline (NA) containing efferents, might induce dilatation of arteries and arteriovenous anastomoses in cephalic (dural and scalp) circulation. This, in turn, can stimulate perivascular sensory afferents of the fifth cranial nerve (V) to cause headache and, possibly, nausea, vomiting and photophobia via putative neurons to the chemoreceptor trigger zone (CTZ) and hypothalamus (HT). In addition, neurogenic inflammation via retrograde release of vasoactive neuropeptides, as well as local ischaemia due to arteriovenous shunting, may accentuate pain sensation. GR43175 and some other antimigraine drugs appear to abort migraine attacks by constricting the dilated cephalic vessels (A). Though it remains to be demonstrated, GR43175 may also have inhibitory influence at the perivascular nerve terminals (B) and CTZ (C), which is outside the blood brain barrier. From Saxena and Ferrari [21].

References

1. Lance JW (1982): *Mechanism and management of headache.* London: Butterworth.
2. Anthony M (1987): Amine metabolism in migraine, pp. 303—329 in: Blau JN (ed), *Migraine, Clinical, therapeutic, conceptual and research aspects.* London: Chapman & Hall.

3. Richardson BP, Engel G, Buchheit K-H, Hoyer D, Kalkman H, Markstein R, Thomson C (1986): Defective serotonergic transmission: A possible cause of migraine and a basis for the efficacy of ergot compounds in the treatment of attacks, pp. 9—21 in: Lance JW (ed), *Recent trends in the management of migraine.* Aulendorf: Editio Cantor.

4. Fozard JR (1987): 5-HT: the enigma variations. *Trends Pharmacol Sci* 8: 501—506.

5. Saxena PR (1987): The arteriovenous anastomoses and veins in migraine research, pp. 581—596 in: Blau JN (ed), *Migraine — Therapeutic, Conceptual and Research Aspects.* Amsterdam: Elsevier.

6. Raskin NH (1988): Headache, 2nd Ed., New York: Churchill Livingstone.

7. Sicuteri F, Testi H, Anselmi B (1961): Biochemical investigations in headache: Increase in hydroxyindoleacetic acid excretion during migraine. *Int. Arch Allergy* 19: 55—58.

8. Curran DA, Hinterberger H, Lance JW (1965): Total plams serotonin, 5-hydroxyindole-acetic acid and p-hydroxy-m-methoxy-mandelic acid excretion in normal and migrainous subjects. *Brain* 88: 997—1010.

9. Curzon G, Theaker P, Phillips B (1966): Excretion of 5-hydroxyindoleacetic acid (5-HIAA) in migraine. *J Neurol Neurosurg Psychiatry* 32: 85—90.

10. Ferrari MD, Odink J, Tapparelli C, Van Kempen MJ, Pennings EJM, Bruyn GW (1989): Serotonin metabolism in migraine. *Neurology* 39: 1239—1242.

11. Somerville BW (1965): Platelet-bound and free serotonin levels in jugular and forearm venous blood during migraine. *Neurology* 26: 41—45.

12. Tandon RN, Sur BK, Nath K (1969): Effect of reserpine injections in migrainous and normal control subjects, with estimations of urinary 5-hydroxyindole acetic acid. *Neurology* 19: 1073—1079.

13. Del Bene E, Anselmi B, Del Bianco PL, Fanciullacci M, Galli P, Salmon S, Sicuteri F (1977): Fenfluramine headache: a biochemical and monoamine receptorial human study, pp. 101—109 in: Sicuteri F (ed), *Headache: New Vistas.* Florence: Biomedical press.

14. Syvalahti E, Kangasniemi P, Ross B (1979): Migraine headache and blood serotonin levels after administration of zimelidine, a selective inhibitor of serotonin uptake. *Curr ther Res* 25: 299—310.

15. MacDonald RA (1956): A study of 356 carcinoids of the gastrointestinal tract. A report of four new cases of the carcinoid syndrome. *Am J Med* 21: 867—878.

16. Edvinsson L, denguerce A, Duverger D, MacKenzie ET, Scatton B (1983): Central serotonergic nerves project to the pial vessels of the brain. *Nature* 306: 55—57.

17. Dhall U, Cowan T, Haven AJ, Burnstock G (1988): Effect of oestrogen and progesterone on noradrenergic nerves and on nerves showing serotonin-like immunoreactivity in the basilar artery of the rabbit. *Brain Res* 422: 335—339.

18. Owman C, Chang J-Y, Hardebo JE (1989): Presence of serotonin in adrenergic nerves of the brain circulation: its role in sympathetic neurotransmission and regulation of cerebral vessel wall. Ch. XVI, This book.

19. Bradley PB, Engel G, Feniuk W, Fozard JR, Humphrey PPA, Middlemiss DN, Mylecharane EJ, Richardson BP, Saxena PR (1986): Proposals for the classification and nomenclature of functional 5-hydroxytryptamine receptors. *Neuropharmacology* 25: 563—576.

20. Humphrey PPA, Feniuk W (1988): Pharmacological characterization of functional neuronal receptors for 5-hydroxytryptamine, pp. 3—19 in: Nobin A, Owman C, Arneklo-Nobin B (eds), *Neuronal messengers in vascular function.* Amsterdam: Elsevier Science Publication.

21. Saxena PR, Ferrari M (1989): 5-Hydroxytryptamine$_1$-like receptor agonists and migraine: Possible impact on the pathophysiology of migraine. *Trends Pharmacol Sci* 10: 200—204.

22. Fozard JR (1989): 5-HT in migraine: Evidence from 5-HT receptor antagonists for a neuronal aetiology, In press, in: Sandler M (ed), *Migraine.* London: Oxford University Press.

23. Loisy C, Beorchia S, Centzone V, Fozard JR, Schechter PJ, Tell GP (1985): Effects on

migraine headache of MDL 72222, an antagonist at neuronal 5-HT receptors. Double-blind, placebo-controlled study. *Cephalalgia* 5: 79—82.

24. Humphrey PPA, Feniuk W, Perren MJ (1989): 5-HT in migraine: evidence with 5-HT$_1$-like receptor agonists for a vascular aetiology, in press in: Sandler M (ed), *Migraine*. London: Oxford University Press.

25. Humphrey PPA, Apperley E, Feniuk W, Perren MJ (1989): A rational approach to identifying a fundamentally new drug in the treatment of migraine. Ch. XXXVII, This book.

26. Saxena PR, Bom AH, Verdouw PD (1989): Characterization of 5-hydroxytryptamine receptors in the cranial vasculature. *Cephalalgia* 9 (Suppl. 9): 15—22.

27. Saxena PR, Verdouw PD (1982): Redistribution by 5-hydroxytryptamine of carotid arterial blood at the expense of arteriovenous blood flow. *J Physiol* 332: 501—520.

28. Bom AH, Verdouw PD, Saxena PR (1989): Carotid haemodynamics in pigs during infusions of 8-OH-DPAT: Reduction in arteriovenous shunting is mediated by 5-hydroxytryptamine$_1$-like receptors. *Br J Pharmacol* 96: 125—132.

29. Bom AH, Verdouw PD, Saxena PR (1989): Reduction of cephalic arteriovenous shunting by ergotamine is not mediated by 5-HT$_1$-like or 5-HT$_2$ receptors. *Br J Pharmacol* 97: 383—390.

30. Meyer JS, Hata T, Imai A (1987): Evidence supporting a vascular pathogenesis of migraine and cluster headache, pp. 265—302 in: Blau JN (ed), *Migraine — Therapeutic, Conceptual and Research Aspects*. Amsterdam: Elsevier.

31. Lauritzen M, Olesen J (1987): Leão's spreading depression, pp. 387—402 in: Blau JN (ed), *Migraine — Therapeutic, Conceptual and Research Aspects*, Amsterdam: Elsevier.

32. Drummond PD, Lance JW (1983): Extracranial vascular changes and the source of pain in migraine headaches. *Ann. Neurol* 13: 32—37.

33. Heyck H (1969): Pathogenesis of migraine. *Res. Clin. Stud. Headache* 2: 1—28.

34. Sherman JL (1963): Normal arteriovenous anastomoses. *Medicine* 92: 247—267.

35. Rowbotham GF, Little E (1965): New concepts on the aetiology and vascularization of meningiomata; the mechanisms of migraine; the chemical process of the cerebrospinal fluid; and the formations of the collections of blood or fluid in the subdural space. *Br J Surg* 52: 21—24.

36. Saxena PR (1989): 5-Hydroxytryptamine receptors and migraine, in press in: Sandler M (ed), *Migraine*. London: Oxford University Press.

37. Brand J, Hadoke M, Perrin VL (1987): Placebo-controlled study of a selective 5-HT$_1$-like agonist, AH25086B, in relief of acute migraine. *Cephalalgia* 7 (Suppl. 6): 402.

38. Doenicke A, Brand J, Perrin VL (1988): Possible benefit of GR43175, a novel 5-HT$_1$-like receptor agonist, for the treatment of severe migraine. *Lancet* 1: 1309—1311.

39. Perrin VL, Färkkilä M, Goasguen J, Doenicke A, Brand J, Tfelt-Hansen P (1989): Overview of initial clinical studies with intravenous and oral GR43175 in acute migraine. *Cephalalgia* 9 (Suppl. 9): 63—72.

40. Perrin VL (1985): Clinical pharmacokinetics of ergotamine in migraine and cluster headache. *Clin Pharmacokin* 10: 334—352.

41. Lataste X (1988): 5-HT$_3$ antagonists as antimigraine compounds. *Abstract, Int. Congr., Cardiovascular Pharmacology of 5-HT*, Oct 4—7, Amsterdam, p. 46.

XXXVII. A rational approach to identifying a fundamentally new drug for the treatment of migraine

P. P. A. HUMPHREY, E. APPERLEY, W. FENIUK and
M. J. PERREN

1. Introduction

As early as about AD 50, Aretaeus of Cappadocia is said to have recognised the symptoms of what is now known as migraine, describing the characteristic unilateral headache associated with nausea and symptom-free periods between attacks. More than two thousand years on we still do not understand the aetiology of this often debilitating disease which afflicts up to 10% of the western world. There is however a lot of circumstantial evidence that somehow the ubiquitous, yet until recently almost enigmatic, biogenic amine, 5-hydroxytryptamine (5-HT), is involved.

As discussed in the preceding chapter, the involvement of 5-hydroxytryptamine (5-HT) was suspected ever since the findings that the urinary excretion of 5-hydroxyindoleacetic acid was increased during a migraine attack [1] and that a headache, claimed to be migrainous, could be initiated by the amine depleting agent, reserpine, in migraineurs but not normal individuals [2, 3]. This appears to correlate with the finding that the platelet serotonin content falls by 30—40% at the onset of a migraine attack [2]. Such observations have led to the view that migraine is a "low 5-HT" syndrome. This could be considered paradoxical in view of the fact that many of the drugs used in the prophylactic treatment of migraine, albeit with modest success, are actually 5-HT_2 receptor antagonists [see 4]. Unless of course one considers that the locus of the disease's lesion is in the central nervous system. Although this may be so, there is compelling evidence to believe that a derangement of the normal function of the cranial vasculature is still the key to the cause of the symptoms of common migraine.

Thus regardless of the putative involvement of 5-HT in the aetiology of migraine, clinical evidence has been provided that generalised vasoconstrictors such as noradrenaline or ergotamine will abort an established migraine attack [5, 6]. Indeed, intravenous 5-HT itself has been shown to terminate a migraine headache [7]. Since 5-HT does not readily cross the blood brain barrier, and since it is a vasoconstrictor of the human extra-cranial circula-

*P.R. Saxena, D.I. Wallis, W. Wouters and P. Bevan (eds), Cardiovascular Pharmacology of
5-Hydroxytryptamine*, pp. 417—431.
© 1990 *Kluwer Academic Publishers, Dordrecht* —

tion, it has been cogently argued that dilation of cephalic (particularly extra-cranial) blood vessels might be involved in the pain of migraine (see preceding chapter; [8]).

2. Research proposal to synthesize selective 5-HT receptor agonists

In the mid 1970's we began to consider potential mechanisms of producing selective vasoconstriction of the extra-cranial circulation. Such a possibility might have seemed remote but for two important pointers in the literature. Firstly an interesting comparative trial of a variety of 5-HT receptor antagonists as migraine prophylactics showed methysergide to be the most effective, despite the fact that it has no more potent an effect as an antagonist at vascular 5-HT_2 or D receptors than the other antagonists examined [9, see 10]. Secondly, Saxena [11] had shown that methysergide has a remarkably selective vasoconstrictor action in the carotid arterial bed when injected intravenously into the anaesthetised dog. Other work from Saxena's group showed that the vasoconstrictor action of 5-HT in the same bed was resistant to blockade by the available 5-HT receptor antagonists, suggesting that a novel 5-HT receptor mechanism might be involved [12]. We therefore set about investigating the nature of carotid vascular 5-HT receptors and particularly concentrated on the pharmacology of methysergide.

2.1 *Methysergide*

In our early studies we were impressed by the finding that methysergide could constrict an extra-cranial vessel of the rabbit, the rabbit isolated perfused ear artery. However, a detailed investigation in our laboratory led us to conclude that methysergide was causing vascular smooth muscle contraction in this preparation by acting as an agonist at α-adrenoceptors [13]. This was of much academic interest but we considered that it was not therapeutically relevant because the concentrations achieved in our experiments, with bolus injections into the perfusate, were high.

We then went on to investigate the more potent vasoconstrictor action of methysergide in anaesthetised dogs. We were able to confirm Saxena's finding [11] of its remarkably selective vasoconstrictor action in the carotid circulation (Figure 1). Thus methysergide (50—250 μg/kg i.v.) decreased flow in the carotid arterial bed with little or no effect on blood pressure or heart rate. Parenthetically, in the femoral artery bed flow actually increased but it was several years before we could explain this paradoxical observation (see below). However, we were able to show at the time that the vaso-constrictor action of methysergide in the carotid artery bed, in which we were most interested, was not antagonised by phentolamine thereby ruling out an action on α-adrenoceptors as we had shown earlier in the rabbit ear

VASCULAR EFFECTS OF INTRAVENOUS METHYSERGIDE

IN THE ANAESTHETISED DOG

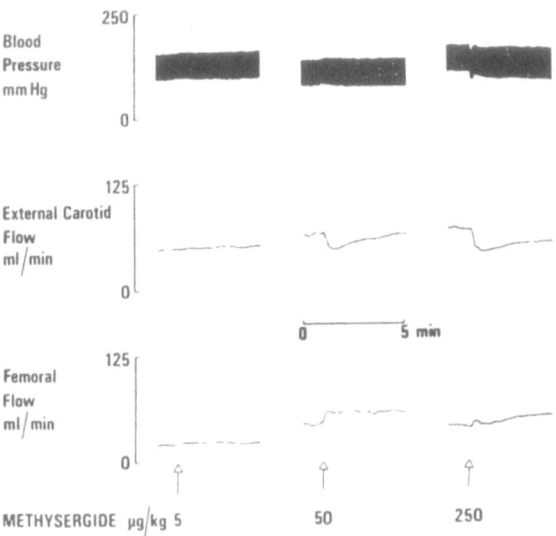

Figure 1. Anaesthetised dog. Flow was recorded in the right common carotid artery (with the internal carotid artery ligated) and in the right femoral artery in the same animal using electromagnetic flow probes. The remarkably selective vasoconstrictor action of methysergide can be seen in the carotid arterial bed with intravenous bolus doses of 50 and 250 μg/kg i.v. (recording from an unpublished experiment performed in 1976). Similar findings had been reported by Saxena earlier [11]. Note that methysergide had little or no effect on blood pressure or heart rate but actually increased blood flow in the femoral bed.

artery preparation (see above; Apperley and Humphrey, unpublished observations). We speculated that a 5-HT receptor might be involved and began to study isolated blood vessels from the external carotid circulation of the dog.

We were disappointed, at first, by our finding that the large arteries from the carotid bed, which we examined *in vitro*, such as the lingual and external carotid artery contained only the ubiquitous 5-HT$_2$ receptor which occurs in most blood vessels. Nevertheless one of the peripheral vessels we examined for comparison, the dog saphenous vein, clearly contained a 5-HT receptor which was not of the 5-HT$_2$ type and was then unknown [14]. Thus, we showed that the contractile action of 5-HT in the dog saphenous vein could not be antagonised by 5-HT$_2$ receptor antagonists [14—16]. Excitingly too, we found that methysergide was a potent contractile agent in the dog saphenous vein and, like 5-HT, its effects could not be antagonised by cyproheptadine in the concentrations which blocked 5-HT$_2$ receptors [14, 15]. The only antagonist we found capable of specifically antagonising 5-HT-

EFFECT OF METHIOTHEPIN AGAINST METHYSERGIDE-INDUCED CONTRACTIONS OF DOG SAPHENOUS VEIN

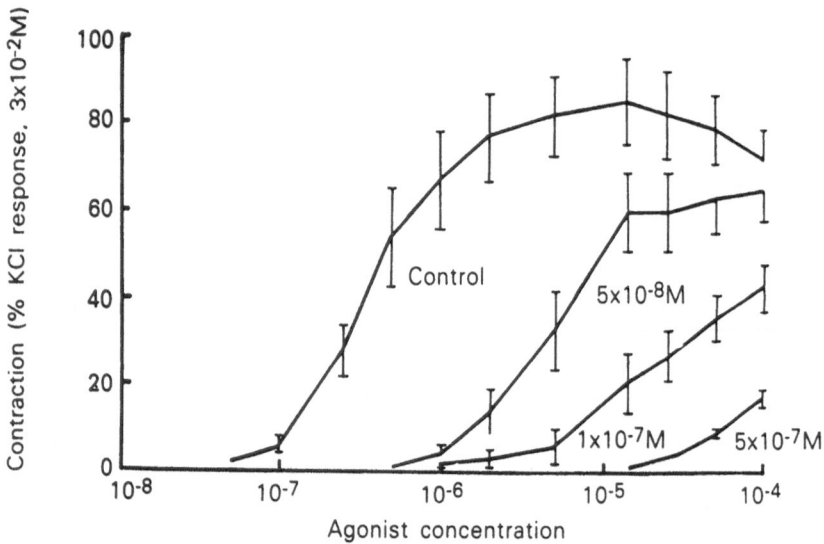

Figure 2. Dog isolated saphenous vein. Molar concentration-effect curves for the contractile action of methysergide are shifted rightwards in a concentration-dependent manner by methiothepin at concentrations of 5×10^{-8}, 1×10^{-7} and 5×10^{-7} M (data from a study unpublished in full but see [17]).

and methysergide-induced contractions in this preparation was methiothepin (Figure 2). The degree of antagonism was similar indicating that both 5-HT and methysergide were acting at a common 5-HT receptor [17]. However, we could not identify this "novel 5-HT receptor" in the extra-cranial circulation in vitro except in the canine auricular artery where sometimes it could be identified, whilst on other occasions we found evidence that it occurred in conjunction with 5-HT$_2$ receptors [15; Apperley & Humphrey, unpublished observations]. We argued that if the novel 5-HT receptor in the dog saphenous vein was the same as the putative "atypical" 5-HT receptor in the carotid circulation then these receptor sites must be largely located in the carotid resistance vessels which were more difficult to study in vitro.

We therefore carried out more experiments in the anaesthetised dog to further examine the vasoconstrictor action of methysergide in vivo. The only way we could obtain reproducible dose-effect curves for methysergide was to inject it close intra-arterially into the carotid artery via the cranial thyroid artery. We were able to show that methysergide's vasoconstrictor action could not be antagonised by a 5-HT$_2$ receptor blocking dose of cyproheptadine (0.1 mg/kg i.v.) but was antagonised by methiothepin (1 mg/kg i.v.) in a specific manner (Figure 3). This convinced us that the dog carotid circulation probably did contain the novel 5-HT receptor we had identified in the dog saphenous vein. We therefore proposed to find a selective agonist

METHYSERGIDE INDUCED VASOCONSTRICTION
IN CAROTID BED OF ANAESTHETISED DOG

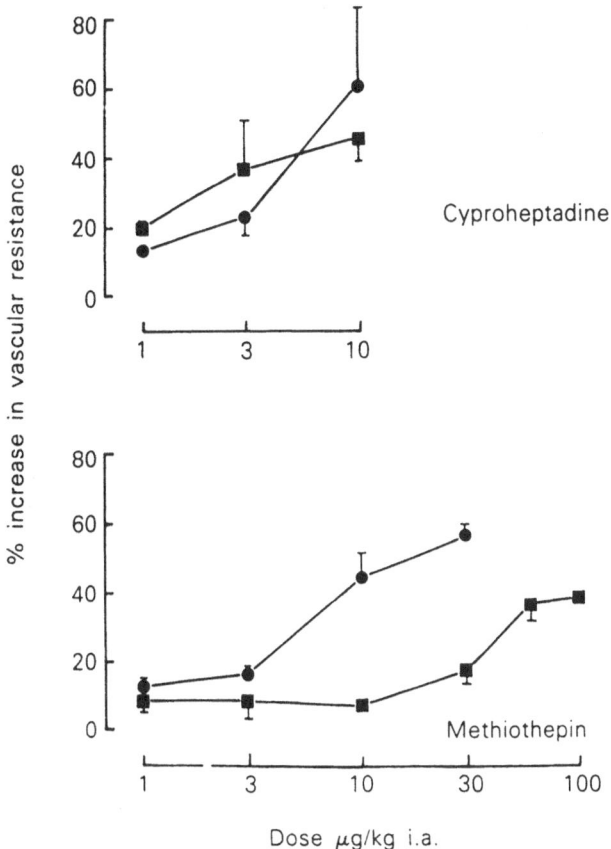

Figure 3. Anaesthetised dog. Flow was measured in the common carotid artery using an electromagnetic flow probe and increases in vascular resistance were calculated as previously described [11, 42]. Dose-response curves for the vasoconstrictor action of methysergide were constructed following its administration intra-arterially into the right common carotid artery via the cranial thyroid artery (●). Note that the dose-response curve for methysergide was shifted to the right by methiothepin (■, 1 mg/kg i.v.) but not by cyproheptadine (■, 0.1 mg/kg). Figure derived from previously unpublished data (each value is the mean ± s.e. mean of observations from four animals).

for this receptor, which we speculated would selectively constrict the canine carotid vascular bed. Our *modus operandi* was the synthesis of tryptamine analogues by our chemists which we then screened for any possible selective agonist actions on the dog saphenous vein 5-HT receptor. In making tryptamine analogues we wanted to avoid the problems associated with the ergots and lysergic acid analogues, which are known to interact with many different receptor types. Thus we know that even methysergide can stimulate

α-adrenoceptors as well as 5-HT receptors (see above) and in the guinea-pig ileum it produces smooth muscle contraction via histamine H_1 receptor activation [18]. Furthermore methysergide is metabolised in vivo to 1-methyl-ergometrine, which also stimulates a variety of different receptors including dopamine D_2 receptors [see 19]. We also hoped by making tryptamine analogues, not only to find a more selective agent, but also to find a full agonist for the novel 5-HT receptor. We argued that methysergide was a partial agonist in the dog saphenous vein [see 15] and that a full agonist might be more effective and actually be efficacious in the treatment of the acute migraine attack unlike methysergide, which is only of value as a prophylactic treatment.

2.2 *5-Carboxamidotryptamine*

One of the first tryptamine analogues we found, which appeared to be a selective agonist for the dog saphenous vein receptor, was 5-carboxamido-tryptamine (5-CT), which potently contracted the canine saphenous vein preparation, but was much weaker in contracting the rabbit isolated aorta, our standard $5\text{-}HT_2$ receptor containing preparation. On this basis we pre-sumed that it would selectively constrict the carotid bed of the anaesthetised dog but were very surprised, and at first disappointed, to find that it actually dilated the carotid bed. We later found that it was also profoundly hypoten-sive in conscious rats, dogs and cats [20—22]. As in the anaesthetised dog, 5-CT also caused extensive vasodilatation in the anaesthetised cat, and the carotid arterial bed was no exception (Figure 4). After extensive studies on isolated blood vessels, we concluded that 5-CT was an extremely potent agonist for the 5-HT receptor mediating smooth muscle relaxation, which had until then been poorly characterised [23—27]. This receptor has now been extensively studied by us in vitro in both the cat saphenous vein and the porcine vena cava and we have found that like the receptor mediating contraction of the dog saphenous vein, it can be blocked by methiothepin [28, 29]. The similarity between the two receptor types has led to their classification in the $5\text{-}HT_1$-like group of receptors defined by Bradley and colleagues [30]. Thus both receptors are potently stimulated by 5-CT and neither are blocked by $5\text{-}HT_2$ or $5\text{-}HT_3$ receptor antagonists but both are blocked by methiothepin. They were given the appellation of $5\text{-}HT_1$-like receptors because they are similar but not identical to any of the known $5\text{-}HT_1$ radioligand binding sites [30]. To this day, 5-CT remains a useful diagnostic agonist to define functional $5\text{-}HT_1$-like receptors. However, we have consistently argued on the basis of both agonist and antagonist data that $5\text{-}HT_1$-like receptors are not homogeneous and that the $5\text{-}HT_1$-like receptor mediating vascular smooth muscle contraction is pharmacologically different to the $5\text{-}HT_1$-like receptor mediating smooth muscle relaxation [31, 32]. We therefore set up screens using isolated pharmacological preparations to

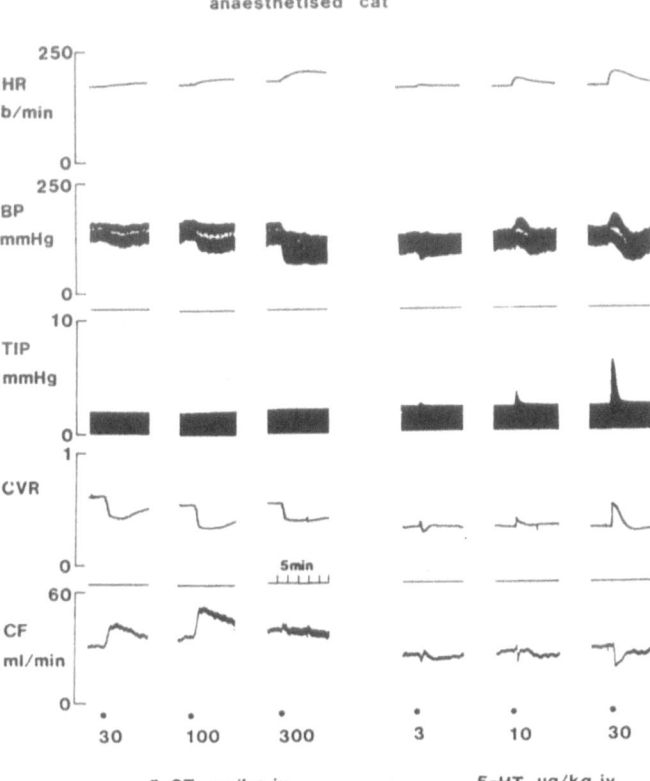

Representative tracing of the effects of 5-CT and 5-HT in the anaesthetised cat

Figure 4. Anaesthetised cat. Mean arterial blood pressure (BP), heart rate (HR) and common carotid flow (CF) were recorded. Common carotid vascular resistance (CVR) was calculated electronically (arbitrary units) and displayed continuously. Intravenous 5-CT has a more selective haemodynamic profile than 5-HT, being devoid of effects mediated via $5-HT_2$ and $5-HT_3$ receptors e.g. bronchoconstriction evinced by the increase in tracheal inflation pressure (TIP), seen only with 5-HT. Note the potent vasodilator effect of 5-CT in the carotid bed and its hypotensive action (reproduced with permission from the British Journal of Pharmacology from [21]).

identify a truly selective agonist for the $5-HT_1$-like receptor in the dog saphenous vein.

2.3 AH25086

After examining many more tryptamine analogues we finally identified AH25086 (3-(2-aminoethyl)-N-methyl-1H-indole-5-acetamide), an agonist which was found to be a potent contractile agent in the dog saphenous vein but which is devoid of agonist activity at $5-HT_2$ and $5-HT_3$ receptors [33,

34]. Importantly too, unlike 5-CT, AH25086 was devoid of agonist activity at the 5-HT$_1$-like receptor mediating smooth muscle relaxation. However AH25086, like 5-CT, did cause inhibition of neurogenically mediated contractions of the dog isolated saphenous vein (35; see Figure 5). This provided good evidence for our previous claim, based initially on the pharmacology of methysergide, that the pre-junctional 5-HT$_1$-like receptor mediating inhibition of noradrenaline release from noradrenergic nerves in the dog saphenous vein is the same as the post-junctional 5-HT$_1$-like receptor mediating contraction, in the same vessel [36, 37]. The presence of these pre-junctional "inhibitory" 5-HT$_1$-like receptors on sympathetic nerves innervating the femoral bed explains the vasodilatator action of methysergide

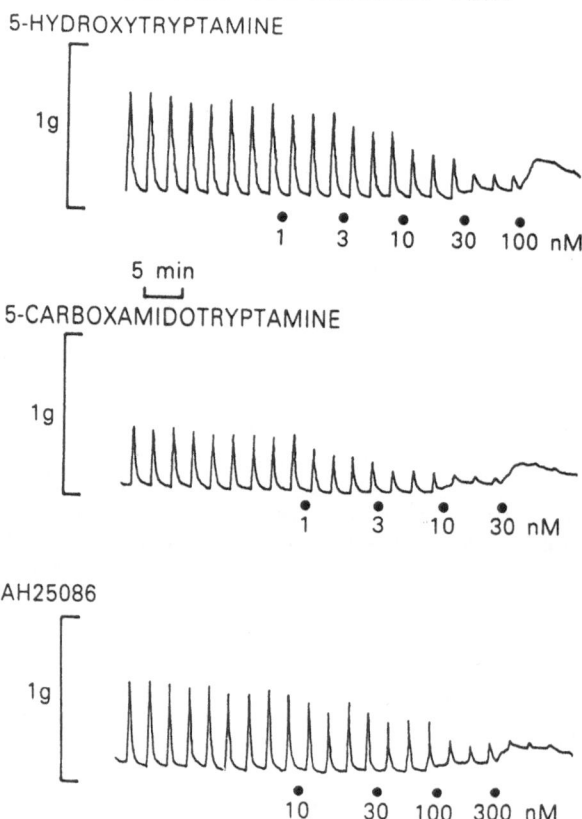

Figure 5. Electrically stimulated dog isolated saphenous vein. The vein preparation was electrically stimulated at 2 Hz as previously described [41]. Note that like 5-HT, 5-CT and AH25086 will also inhibit the neurogenically mediated twitches without affecting tone induced by the continuous presence of an exogenous spasmogen such as methoxamine (latter data not shown). This pre-junctional action of 5-HT has been shown to result from inhibition of noradrenaline release in response to nerve stimulation [36].

we had observed years earlier in this bed (see above). Thus when there is a high sympathetic drive to the femoral vasculature, activation of the prejunctional 5-HT receptor produces a sympatholytic effect [38].

As anticipated, low doses of AH25086 dilated the femoral bed of the dog in vivo, but unlike 5-CT, it did not cause a generalised vasodilatation and hypotension (unpublished observations). Indeed when injected intravenously into the anaesthetised dog the predominant effect of AH25086 is a pronounced vasoconstrictor action in the carotid arterial bed with little effect on blood pressure, heart rate or total peripheral resistance [35]. It would appear that the 5-HT$_1$-like receptors for which AH25086 is selective are remarkably localised. In the anaesthetised cat too, AH25086 has a very selective vasoconstrictor action which we were able to show was confined not just to the carotid circulation but *within* the carotid circulation. Thus, its effect on carotid blood flow could be explained almost entirely on the basis of a vasoconstrictor action of AH25086 on carotid arteriovenous anastomoses or shunt vessels. Interestingly methysergide had only a small effect on shunt vessels in these experiments, presumably because, unlike AH25086, it behaves as a partial agonist at the 5-HT$_1$-like receptors typified in the dog saphenous vein [see 35].

The selective vasoconstrictor profile of AH25086 was such that we were keen to have the compound examined in human volunteers. Its acceptable tolerability led to its clinical evaluation, when preliminary studies by the intravenous route suggested that it was very effective in aborting all the symptoms of the acute migraine attack [39, 40]. However, AH25086 was not suitable for full development and GR4317 (3-(2-(dimethylamino)ethyl)-N-methyl-1H-indole-5-methanesulphonamide) was finally identified as a better drug candidate, being suitable for oral as well as parenteral administration.

2.4 *GR43175*

GR43175 has a pharmacological profile in vitro which is similar to that of AH25086. Thus GR43175 is a very selective agonist for the 5-HT$_1$-like receptor located both pre- and post-junctionally in the dog saphenous vein, being about five times less potent than 5-HT [41]. Experiments carried out both in vitro and in vivo have ruled out the possibility of an action of GR43175 on a variety of other non-5-HT receptor types [41, 42; unpublished observations].

In the anaesthetised dog, GR43175 is a potent and selective vasoconstrictor of the carotid arterial bed, 50% of the maximum vasoconstrictor effect occurring at 35—40 μg/kg i.v. [42]. Experiments in the anaesthetised cat indicate that its carotid vasoconstrictor action, like that of AH25086, is localised to the arteriovenous anastomoses or shunt vessels where it reduced flow [43]. In contrast, the proportion of carotid blood flow distributed to the capillary beds of the brain and extra-cellular structures actually increased a little following GR43175 [43]. More detailed haemodynamic measurements in cats and dogs with radiolabelled microspheres and flow probes have provided further evidence for the remarkably selective vasoconstrictor action of GR43175, with no evidence of any vasoconstrictor action which might compromise the blood supply to any of the major organs including the brain, heart, liver and kidney (see Figure 6) [43, 44]. In this respect, and many others, GR43175 cannot be compared with ergotamine which has a generalised vasoconstrictor action.

It has been shown by Saxena, and ourselves, that ergotamine can, by careful choice of the dose, produce a selective vasoconstriction of carotid shunt vessels. However, increasing the dose leads to a generalised vasoconstriction in all the arterial beds [43, 45]. In marked contrast, even very high doses of GR43175 (up to 1 mg/kg i.v.) do not produce any significant vasoconstriction in any of the arterial beds we have examined including, for example in the dog, the coronary, vertebral and mesenteric beds [42, 43]. However in the femoral artery bed low doses of GR43175 produce vasodilatation, presumably by the pre-junctional mechanism discussed above, whilst higher doses (100 μg/kg i.v. and above) produce some vasoconstric-

SELECTIVE VASOCONSTRICTOR ACTION OF GR43175 IN THE CANINE CAROTID BED

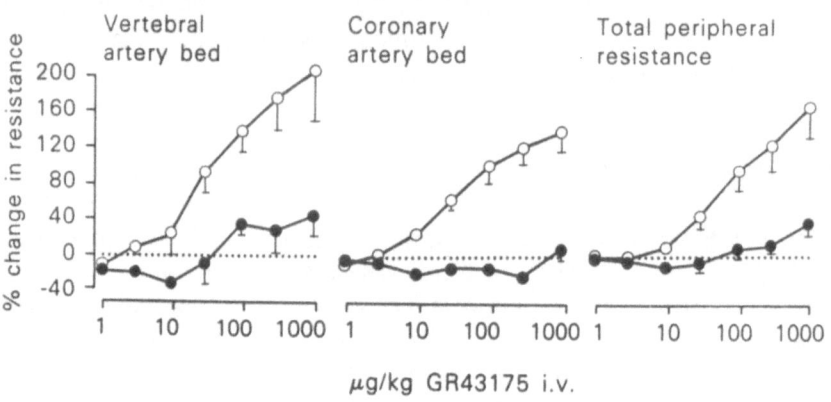

μg/kg GR43175 i.v.

Figure 6. Comparison of the effect of GR43175 on carotid arterial vascular resistance (○) with its effect in other vascular beds (●) in anaesthetised beagle dogs. Either vertebral artery blood flow or coronary artery blood flow was recorded in the same animal as common carotid blood flow, using electromagnetic flow probes. In other experiments common carotid blood flow was recorded in conjunction with ascending aortic flow in order to obtain an estimate of total peripheral vascular resistance. The resistance changes calculated are the mean with s.e. mean indicated by the vertical bars (reproduced, with permission from the British Journal of Pharmacology, from [42]).

tion. We have speculated that this latter observation reflects the presence of significant flow through shunt vessels which are known to be present in canine foot pads and which contain 5-HT$_1$-like receptors mediating constriction as in the carotid circulation [see ref. 42]. Interestingly in man, measurement of arm to toe blood pressure gradients have provided no evidence for a vasoconstrictor action of GR43175 on leg arteries, which is in marked contrast to the effects of a clinical dose of ergotamine [46]. It is evident that ergotamine has a generalised vasoconstrictor action mediated via activation of a number of different receptor types [see 47]. Ironically, however, recent studies indicate that ergotamine does *not* mediate closure of carotid shunt vessels in either the pig or cat by activation of 5-HT$_1$-like receptors [48]. All the evidence clearly points to the fact that GR43175 is not a "selective ergotamine" as has been suggested [49].

3. Clinical evaluation of GR43175

Given the very selective pharmacological profile of GR43175, and our earlier experience with AH25086, we were keen to have it evaluated in the migraine clinic. Experiments in animals suggested that it would be active not only by the intravenous route but also when administered subcutaneously and orally (unpublished observations). GR43175 was therefore investigated initially in volunteers and then migraineurs by intravenous injection as a bolus or by infusion. Having confirmed that it was effective in the treatment of the acute attack in an open study [50], the clinical evaluation has now been extended to subcutaneous and oral formulations of GR43175. The initial findings demonstrate that the drug is effective by these routes as well, in aborting all the symptoms of established severe migraine attacks [51]. Clearly these findings need to be confirmed but there is already much interest amongst scientific and clinical investigators about its possible mode of action. We have evidence in animals that GR43175 has no analgesic activity and that it does not penetrate into the central nervous system to any marked degree [52]. We have proposed that evidence to date is consistent with the view that it is the vasoconstrictor action of GR43175 which is therapeutically important [35, 44]. Whether the locus of this action is at the level of carotid shunt vessels or perhaps the meningeal circulation remains to be seen [see 35 and 44 for discussion of this point]. Nevertheless, the discovery of GR43175 is consistent with our original research proposal that vasoconstrictors are effective in the acute treatment of a migraine attack and has once again raised the level of interest in the "vascular" theories of migraine. Perhaps, after all, the final common pathological event in migraine and other types of vascular headache is a severe but reversible (neurogenically mediated?) derangement of blood flow at a yet to be precisely identified locus within the cephalic circulation.

4. Concluding remarks

We have described about fifteen years of research on vascular 5-HT receptors in our laboratories, which focused on the possibility that 5-HT receptors on some blood vessels in the head might be different. This turned out to be so and we have therefore attempted to exploit this difference presented by nature.

The pharmacological twists in the trail which led to the development of GR43175 have been outlined. Some of the scientific clues came from the pharmacology of the ergots which act at a variety of different types of receptor. Ironically however, ergotamine does not appear to stimulate the one 5-HT receptor sub-type through which we believe GR43175 mediates its antimigraine action. Hopefully the much greater selectivity of GR43175 both at the level of amine receptors, and within the vasculature as a whole, will provide a much safer type of drug for the treatment of the acute attack. With better bioavailability than that of ergotamine, GR43175 holds the promise of an oral treatment which will abort the majority of severe attacks [53—55].

Acknowledgement

We are extremely grateful to Mrs. Rosemary Cockburn who so competently typed and helped to prepare this manuscript.

References

1. Sicuteri F, Testi A, Anselmi B (1961): Biochemical investigations in headache: Increase in the hydroxyindoleacetic acid excretion during migraine attacks. *Int Arch Allergy* 19: 55—58.
2. Anthony M, Hinterberger H, Lance JW (1967): Plasma serotonin in migraine and stress. *Arch Neurol* 16: 544—552.
3. Carroll JD, Hilton BP (1974): The effects of reserpine injection on methysergide treated control and migrainous subjects. *Headache* 14: 149—156.
4. Fozard JR (1982): Mechanism of the hypotensive effect of ketanserin. *J Cardiovasc Pharmacol* 4: 829—838.
5. Graham JR, Wolff HG (1938): Mechanism of migraine headache and action of ergotamine tartrate. *Archs Neurol Psychiat, Chicago* 39: 737.
6. Wolff HG (1963): *Headache and other head pain.* London: Oxford University Press.
7. Kimball RW, Friedman AP, Vallejo E (1960): Effect of serotonin in migraine patients. *Neurology* 10: 107—111.
8. Lance JW (1973): *The mechanism and management of headache.* Second Edition, London: Butterworth Publishers.
9. Lance JW, Anthony M, Somerville B (1970): Comparative trial of serotonin antagonists in the management of migraine. *Br Med J* 2: 327—330.
10. Humphrey PPA, Feniuk W, Watts AD (1982): Ketanserin — a novel hypertensive drug? *J Pharm Pharmacol* 34: 541.

11. Saxena PR (1974): Selective vasoconstriction in carotid vascular bed by methysergide: Possible relevance to its antimigraine effect. *Eur J Pharmacol* 27: 99—105.

12. Saxena PR (1972): The effects of antimigraine drugs on the vascular responses by 5-hydroxytryptamine and related biogenic substances on the external carotid bed of dogs: possible pharmacological implications to their antimigraine action. *Headache* 12: 44—54.

13. Apperley E, Humphrey PPA, Levy GP (1976): Receptors for 5-hydroxytryptamine and noradrenaline in rabbit isolated ear artery and aorta. *Br J Pharmacol* 58: 211—221.

14. Apperley E, Humphrey PPA, Levy GP (1977): Two types of excitatory receptor for 5-hydroxytryptamine in dog vasculature? *Br J Pharmacol* 61: 465P.

15. Apperley E, Feniuk W, Humphrey PPA, Levy GP (1980): Evidence for two types of excitatory receptor for 5-hydroxytryptamine in dog isolated vasculature. *Br J Pharmacol* 68: 215—224.

16. Feniuk W, Humphrey PPA, Perren MJ, Watts AD (1985): A comparison of 5-hydroxy-tryptamine receptors mediating contraction in rabbit aorta and dog saphenous vein. Evidence for different receptor types obtained by use of selective agonists and antagonists. *Br J Pharmacol* 86: 697—704.

17. Apperley E, Humphrey PPA (1986): The interaction of 5-hydroxytryptamine and methysergide with methiothepin at "5-HT$_1$-like" receptors in dog saphenous vein. *Br J Pharmacol* 87: 131P.

18. Gunning SJ, Bunce KT, Humphrey PPA (1988): Methysergide contracts guinea-pig ileum via histamine H$_1$ receptors. *Br J Pharmacol* 93: 238P.

19. Berde B, Schild HO (Eds) (1978): *Ergot alkaloids and related compounds.* Berlin: Springer-Verlag.

20. Dalton DW, Feniuk W, Humphrey PPA (1986): An investigation into the mechanisms of the cardiovascular effects of 5-hydroxytryptamine in conscious normotensive and doca-salt hypertensive rats. *J Auton Pharmacol* 6: 219—228.

21. Connor HE, Feniuk W, Humphrey PPA, Perren MJ (1986): 5-Carboxamidotryptamine is a selective agonist at 5-hydroxytryptamine receptors mediating vasodilatation and tachycardia in anaesthetized cats. *Br J Pharmacol* 87: 417—426.

22. Feniuk W, Humphrey PPA, Hunt AAE (1985): The haemodynamic profile and mechanism of the hypotensive action of 5-carboxamidotryptamine in conscious dogs. *Br J Pharmacol* 85: 310P.

23. Eyre P (1975): Atypical tryptamine receptors in sheep pulmonary vein. *Br J Pharmacol* 55: 329—333.

24. Feniuk W, Humphrey PPA, Watts AD (1983): 5-Hydroxytryptamine-induced relaxation of isolated mammalian smooth muscle. *Eur J Pharmacol* 96: 71—78.

25. Feniuk W, Humphrey PPA, Watts AD (1984): 5-Carboxamido-tryptamine — a potent agonist at 5-hydroxytryptamine receptors mediating relaxation. *Br J Pharmacol* 82: 209P.

26. Trevethick MA, Feniuk W, Humphrey PPA (1984): 5-Hydroxytryptamine-induced relaxation of neonatal porcine vena cava *in vitro*. *Life Sci* 35: 477—486.

27. Trevethick MA, Feniuk W, Humphrey PPA (1986): 5-Carboxamidotryptamine: a potent agonist mediating relaxation and elevation of cyclic AMP in the isolated neonatal porcine vena cava. *Life Sci* 38: 1521—1528.

28. Sumner MJ, Humphrey PPA, Feniuk W (1987): Characterisation of the 5-HT$_1$-like receptor mediating relaxation of porcine vena cava. *Br J Pharmacol* 92: 574P.

29. Sumner MJ, Feniuk W, Humphrey PPA (1989): Further characterisation of the 5-HT receptor mediating vascular relaxation and elevation of cyclic AMP in isolated porcine vena cava. *Br J Pharmacol* 97: 292—300.

30. Bradley PB, Engel G, Feniuk W, Fozard JR, Humphrey PPA, Middlemiss DN, Mylecharane EJ, Richardson BP, Saxena PR (1986): Proposals for the classification and nomenclature of functional receptors for 5-hydroxytryptamine. *Neuropharmacology* 25: 563—576.

31. Humphrey PPA (1984): Peripheral 5-hydroxytryptamine receptors and their classification. *Neuropharmacology* 23: 1503—1510.

32. Humphrey PPA, Feniuk W (1987): Classification of functional 5-hydroxytryptamine receptors, pp. 277—280 in: Rand MJ, Raper (eds), *Pharmacology, International Congress Series 750 (Proceedings of Xth International Congress of Pharmacology — I.U.P.H.A.R.)*. Netherlands: Elsevier Science Publishers.

33. Feniuk W, Humphrey PPA (1989): Mechanisms of 5-hydroxytryptamine-induced vaso-constriction, pp. 100—122, in Fozard JR (ed), *The Peripheral Actions of 5-Hydroxy-tryptamine*. London: Oxford University Press.

34. Humphrey PPA, Feniuk W (1989): The sub-classification of functional 5-HT$_1$-like receptors, in press in: Mylecharane EJ, Angus JA, de la Lande IS, Humphrey PPA (eds), *Serotonin (Proceedings of the Heron Island Meeting, September 1987)*. London: Mac-millan Press Limited.

35. Humphrey PPA, Feniuk W, Perren MJ (1989): 5-HT in migraine: Evidence with 5-HT$_1$-like receptor agonists for a vascular aetiology, in press in: Sandler M, Collins G (eds), *Migraine, A spectrum of ideas*. London: Oxford University Press.

36. Watts AD, Feniuk W, Humphrey PPA (1981): A pre-junctional action of 5-hydroxy-tryptamine and methysergide on noradrenergic nerves in dog isolated saphenous vein. *J Pharm Pharmacol* 33: 515—520.

37. Feniuk W, Humphrey PPA, Watts AD (1981): Further characterisation of pre- and post-junctional receptors for 5-hydroxytryptamine in isolated vasculature. *Br J Pharmacol* 73: 191P—192P.

38. Feniuk W, Humphrey PPA, Watts AD (1981): Modification of the vasomotor actions of methysergide in the femoral arterial bed of the anaesthetised dog by changes in sympathetic nerve activity. *J Auton Pharmacol* 1: 127—132.

39. Doenicke A, Siegel E, Hadoke M, Perrin VL (1987): Initial clinical study of AH25086B (5-HT$_1$-like agonist) in the acute treatment of migraine. *Cephalalgia* 7(6): 438—439.

40. Brand J, Hadoke M, Perrin VL (1987): Placebo controlled study of a selective 5-HT$_1$-like agonist, AH25086B, in relief of acute migraine. *Cephalalgia* 7(6): 402—403.

41. Humphrey PPA, Feniuk W, Perren MJ, Connor HE, Oxford AW, Coates IH, Butina D (1988): GR43175, a selective agonist for the 5-HT$_1$-like receptor in dog isolated saphenous vein. *Br J Pharmacol* 94: 1123—1132.

42. Feniuk W, Humphrey PPA, Perren MJ (1989): The selective carotid arterial vaso-constrictor action of GR43175 in anaesthetised dogs. *Br J Pharmacol* 96: 83—90.

43. Perren MJ, Feniuk W, Humphrey PPA (1989): The selective closure of feline carotid arteriovenous anastomoses by GR43175. *Cephalalgia* 9 (Suppl. 9): 41—46.

44. Humphrey PPA, Perren MJ, Feniuk W, Oxford AW (1989): The pharmacology of the novel 5-HT$_1$-like receptor agonist GR43175. *Cephalalgia* 9 (Suppl. 9): 23—33.

45. Johnston BM, Saxena PR (1978): The effect of ergotamine on tissue blood flow and the arteriovenous shunting of radioactive microspheres in the head. *Br J Pharmacol* 63: 541—549.

46. Neilsen TH, Tfelt-Hansen P (1989): Lack of effect of GR43175 on peripheral arteries in man. *Cephalalgia* 9 (Suppl. 9): 93—95.

47. Feniuk W, Humphrey PPA, Perren MJ (1989): GR43175 does not share the complex pharmacology of the ergots. *Cephalalgia* 9 (Suppl. 9): 35—39.

48. Saxena PR, Bom AH, Verdouw PD (1989): Characterization of 5-hydroxytryptamine receptors in the cranial vasculature. *Cephalalgia* 9 (Suppl. 9): 15—22.

49. Fozard JR (1987): 5-HT: The enigma variations. *Trends Pharmacol Sci* 501—506.

50. Doenicke A, Brand J, Perrin VL (1988): Possible benefit of GR43175, a novel 5-HT$_1$-like receptor agonist, for the acute treatment of severe migraine. *Lancet* 1: 1309—1311.

51. Perrin VL, Färkkilä M, Goasguen J, Doenicke A, Brand J, Tfelt-Hansen P (1989): Overview of initial clinical studies with intravenous and oral GR43175 in acute migraine. *Cephalalgia* 9 (Suppl. 9): 63—72.

52. Humphrey PPA, Feniuk W, Perren MJ, Oxford AW, Brittain RT (1989): Sumatriptan Succinate. *Drugs of the Future* 14(1): 35—39.

53. Dallas FAA, Dixon CM, McCulloch RJ, Saynor DA (1989): The kinetics of ^{14}C-GR43175 in rat and dog. *Cephalalgia* 9 (Suppl. 9):53—56.
54. Fowler PA, Thomas M, Lacey LF, Andrew P, Dallas FAA (1989): Early studies with the novel 5-HT$_1$-like agonist GR43175 in healthy volunteers. *Cephalalgia* 9 (Suppl. 9): 57—62.
55. Doenicke A, Melchart D, Bayliss EM (1989): Effective improvement of symptoms in patients with acute migraine with GR43175 dispersible tablets. *Cephalalgia* 9 (Suppl. 9): 89—92.

XXXVIII. Treatment of migraine with drugs related to 5-hydroxytryptamine

P. TFELT-HANSEN and T. H. NIELSEN

1. Introduction

The 5-hydroxytryptamine (5-HT) antagonist methysergide was introduced in the prophylaxis of migraine in 1959 [1] and later proved to be quite effective [2]. Ergotamine, one of the traditional drugs used in the treatment of migraine attacks, was later found to act on 5-HT receptors [3]. Recently GR43175, a 5-HT_1-like receptor agonist, has been introduced as a new treatment for migraine attacks [4].

The pathophysiology of migraine remains an enigma, but the efficacy of drugs related to 5-HT in the treatment of migraine apparently lends support to the involvement of 5-HT in the pathophysiology of migraine. However, the use of pharmacological evidence obtained in animal studies to support a pathophysiological theory in man might be treacherous, partly because of differences in pharmacokinetics, partly because of differences in the pharmacodynamic parameters available for investigations.

In this chapter aspects of the pharmacology of methysergide and ergotamine with relevance to migraine therapy and pathophysiology will be reviewed. Moreover, early clinical experience with GR43175 will be presented (for a review of pharmacological background see [4]).

2. Methysergide

2.1 Therapeutic use

Methysergide is of proven efficacy in the prophylaxis of migraine [2] and, in our opinion, it is one of the most effective drugs for this purpose. The clinical use of methysergide is, however, hampered by the fibrotic side effects occurring after chronic use. These side effects can possibly be minimized by withdrawing the drug for 2 months every 6 months or for 1 month every 4

P.R. Saxena, D.I. Wallis, W. Wouters and P. Bevan (eds), Cardiovascular Pharmacology of 5-Hydroxytryptamine, pp. 433—441.

434   *P. Tfelt-Hansen and T. H. Nielsen*

months. For this reason methysergide cannot be considered as a drug of first choice.

Methysergide was introduced in pharmacotherapy as a specific 5-HT antagonist [1, 5]. Later, when it was difficult to understand why a 5-HT antagonist should be effective in migraine, "a low 5-HT syndrome', it was suggested that methysergide could be beneficial in migraine by a selective vasoconstriction in the carotid vascular beds [6, 7]. These animal studies indicated the presence of atypical 5-HT receptors in the carotid bed and this subsequently led to the development of a completely new class of drugs, 5-HT_1-like agonists [4]. In addition to its use in migraine therapy and pharmacology, methysergide was considered for many years as the most potent 5-HT antagonist, that could be administered to man. It was used as an experimental tool to investigate the role of 5-HT in endocrinological regulation and certain CNS functions.

Recent pharmacokinetic studies in man have demonstrated that methysergide is probably only a "prodrug"; its main metabolite is methylergometrine. In the following these pharmacokinetic results, which have important impact on the rationale for transferring animal results to man, and which might explain some curios pharmacodynamic results in man, will be reviewed.

2.2 *Pharmacokinetics of methysergide*

Methysergide was originally synthesized from methylergometrine by adding a methyl group and in the first paper on methysergide [5] it is suggested that methysergide may be demethylated to methylergometrine to some extent in rats. This demethylation to methylergometrine probably explains the small uterotonic effect observed with methysergide [5]. Later, another study using fluorescence detection of the drugs in urine confirmed demethylation of methysergide to methylergometrine [8]. However, these semi-quantative results seem to have been largely forgotten.

With a recently developed high performance liquid chromatographic method with fluorescence detection we measured methysergide and methyl-ergometrine in plasma after intravenous (Figure 1) and oral (Figure 2) administration of methysergide [9]. It was established that methysergide is quickly cleared from plasma (t1/2: approximately 50 min), with simultaneous appearance of methylergometrine (t1/2: approximately 200 min). After i.v. administration the area under the curves (AUC) of the two drugs was similar (Figure 1). However, it is interesting to note that after oral administration of methysergide (bioavailability 13%) the AUC for methylergometrine was 10 times greater than the AUC for methysergide (Figure 2). Similarly, in rats 10 mg/kg methysergide resulted in concentrations of 61 ng/ml for methyl-ergometrine and 8 ng/ml for methysergide after oral administration (unpublished observations). After i.v. injection of the same dose of methysergide to rats methylergometrine was hardly detectable (Bredberg, personal communication).

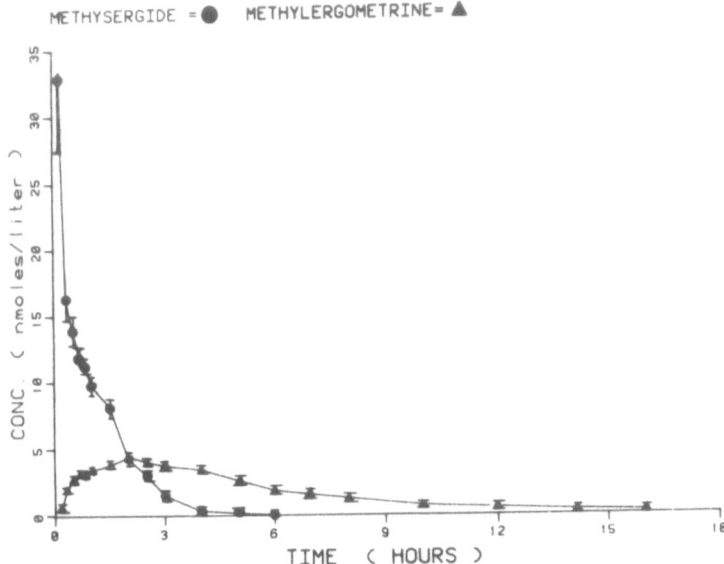

Figure 1. Plasma concentrations of methysergide and methylergometrine after 1 mg methysergide i.v. (Reproduced from |9| with permission from the publisher).

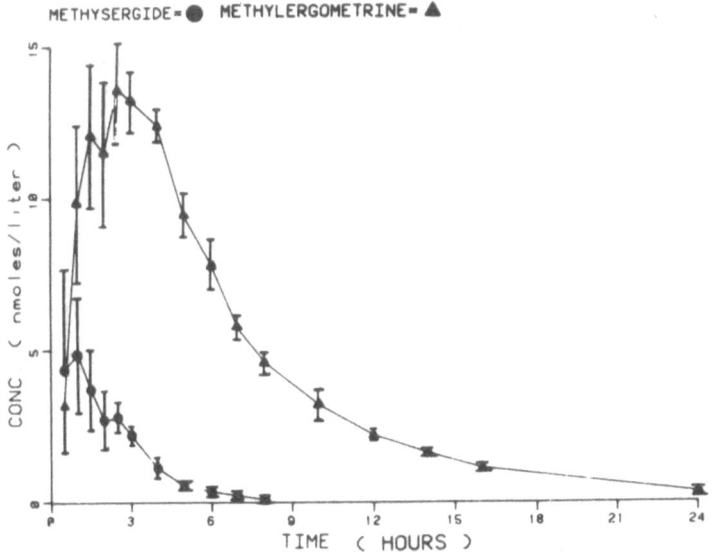

Figure 2. Plasma concentrations of methysergide and methylergometrine after 2 mg methysergide given orally as tablets. Note the difference from the scale in Figure 1 (Reproduced from |9| with permission from the publishers).

2.3 Pharmacology of methysergide and methylergometrine

The activity profiles of methysergide and methylergometrine, in comparison with those of bromocriptine and lysergide (LSD), are shown in Table 1 [10]. Based on these results, bromocriptine is the most selective dopamine agonist, methysergide the most selective 5-HT antagonist, whereas both methylergometrine and LSD have actions on several receptors. Methylergometrine thus has a strong uterotonic effect (its normal therapeutic use) and some 5-HT antagonistic effect and dopamine agonist effect. In a probably more relevant model for 5-HT antagonistic effect, the human temporal artery in vitro, methylergometrine was found 40 times more potent as a 5-HT antagonist than methysergide [11].

The dopaminergic agonistic effect of methylergometrine probably explains that whereas methysergide, when administered by the parenteral route, has minimal dopaminergic activity (see Table 1), its oral administration in human volunteers results in a significant decrease in plasma prolactin [12]. This is due to conversion of methysergide to methylergometrine (see Figure 1 and 2).

As mentioned above methysergide in rather high i.v. bolus doses (20—640/μg/kg) was found to have a selective vasoconstrictor effect on the carotid vascular bed in dogs [6] and, in a later study, high i.v. doses (50—350/μg/kg) of methysergide constricted arteriovenous anastomoses in the carotid vascular bed in pigs [7]. In contrast, 350/μg/kg methysergide orally for six days did not influence carotid blood flow [7]. The discrepancy is probably due to the fact that after i.v. administration methysergide is present in high concentrations in plasma, but after oral administration methysergide is converted to methylergometrine. Therefore, the pharmacokinetic behavior

Table 1. Pharmacological profiles of bromocriptine, methylergometrine, methysergide and LSD (most active compound in each test = 1000).

Activity	Bromocriptine	Methylergometrine	Methysergide	LSD
Blockade of 5-HT-induced contraction of isolated rat uterus	3	250	1000	250
Rabbit uterus contraction in situ (i.v).	0	1000	40	670
Dopaminergic stereotype behaviour in rats (i.p.)	630	310	<1	1000
Contralateral turning behaviour in 6-hydroxy-dopamine treated rats	1000	400	<1	750

Modified from [10].

of methysergide questions the relevance of the selective vasoconstrictor effect of methysergide in the clinical efficacy of the drug in migraine. Thus, for future animal studies the use of the oral route of administration for methysergide or alternatively the use of parenteral methylergometrine are recommended.

3. Ergotamine

3.1 *Therapeutic use and pharmacology*

Initially, ergotamine was introduced in the treatment of migraine attacks as an alpha-adrenoceptorblocker 60 years ago and is still the drug of choice for the treatment of moderate to severe migraine attacks. However, in 1938 increased pulsations of the superficial temporal artery were noted during attacks of migraine and the time course of the beneficial effect of ergotamine in migraine parallelled the decrease in pulsations [13]. This implied that ergotamine exerts its therapeutic effect in migraine by constriction of these vessels. Recently, however, it has been suggested that ergotamine exerts its effect in migraine by an effect on the brain stem [14] or on perivascular neurogenic inflammation [15]. Ergotamine is a vasoconstrictor and in animals a relatively selective vasoconstriction in cranial vasculature has been found [16]. This effect of ergotamine has been shown to be due to a closure of arteriovenous anastomoses in the extracerebral circulation [17] but the receptor involved remains unidentified [18]. It is, however, uncertain if arteriovenous anastomoses are involved in migraine pain [19] and ergotamine does not affect cerebral blood flow [20] in humans.

3.2 *Pharmacokinetics and pharmacodynamics in man*

A summary of the pharmacokinetic properties of ergotamine are presented in Table 2. The drug is quickly cleared from the blood after i.v. and i.m. injections with a half life of 2 hours [21]. The oral and rectal bioavailability is only a few per cent [22] resulting in plasma concentrations of ergotamine at or below the detection limit of 0.1 ng/ml in most cases. Due to the poor, and variable bioavailability, one has to "tailor" the dose of ergotamine for individual patient by trial and error.

Although ergotamine is described as a "general" vasoconstrictor, the sensitivity of the different parts of the vascular system varies considerably. Thus using a combined pharmacokinetic-pharmacodynamic model the theoretical steady-state EC_{50} of ergotamine for the pressor (arteriolar effect) and arterial vasoconstrictor response were 1.52 and 0.24 ng/ml, respectively [23]. These results are supported by the fact that increases in arterial pressure are observed during a few hours after parenteral ergotamine (concentrations

Table 2. Pharmacokinetics of ergotamine.

Route of administration	Dose (mg)	Appears quickly in blood	Bioavailability[a]
Intravenous	0.25—0.5	yes	100%
Intramuscular	0.5	yes	47%
Oral	2	no	1—2%[b]
Rectal suppositories	2	no	1—3%
Rectal solution	2	yes	1—3%

[a], Bioavailability could only be calculated for the intramuscular route. For the other routes, estimates are given; [b], below detection limit of 0.1 ng/ml. Data from [21, 22].

above 1 ng/ml) but not after suppositories (concentrations near 0.1 ng/ml). In contrast, ergotamine-induced arterial vasoconstriction lasts at least 24 hours after administration by either route [23]. In clinical practice migraine is treated successfully with ergotamine by oral or rectal route which result in very low plasma concentrations. We must therefore assume that the "therapeutic concentrations" of ergotamine are probably without any effect on the resistance vessels.

4. GR43175

4.1 *Pharmacology*

Atypical 5-HT receptors (later named as 5-HT$_1$-like receptors) were identified in the carotid vasculature, as mentioned above, by experiments with methysergide [7]. Subsequently, a selective agonist of these 5-HT$_1$-like receptors, GR43175, was developed and this drug has so far been promising in the treatment of migraine attacks [4]. Only one point in the developement of this new drug needs to be mentioned here: the carotid vasoconstrictor action of GR43175 is, as found earlier with methysergide [7] and ergotamine [17], predominantly at the level of ateriovenous anastomoses [4]. These arteriovenous shunts, as mentioned before, may not be involved in the pathophysiology of migraine [19]. How can GR43175 then be effective in migraine? 5-HT$_1$-like receptors have also been recently identified in human basilar arteries [24] and it may be that GR43175 constricts dilated cerebral, meningeal or extracranial arteries to releive pain. In contrast to ergotamine [23], GR43175 (2 mg, i.v.) has no vasoconstrictor effect on leg arteries [25].

4.2 *Clinical results*

In open dose-ranging studies [26—28] GR43175 has been administered to migraine patients by several routes: intravenous bolus and infusion, subcutaneous injection, and dispersible tablets. Furthermore, one small double blind trial with i.v. GR43175 has been performed [27].

In an i.v. open dose-ranging study 34 patients were treated for 46 migraine attacks [26]. With the highest dose of 2 mg GR43175 infused over 10 min in 25 migraine attacks, improvement in headache severity was reported as follows: from a severe headache to no headache in 17 attacks (71%); from a severe to a mild headache in 7 attacks; and from a moderate to a mild headache in 1 attack. Symptoms were relieved rapidly, with optimum responses occuring within 10 to 20 min of starting the infusion and symptoms did not recur. Side effects, including a feeling of heaviness or pressure in various parts of the body and, occasionally, a feeling of warmth or tingling, were reported in 60% of attacks treated with the 2 mg dose. These side effects were mild and short-lived.

GR43175 was administered subcutaneously to 111 migraine patients with moderate or severe headaches in a series of open dose-ranging studies [28]. A dose-related increase in response rate from 33% with 1 mg to 96% with 4 mg GR43175 was observed. Side effects were minor and transient. In one center, 10 patients treated with 2—3 mg doses were investigated especially for recurrence within 24 h: 5 patients experienced a recurrence of their migraine attack 4 to 15 h after the initial successful treatment. Thus the problem of recurrence should be investigated in future trials with GR43175.

So far only 45 patients have received GR43175 as dispersible tablets in open dose-ranging studies [27]. Doses of 70—280 mg have shown efficacy rates in the range of 70—85% by 2 hours. Large controlled double-blind studies are in progress to evaluate GR43175 for use by this most convenient route of drug administration.

Finally, the results of a small double blind trial in 30 patients treated with either 64 μg/kg GR43175 or placebo as an intravenous bolus are shown in Table 3 [27]. Headache severity (none, mild, moderate or severe) was rated

Table 3. The effect of i.v. GR43175 (64 μg/kg) or placebo on migraine attacks in a double blind trial in 30 migraine patients.

	GR43175		Placebo	
	Pretreatment	20 min after treatment	Pretreatment	20 min after treatment
Headache				
Severe	14	1	12	11
Moderate	1	0	3	2
Mild	0	7	0	2
None	0	7	0	0
Nausea	15	2	14	11
Vomiting	6	0	11	5

before and 20 min after injections, as were associated symptoms such as nausea, vomiting and photophobia. A good response was defined as a complete relief of headache or a decrease in headache to a mild severity and this occurred in 14 of 15 patients (93%) treated with GR43175 and in only 2 of 15 patients (13%) treated with placebo ($p < 0.05$). Non-responders in the latter group were subsequently treated openly with GR431745, and 92% responded.

4.3 Conclusion

The novel $5\text{-}HT_1$-like agonist, GR43175, is a selective vasoconstrictor of the carotid vascular bed and the results obtained so far mainly in open dose-ranging studies on the treatment of migraine attacks are promising. These early clinical experiences with GR43175 should for the monent be regarded as "extensive pilot studies", which need confirmation in controlled double-blind trials. If proven effective in such trials, which are currently in progress, GR43175 could be an important tool in investigations of the pathogenesis of migraine.

References

1. Sicuteri F (1959): Prophylactic and therapeutic properties of 1-methyl-lysergic acid butanolamide in migraine. *Int Arch Allergy* 15: 300—307.
2. Pedersen E, Moller CE (1966): Methysergide in migraine prophylaxis. *Clin Pharmacol Ther* 7: 520—526.
3. Müller-Scweinitzer E (1976): Evidence for stimulation of 5-HT receptors in canine saphenous arteries by ergotamine. *Naunyn-Schmiedeberg's Arch Pharmacol* 295: 41—44.
4. Humphrey PPA, Feniuk W, Perren MJ, Connor, HE, Oxford AW (1989): The pharmacology of the novel $5\text{-}HT_1$-like receptor agonist GR43175. *Cephalalgia* 9 (Suppl. 9): 23—33.
5. Fanchamps A, Doepfner W, Weidman H, Cerletti A (1960): Pharmakologische Charakterisierung von Deseril, einem Serotonin-Antagonisten. *Schweiz Med Wschr* 51: 1040—1046.
6. Saxena PR (1974): Selective vasoconstriction in carotid vascular bed by methysergide: possible relevance to its antimigraine effect. *Eur J Pharmacol* 27: 99—105.
7. Saxena PR, Verdouw PD (1984): Effects of methysergide and 5-hydroxytryptamine on carotid blood flow distribution in pigs: further evidence for the presence of atypical 5-HT receptors. *Br J Pharmac* 82: 817—826.
8. Bianchine JR (1968): Metabolism of methysergide (MS) in the rabbit and man. *Fed Proc* 27: 238.
9. Bredberg U, Eyjolfdottir GS, Paalzow L, Tfelt-Hansen P, Tfelt-Hansen V (1986): Pharmacokinetics of methysergide and its metabolite methylergometrine in man. *Eur J Clin Pharmacol* 30: 75—77.
10. Berde B, Stürmer E (1978): Introduction to the pharmacology of ergot alkaloids and related compounds as a basis of their therapeutic application, pp. 1—28 in: Berde B, Schild HO (eds), *Ergot alkaloids and related compounds. Handbook Exp Pharmacol* 49.
11. Tfelt-Hansen P, Jansen I, Edvinsson L (1987): Methylergometrine antagonizes 5 HT in the temporal artery. *Eur J Clin Pharmacol* 33: 77—79.

12. Flückiger E, del Pozo E (1978): Influence on the endocrine system pp. 615—690 in: Berde B, Schild HO (eds), *Ergot alkaloids and related compounds. Handbook Exp Pharmacol* 49.
13. Graham JR, Wolff HG (1938): Mechanism of migraine headache and action of ergotamine tartrate. *Arch Neurol Psychiatr* 39: 737—763.
14. Raskin NH (1981): Pharmacology of migraine. *Ann Rev Pharmacol Toxicol* 21: 463—478.
15. Markowitz S, Saito K, Moskowitz MA (1988): Neurogenically mediated plasma extravasation in dura mater: Effect of ergot alkaloids. A possible mechanism of action in vascular headache. *Cephalalgia* 8: 83—91.
16. Saxena PR, de Vlaam-Schluter GM (1974): Role of some biogenic substances in migraine and relevant mechanism in antimigraine action of ergotamine-studies in an experimental model for migraine. *Headache* 13: 142—163.
17. Johnston BM, Saxena PR (1978): The effect of ergotamine on tissue blood flow and the arteriovenous shunting of radioactive microspheres in the head. *Br J Pharmacol* 63: 541—549.
18. Bom AH, Heiligers J, Saxena PR, Verdouw, PD (1989): Ergotamine-induced reduction in arteriovenous shunting is not mediated by 5-HT$_1$-like or 5-HT$_2$ receptors. *Br J Pharmacol* 97: 383—390.
19. Olsen TS, Olesen J (1988): Regional cerebral blood flow in migraine and cluster headache, pp. 377—391 in: Olesen J, Edvinsson L (eds), *Basic mechanisms of headache.* Amsterdam: Elsevier.
20. Andersen AR, Tfelt-Hansen P, Lassen NA (1987): The effect of ergotamine and dihydroergotamine on cerebral blood flow in man. *Stroke* 18: 120—123.
21. Ibraheem JJ, Paalzow L, Tfelt-Hansen P (1982): Kinetics of ergotamine after intravenous and intramuscular administration to migraine sufferers. *Eur J Clin Pharmacol* 23: 235—240.
22. Ibraheem JJ, Paalzow L, Tfelt-Hansen P (1983): Low bioavailability of ergotamine tartrate after oral and rectal administration in migraine sufferers. *Br J Clin Pharmacol* 16: 695—699.
23. Tfelt-Hansen P (1986): The effect of ergotamine on the arterial system in man. *Acta Pharmacol Toxicol* 59 suppl. 3: 1—30.
24. Parsons AA, Whalley ET (1989): Characterization of the 5-HT receptor which mediates contraction of the human basilar artery. *Cephalalgia* 9 (Suppl 9): 47—51.
25. Nielsen TH, Tfelt-Hansen P (1989): Lack of effect of GR43175 on peripheral arteries in man. *Cephalalgia* 9 (Suppl. 9): 93—95.
26. Doenicke A, Brand J, Perrin VL (1988): Possible benefit of GR43175, a novel 5-HT$_1$-like receptor agonist, for the acute treatment of severe migraine. *Lancet* 1: 1309—11.
27. Perrin VL, Färkkilä M, Goasguen J, Docnicke A, Brand J, Tfilt-Hansen P (1989): Overview of initial clinical studies with intravenous and oral GR43175 in acute migraine. *Cephalalgia* 9 (Suppl. 9): 63—72.
28. Tfelt-Hansen P, Brand J, Dano P, Doenicke A, Findley LJ, Iversen HK, Melchart D, Sahlender HM (1989): Early clinical experience with subcutaneous GR43175 in acute migraine: an overview. *Cephalalgia* 9 (Suppl 9): 63—72.

Blood Platelets

XXXIX. The human platelet 5-HT$_2$-receptor: an up-date

D. DE CHAFFOY DE COURCELLES and F. DE CLERCK

1. Platelet activation

1.1 Functional aspects

Platelets are oval discs 2 to 3 μm in diameter, circulating in the blood. They can adhere to damaged blood vessel walls (adhesion) and stick to each other (aggregation). Platelets contain α-granules, dense bodies, lysosomes, mito-chondria and glycogen particles. Three different channel-like structures have been identified: an open canalicular system, a dense tubular system and circumferential microtubules. The platelet plasma membrane resembles, in structure as well as in function, that of cells of other tissue. In the sub-membrane area, platelets have microtubules which support their discoid shape and microfilaments which contain contractile proteins involved in the platelet release reaction. Such a release reaction is provoked by platelet stimulation with excitatory agonists. This results in the appearance in the extracellular space of the content of the granules, the dense bodies and the lysosome-like particles. The α-granules contain secretable platelet proteins, such as fibrinogen, β-thromboglobulin, platelet factor-4 and cationic pro-teins. The dense bodies mainly contain ATP, ADP, calcium and serotonin. The lysosome-like particles contain acid hydrolases. The extent of secretion of the contents of these different subcellular particles depends upon the nature and the concentration of the challenging agonist. Platelets also biosynthetize and release metabolites from arachidonic acid (see also section 1.2).

The primary platelet response, upon contact with an agonist, is a shape change which occurs within seconds of the stimulus. Platelets loose their discoid shape and pseudopods become apparent on a sphere-like cell. The shape change reaction is elicited by all platelet agonists except epinephrine, and does not require extracellular Ca^{2+} nor cell-to-cell contact. The second functional response consists of cell-to-cell sticking or aggregation; in contrast to the shape change reaction, it requires extracellular Ca^{2+} and cell-to-cell

P.R. Saxena, D.I. Wallis, W. Wouters and P. Bevan (eds), Cardiovascular Pharmacology of 5-Hydroxytryptamine, pp. 445—457.

contact. The sequence of onset of these various platelet responses is usually: shape change, aggregation, and release of intragranular products from the dense bodies, α-granules, and lysosomes. Together with metabolites of arachidonic acid, the intragranular platelet-release products create a "positive feedback loop" [1] and recruit additional cells to form an irreversible aggregate [1—3]. The complete sequence of a platelet reaction has been defined as the "*basic platelet reaction*" [1]. Mammalian blood platelets are activated from resting into aggregating/secreting cells by a large variety of excitatory agonists. They include platelet-derived products (ADP, 5-hydroxy-tryptamine (5-HT), prostaglandin endoperoxides, or thromboxane A_2), pressor hormones (adrenaline, noradrenaline, vasopressin, angiotensin II and dopamine), connective tissue components of the vascular wall (collagen or basement membrane constituents), activated plasma coagulation or fibrinolysis factors (thrombin, plasmin or fibrinogen-fibrin degradation products), as well as products formed under pathological conditions (e.g. antigen-antibody complexes, aggregated gammaglobulin, platelet-activating factor). Depending upon the stage (shape change, reversible or irreversible aggregation, arachidonate metabolism, secretion) to which platelets react upon contact with a single stimulus, agonists have been classified into strong (thrombin, collagen), intermediate (ADP, epinephrine) or weak (5-HT) platelet stimuli (see Table 1).

Table 1. Functional events on activation of human platelets.

| Agonist | Shape change | Aggregation | AA metabolism | Granule secretion | |
				α-	Dense-
Thrombin	+++	+++	+++	+++	+++
Collagen	++	++	++	++	++
PAF	++	++	++	++	++
PG endoperoxides-TXA$_2$	+++	+++	+++	+++	+++
ADP	++	++	++	+	+
Epinephrine		+	+	+	+
Serotonin	++	+			

1.2 *Signal transduction*

Platelet stimuli operate through specific receptors on the platelet surface membrane. Subsequent to the formation of an agonist-receptor complex, the signal transducing system translates the extracellular message into intra-cellular signals which will activate the complex biochemical machinery, leading to the functional platelet response. Most of the excitatory agonists of platelets induce an activation of phospholipase C and a rise in intracellular Ca^{2+} [4]. Although the direct evidence is poor, it is believed that one of the primary steps following receptor occupancy is the activation of phosphatidy-linositol, 4,5 bisphosphate (PIP$_2$)-specific phospholipase C, leading to the formation of diacylglycerol and inositol-trisphosphate (IP$_3$). Diacylglycerol activates protein kinase C [5] and IP$_3$ can mobilize Ca^{2+} from the dense tubular system [6, 7]. Whether IP$_3$ is important in platelet activation is still a matter of debate; indeed, upon activation, intracellular Ca^{2+} is released on a msec time-scale when formation of IP$_3$ is not yet apparent [8, 9]. Most of the increase of intracellular Ca^{2+} is due to influx from the extracellular space [10–12]. Diacylglycerol (DAG) and protein kinase C have unequivocally been shown to play a crucial role in provoking the aggregation/secretion reaction [5, 12–14]. Furthermore, the enzyme plays a role in terminating the primary steps in signal transduction, such as inhibition of phospholipase C (or its coupling to excitatory receptors) [12, 15, 16] and the stimulation of Ca^{2+}-efflux [12, 17, 18]. The major substrate of platelet protein kinase C is a 40 kDa protein whose function is still under investigation. Diacylglycerol is not only formed from PIP$_2$, but also from other phospholipids, in particular PI [19]. Apart from phospholipase C, phospholipase A$_2$ plays a crucial role in transducing the extracellular signal. For example, thrombin- and collagen-receptors are linked to this enzyme [4, 20], which catalyses the liberation of arachidonic acid from phospholipids. Furthermore, increases in cytoplasmic Ca^{2+} activate phospholipase A$_2$ [21]. Arachidonic acid is rapidly metabolized into cyclooxygenase and lipoxygenase products. Of the former, the prosta-glandin endoperoxides (PGENDs), PGG$_2$ and PGH$_2$ and their metabolite, thromboxane A$_2$, are potent platelet activators [22, 23]. Arachidonic acid and/or its metabolites might play an important role as second messengers; indeed, like IP$_3$ and DAG, they can mediate the release of Ca^{2+} from intracellular stores [24, 25] and activate protein kinase C [26, 27].

Although most of the excitatory platelet agonists have either phospholi-pase C and/or phospholipase A$_2$ in their signal transducing pathway, alterna-tive mechanisms for platelet activation may exist which operate indepen-dently from these enzymes [4]. This seems to be particularly the case for adrenaline- and ADP-induced platelet reactions for which the transducing pathways are still controversial [28–31].

It is suggested that a number of platelet excitatory agonists such as epinephrine, ADP, vasopressin, PGENDs, platelet activating factor (PAF) and thrombin, are negatively coupled to adenylate cyclase [32–34]. At least for vasopressin, PGENDs, PAF and low concentrations of thrombin, this phenomenon can be explained by an inhibitory effect of protein kinase C on the stimulation of adenylate cyclase [35]. In resting platelets, cAMP levels are low; it follows that negative coupling as such cannot provoke the secretion and aggregation response.

2. Platelet activation by 5-HT

2.1 Functional aspects

5-HT, biosynthetized from tryptophan by the enterochromaffin cells in the gastrointestinal tract, is taken up by circulating platelets from the surrounding plasma by an active, carrier-mediated transport system and, to a lesser extent, by passive diffusion; the energy-requiring uptake is a saturable process requiring Na^+ and Cl^- ions, directly coupled to K^+ efflux. Apart from uptake and storage by the platelets, 5-HT activates these cells by interacting with 5-HT_2 receptors on the platelet plasma membrane.

In human and rabbit platelets, 5-HT induces transient and reversible aggregation in citrated, platelet-rich plasma (Figure 1). In a small percentage of healthy volunteers and in a substantial number of cardiovascular patients, irreversible, release-associated platelet aggregation is observed [36]. In cat, sheep and pig platelets, activation by 5-HT results in irreversible aggregation and an associated release reaction [37—39].

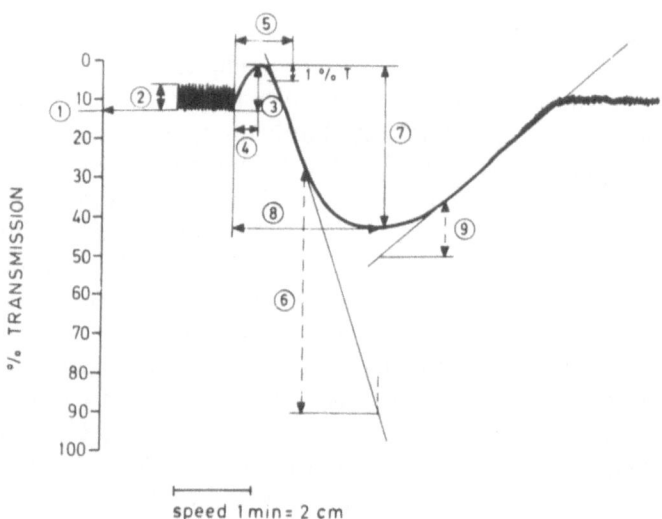

Figure 1. Serotonin-induced shape change and aggregation, a turbidimetric aggregation tracing.

Definition of parameters used for the evaluation of the first wave of aggregation.

(1) Initial light transmission (T time $0'$) in % T; (2) Amplitude of baseline oscillations in stirred platelet-rich plasma (P.R.P.) in % T; (3) Shape change (S.C.) in Δ % T; (4) Time to maximal shape change (Time S.C.) in sec; (5) Aggregation induction time (A.I.T.), i.e. time between addition of agonist and increase by 1 % T after the curve has passed through S.C., in sec; (6) Aggregation velocity or slope (Slope Aggr.) in Δ % T/min; (7) Aggregation maximum (Max) in Δ % T; (8) Reaction time (R.T.) to reach the Max in sec; (9) Disaggregation velocity or slope (Slope Desaggr.) in Δ % T/min.

Derived from De Clerck, F. (36) with permission.

2.2 Signal transduction

On the human platelet, the receptors for 5-HT resemble the 5-HT$_2$-type as defined by radioligand binding studies using [³H]LSD as a probe [40]. Thus, 5-HT antagonists like ketanserin and spiperone are potent inhibitors of [³H]LSD binding (nM range), while 5-HT displaces the probe in the micromolar range.

Evidence for the involvement of phospholipase C in the signal transducing system coupled to the 5-HT$_2$ receptor was found in platelets prelabelled with [³²P]orthophosphate. When stimulated with serotonin, rapid increases in [³²P]phosphatidic acid (PA) and [³²P]40kDa protein are apparent (Figure 2). Diacylglycerol is the endogenous activator of platelet protein kinase C, which has 40kDa-protein as its major substrate, while endogenous diacylglycerol is rapidly phosphorylated to PA by diacylglycerol kinase. Therefore, these data indicate a 5-HT-induced activation of phospholipase C. Further evidence for the involvement of this enzyme is that platelets prelabelled with [³H]arachidonic acid show formation of [³H]diacylglycerol within 10 seconds after stimulation with 5-HT [41].

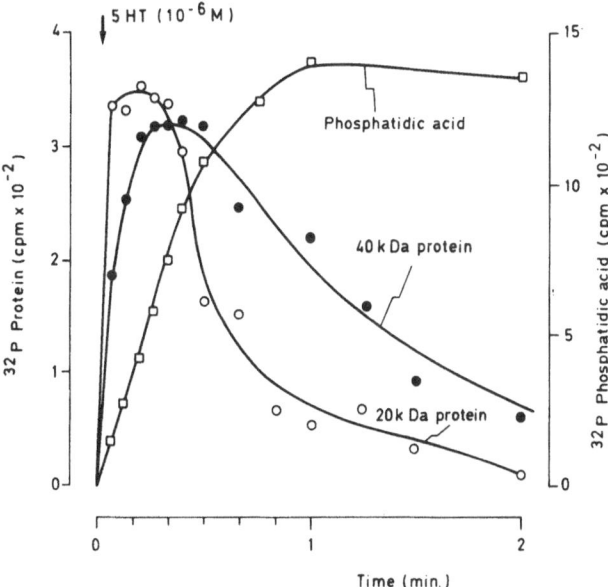

Figure 2. Serotonin-induced changes in phosopholipase C, protein kinase C and myosin light chain kinase activity.

Time course of increase in phosphorylation. Isolated human platelets prelabelled with [³²P]orthophosphate were stimulated with 10^{-6} M 5-HT. (○) ³²P-labelled 20 kDa protein = myosin light chain, (●) [³²P]labelled 40 kDa protein = major substrate for protein kinase C, (□) [³²P]phosphatidic acid as an indirect measure for phospholipase C activation.

Derived from de Chaffoy de Courcelles et al. (40) with permission.

5-HT also induces a rapid increase in intracellular Ca^{2+}, as measured with fluorescent probes [42] or by measuring the increase in phosphorylation of the myosin light chain (Figure 2). This protein is phosphorylated by myosin light chain kinase, which is a Ca^{2+}-calmodulin sensitive enzyme. Although the increase in Ca^{2+} can be seen in the absence of extracellular Ca^{2+}, most of the 5-HT-induced Ca^{2+}-increase when the extracellular Ca^{2+} is in the physiological range, is caused by influx (P. Roevens, personal communication). IP_3 had been shown to mobilize Ca^{2+} from the dense tubular system [6, 7]. However, 5-HT-induced IP_3 formation is minor and much slower than Ca^{2+}-mobilization and DAG formation [43]. A causal relationship between IP_3 formation and intracellular Ca^{2+}-mobilization is therefore not apparent. Furthermore, the mechanism for 5-HT-stimulated Ca^{2+}-influx remains unsolved.

Although 5-HT-stimulated formation of [^{3}H]inositol phosphates was found in prelabelled platelets [43], these data show no evidence for coupling of the receptor to inositolphospholipid-specific phospholipase C. 5-HT induces changes in inositolphospholipid metabolism, but they are probably explained by an increased interconversion [43]. In view of recent findings that receptor activation might lead to activation of non-inositolphospholipid-specific phospholipase C [44, 45] and a role for these phospholipids in processes not directly related to signal transduction [46], the involvement of inositolphospholipids-specific phospholipase C as a primary step in the signal transducing system coupled to the platelet 5-HT receptor remains to be proven. Human platelet activation by 5-HT does not induce liberation of arachidonic acid or formation of its metabolites; neither phospholipase A_2 nor diacylglycerol lipase activity are necessary to evoke the functional responses [47—49].

Since [^{32}P]PA formation is the most reliable step for quantifying receptor activation of the signal transducing system, this assay was used for pharmacological identification. The inhibitory potencies of different drugs on serotonin-induced [^{32}P]PA formation were comparable with their effects both on affinity for 5-HT$_2$ binding sites and on 5-HT-induced aggregation of human platelets (Figure 3). Furthermore, a close correlation was found between the 5-HT concentration-dependent effects on PA formation and on the slope of aggregation (Figure 4). These data point to activation of phospholipase C as a part of the molecular link between receptor occupation and the physiological response.

3. An important role for 5-HT in amplifying the platelet excitatory response

3.1 *Functional aspects*

As they take part in the formation of a haemostatic plug or an arterial

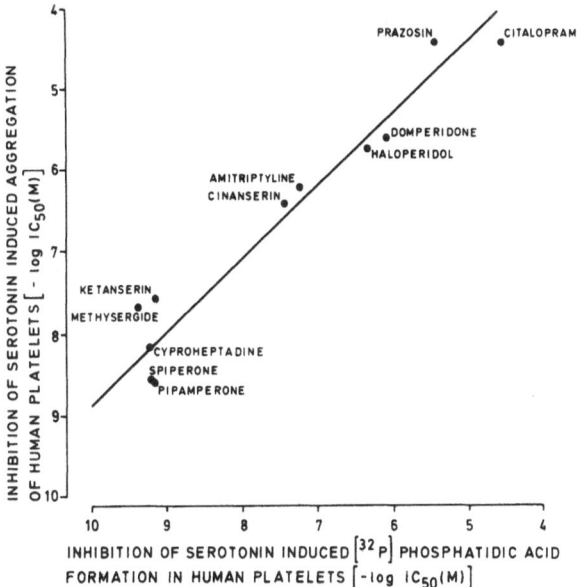

Figure 3. Correlation between drug potencies to inhibit serotonin-induced [^{32}P]PA formation and serotonin-induced aggregation of human platelets.
   Derived from de Chaffoy de Courcelles et al. (41).

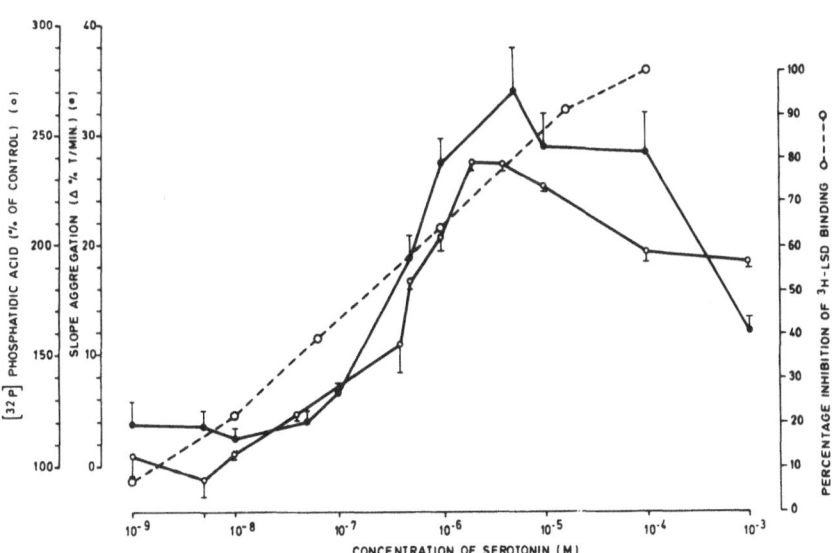

Figure 4. Concentration-response curves for serotonin on: ○, [^{32}P]PA formation; ●, Aggregation; and ---, inhibition of ^{3}H-LSD binding.
   Derived from de Chaffoy de Courcelles et al. (41).

thrombus, platelets are exposed to a multitude of agonists, generated in various concentrations from different sources to act *in concert* and to potentiate each other's effects on the same target cells. Through such amplification mechanisms, the functional response is more complete than predictable from the potency of the single interacting agonists. Amplification interactions between various agonists have long been recognized in platelet research. The phenomenon has been demonstrated for interactions between adrenaline and thrombin, collagen, serotonin, ADP, PAF and angiotensin II [50—55], and for ADP with arachidonic acid [56, 57]. Such synergisms are found mainly in platelet-rich plasma, but occur also in whole blood [58—60]. Similarly, intravascular platelet aggregation in vivo is potentiated when pairs of agonists are combined in intravenous infusions [47, 61, 67]. Indications that amplification mechanisms are operative in haemostatic and thrombotic processes in vivo in experimental animals have been obtained, using pharmacological dissection with compounds blocking specific receptors for platelet agonists. In particular, the application of compounds (e.g. ketanserin) blocking platelet $5-HT_2$ receptors [48, 63] demonstrated an unexpectedly important contribution of 5-HT to the platelet-vessel wall interactions during haemostasis and arterial thrombosis, even in species in which the monoamine by itself produced little platelet activation.

In vitro, 5-HT amplifies the reaction of human platelets to several agonists. The monoamine preconditions the platelets to respond strongly to a low concentration of a second stimulus (e.g. ADP, collagen, epinephrine, norepinephrine, U46619) [47, 51, 52]. The potency of 5-HT as an amplifier is particularly evident when multiple agonists are used to challenge the platelets (Figure 5).

Serotonergic amplification of platelet reactions requires continuous activation of receptors for the process to proceed to completion. Irrespective of the nature of the second interacting agonist, the synergistic action of 5-HT on the platelet is prevented or reversed by specific $5-HT_2$ receptor antagonists [52, 64].

3.2 *At signal transduction level*

The potentiating effect of 5-HT, relative to the single agonist, occurs at an early stage after platelet activation, i.e. the shape-change reaction and on the rate and intensity of the first wave of platelet aggregation [64, 65]. Molecular evidence suggesting this was obtained from experiments in which synergistic effects between adrenaline and 5-HT were analysed at the level of signal transduction [42, 66]. In platelets prelabelled with [32P]orthophosphate, adrenaline — when given alone — had no apparent effect on [32P]PA formation (Figure 6). 5-HT stimulated [32P]PA formation; when given together with adrenaline, the monoamine has an obvious amplifying effect (Figure 6). Essentially similar observations were made for the aggregation response and when intracellular Ca^{2+} was measured using Quin-2 as a

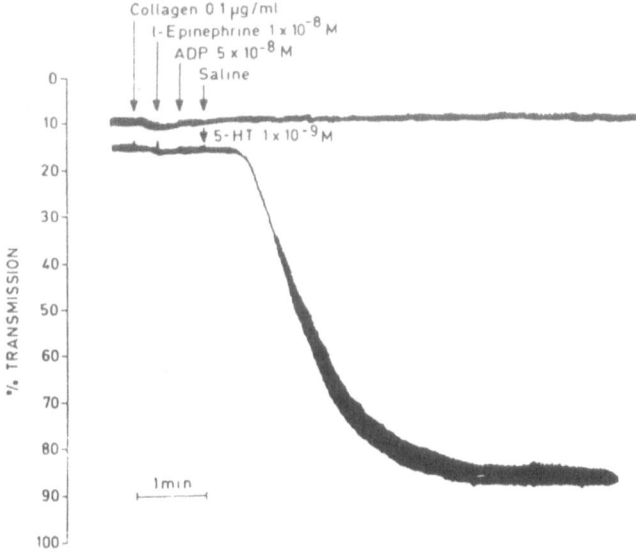

Figure 5. Amplification effect of 5-HT on platelet aggregation. Synergism between collagen, epinephrine, ADP and serotonin in producing full aggregation/release of human platelets in citrated plasma. An ineffective cocktail of low concentrations of collagen (0.1 μg/ml), epinephrine (10^{-8} M) and ADP (5×10^{-8} M) produces a full platelet reaction upon addition of a low concentration of serotonin (5-HT 10^{-9} M).

    Derived from De Clerck et al. (64).

fluorescent probe [42, 66]. In both assays, the amplifying effect occurs in a concentration-dependent manner for both agonists [66]. Furthermore, the combined effect of 5-HT and adrenaline is completely abolished by ketanserin at the same dose range as the effect of 5-HT alone (Figure 6).

    Since radioligand-binding data using membranes from platelets, treated with either 5-HT or adrenaline, revealed changes neither in the maximal binding capacity nor in the affinity of the 5-HT₂ receptor or the α_2-adrenoceptor [66], it follows that the amplifying effect of serotonin in platelet function might occur at the level of signal transduction.

4. Conclusion

The human platelet is a useful model for studying the 5-HT₂ receptor. Using radioligand-binding techniques, the characteristics of the receptor and its regulation can be studied in vitro and ex vivo. Furthermore, the platelet displays a well defined functional response to 5-HT; this phenomenon thus enables researchers to verify the functional repercussions of different manipulations. In addition, chemical quantification of the primary biochemical responses, which form part of the signal transducing system, can unmask

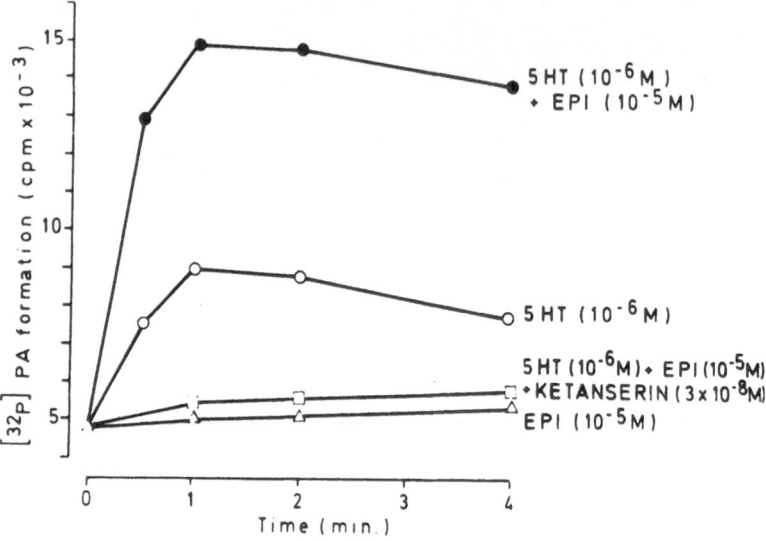

Figure 6. Synergistic effects of serotonin and epinephrine on human platelet phospholipase C.

Platelets prelabelled with [³²P]orthophosphate for 70 min were stimulated with serotonin (5-HT), or epinephrine (EPI), or a mixture of 5-HT and EPI, or a mixture of 5-HT and EPI after preincubation for 10 min with ketanserin. At the times indicated, duplicate samples were taken. Results are representative for 5 separate experiments.

Derived from de Chaffoy de Courcelles et al. (42).

mechanisms involved in the pharmacological alteration of functional platelet responses.

References

1. Holmsen H (1977): Prostaglandin endoperoxide-thromboxane synthesis and dense granule secretion as positive feedback loops in the propagation of platelet responses during "the basic platelet reaction". *Thromb Haemost* 38: 1030–1041.
2. Vargaftig BB, Chignard M, Benveniste J (1981): Present concepts on mechanisms of platelet aggregation. *Biochem Pharmacol* 30: 263–271.
3. Zucker MB, Nachmias VT (1985): Platelet activation. *Arteriosclerosis* 5: 2–18.
4. Lapetina E (1987): Inositide-dependent and independent mechanisms in platelets activation, pp. 287–310 in: Putney Jr JW (ed), *Phosphoinositides and receptor mechanisms*. New York: Alan R. Liss, Inc.
5. Nishizuka Y (1984): Turnover of inositol phospholipids and signal transduction. *Science* 225: 1365–1370.
6. O'Rourke FA, Halenda SP, Zavoico GB, Feinstein MB (1985): Inositol 1,4,5-trisphosphate releases Ca^{2+} from a Ca^{2+}-transporting membrane vesicle fraction derived from human platelets. *J Biol Chem* 260: 956–962.
7. Authi KS, Crawford N (1985): Inositol 1,4,5-trisphosphate-induced release of sequestered Ca^{2+} from highly purified human platelet intracellular membranes. *Biochem J* 230: 247–253.
8. Sage SO, Rink TJ (1987): The kinetics of changes in intracellular calcium concentration in fura-2-loaded human platelets. *J Biol Chem* 262: 16364–16369.

9. Sage SO, Rink TJ (1986): Kinetic differences between thrombin-induced and ADP-induced calcium influx and release from internal stores in fura-2-loaded human platelets. *Biochem Biophys Res Commun* 136: 1124—1129.

10. Hallam TJ, Rink TJ (1985): Agonists stimulate divalent cation channels in the plasma membrane of human platelets. *FEBS* 186: 175—179.

11. Sage SO, Rink TJ (1986): Effects of ionic substitution on $[Ca^{2+}]_i$ rises evoked by thrombin and PAF in human platelets. *Eur J Pharmacol* 128: 99—107.

12. de Chaffoy de Courcelles D, Roevens P, Van Belle H, Kennis L, Somers Y, De Clerck F: The role of endogenously formed diacylglycerol in the propagation and termination of platelet activation. A biochemical and functional analysis using the novel diacylglycerol kinase inhibitor, R 59 949. *J Biol Chem* in press.

13. Kaibuchi K, Takai Y, Sawamura M, Hoshijima M, Fujikura T and Nishizuka Y (1983): Synergistic functions of protein phosphorylation and calcium mobilization in platelet activation. *J Biol Chem* 258: 6701—6704.

14. Rink TJ, Sanchez A, Hallam TJ (1983): Diacylglycerol and phorbol ester stimulate secretion without raising cytoplasmic free calcium in human platelets. *Nature* 305: 317—319.

15. MacIntyre DE, McNicol A, Drummond AH (1985): Tumour-promoting phorbol esters inhibit agonist-induced phosphatidate formation and Ca^{2+} flux in human platelets. *FEBS* 180: 160—164.

16. Watson SP, Lapetina EG (1985): 1,2-Diacylglycerol and phorbol ester inhibit agonist-induced formation of inositol phosphates in human platelets: possible implications for negative feedback regulation of inositol phospholipid hydrolysis. *Proc Natl Acad Sci USA* 82: 2623—2626.

17. Pollock WK, Sage SO, Rink TJ (1987): Stimulation of Ca^{2+} efflux from fura-2-loaded platelets activated by thrombin or phorbol myristate acetate. *FEBS* 210: 132—136.

18. Rink TJ, Sage SO (1987): Stimulated calcium efflux from fura-2-loaded human platelets. *J Physiol* 393: 513—524.

19. Wilson DB, Neufeld EJ, Majerus PW (1985): Phosphoinositide interconversion in thrombin-stimulated human platelets. *J Biol Chem* 260: 1046—1051.

20. Siess W, Cuatrecasas P, Lapetina EG (1983): A role for cyclooxygenase products in the formation of phosphatidic acid in stimulated human platelets. *J Biol Chem* 258: 4683—4686.

21. Billah MM, Lapetina EG, Cuatrecasas P (1980): Phospholipase A₂ and phospholipase C activities of platelets. Differential substrate specificity, Ca^{2+} requirements, pH dependency and cellular localization. *J Biol Chem* 255: 10227—10231.

22. Gerrard JM, Peterson DA, White JG (1981): Calcium mobilization, pp. 407—436 in: Gordon JL (ed), *Platelets in biology and pathology-2.* Amsterdam: Biomedical Press.

23. MacIntyre DE (1981): Platelet prostaglandin receptors, pp. 211—248 in Gordon JL (ed), *Platelets in biology and pathology-2.* Amsterdam: Biomedical Press.

24. Chan KM, Turk J (1987): Mechanism of arachidonic acid-induced Ca^{2+} mobilization from rat liver microsomes. *Biochim Biophys Acta* 928: 186—193.

25. Wolf BA, Turk J, Sherman WR, McDaniel ML (1986): Intracellular Ca^{2+} mobilization by arachidonic acid. *J Biol Chem* 261: 3501—3511.

26. Nishikawa M, Hidaka H, Shirakawa S (1988): Possible involvement of direct stimulation of protein kinase C by unsaturated fatty acids in platelet activation. *Biochem Pharmacol* 37: 3079—3089.

27. Sekiguchi K, Tsukuda M, Ogita K, Kikkawa U, Nishizuka Y (1987): Three distinct forms of rat brain protein kinase C: differential response to unsaturated fatty acids. *Biochem Biophys Res Commun* 145: 797—802.

28. Daniel JL, Dangelmaier CA, Selak M, Smith JB (1986): ADP stimulates IP₃ formation in human platelets. *FEBS* 206: 299—303.

29. Fisher GJ, Bakshian S, Baldassare JJ (1985): Activation of human platelets by ADP

causes a rapid rise in cytosolic free calcium without hydrolysis of phosphatidylinositol-4,5-bisphosphate. *Biochem Biophys Res Commun* 129: 958–964.

30. Figures WR, Scearce LM, Wachtfogel Y, Chen J, Colman RF and Colman RW (1986): Platelet ADP receptor and α_2-adrenoreceptor interaction. *J Biol Chem* 261: 5981–5986.

31. Siess W, Weber PC (1984): Activation of phospholipase C is dissociated from arachidonate metabolism during platelet shape change induced by thrombin or platelet-activating factor. *J Biol Chem* 259: 8286–8292.

32. Vanderwel M, Lum DS, Haslam RJ (1983); Vasopressin inhibits the adenylate cyclase activity of human platelet particulate fraction through V_1-receptors. *FEBS Lett* 164: 340–344.

33. Williams KA, Haslam RJ (1984): Effects of NaCl and GTP on the inhibition of platelet adenylate cyclase by 1-0-octadecyl-2-0-acetyl-sn-glyceryl-3-phosphorylcholine (synthetic platelet-activating factor). *Biochim Biophys Acta* 770: 216–223.

34. Avdonin PV, Svitina-Ulitina IV, Letin VL, Tkachuk VA (1985): Interaction of stable prostaglandin endoperoxide analogs U46619 and U44069 with human platelet membranes: coupling of receptors with high-affinity GTPase and adenylate cyclase. *Thromb Res* 40: 101–112, 1985.

35. Williams KA, Murphy W, Haslam RJ (1987): Effects of activation of protein kinase C on the agonist-induced stimulation and inhibition of cyclic AMP formation in intact human platelets. *Biochem J* 243: 667–678.

36. De Clerck F (1988): Human platelet aggregation induced by 5-hydroxytryptamine: a methodological study. *Hematol Rev* 2: 197–262.

37. Michal F, Penglis F (1969): Inhibition of serotonin-induced platelet aggregation in relation to thrombus production. *J Pharmacol Exp Ther* 166: 276–284.

38. Drummond AH, Gordon JL (1974): Platelet release reaction induced by 5-hydroxytryptamine. *J Physiol* 240: 39P–40P.

39. Gordon JL, Drummond AH (1975): Irreversible aggregation of pig platelets and release of intracellular constituents induced by 5-hydroxytryptamines. *Biochem Pharmacol* 24: 33–6.

40. de Chaffoy de Courcelles D, Roevens P, Van Belle H (1984): Stimulation by serotonin of 40 kDa and 20 kDa protein phosphorylation in human platelets. *FEBS* 171: 289–292.

41. de Chaffoy de Courcelles D, Leysen JE, De Clerck F, Van Belle H, Janssen PAJ (1985): Evidence that phospholipid turnover is the signal transducing system coupled to serotonin-S_2 receptor sites. *J Biol Chem* 260: 7603–7608.

42. de Chaffoy de Courcelles D, Roevens P, Van Belle H, De Clerck F (1987): The synergistic effect of serotonin and epinephrine on the human platelet at the level of signal transduction. *FEBS* 219: 283–288.

43. de Chaffoy de Courcelles D, Roevens P, Wynants J, Van Belle H (1987): Serotonin-induced alterations in inositol phospholipid metabolism in human platelets. *Biochim Biophys Acta* 927: 291–302.

44. Cabot MC, Welsh CJ, Zhang Z, Cao H, Chabbott H, Lebowitz M (1988): Vasopressin, phorbol diesters and serum elicit choline glycerophospholipid hydrolysis and diacylglycerol formation in nontransformed cells: transformed derivatives do not respond. *Biochim Biophys Acta* 959: 46–57.

45. Irving HR, Exton JH (1987): Phosphatidylcholine breakdown in rat liver plasma membranes. *J Biol Chem* 262: 3440–3443.

46. de Chaffoy de Courcelles D (In press): Is there evidence for a role of the phosphoinositol-cycle in the myocardium?

47. De Clerck F, Herman AG (1983). 5-Hydroxytryptamine and platelet aggregation. *Fed Proc* 42: 228–232.

48. De Clerck F, Van Nueten JM, Reneman RS (1984): Platelet-vessel wall interactions: implication of 5-hydroxytryptamine. A review. *Agents Actions* 15: 612–626.

49. De Clerck F, Xhonneux B, Leysen J, Janssen PAJ (1984): Evidence for functional 5-HT receptor sites on human blood platelets. *Biochem Pharmacol* 33: 2807—2811.
50. Ardlie NG, Cameron HA, Garrat J (1984): Platelet activation by circulating levels of hormones: a possible link in coronary heart disease. *Thromb Res* 36: 315—322.
51. Baumgartner HR, Born GVR (1968): Effects of 5-hydroxytryptamine on platelet aggregation. *Nature* 218: 137—141.
52. De Clerck F, David JL, Janssen PAJ (1982): Inhibition of 5-hydroxytryptamine-induced and -amplified human platelet aggregation by ketanserin (R 41 468), a selective 5-HT₂-receptor antagonist. *Agents Actions* 12: 388—397.
53. Grant JA, Scrutton MC (1980): Positive interaction between agonists in the aggregation response of human blood platelets: interaction between ADP, adrenaline and vasopressin. *Br J Haematol* 44: 109—125.
54. Huang EM, Detweiler TC (1981): Characteristics of the synergistic actions of platelet agonists. *Blood* 57: 685—691.
55. Nakanishi M, Imamura H, Goto K (1971): Potentiation of ADP-induced platelet aggregation by collagen and its inhibition by a tetrahydrotheino-pyridine derivative. *Biochem Pharmacol* 20: 2116—2118.
56. Kinlough-Rathbone RL, Packham MA, Mustard JF (1977): Synergism between platelet aggregating agents: the role of the arachidonate pathway. *Thromb Res* 11: 567—580.
57. Silver MJ, Smith JB, Ingerman L, Kolsis JJ (1973): Arachidonic acid-induced human platelet aggregation and prostaglandin formation. *Prostaglandins* 4: 863—876.
58. Bushfield M, Lumley P, MacIntyre De (1986): Synergistic activation of human platelets in whole blood. *Br J Pharmacol* 89: 855P.
59. De Clerck F, Somers Y, Van Gorp L (1984): Platelet-vessel wall interactions in haemostasis: implication of 5-hydroxytryptamine. *Agents Actions* 15: 627—635.
60. Setiabudy-Dharma R, Funahara, Y (1986): Enhancement of collagen-induced aggregation of platelets in whole blood. *Thromb Res* 48: 621—634.
61. Doni MG, Aragno R (1977): Effect of catecholamine on ADP aggregation of rat platelets in vivo. *Experientia* 33: 1331—1332.
62. Holmes IB (1979): Potentiating effect of adrenaline on adenosine diphosphate-induced reduction in rabbit circulating platelet count: inhibition by dihydroergotamine. *Thromb Haemost* 42: 641—648.
63. Van Nueten JM, Janssen PAJ, Symoens J, Janssens WJ, Heykants J, De Clerck F, Leysen JE, Van Cauteren H, Vanhoutte PM (1987): Ketanserin, pp. 1—56 in: Scriabine A (ed), *New cardiovascular drugs*. New York: Raven Press.
64. De Clerck F, Xhonneux B, de Chaffoy de Courcelles D. (1988): Functional expression of the amplification reaction between serotonin and epinephrine on platelets. *J Cardiovasc Pharmacol* 11 (Suppl. 1): S1—S5.
65. Michal F, Motamed M (1976): Shape change and aggregation of blood platelets: interaction between the effect of adenosine diphosphate, 5-hydroxytryptamine and adrenaline. *Br J Pharmacol* 56: 209—218.
66. de Chaffoy de Courcelles D, Roevens P, De Clerck F (1988): The synergistic effect of serotonin and epinephrine at the level of signal transduction. *J Cardiovasc Pharmacol* 11 (Suppl. 1): S107—S110.
67. De Clerck F, de Chaffoy de Courcelles D (1987): Amplification mechanisms in platelet activation, in: Meyer F, Marche P (eds), *Blood cells and arteries in hypertension and atherosclerosis*. New York: Raven Press.

XXXX. ICI 170809, A selective 5-hydroxytryptamine antagonist, inhibits human platelet aggregation *in vitro* and *ex vivo*

THOMAS P. BLACKBURN, STEPHEN J. HAWORTH, CAROL L. JESSUP, PAMELA B. MORTON and CHRISTINE WILLIAMS

1. Introduction

In vitro 5-hydroxytryptamine (5-HT) causes both a shape change and aggregation of human platelets. Few studies have been reported on 5-HT-induced platelet aggregation in patients with peripheral or cerebrovascular disease, although these patients have been reported to have enhanced platelet activity [1—6] and show hyperaggregability in response to known aggregating agents [7—9].

The aim of this study was to assess the antagonist potency of [2(2-dimethylamino-2-methylpropylthio)-3-phenylquinoline] (ICI 170,809) a selective $5-HT_2$ receptor antagonist [10], on 5-HT-induced platelet aggregation in normal volunteers. The antagonist potency of ICI 170,809 at human platelet receptors was determined both in vitro and ex vivo after administration of a single oral dose of the drug.

2. Methods

2.1 *Preparation of platelet rich and platelet poor plasma*

Human volunteers were bled from an antecubital vein into tubes containing trisodium citrate solution (3.2% w/v. 1 part to 9 parts whole blood). Platelet rich plasma (PRP) and platelet poor plasma (PPP) were prepared by centrifugation (200 g × 15 min and 15,000 g × 2 min respectively).

2.2 *In vitro platelet aggregation*

Platelet aggregation was measured using a Payton aggregometer. Aliquots (250 μl) of PRP were stirred (900 rpm) and incubated (37 °C) for 60 seconds in an aggregometer before either ICI 170,809 or vehicle was added.

P.R. Saxena, D.I. Wallis, W. Wouters and P. Bevan (eds), Cardiovascular Pharmacology of 5-Hydroxytryptamine, pp. 459—463.
© 1990 *Kluwer Academic Publishers, Dordrecht —*

Platelets were incubated for a further 60 seconds and a single concentration of 5-HT was then added. This procedure was repeated using a range of concentrations of 5-HT (5×10^{-9} to 5×10^{-5} M). The extent of aggregation was measured and expressed as a percentage of the maximum obtained with vehicle controls.

2.3 Ex vivo platelet aggregation

Aliquots of PRP (250 μl) were incubated for 120 seconds in an aggregometer (900 rpm, 37 °C) before concentrations of 5-HT (5×10^{-9} to 5×10^{-5} M) were added.

2.4 Volunteer study design

The volunteer study was a double blind randomised cross-over design in which seven male volunteers (18—45 years, body weight 63—91 kg) received ICI 170,809 on three occasions and placebo on another; the interval between study periods was 7 days. ICI 170,809 was administered orally as one of four doses [3, 7, 15 or 30 mg) to volunteers who had fasted overnight. Platelet sensitivity to 5-HT, measured as the extent of aggregation, was determined on three separate occasions before and 2, 5, 8 and 24 hours after oral administration of ICI 170,809 or placebo. The extent of 5-HT induced aggregation in the presence of either ICI 170,809 or placebo was expressed as a percentage of the mean of the maximum aggregation responses obtained on three occasions prior to dosing.

3. Results

3.1 In vitro platelet aggregation

5-HT induced a concentration-dependent aggregation in platelets from normal subjects over the concentration range 8×10^{-7} M to 2×10^{-5} M, with an EC_{50} of 5.93 ($\pm$ 0.65) $\times 10^{-7}$ M, n = 8. ICI 170,809 (1×10^{-7} M and 4×10^{-7} M) caused a rightward shift of the 5-HT effect curve, and reduced the extent of the maximum achievable aggregation. These same antagonist concentrations caused significant blockade of 5-HT (1×10^{-5} M) responses yielding mean ($\pm$ s.e.) percentage inhibition of 58.3 ($\pm$ 4.5)% (n = 8) and 77.5 ($\pm$ 2.1)% (n = 7) respectively.

3.2 Ex vivo platelet aggregation

When dosed orally to human volunteers ICI 170,809 (3 mg) did not signifi-

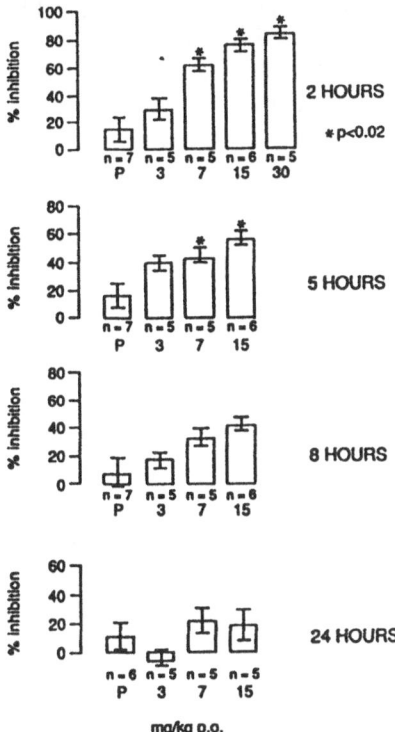

Figure 1. Effect of ICI 170,809: 3, 7, 15 or 30 mg/kg p.o. and placebo on 5-HT induced platelet aggregation 2, 5, 8 and 24 hours after single oral dose.

cantly (P > 0.05) modify *ex vivo* platelet aggregation. The drug, at higher doses (7, 15 and 30 mg), caused inhibition (mean % ± s.e., n ⩾ 5) of 5-HT-induced platelet aggregation at 2 hours of 59.5 ± 4.6, 73.8 ± 4.2 and 82.4 ± 4, respectively, which was significantly different (P < 0.05) from placebo. This activity persisted for 5 hours with the 7 and 15 mg doses (mean % inhibition ± s.e., n ⩾ 5; 42.4 ± 4.8 and 54.6 ± 4.2, respectively) (Figure 1).

4. Discussion

In a double blind randomised study to measure the ability of ICI 170,809 to inhibit 5-HT-induced aggregation in human platelets, the drug was demonstrated to be a potent, orally active compound with a minimum effective oral dose in human volunteers of 0.1 mg/kg.

Controversy still exists about the exact role of platelets in the pathogenesis of a number of cardiovascular diseases. Peripheral arterial vasospasms, subsequent to platelet activation, appear to be mediated in part by 5-HT and can be effectively reduced by ketanserin, a specific 5-HT$_2$ receptor antagonist [11]. In animal studies post-thrombotic peripheral collateral circulation could be significantly restored by treatment with ketanserin [12, 13] and the 5-HT-induced reduction of blood supply through the collateral system could be effectively counteracted by pretreatment with ketanserin [13, 14]. Since 5-HT appears to be an active component of platelet mediated vasospasm [11, 15] ICI 170,809, like ketanserin, might well interrupt the vicious circle of 5-HT-induced platelet aggregation and subsequent vasoconstriction (post-ischaemic vasoconstriction) in cardiovascular disease where platelet function is compromised.

5. Conclusions

In vitro, ICI 170,809 (1×10^{-7} M and 4×10^{-7} M), significantly inhibited 5-HT-induced aggregation by 58 and 77% respectively, whilst the minimum effective dose *ex vivo* was 0.1 mg.kg^{-1} p.o. These results suggest that ICI 170,809 has potential to modulate the vasospastic effects of 5-HT released from platelets during trauma.

References

1. Handin RI, McDonough M, Lesch M (1978): Elevation of platelet factor four in acute myocardial infarction: measurements by radioimmunoassay. *J Lab clin Med* 91: 340—349.
2. Green LH, Scroppian E, Handin RI (1980): Platelet activation during exercise-induced myocardial ischaemia. *New Engl J Med* 302: 193—197.
3. Schwartz MB, Hangier J, Timmons S, Freisinger GC (1980): Platelet aggregates in ischaemic heart disease. *Thromb Haemostasis* 434: 185—188.
4. Baele G, Bogaerts H, Clements DL, Pannier R, Barbier F (1981): Platelet activation during treadmill exercise in patients with chronic peripheral arterial disease. *Thromb Res* 23: 215—223.
5. Rotmensch HH, Vlasses PH, Carpentier KL, D'Amelia LF, Swanson BN, Ferguson RK (1983): Plasma platelet products and exercise-induced myocardial ischaemia. *J Lab clin Med* 102: 63—69.
6. De Cree J, Leempoels J, Demoen B, Roels V, Verhaegen H (1985): The effects of ketanserin, a 5-HT$_2$-receptor antagonist, on 5-hydroxytryptamine-induced irreversible platelet aggregation in patients with cardiovascular diseases. *Agents and Actions* 16: 5, 313—317.
7. Steele PP, Welly HS, Davies H, Genton E (1973): Platelet function studies in coronary artery disease. *Circulation* 48: 1194—1200.
8. Dreyfuss F, Zahavi J (1973): Adenosine diphosphate-induced platelet aggregation in myocardial infarction and ischaemic heart disease. *Atherosclerosis* 17: 107—120.
9. Salky M, Dugdale M (1973): Platelet abnormalities in ischaemic heart disease. *Am J Cardiol* 32: 612—617.
10. Blackburn TP, Thornber CW, Pearce RJ, Cox B (1988): *In vitro* pharmacology of ICI 170,809 — A new 5-HT$_2$ antagonist. *FASEB Journal* 2(5): A1404, 6441.
11. De Clerck F, Van Neuten JM (1982): Platelet-mediated vascular contractions: Inhibition of the serotonergic component by ketanserin. *Thromb Res* 27: 713—723.

12. Nevelsteen A, Loots W, De Clerck F, De Gryse A (1984): Restoration of post-thrombotic peripheral collateral circulation in the cat by ketanserin, a selective 5-HT$_2$ receptor antagonist. *Archs int Pharmacodyn Ther* 270: 268—279.

13. Blackshear JL, Orlandi S, Garnic JD, Hollenberg NK (1983): Serotonin induces large artery spasm *in vivo* via 5-HT$_2$ receptors. *Circulation* 68: III-197, Abs. 798.

14. Verheyen V, Vlaminckx E, Lauwers F, Van Den Broeck C, Wouters L (1984): Serotonin-induced blood flow changes in the rat hind legs after unilateral ligation of the femoral artery. Inhibition by the S$_2$-receptor antagonist ketanserin. *Archs int Pharmacodyn Ther* 270: 280—294.

15. Hollenberg NK (1988): Serotonin and vascular responses. *Ann Rev Pharmacol Toxicol* 28: 41—59.

Subject index

466

Developments in Cardiovascular Medicine

1. Ch.T. Lancée (ed.): *Echocardiology*. 1979   ISBN 90–247–2209–8
2. J. Baan, A.C. Arntzenius and E.L. Yellin (eds.): *Cardiac Dynamics*. 1980
                                                                ISBN 90–247–2212–8
3. H.J.Th. Thalen and C.C. Meere (eds.): *Fundamentals of Cardiac Pacing*. 1979
                                                                ISBN 90–247–2245–4
4. H.E. Kulbertus and H.J.J. Wellens (eds.): *Sudden Death*. 1980 ISBN 90–247–2290–X
5. L.S. Dreifus and A.N. Brest (eds.): *Clinical Applications of Cardiovascular Drugs*.
   1980   ISBN 90–247–2295–0
6. M.P. Spencer and J.M. Reid: *Cerebrovascular Evaluation with Doppler Ultrasound*.
   With contributions by E.C. Brockenbrough, R.S. Reneman, G.I. Thomas and D.L.
   Davis. 1981   ISBN 90–247–2384–1
7. D.P. Zipes, J.C. Bailey and V. Elharrar (eds.): *The Slow Inward Current and Cardiac
   Arrhythmias*. 1980   ISBN 90–247–2380–9
8. H. Kesteloot and J.V. Joossens (eds.): *Epidemiology of Arterial Blood Pressure*. 1980
                                                                ISBN 90–247–2386–8
9. F.J.Th. Wackers (ed.): *Thallium-201 and Technetium-99m-Pyrophosphate. Myocardial Imaging in the Coronary Care Unit*. 1980   ISBN 90–247–2396–5
10. A. Maseri, C. Marchesi, S. Chierchia and M.G. Trivella (eds.): *Coronary Care Units*.
    Proceedings of a European Seminar, held in Pisa, Italy (1978). 1981
                                                                ISBN 90–247–2456–2
11. J. Morganroth, E.N. Moore, L.S. Dreifus and E.L. Michelson (eds.): *The Evaluation of
    New Antiarrhythmic Drugs*. Proceedings of the First Symposium on New Drugs and
    Devices, held in Philadelphia, Pa., U.S.A. (1980). 1981   ISBN 90–247–2474–0
12. P. Alboni: *Intraventricular Conduction Disturbances*. 1981 ISBN 90–247–2483–X
13. H. Rijsterborgh (ed.): *Echocardiology*. 1981   ISBN 90–247–2491–0
14. G.S. Wagner (ed.): *Myocardial Infarction*. Measurement and Intervention. 1982
                                                                ISBN 90–247–2513–5
15. R.S. Meltzer and J. Roelandt (eds.): *Contrast Echocardiography*. 1982
                                                                ISBN 90–247–2531–3
16. A. Amery, R. Fagard, P. Lijnen and J. Staessen (eds.): *Hypertensive Cardiovascular
    Disease*. Pathophysiology and Treatment. 1982   IBSN 90–247–2534–8
17. L.N. Bouman and H.J. Jongsma (eds.): *Cardiac Rate and Rhythm*. Physiological,
    Morphological and Developmental Aspects. 1982   ISBN 90–247–2626–3
18. J. Morganroth and E.N. Moore (eds.): *The Evaluation of Beta Blocker and Calcium
    Antagonist Drugs*. Proceedings of the 2nd Symposium on New Drugs and Devices,
    held in Philadelphia, Pa., U.S.A. (1981). 1982   ISBN 90–247–2642–5
19. M.B. Rosenbaum and M.V. Elizari (eds.): *Frontiers of Cardiac Electrophysiology*.
    1983   ISBN 90–247–2663–8
20. J. Roelandt and P.G. Hugenholtz (eds.): *Long-term Ambulatory Electrocardiography*.
    1982   ISBN 90–247–2664–6
21. A.A.J. Adgey (ed.): *Acute Phase of Ischemic Heart Disease and Myocardial
    Infarction*. 1982   ISBN 90–247–2675–1
22. P. Hanrath, W. Bleifeld and J. Souquet (eds.): *Cardiovascular Diagnosis by
    Ultrasound*. Transesophageal, Computerized, Contrast, Doppler Echocardiography.
    1982   ISBN 90–247–2692–1

Developments in Cardiovascular Medicine

43. S. Sideman and R. Beyar (eds.): [3-D] *Simulation and Imaging of the Cardiac System.* State of the Heart. Proceedings of the International Henry Goldberg Workshop, held in Haifa, Israel (1984). 1985   ISBN 0–89838–687–X

44. E. van der Wall and K.I. Lie (eds.): *Recent Views on Hypertrophic Cardiomyopathy.* Proceedings of a Symposium, held in Groningen, The Netherlands (1984). 1985   ISBN 0–89838–694–2

45. R.E. Beamish, P.K. Singal and N.S. Dhalla (eds.), *Stress and Heart Disease.* Proceedings of a International Symposium, held in Winnipeg, Canada, 1984 (Vol. 1). 1985   ISBN 0–89838–709–4

46. R.E. Beamish, V. Panagia and N.S. Dhalla (eds.): *Pathogenesis of Stress-induced Heart Disease.* Proceedings of a International Symposium, held in Winnipeg, Canada, 1984 (Vol. 2). 1985   ISBN 0–89838–710–8

47. J. Morganroth and E.N. Moore (eds.): *Cardiac Arrhythmias.* New Therapeutic Drugs and Devices. Proceedings of the 5th Symposium on New Drugs and Devices, held in Philadelphia, Pa., U.S.A. (1984). 1985   ISBN 0–89838–716–7

48. P. Mathes (ed.): *Secondary Prevention in Coronary Artery Disease and Myocardial Infarction.* 1985   ISBN 0–89838–736–1

49. H.L. Stone and W.B. Weglicki (eds.): *Pathobiology of Cardiovascular Injury.* Proceedings of the 6th Annual Meeting of the American Section of the I.S.H.R., held in Oklahoma City, Okla., U.S.A. (1984). 1985   ISBN 0–89838–743–4

50. J. Meyer, R. Erbel and H.J. Rupprecht (eds.): *Improvement of Myocardial Perfusion.* Thrombolysis, Angioplasty, Bypass Surgery. Proceedings of a Symposium, held in Mainz, F.R.G. (1984). 1985   ISBN 0–89838–748–5

51. J.H.C. Reiber, P.W. Serruys and C.J. Slager (eds.): *Quantitative Coronary and Left Ventricular Cineangiography.* Methodology and Clinical Applications. 1986   ISBN 0–89838–760–4

52. R.H. Fagard and I.E. Bekaert (eds.): *Sports Cardiology.* Exercise in Health and Cardiovascular Disease. Proceedings from an International Conference, held in Knokke, Belgium (1985). 1986   ISBN 0–89838–782–5

53. J.H.C. Reiber and P.W. Serruys (eds.): *State of the Art in Quantitative Cornary Arteriography.* 1986   ISBN 0–89838–804–X

54. J. Roelandt (ed.): *Color Doppler Flow Imaging and Other Advances in Doppler Echocardiography.* 1986   ISBN 0–89838–806–6

55. E.E. van der Wall (ed.): *Noninvasive Imaging of Cardiac Metabolism.* Single Photon Scintigraphy, Positron Emission Tomography and Nuclear Magnetic Resonance. 1987   ISBN 0–89838–812–0

56. J. Liebman, R. Plonsey and Y. Rudy (eds.): *Pediatric and Fundamental Electrocardiography.* 1987   ISBN 0–89838–815–5

57. H.H. Hilger, V. Hombach and W.J. Rashkind (eds.), *Invasive Cardiovascular Therapy.* Proceedings of an International Symposium, held in Cologne, F.R.G. (1985). 1987   ISBN 0–89838–818–X

58. P.W. Serruys and G.T. Meester (eds.): *Coronary Angioplasty.* A Controlled Model for Ischemia. 1986   ISBN 0–89838–819–8

59. J.E. Tooke and L.H. Smaje (eds.): *Clinical Investigation of the Microcirculation.* Proceedings of an International Meeting, held in London, U.K. (1985). 1987   ISBN 0–89838–833–3

Developments in Cardiovascular Medicine

Developments in Cardiovascular Medicine

78. M.M. Scheinman (ed.): *Catheter Ablation of Cardiac Arrhythmias*. Basic Bioelectrical Effects and Clinical Indications. 1988   ISBN 0–89838–967–4
79. J.A.E. Spaan, A.V.G. Bruschke and A.C. Gittenberger-De Groot (eds.): *Coronary Circulation*. From Basic Mechanisms to Clinical Implications. 1987
                                                                    ISBN 0–89838–978–X
80. C. Visser, G. Kan and R.S. Meltzer (eds.): *Echocardiography in Coronary Artery Disease*. 1988   ISBN 0–89838–979–8
81. A. Bayés de Luna, A. Betriu and G. Permanyer (eds.): *Therapeutics in Cardiology*. 1988   ISBN 0–89838–981–X
82. D.M. Mirvis (ed.): *Body Surface Electrocardiographic Mapping*. 1988
                                                                    ISBN 0–89838–983–6
83. M.A. Konstam and J.M. Isner (eds.): *The Right Ventricle*. 1988 ISBN 0–89838–987–9
84. C.T. Kappagoda and P.V. Greenwood (eds.): *Long-term Management of Patients after Myocardial Infarction*. 1988   ISBN 0–89838–352–8
85. W.H. Gaasch and H.J. Levine (eds.): *Chronic Aortic Regurgitation*. 1988
                                                                    ISBN 0–89838–364–1
86. P.K. Singal (ed.): *Oxygen Radicals in the Pathophysiology of Heart Disease*. 1988
                                                                    ISBN 0–89838–375–7
87. J.H.C. Reiber and P.W. Serruys (eds.): *New Developments in Quantitative Coronary Arteriography*. 1988   ISBN 0–89838–377–3
88. J. Morganroth and E.N. Moore (eds.): *Silent Myocardial Ischemia*. Proceedings of the 8th Annual Symposium on New Drugs and Devices (1987). 1988
                                                                    ISBN 0–89838–380–3
89. H.E.D.J. ter Keurs and M.I.M. Noble (eds.): *Starling's Law of the Heart Revisted*. 1988   ISBN 0–89838–382–X
90. N. Sperelakis (ed.): *Physiology and Pathophysiology of the Heart*. (Rev. ed.) 1988
                                                                    ISBN 0–89838–388–9
91. J.W. de Jong (ed.): *Myocardial Energy Metabolism*. 1988   ISBN 0–89838–394–3
92. V. Hombach, H.H. Hilger and H.L. Kennedy (eds.): *Electrocardiography and Cardiac Drug Therapy*. Proceedings of an International Symposium, held in Cologne, F.R.G. (1987). 1988   ISBN 0–89838–395–1
93. H. Iwata, J.B. Lombardini and T. Segawa (eds.): *Taurine and the Heart*. 1988
                                                                    ISBN 0–89838–396–X
94. M.R. Rosen and Y. Palti (eds.): *Lethal Arrhythmias Resulting from Myocardial Ischemia and Infarction*. Proceedings of the 2nd Rappaport Symposium, held in Haifa, Israel (1988). 1988   ISBN 0–89838–401–X
95. M. Iwase and I. Sotobata: *Clinical Echocardiography*. With a Foreword by M.P. Spencer. 1989   ISBN 0–7923–0004–1
96. I. Cikes (ed.): *Echocardiography in Cardiac Interventions*. 1989
                                                                    ISBN 0–7923–0088–2
97. E. Rapaport (ed.): *Early Interventions in Acute Myocardial Infarction*. 1989
                                                                    ISBN 0–7923–0175–7
98. M.E. Safar and F. Fouad-Tarazi (eds.): *The Heart in Hypertension*. A Tribute to Robert C. Tarazi (1925–1986). 1989   ISBN 0–7923–0197–8
99. S. Meerbaum and R. Meltzer (eds.): *Myocardial Contrast Two-dimensional Echocardiography*. 1989   ISBN 0–7923–0205–2

Developments in Cardiovascular Medicine